APPLICATION of MEASUREMENT
to Health and Physical Education

FIFTH EDITION

APPLICATION of MEASUREMENT
to Health and Physical Education

H. HARRISON CLARKE

Research Professor Emeritus
University of Oregon

Prentice-Hall, Inc., Englewood Cliffs, New Jersey

Library of Congress Cataloging in Publication Data

CLARKE, HENRY HARRISON (date)
    Application of measurement to health and physical
education.

    Includes bibliographies.
    1. Physical fitness—Testing.   I. Title.
GV436.C49 1976   613.7   75–29402
ISBN 0–13–039024–0

Printed in the United States of America

10   9   8   7   6   5   4   3   2   1

PRENTICE-HALL INTERNATIONAL, INC., *London*
PRENTICE-HALL OF AUSTRALIA PTY. LIMITED, *Sydney*
PRENTICE-HALL OF CANADA, LTD., *Toronto*
PRENTICE-HALL OF INDIA PRIVATE LIMITED, *New Delhi*
PRENTICE-HALL OF JAPAN, INC., *Tokyo*
PRENTICE-HALL OF SOUTHEAST ASIA PTE. LTD., *Singapore*

TO MY WIFE

Florence Osborn Clarke

PART ONE
Fundamental Considerations
of Measurement

Contents

PART TWO
Physical Fitness

*specific test
don't need*

PART THREE
Social Efficiency

PART FOUR
Physical Education Skills and Appreciations

PART FIVE
Administrative Problems

Illustrations

Tables

The Fifth Edition of *Application of Measurement to Health and Physical Education* constitutes a thorough revision of the preceding text. It has been brought up to date in all respects with the most recent knowledge about tests available. New tests have been added and old ones reassessed in light of current information.

Every effort has been made to make this a practical and functional publication. Now 119 tests and test batteries may be *given* and *scored* directly from the text. In addition, 151 other tests are described, evaluated, and their sources provided. To indicate the many test items described in the test batteries would greatly increase the number of devices included in the book. New illustrations have been added to further enhance the material.

In this, as in the fourth edition, a special effort was made to make the book more useful to health educators. To accomplish this purpose, Dr. Robert E. Kime, Professor of Health Education, and Dr. Lorraine G. Davis, Assistant Professor of Health Education at the University of Oregon assisted materially in making suggestions, providing objectives, preparing materials, and evaluating tests in this field.

As was true for other editions of this text, the approach to measurement is in terms of improved health and physical education services. Measurement is presented as a means of enabling health and physical educators to serve pupils better than would otherwise be possible. Measurement is utilized to make health and physical education effective forces in the curriculum from elementary school through college.

Tests are considered in relation to specific educational objectives, so that their utility in meeting a given objective is shown. Thus, tests designed to meet the physical fitness objective are grouped together, as are those intended to meet the social objective and those directed toward recreational and cultural objectives. Not only are tests in each of these areas presented and evaluated, but the procedures and methods employed to meet each objective are considered. Thus, emphasis is placed on the *use* of test results; *the application of measurement.*

Too frequently, measurement has been considered an academic appendage of health and physical education programs, the province primarily of the research worker and of the individual intellectually oriented. Often measurement has been discussed on a purely technical basis with slight emphasis on the use of tests and practically none on necessary procedures for applying test results. Actually, measurement should be vital to health and physical education programs; teachers in these fields should turn to it as readily and naturally as they turn to the various activities of their programs. It should be a dynamic force in these programs. Through the intelligent use of measurement, health and physical education can take their places as indispensible phases of the educational process.

The current trends of health and physical education, a consideration of the desirable qualities to measure, and an explanation of definite administrative procedures to use in putting tests into practical use will be found in Part One. In the first chapter is an orientation to the place of physical education in our culture. In the second chapter, criteria for selecting tests from a scientific point of view are considered, so

Preface

that health and physical educators may be prepared to evaluate tests for themselves.

A separate part of the text is devoted to each of the objectives of health and physical education. The importance of each objective, the educational and administrative procedures for its realization, the various phases of physical fitness testing are presented in Part Two. In Part Three, social efficiency and motor ability tests are described, evaluated, and their uses indicated. A similar presentation is made for skill and knowledge tests in Part Four. Part Five is devoted to administrative problems and the process of inaugurating measurement programs.

Appendix A includes statistical procedures essential for the construction of tests. Scoring tables necessary to the use of tests described throughout the text appear in Appendix B.

The writer wishes to express his gratitude to the many authors and publishers who have so generously permitted use of their materials.

H. H. C.

APPLICATION of MEASUREMENT
to Health and Physical Education

PART ONE

FUNDAMENTAL CONSIDERATIONS OF MEASUREMENT

The physical and health educators' approaches to measurement should be in terms of improved service to students. Teachers with vision and will to work have little enough time to accomplish what they are trained for—that is, to contribute significantly to the growth and development of individuals in their care. Each person is a unique problem, with his own peculiar background and capabilities, differing from others in innumerable ways. A fundamental function of physical and health educators is *to understand each person's needs* in order to give adequate guidance and to adapt programs to meet needs.

If these functions are to be accomplished efficiently, measurement is indispensable, for orderly progress cannot be achieved without the guidance that intelligent use of measurement provides. By utilizing measurement properly, the educator may fulfill his destiny, giving the service that he should be qualified to give.

Successful measurement, then, involves defining and measuring the truly important outcomes of physical education and health education—that is, the abilities, needs, and capacities of individual pupils. The only justification of a testing program

Approach to Measurement

of any kind in the schools is that it insures and enhances students' education. Of course, testing does not take the place of teaching. It does, however, make teaching more definite and concrete, and can itself be a highly effective teaching device. The purposes of this chapter are to outline such an approach to measurement and to indicate a practical basis for the selection of tests.

PHYSICAL EDUCATION AND MEASUREMENT

Early Measurement

Physical education has a rich heritage in measurement and evaluation. Since the early work of Edward Hitchcock at Amherst College in 1861, research leading to the construction of evaluation instruments has been a consuming interest of many workers in the field. Tests in some areas of physical education are much more numerous and better constructed than in others. The history of physical education reveals the reason, for measurement emphases have been closely associated with the changing role of physical education in our society. The direction of measurement over the years has reflected the changing philosophy and objectives of this field.

Early Influences. The earliest physical education in the United States was patterned after European systems, especially the German and Swedish. Although parts of these systems still exist and are of great value to physical education, none of them were generally adopted. A new country was being explored, settled, and developed; a new and powerful nation was being created; a new culture was evolving. It was to be expected that physical education would eventually reflect and support this unfolding culture. Although certain beginnings can be traced to this earlier

3

period, the emergence of a culturally oriented physical education was not generally apparent until after World War I.

Between the Civil War and World War I, the primary objective of physical education was physical fitness. Most pioneer leaders of this era were trained in medicine. These men and women were attracted to the field because of the potential health or preventive medicine values of proper physical activity. They gave major direction to physical education for a half century during its formative years.

Among the professional leaders of this period were many who were interested in research. These pioneers early turned their attention toward studying the effectiveness of their programs and constructing tests to evaluate results. In keeping with their objectives, tests were designed to measure aspects of physical fitness. The earliest form of such testing was anthropometry, based upon the theory that emphasis should be placed on bodily symmetry and proportion with exercise prescribed to affect muscle size. For example, in his earliest work, Hitchcock,[1] who introduced the science of anthropometrics into physical education, utilized tests of height, weight, various breadths and girths, and vital capacity. Later, due to the research of Dudley A. Sargent, indicating that "capacity" of the muscles should be given value in judging an individual's fitness, interest changed to strength and its measurement. With the invention of the ergograph by Mosso and its use to study muscle fatigue and the efficiency of the circulatory system, still another shift in measurement occurred to determine the efficiency of the cardiovascular system. The measurement emphasis during this period was consistent with the physical fitness objective. The changes in the actual types of tests utilized

[1]J. Edmund Welch, *Edward Hitchcock, M.D.: Founder of Physical Education in the College Curriculum.* Montgomery, West Virginia: The Author, West Virginia Institute of Technology, 1966.

were the results of increased knowledge and understanding of the factors involved.

Organismic Concept. The concept of organismic totality was gaining favor in man's beliefs. Milestones in the growth of this concept were: the Athenian education of the fifth century B.C., which recognized the need for balance in the mental, social, and physical education of the individual; the expressions of Locke, Rousseau, and other European philosophers that in a sane body lies a sane mind, a thought voiced later by Horace Mann, Henry Barnard, and Herbert Spencer; the early observations of physical educators that the care and development of the body contributes to the individual's mental, emotional, and social effectiveness; the experimentation of psychologists, such as James, Thorndike, and more recently Harold E. Jones and Willard C. Olson, who demonstrated the interaction of basic forces in the individual; and the dramatic findings of physicians that the "whole man" must be treated, not just the disease or the disability.

The cumulative impact of evidence verifying the organismic concept led to enlarged functions of physical education after World War I. It also set the stage for an expansion in research with new emphases in measurement, inevitable concomitants of changing philosophies and objectives.

Factors Shaping Modern Practice

Modern physical education dates from the early 1920s, when it became an integral part of education. The leadership shift was to men and women prepared as educators. The objectives showed recognition of physical education as a part of the educational process. In the period of transition, great difficulty was encountered in making necessary adjustments and thinking through, adopting, and putting into practice effective education procedures. At the same time, to further

medical
& fitness
recreation
life-time sports

complicate the situation, physical education was undergoing tremendous expansion throughout the United States. While many factors shaped modern practice in physical education, six especially significant ones have been selected for consideration here.

Educational Balance. As mentioned above, new objectives were recognized as physical education struggled for a place in the educational curricula of schools and colleges. Initially, however, physical educators were prone to go to extremes in promoting their favorite objective—be it physical fitness, character development, or preparation for leisure pursuits. In practice, some programs were all sports and games designed to develop desirable personal and social behavior patterns; other programs catered almost entirely to the teaching of sports skills for leisure use; in still others, mass drills and apparatus exercises were dominant as the development and coordination of the body were stressed.

At the beginning, there was also a tendency on the part of some influential leaders to abandon the biological heritage of physical education. The understandings and tested practices of fifty years were frequently rejected in the rush to adopt new ideas and procedures. In general, improvement of physical fitness became a concomitant of an activity program designed to realize other objectives. The results of this repudiation of the historic role of physical education found our youth to be no better off physically in World War II than they had been in the previous world war.

Too often during this period, an "either-or" attitude was adopted. Intolerance and immature judgment marked many professional arguments. World War II had a leavening influence, for, following it, there was a tendency to seek for educational balance, so that physical education could make its fullest contribution to the lives of everyone. As the late dean of

physical education researchers, C. H. McCloy,[2] wrote: "I have always felt that a well-equipped physical educator would have room in his mind for a reasonably large number of objectives, of ideas, and of questions—and that the addition of some new idea should simply mean some careful rearrangements—but that the *good* ideas, even though they dated back 4,000 years to the Egyptians and the Chinese—should still be welcomed, constantly experimented with and improved—and put to use."

Eleanor Metheny has written, as a consequence of the proliferation of stated objectives, confusion results concerning the total potential of physical education today. "Too many objectives, particularly if they are not clearly defined and even more particularly if the relationships among them are not clearly understood, can be self-defeating. If we try to be all things to all men, we shall end up doing little if anything for any of them. And so we need to continually examine and re-examine our objectives—their sources, implications, and relations—to keep them in perspective."[3]

Educating for Democracy. In this century, our democratic belief met its first great challenge with the rise of fascism and national socialism in Italy and Germany, culminating in World War II in which the democracies were forced to defend their ideals of government. Today, communism constitutes a similar challenge. If belief in democracy is to survive, it must be essentially the result of informed public understanding and action. Schools and colleges should not only be dispensers of knowledge pertaining to democratic concepts, but should be laboratories in democratic living. Leaders in physical education are alive to this prob-

[2]C. H. McCloy, "Why Not Some Physical Fitness?", *The Physical Educator,* **13,** No. 3 (October 1956), 83.

[3]Eleanor Metheny, "Man Is Bio-Psycho-Philosophical Organism Capable of Voluntary Movement," *The Physical Educator,* **16,** No. 3 (October 1959), 83.

lem, as it relates to their field, as evidenced by many recent publications. The processes of democracy, as revealed in research in group dynamics, are being studied and applied to physical education. The need to determine the physical educator's contribution to education in a democracy is essential and constitutes a forceful challenge for the future of the field.

Turbulence in American education today is caused by new social trends and forces. The need to develop international and interracial understandings has added new dimensions to education. The women's "liberation" movement has necessitated a reappraisal of practices in physical education and athletics for women. Leaders in physical education have made strong efforts to deal with such problems. Among the noteworthy examples of these efforts are: the National Conference on the Interpretation of Physical Education,[4] which presented a series of basic beliefs agreed to in principle by leaders of the profession; and the prepared pamphlet, *This Is Physical Education*,[5] published by the Physical Education Division of the American Association for Health, Physical Education, and Recreation, which provides an interpretation of physical education through a description of its broader and deeper understandings.

Individual Needs. Physical educators are well aware that males and females differ from each other in many ways and that these differences affect their physical education performances. However, recent studies[6] have quantified the nature, extent, and significance of such differences as related to physical education and athletics. For example, a 12-year longitudinal growth study was conducted in the Medford, Oregon public schools, in which the same boys were tested annually within two months of their birthdays from age seven years until they graduated from high school.[7] Taking a single age, 14 years, the ranges of some of the tests were: skeletal age, 80 months; weight, 115 pounds; leg lift strength, 1375 pounds; and Physical Fitness Index (strength relative to age and weight), 131. Further, these differences were shown to have great significance in the abilities of boys to participate in physical education and athletic activities, in recognition by their peers, in personal-social relationships, and in mental accomplishments. The totality of the individual was demonstrated. Thus, each child brings more than his body to the gymnasium, the playground, and the athletic field; he also brings his mind, his emotions, and his unique personal and social traits.

As a consequence of these differences, the individual needs of some may be pronounced. Insofar as activities and methods and the qualifications of personnel permit, physical education should meet the needs of those who are handicapped in some respect, those who have functional defects or deficiencies amenable to improvement through exercise, or those who possess other inadequacies which interfere with their successful participation in the diversified and vigorous activities of the general program.

Presidential Concern. Oberteuffer[8] has pointed out that the United States is now in the fourth discernible period in the twentieth century of intensified interest in

[4]*Report of the National Conference on Interpretation of Physical Education* (Chicago: The Athletic Institute, 1961).

[5]*This is Physical Education* (Washington: American Association for Health, Physical Education, and Recreation, 1965).

[6]H. Harrison Clarke, "Individual Differences, Their Nature, Extent, and Significance," *Physical Fitness Research Digest,* President's Council on Physical Fitness and Sports, **3,** No. 4 (October 1973).

[7]H. Harrison Clarke, *Physical and Motor Tests in the Medford Boys' Growth Study* (Englewood Cliffs, N.J.: Prentice-Hall, 1971).

[8]Delbert Oberteuffer, "The Role of Physical Education in Health and Fitness," *American Journal of Public Health,* **52,** No. 7 (July 1962), 1155.

the role of physical education in physical fitness. These periods are: (a) Theodore Roosevelt's advocacy of the vigorous life to make this nation strong; (b) draft statistics following World War I, which shocked legislatures throughout the land into passing state laws requiring physical education in the schools; (c) the all-out effort during World War II to prepare the population to wage total war, initiated by Franklin D. Roosevelt; and (d) since 1955, when Dwight D. Eisenhower and, later, other presidents took executive actions to establish and continue a President's Council on Physical Fitness and Sports. President Eisenhower's concern was with the development and maintenance of a physically vigorous and emotionally stable citizenry as essential for national survival. However, President Kennedy associated it with a broader need when he stated, ". . . we do know what the Greeks knew: that intelligence and skill can only function at the peak of their capacity when the body is healthy and strong; that hardy spirits and tough minds usually inhabit sound bodies."[9]

The latest period of intensified interest in physical fitness was triggered by the results of a minimal test of muscular fitness with which Dr. Hans Kraus and associates compared United States children with children from Austria, Italy, and Switzerland, much to the discredit of American youth. Similar surveys with Kraus' and other tests followed with comparable results. The President's Council on Physical Fitness and Sports took dynamic action to alert the public to the national danger resulting from this situation; a tremendous push for physical fitness emphasis in the schools and colleges of the country ensued.

Starting primarily as a public relations agency in the late 1950s, the Council extended its services to Americans of all ages and provided materials for the conduct of proper physical fitness programs. National influence was exerted on physical fitness efforts in schools and colleges, youth serving agencies, community recreation centers, business and industry, and the adult population at large. Among continuing projects conducted by the Council are: regional physical fitness clinics and medical symposia; publication of brochures, manuals, and a quarterly *Physical Fitness Research Digest;* preparation of promotional and instructional films; a Presidential Physical Fitness Awards program for boys and girls; and a Presidential Sports Award program for adults. In 1973, the Council received a President's Citation from the American Association for Health, Physical Education, and Recreation for informing the American public of the need for maintaining health through physical activity.[10]

Rise of Spectator Sports. A tremendous cultural phenomenon of our time is the rise of spectator sports. Literally millions of people annually watch school, college, and professional sports contests from the stands; millions more view many of these same contests from in front of television sets or listen to their accounts on the radio. Nearly every cross-roads hamlet in the nation has its school athletic teams; partisan fans support these teams in their contests against those of neighboring schools. Frequently, area, district, and state championships are organized; spectator interest and attendance constantly mount as the championship level is reached. Colleges and universities have their conference championships, bowl games, and rated teams and players; the paid attendance of spectators place many athletic departments in the realm of big business.

The rise of spectator sports has had marked effects, both positive and negative, on school and college physical educa-

[9]John F. Kennedy, "The Soft American," *Sports Illustrated,* **13,** No. 25 (December 25, 1960), 15.

[10]H. Harrison Clarke, "President's Council on Physical Fitness and Sports," *The Academy Papers,* No. 8, 1974.

tion programs. On the negative side, the drive to field the best possible athletic teams has often pre-empted personnel, attention, facilities, time allotment, and budget. On the positive side, it has stimulated athletic participation, engendered support for physical education, and created interest in the activities of the physical education program. It has also frequently contributed financially to the construction of improved athletic facilities, which are shared by the physical education program. As the realization becomes clear that a strong physical activity program for all students contributes dynamically to improved athletic teams, increased support is readily realized for physical education.

Implications for Measurement and Evaluation

As noted before, measurement and evaluation always show relationship to purposes to be achieved. It may therefore be expected that more and better instruments will have been developed to determine achievement of older objectives than there has been time to develop in relation to newer goals. The construction of tests in various phases of physical fitness has been in process for a century. A wide research experience and valid instruments are at hand, augmented by materials developed by scientists in physiology and related fields. On the other hand, tests of personality, social adjustment, and peer status are of recent origin, and only limited research and the construction of relatively crude instruments have so far been possible. A considerable time lag is inevitable between new program emphases and the construction of adequate instruments to evaluate their outcomes.

As inferred, then, a consideration of measurement impels one to philosophical analyses. Therefore, in order to select tests, the teacher must first decide what to test, which requires that he first select aims and objectives. To do otherwise would be

to place the cart before the horse or to start a journey without knowing either the direction or the destination. The physical educator without definite aims and objectives and without well-thought-out procedures for realizing them is in an untenable position. Thus, no testing project should be undertaken unless it is part of an attack upon a clearly defined educational problem, the solution of which can be aided materially by the use of tests. This means that tests should not be given merely for the sake of testing, but only when there is some definite object in view. *The follow-up program—the use of test results for program modification in order to serve the pupil better than would otherwise be possible—is the real justification for the administration of tests.*

The following three questions should be answered by all physical educators planning physical education programs: (a) What are the objectives of my physical education program? (What am I trying to accomplish in physical education, anyway?) (b) What procedures shall I follow in meeting these objectives? (How am I going to do it?) (c) What types of tests are needed to make my program effective and later to determine results? (What tests will help me to do it and show that it has been done?) These questions indicate the logical sequence of steps to be followed in the establishment of any rational physical education program.

The scientific or measurement approach to program planning is the only way the teacher has of insuring against waste. The physical educator who does not measure dissipates much of his efforts. If he does not test to determine the physical needs of individuals, how can he plan a program to meet those needs, and how will he know that they have been met? Can he show how his teaching is benefiting his pupils? In what ways and how much? Can he prove that certain phases of his teaching are not definitely harmful? Can he demonstrate how well an activity has been learned? Could he defend his physical education program against an investigation by administrative officials—except through verbal rationalization?

INTEREST IN HEALTH EDUCATION MEASUREMENT[11]

Early Measurement

The scientific revelations of Pasteur in France, Koch in Germany, and Metchnikoff in Russia during the nineteenth century stimulated public thought about personal health as related to disease. These European advances, supported by American scientists, led to widespread acceptance of the importance of health knowledge to environmental control of disease in this country.

In 1829, William A. Alcott established the need for improving the hygiene of schools in his publication, *Construction of School Buildings.*[12] In 1837, Horace Mann pointed to the need for health instruction in the public schools.[13] Many schools had begun medical inspection of children by the year of 1894. Thus, the three phases of the modern school health program, namely, healthful school environment, health instruction, and health services, had their beginnings in the United States during the nineteenth century. Health education is defined as follows.

Health education is a process with intellectual, psychological, and social dimensions relating to activities which increase the abilities of people to make informed decisions affecting their personal, family, and community well being. This process, based on scientific principles, facilitates learning and behavioral change in both personnel and consumers, including children and youth.[14]

Health is, therefore, a multifaceted discipline which encompasses the entire being and has to do with living. It includes school and community programs to improve the quality of life.

Early measurement techniques generally compared existing programs to recommended practices for the three phases of the complete school health program. As early as 1911, however, Luther H. Gulick[15] speaking before the Congress of the American School Hygiene Association, stated that a fundamental need in school hygiene was for the definite measurement of results. Gulick urged that the greatest need of education itself was neither authority nor philosophy, but specific methods of testing the effects of present systems and practices. Evaluation of health education in the past focused on the recognition and learning of facts. Present trends include assessing concepts and attitudes and determining behavior patterns.

Factors Shaping Modern Practice

The results of the compulsory examinations of prospective draftees during World War I presented the first opportunity for the public to view the general physical status of young men. They realized that half of the many defects discovered might have been corrected if recognized during the school years. This strengthened the position of health education in the schools.

During the 1920s, the term "health ser-

[11]Acknowledgments for the preparation of this section and the section on "Objectives of Health Education" are made to Dr. Robert E. Kime, Professor of Health Education, and Dr. Lorraine G. Davis, Assistant Professor of Health Education, both of University of Oregon.

[12]William A. Alcott, "Essays on the Construction of School Houses," *Lectures Before the American Institute of Instruction,* Vol. II (Baltimore: Hilliard, Gray, Little, and Wilkins, 1932).

[13]Horace Mann, *First Annual Report of the Secretary of the Board of Education* (Boston: Dutten and Wentworth, 1838).

[14]*Report of the Joint Committee on Health Education Terminology, President's Committee on Health Education, Final Report,* March 15, 1973.

[15]Luther H. Gulick, "Measurement as Applied to School Hygiene," *American Physical Education Review,* **16,** No. 4 (April 1911), 239–41.

vice" came into use to designate the broader responsibilities of the school toward the student.[16] Within this concept, boys and girls were evaluated with respect to their total health, including annual medical examinations, daily teacher observation, height and weight status, vision and hearing screening tests, and dental examinations. The Malden, Massachusetts school health project conducted by Claire E. Turner[17] in 1922 did much to support general school health and health instruction. Over a period of two years, he experimented with health education procedures in the fourth, fifth, and sixth grades. His experimental groups proved superior to the control groups in growth, health status, and health habits.

Following World War II, a great deal of interest in health education was evident. Instruments were developed that enabled evaluation of the school plant and facilities to insure a healthful school environment. Health knowledge tests were constructed and instruments were developed to assess health attitudes and habits. The instructional curriculum was constantly improved and new techniques of health-habit motivation were examined and utilized. In the 1950s and 1960s, measurement in the health field became increasingly related to the crises of the so-called sexual revolution, the drug scene, and a venereal disease epidemic. These crises influenced health education and were manifested in the measurement of the young person's knowledge about them.

These concerns have continued and, now, with the economic crises, accountability is a major issue in education and all areas of life. With the need to "prove" worth or increases in knowledge or improvements in attitudes for purposes of maintaining or expanding programs, evaluation in health education has become especially important. This observation is especially crucial since health education is a recent addition to academic offerings by the schools.

A movement is in progress to make health education practical for students, now and through a lifetime. Measurement has become an essential part of this movement; a drive is evident to utilize tests for comparative purposes nationwide. A major problem found in health education is that by the nature of the subject area the content is constantly changing through research in health and medical science, so it must be updated regularly. Health education is still in the developmental stages, but, in many schools, has finally received separate recognition as a required academic subject. Continuous measurement and evaluation has led to better programs and will continue to point the way for progress in the future.

OBJECTIVES OF PHYSICAL EDUCATION

In considering physical education objectives, the individual should be regarded as an indivisible unit, acting and reacting as an integrated whole. Man cannot sensibly be divided into separate compartments. His muscles, internal organs, blood, and mind contribute to functional unity. Strength, at least its application to one's activities, depends no less on character than on muscles and on the quantity and quality of blood circulating through these muscles; and the quantity and quality of the blood depends on the efficiency of the other organs of the body. Without the help of the heart, the nervous system, the liver, the thyroid, and all the other glands, the muscles of the greatest athlete in the world would remain impotent. A healthy mind is necessary too. No soldier has ever been really great if not led by faith in himself, in the cause for which he fought, in his leaders, and in his country. To fight, or

[16]Deobold B. VanDalen, Elmer D. Mitchell, and Bruce L. Bennett, *A World History of Physical Education: Cultural, Philosophical, Comparative* (Englewood Cliffs, N.J.: Prentice-Hall, 1953), p. 445.

[17]Claire E. Turner, *Principles of Health Education* (New York: D. C. Heath, 1939), pp. 38–64.

even merely to work in time of stress, requires more than well-trained muscles.

Furthermore, all physiological activities contain mental elements and effects, and all mental elements are bound to organic functions. It is now generally accepted by scientists that body disturbances create psychic disturbances and psychic disturbances create body disturbances. The more informed people become concerning symptoms of stress and strain, the more difficult it becomes to determine whether physical symptoms are due mainly to emotional disturbances or to physical causes. In fact, the whole question of resistance to disease is bound up with the emotional resilience of the individual. For example, the physical changes that take place under the influence of fear are familiar phenomena: effects on the skin, the respiratory system, the heart, the digestive-eliminative functions, and so on. Actually, no comprehensive evaluation of the individual is possible unless a thorough physical examination has been made and any symptoms of emotional upsets explored—especially if, after a reasonable time, the condition does not respond to physical remedies. Many people have carried the physical symptoms of mental disturbances to the point where they have undergone painful treatment and even hospitalization and surgery.[18]

In like manner, physical abnormalities have often been the cause of mental, social, and emotional difficulties. To cite a homely illustration, an individual cannot perform his best mental work (nor is he such a social being) when he has a splitting headache or is suffering from indigestion. In treating mental patients, psychologists routinely investigate physical conditions as sources of the ailment as regularly as— and even before—they seek obscure psychological reasons. Thus, a regular phase of the corrective treatment applied to truancy offenders by Children's Courts is the correction of any physical defects found. Likewise, intelligent parents consider physical reasons as possible causes of emotional upsets in their children. An important responsibility of the school health service is the discovery and elimination of physical defects in children in order that they may benefit from their education and be better able to take their places in society after graduation.

All these possibilities illustrate the necessity for considering human beings as entities rather than as dichotomies of physical and mental forces. The pupil, then, must not be separated into "body" and "mind," but should be regarded as a complicated and precise mechanism, the effective and unimpaired action and interaction of all the parts being essential for the well-being of the individual as a whole. Therefore, every instructor must be concerned for the body, the mind, and the spirit of his pupils.

From the administrative point of view, however, the *determination* of physical education objectives in terms of the major contribution to each field in the growth and development of the child—such as physical, mental, and social—is the only reasonable way of clearly stating the purposes to be attained in this field. Such designations should be considered as a method of analysis, not as mutually exclusive categories.

Physical education is identical with other kinds of education so far as its aims and purposes are concerned. As expressed by Champlin:[19] "*Personal and social developments in terms of all-round fitness to live the good life in our democracy* are its objectives." This means physical fitness, social efficiency (including moral and spiritual qualities), recreational competency, and the cultural appreciations to serve others

[18]Edward Lies, "Physical Aspects of Emotional Problems," *Child Study,* **18,** No. 1 (Fall 1950), 3.

[19]Ellis H. Champlin, "Physical Education and the Good Life," *Springfield College Bulletin* (November 1955).

and the nation and to enjoy the satisfactions of responsible, democratic citizenship. The great difference from other programs of education is that the medium employed to educate is physical activity with its associated understandings, skills, attitudes, and behavior patterns.

PHYSICAL FITNESS: *The ability to carry out daily tasks with vigor and alertness, without undue fatigue, and with ample energy to enjoy leisure-time pursuits and to meet unusual situations and unforeseen emergencies.*

Thus, physical fitness is the ability to last, to bear up, to withstand stress, and to persevere under difficult circumstances where an unfit person would give up. Physical fitness is the opposite to being fatigued from ordinary efforts, to lacking the energy to enter zestfully into life's activities, and to becoming exhausted from unexpected, demanding physical exertion.

Organically, man is a muscular creature. Thus, children, as well as their teachers and parents, are meant to be physically active. They possess an organism designed for movement with the neuromuscular mechanisms which will produce movement of infinite variety and magnitude. When children succumb to a state of physical inactivity, as from disease, or give way to the lazy ease and comfort of modern living, they pay a price in decreased efficiency in every part. Remove physical activity from life and atrophy not only of size but of function results. Experience becomes limited. Muscles become small and weak and fatigue easily.

The definition given implies that physical fitness is more than "not being sick" or merely "being well." It is different from resistance to or immunity from disease. It is a positive quality, extending on a scale from death to "abundant life." All living individuals, thus, have some degree of physical fitness, which varies considerably in different people and in the same person

from time to time. In accordance with this concept, children who are not sick, who are free from defects and handicaps, and who are adequately nourished, may still exhibit physical deficiencies. Such deficiencies may be observed in pupils who are lacking in circulatory endurance; they may also have postural defects and inadequate body flexibility.

Physical fitness, therefore, is an essential quality in man. School children, as well as their parents, may not need the muscular development and strength required of their pioneering forefathers, whose very lives often depended upon them; but, in intellectual as in physical work, a sound heart and lungs, good digestion, and a vigorous, well-developed physique are still great assets for effective accomplishment and for living a satisfying life.

SOCIAL EFFICIENCY: *The development of desirable standards of conduct and the ability to get along with others.*

The term "social efficiency" indicates those traits usually included in the concepts of character and personality. It involves human relationships. It has a definite social implication, since in our democratic society, the effects of one's actions upon others are of primary concern.

"Character" was once thought of as morality, and "personality" as the impression the individual makes upon others. According to this belief, one could have a "sterling" character and still be thoroughly disliked. A "pleasing" personality, on the other hand, indicated readiness in favorably impressing others, regardless of the fact that the possessor of the personality might be a complete scoundrel. With the emphasis in education today upon the social aspect of living, resulting from men's interdependence, the definition of character has been extended to include these relationships, and the concept of personality has been defined to include morality. The attempt has been to redefine both "character" and "personality" as all-inclusive terms embracing both individual and social behavior. The concept is dependent upon: (a) individual traits, such as courage, initiative, morality, perseverance, and self-control; (b) group traits, such as sympathy, courtesy (sportsmanship), honesty, co-operation, and loyalty; and (c) their interrelations for the common good. *A socially efficient individual is one who functions harmoniously within himself, in his relationship with others, and as a member of the society of which he is a part.*

Participation in many physical education activities necessitates numerous person-to-person contacts; when properly directed, these contacts result in and promote desirable social relationships. They are real to the child—they have meaning; decisions must be made that affect not only the child himself but others participating in the activity. When the social studies teacher stresses the duty of the citizen to vote, this duty is, on the whole, a relatively abstract concept, and its reality is not experienced by school children for some time to come. When one boy shoves an opponent in a basketball game, the effect is immediately felt; it is a concrete situation that is meaningful to him, to the boy shoved, and, in varying degrees, to all members of both teams. Physical activities, therefore, *properly presented and conducted,* develop traits basic to future civic behavior—traits that are fundamental to the social development of the individual—courage, co-operation, persistence, initiative, resourcefulness, and will power; respect for the rights of others, for authority, and for the rules of the game; also, self-respect, loyalty, justice, self-confidence, sacrifice of self for the good of the group, aggressiveness, followership, and leadership. The transfer of such traits to other school activities and to life situations, especially if the total interest of the pupil is stressed throughout, may well occur.

Social efficiency also embraces moral and spiritual values. The Educational Poli-

cies Commission[20] has defined these values as those which, when applied in human behavior, "exalt and refine life and bring it into accord with the standards of conduct that are approved in our democratic culture." Many of these values find political expression in the Constitution and Bill of Rights. Among these are: the supreme importance of the individual personality, moral responsibility for one's conduct, voluntary co-operation through common consent, devotion to truth, respect for excellence, moral equality, pursuit of happiness, and emotional and spiritual experiences transcending the materialistic aspects of life. The student can learn to compare the worth of one desire as it conflicts with another, or his own desires as they conflict with those of other people. He can do this by facing athletic situations which involve a moral choice among competing courses of action, by thought and discussion about the possible results of one course of action as weighed against another, and by later re-examination of the results.

RECREATIONAL COMPETENCY: *The improvement and betterment of man through creative, wholesome, and imaginative leisure-time living patterns.*[21]

Changing conditions of modern living have greatly increased the need for recreative activities. Today, men do not engage in a wide variety of activities in their work, but often repeat the same movement to distraction. Then, bodies and minds require change—not only for pleasure, but even more to re-create their vitality and capacity for enjoyment. In large measure, too, the demands upon the worker's physical and mental energies are less than before, but as a rule the nervous tension is

[20]Educational Policies Commission, *Moral and Spiritual Values in the Public Schools* (Washington: National Education Association, 1951).

[21]Lynn S. Rodney, *Administration of Public Recreation* (New York: Ronald Press, 1964), p. 4.

greater, due to the mechanization of industry. Laborsaving devices have cut down the amount of work required in the home, drudgery is reduced, and children who formerly had many chores about the house now find few tasks to perform.

That the American people are utilizing their free time for recreational pursuits is clearly evident. Chase[22] estimated that in 1927, out of a national income of 92 billion dollars, the American people expended 21 billions upon leisure-time activities and for commodities consumed during leisure. By 1950, Dewhurst[23] estimated that approximately twice this amount was being spent for one purpose or another by the American public in the pursuit of recreational interests. Pendergast[24] indicated that the average American in 1962 has more leisure than working hours in a year; his calculation gives about 2175 leisure hours annually as compared to 1960 hours of paid work. In 1973, Nanus and Adelman[25] predicted that the following leisure-related events would occur by 1980, based on a manpower study of the U.S. Department of Labor: average work week reduced to 32 hours; 30-day work vacations for at least half of all employees; and average age of retirement around 60 years. To meet adequately the modern demand for participation in wholesome recreational activities is a stupendous task, which will become increasingly pressing as time goes on.

Recreation is obviously a very broad field, including all those numerous activities that adults and children engage in for the pleasure, satisfaction, and benefits that

can be derived from them. Physical education can contribute to the development of one's recreational competency, especially through play, games, and sports.

Culture: *The enrichment of human experience through physical activities that lead to a better understanding and appreciation of the environment in which people find themselves.*

Traditionally, culture has been thought of as confined to the classical areas of human thought: literature, philosophy, art, and music. Only infrequently since the time of the early Greeks has physical education been considered to possess cultural potentialities. This lack of recognition is due in part to the general concept of culture still prevailing in the minds of educators in general, and in part to a similar lack of recognition by physical educators themselves. There are, however, great cultural potentialities in physical education.

A broad definition of "culture" is: *one's stock of appreciation, including all aspects of living that will improve one's understanding and enjoyment of those objects, people, and events that make up his environment, both local and world-wide.* Many activities included in the physical education program are cultural—in fact, any worthwhile activity executed skillfully enough to help pupils to understand each other and the world. For example, the grace, rhythm, and creative expression of the dance, together with its association with the present and past in this and other countries, its racial and folklore significance—these are truly and highly cultural. An understanding and appreciation of the human body, both biologically and aesthetically, is cultural. Appreciations of skilled performance on the part of others, be they amateurs or professionals, are cultural. The historical backgrounds of such age-old physical skills as archery, fencing, boxing, wrestling, and track and field events are cultural. Play and sport have been prominent in man's heritage, traced back to his earliest consciousness; they are included in his cul-

---

[22]Charles A. Beard, *Whither Mankind* (New York: Longmans, Green & Co., 1928), Ch. 14.

[23]J. Frederic Dewhurst, *America's Needs and Resources: A New Survey* (New York: Twentieth Century Fund, 1955), p. 348.

[24]Joseph Pendergast, "The Place of Recreation in Modern Living," *Journal of Health, Physical Education, and Recreation* **33,** No. 6 (September 1962), 22.

[25]Burt Nanus and Harvey Adelman, "Forecast for Leisure," *Journal of Health, Physical Education, and Recreation,* **44,** No. 1 (January 1973), 61.

tural perspective and they have complemented his search for understanding and meaning in life.

Although not categorized as cultural, Nixon and Jewett[26] included as one of their objectives of physical education to develop a basic understanding and appreciation of human movement. Included under this broad objective were: the development of understanding and appreciation of the deeper, more significant human meanings and values acquired through idea-directed movement experience; an appreciation of human movement as an essential non-verbal mode of human experience; and the development of key concepts through volitional movements and closely related non-verbal learning activities.

In writing on a contemporary view of sport, Miller and Russell[27] show that the theme of sport has crept into the dialogue of many disciplines. It is evident in psychology, with man's search for self; in philosophy, with the attempt to clarify man's relations with reality; in sociology, with serving as a locus for man's relationships with other men; in the arts, as prominent vehicles for creative expression; in education, with its impact on learning. Sport pervades the American way of life. The authors state: "At a time that is characterized by instant change, the flurries of flights to the moon, the sounds of intercontinental aircraft rushing past with fleeting intensity, sport seems to remain a mission of permanence—inexhaustibly vital, immortally versatile."

Emphasis for Girls and Women

Many great educators since Aristotle have suggested the complete separation of educational aims and objectives for men

and women. However, in recent decades there has been a drastic increase in civil, vocational, and intellectual freedom for women, and this trend is still progressing, actually at an accelerated pace. Aside from definite biological differences, the educational and physiological needs of women are converging with those of men. Thus, the generalization may be advanced that the aims and objectives of education and physical education are essentially the same for boys and girls, differing primarily in emphases and details.

To illustrate the emphases recognized by women, Jane Shaw,[28] in a study of reasons for participation in a YWCA physical education program as expressed by out-of-school girls and women, found that they came to the gymnasium because they were not satisfied with their lives as they were living them; they felt that something was lacking and sincerely wanted to better themselves. Reasons given for YWCA participation were as follows.

1. To reduce.

2. To gain weight.

3. To correct posture or some figure fault.

4. To learn to relax and take things easy after working all day in an office.

5. To learn skills, such as tennis, swimming, and so forth, so that they could play them on their vacation and in their spare time.

6. To learn social dancing so that they would become more popular and have more dates.

7. To participate in a recreation program.

8. To seek company, a desire brought on by lack of companionship.

After this analysis of felt needs, and after subsequent interviews with many of the women, the following physical education objectives were proposed.

1. Physical fitness: Organic vigor and efficiency, knowledge of requirements for healthful liv-

[26]John E. Nixon and Ann E. Jewett, *An Introduction to Physical Education,* 7th Ed. (Philadelphia: W. B. Saunders 1969), p. 90.

[27]Donna Mae Miller and Kathryn R. E. Russell, *Sport: A Contemporary View* (Philadelphia: Lea & Febiger, 1971), p. vii.

[28]Jane Shaw, "Expressed Objectives of Physical Education by Girls and Women." Unpublished study, Syracuse University.

ing, nutrition, exercise, and rest; relaxation; correction of physical defects; and preparation for motherhood.

2. Personal appearance and beauty: Development of a beautiful and graceful body; development of good posture and physical poise; elimination of physical defects affecting appearance; knowledge and care of hair, complexion, nails, and so forth; and knowledge of appropriate, healthful, and becoming clothing.

3. Human relationships: Opportunity to make friends; development of democratic conduct and ideals; opportunity for a rich and varied social life; development of consideration for the well-being of others; development of courtesy, co-operation, and sportsmanship; and development of social skills that will add to their popularity and social adjustment.

4. Recreational skills: Development of many skills that will be useful as leisure-time activities, and enjoyment of those skills and games of a recreational nature.

5. Appreciations: Appreciation of rhythm and music; appreciation of beauty, grace, and poise; appreciation of art, skill, and achievement; appreciation of ability in others; appreciation of personality; and appreciation of freedom and democracy.

Robinson[29] has taken strong issue with the concept that participation in physical activity and sports by girls and women detracts from their femininity. He contends that the belief has been fostered by a cultural emphasis of women as attractive objects and by a belief that sport was a male domain. He hypothesizes logically that when muscles are well conditioned, one's appearance is also enhanced: with an improvement in muscle tone, the firm clean lines of a well-proportioned and attractive body are revealed; muscles which have minimal exercise tend to be flaccid, having poor tone which adds to the flabby appearance of ever present adipose tissue. The author concludes "We should learn to accept strength in women as being as in-

trinsic to femininity as it is to masculinity, just as we accept kindness as much a part of the male role as it is of the female role."

Thus, the values of physical education which women recognize as essential, correspond well with the stated objectives propounded in this text. Certainly, the physical, emotional, and social stresses of modern life strike both sexes indiscriminately. Strength and endurance are needed by both sexes. Boys may have a more immediate application for these qualities to athletic participation; however, many working housewives have need for a greater absolute level of physical fitness than do their sedentary husbands. While body poise and grace are recognized as immediately desirable traits for girls and women, they might actually be cited as prime criteria for good motor performance in both men's and women's activities. Even "beauty," if replaced by a term to indicate the idea of "attractive physical appearance," appears as a vital need for both men and women.

OBJECTIVES OF HEALTH EDUCATION

The responsibility of the school in meeting the health needs of all students has been clearly stated in publications concerning general aims of education. An early influential statement of aims was the 1918 report by the Commission on the Reorganization of Secondary Education.[30] Health was placed first in its list of seven cardinal principles of education. The 1938 report of the Educational Policies Commission[31] described the health educated person as one who understands the basic facts about

[29]Paul D. Robinson, "Physical Activity and Femininity," *British Journal of Physical Education,* **4,** No. 4 (July–August 1973), 59.

[30]Commission on the Reorganization of Secondary Education, Cardinal Principles of Education, Bulletin 1918, No. 35 (Washington: Superintendent of Documents, Government Printing Office, 1918).

[31]National Education Association and Association of School Administrators, *The Purposes of Education in American Democracy* (Washington: Educational Policies Commission, 1938).

health and disease, who protects his own health and the health of his dependents, and who works to improve the health of his community.

An individual must increasingly accept responsibility for making wise choices to protect his health and the health status of the family. In 1973, the Oregon state health specialists proposed two sets of goals to provide direction for the scope and content of health education in the schools of the state; one goal was for over-all health education and the other was for the health education program.[32]

The health education goals are as follows.

1. Mental Health: The student will possess the knowledge attitudes and skills to foster individual, family, and community mental health needs.

2. Community Health: The student will be able to accept responsibilities for promoting the health of the local, national, and international community by exploring occupational opportunities in health agencies and by utilizing the services of these groups.

3. Physical Health: The student will possess the basic knowledge, skills, and attitudes necessary to develop and maintain optional individual physical health and foster that of others.

4. Safe Living: The student will be able to apply his knowledge and skills to promote safe living.

The health program goals are as follows.

1. The student has positive feelings about himself and other people.

2. The student has the knowledge and skills needed to insure the physical and mental health of himself and others.

3. The student makes decisions and acts in ways which contribute to good personal and community health.

4. The student has a basic knowledge of human growth and development.

[32]*Tri-County Course Goals Project,* Health Specialists, Oregon State Department of Education, Salem, Oregon, 1973.

5. The student has knowledge and skills relative to safe living, accident prevention, and emergency care.

6. The student knows the purposes served by the family in providing psychological security to its members.

7. The student knows the major local, national, and global health problems, and some of the ways in which they might be solved.

8. The student is familiar with, is able to evaluate and use material and services provided by individuals and/or organizations dedicated to solving health problems.

9. The student is knowledgeable about career opportunities in health and allied fields.

The objective of health education is to assist the student to attain and maintain optimal physical, mental, and social health. In the school health program, the immediate objectives are determined by current needs of the students. Objectives in different grade levels vary somewhat due to differences in the maturity and intellectual capacity of the students. Basically, the objectives at the elementary school level are to instill good health attitudes and habits. At the secondary school level, the objectives are to assist students to realize personal responsibilities to maintain their own health. For the college student, objectives expand toward developing a critical analysis of personal and community health in hope of bettering the future of society.

The major purpose of a school health education program is to improve and maintain the health of students. The areas included in school health education are healthful environment, health instruction, and health services. The health program should include inspection and supervision of the physical, mental, emotional, and social environments of pupils during their stay in the public schools. It also includes health instruction in the areas of nutrition, accident prevention, personal and community health, recreation, and physical education. The health needs of individual pupils should be discovered and brought to the attention of parents as soon as possible.

The World Health Organization[33] has also established objectives for health education, which serve as overall guidelines for the world. They are as follows.

1. To intensify . . . concrete and effective action to ensure that children and young people receive a multidisciplinary health education, which is of particular importance for the development of future generations;

2. To explore and promote new approaches for tackling and solving in an appropriate way the problems posed by the health education of mothers, children, and young people in order to take care of their health and of their protection against the harmful factors of modern life;

3. To support actively the basic right to health of the child and the adolescent and to promote by suitable means the improvement of the legislative provisions, together with other concrete actions aimed at ensuring a healthy future for the rising generations;

4. To invite other organizations . . . and through these . . . national health agencies, volunteer organizations, and parents, to participate actively in the implementation of activities for the health education of children and young people.

SELECTION OF TESTS

Tests in health and physical education may be used for many purposes. All purposes, however, focus in one all-encompassing aim: to realize educational objectives; to serve students better than would otherwise be possible. If the preceding discussion in this chapter is sound, therefore, physical educators will then logically devise procedures, select activities, and adopt methods to develop physical fitness, social efficiency, recreational competency, and cul-

tural appreciations adapted to the separate needs of students.

Procedures for meeting each of the physical education objectives will be contained in Chapters 3, 10, and 13, which introduce the various types of tests. Examples of the manner in which physical education tests may be selected on the basis of educational procedures are given as follows.

1. If individual physical fitness needs are to be met, tests measuring essential elements of physical fitness are necessary—in order to select those with such needs, to follow their progress, and to know when needs have been met.

2. If maintenance of physical fitness on the part of all students is desired, again tests measuring essential elements of this quality are needed as a periodic check on fitness status.

3. If nutritional status or physiological efficiency of pupils is to be given special attention, appropriate tests in these areas should be selected.

4. If pupils with postural defects are to be selected for inclusion in remedial classes, a test of this quality is obviously necessary.

5. If pupils with postural and/or orthopedic defects have weaknesses of various muscle groups, strength tests of the involved muscles are needed.

6. If homogeneous grouping of pupils for participation in the broad physical education program is considered desirable for pedagogical purposes or to provide a desirable setting for the development of personal-social relationships, general motor ability tests might well prove helpful.

7. If pupils with tendencies toward social maladjustment or who are generally rejected by their peers are to be discovered and helped, personality tests, behavior rating scales, and peer-status instruments will prove advantageous.

8. If emphasis is to be placed upon the general development of athletic ability, tests of general motor capacity and ability will be found most useful.

9. If homogeneous grouping by specific skill ability is desired, appropriate skill tests and achievement scales are necessary.

[33]World Health Organization, *Official Records of the WHO,* No. 217 (Geneva, 47th Annual Conference of WHO, 1974), p. 13.

10. If skill in and understanding of specific physical education activities are sought, skill tests, knowledge tests, and attitude scales may be selected.

11. If pupils are to be motivated toward whole hearted and enthusiastic participation in physical education activities, follow-up testing with tests of basic physical and motor traits and the use of self-testing procedures will prove effective.

12. If pupils are to be graded in health and physical education, objective evidence in arriving at the grades will be of special significance to pupils and parents.

13. If reports of pupil progress are to be prepared for administrators, boards of education, and the public, the most essential physical and social growth factors should be measured.

In considering the selection of actual tests that will be used in the physical education program, two points should be borne in mind. First, only those tests should be selected that will aid in making physical education effective. Second, only the best tests available for the job intended should be used. The use of poorly constructed or empirical tests, when scientifically constructed tests are available, is little less than folly and decidely a waste of time. If important decisions are to be made concerning the pupil's physical fitness, personal-social status, and the like, the physical educator should be as sure as he can be that he is right.

Conclusions

The regular use of measurement is one of the most distinctive marks of the professional viewpoint in any human activity. This statement applies particularly to engineering, medicine, and education, and perhaps most to physical education, which affects pupils so immediately and so profoundly in their most impressionable years. Educational tests and the programs resulting from their use in physical education are coming to be regarded as

synonymous with good teaching practice, for it is only through measurement that the effects of teaching can be determined at all—that progress can be known. Therefore, the physical educator contemplating the inauguration of any program should turn to measurement as a matter of course. It is not too much to say that the use of measurement in physical education may be considered as a prerequisite to the professional growth of the educator.

But although the progressive physical educator should use tests, his attitude toward testing should be both liberal and critical. A liberal viewpoint will allow him to use imperfect tests if and when they are the best available at the moment, in the hope that through their greater use better tests will eventually result. A critical viewpoint prevents him from being satisfied with present tests and insures a demand for progressively better tests.

Selected references

Clarke, H. Harrison, "Individual Differences, Their Nature, Extent, and Significance," *Physical Fitness Research Digest*, President's Council on Physical Fitness and Sports, **3,** No. 4 (October 1973).

Clarke, H. Harrison, *Physical and Motor Traits in the Medford Boys' Growth Study.* Englewood Cliffs, N.J.: Prentice-Hall, Inc., 1971.

Clarke, H. Harrison and Franklin B. Haar, *Health and Physical Education for the Elementary School Classroom Teacher.* Englewood Cliffs, N.J.: Prentice-Hall, Inc., 1964.

McCloy, C. H., "Why Not Some Physical Fitness?" *The Physical Educator*, **13,** No. 3 (October 1956), 83.

Metheny, Eleanor, "Man Is a Bio-Psycho-Philosophical Organism Capable of Voluntary Movement," *The Physical Educator*, **16,** No. 3 (October 1959), 83.

Robinson, Paul D., "Physical Activity and Femininity," *British Journal of Physical Education*, **4,** No. 4 (July–August 1973), 59.

ROGERS, FREDERICK RAND, *Dance: A Basic Educational Technique.* New York: The Macmillan Company, 1941, Ch. 1.

SARGENT, DUDLEY A., "Twenty Years of Progress in Efficiency Tests." *American Physical Education Review,* **18,** No. 7 (October 1913), 452.

This is Physical Education. Washington: American Association for Health, Physical Education, and Recreation, 1965.

CHAPTER 2

Measurement is neither a new nor an uncommon phenomenon. In all walks of life measurement is used. In fact, if all our various testing devices were suddenly destroyed, contemporary civilization would collapse like a house of cards.

For ages the ingenuity of man has been directed toward the control of his environment. His procedures have evolved from pure trial and error, and even chance, through intelligent appraisal of existing knowledge and a thoughtful consideration and testing of likely hypotheses, to the marvelous method of modern science, which measures weights in millionths of a pound, distinguishes among thousands of colors and shades, calculates time even in millionths of a second, and so forth. Aristotle was one of the first great scientists. Since his time, man's quantitative conquest of nature has expanded not only into all branches of physics and chemistry, but into organic and psychological phenomena as well. Education, and even more recently physical education, are but relative newcomers to the scientific procedure. It is safe to predict that the future effectiveness of education and physical education will be proportionate to the refinement and use of testing instruments available in these fields.

Test Evaluation

FUNCTION OF MEASUREMENT

Reduced to its simplest terms, the function of measurement is *to determine status*. Status must be determined before conclusions concerning the thing measured can be drawn and before comparisons can be made. In this concept, several factors are involved.

Status

By measurement the status of the quality to be measured is determined. For example, the distance an athlete can jump may be measured with a steel tape; the speed he can run, with a stop watch; the amount he weighs, with scales; and the capacity of his lungs, with a spirometer. In each case, a quantitative measure indicates the status of the quality involved in terms of feet and inches, minutes and seconds, pounds, and cubic inches, respectively. Status is determined by the surveyor with level and compass, by the photographer with photoelectric cell, by the mechanic with vernier calipers, and by the bacteriologist with microscope. To determine status, therefore, is the function of measurement.

Comparison

After the status of a person is known with reference to a particular quality as measured, comparisons can be made with others in his group, with norms, with standards, and with himself at different points in time. To illustrate these comparisons, the testing of body weight is used as an example. A boy's weight, his status, may be 200 pounds. When compared with others in his group, this weight may be among the highest of those taking the test. When compared with a norm based upon his sex, age, and height—which, let us say is 160 pounds—he is found to be 40 pounds, or 25 percent, overweight. Compared with national standards, this 25 per-

21

cent overweight is classified as obese. As his weight is high, he is given treatment through appropriate diet and exercise, with the result that his weight is lowered to 180 pounds, an improvement of 20 pounds. Thus, the round of measurement possibilities on an individual basis is complete. Similar processes are possible for groups.

The fact that the amount of change in status can be determined by measuring the same individual or individuals after a lapse of time is a highly important factor in physical education, for it becomes possible to measure the progress of the individual, the group, and the school, so that program and teacher efficiency are in turn rendered measurable. These measures of progress are also the basis for research.

CRITERIA OF TESTS

After the physical educator has decided upon the objectives of his program, after he has devised administrative and educational procedures to realize these objectives, and after he has determined the type of tests he will need for their full realization, he is ready to select the specific tests to be utilized for each essential task to be performed. In order to make satisfactory selections, *he should evaluate available tests in terms of their scientific attributes.* To do this, he should answer questions concerning each test considered, in order to be able to choose the best and the most useful for the job to be done. For example, (a) does the test measure the quality for which it is to be used? *(validity)*; (b) can the test be administered accurately? *(reliability, objectivity)*; (c) can the test scores be interpreted in terms of relative performance? *(norms, standards)*; (d) is the test economical? *(cost of instruments, economy of time)* An understanding of these terms is essential before tests can be intelligently evaluated and wise choices made.

Test construction is based upon the use

of *statistics*—mathematical procedures showing relationship between variables. Investigators utilize statistics in the analysis of their measurement scores. Thus, a knowledge of statistics is necessary in order to understand and evaluate their researches. A presentation of statistical processes appears in Appendix A.

VALIDITY OF TESTS

A *valid* test is one that measures what it is used to measure. The need for this quality in a test is so obvious as to preclude argument. To use a test to measure something for which it is not intended is absurd. We do not weigh a person in order to determine his height, nor do we use a barometer to determine temperature. On the contrary, if we wish to know a person's weight, we use scales that measure weight; if we wish to know his temperature, we use a thermometer that measures heat.

Certain relationships can be readily seen. We know that scales measure weight; a stop watch, time; a steel tape, distance; and a thermometer, heat. And yet, originally, the validity of these measures had to be established. How do we know that the scales measure weight? That the thermometer measures temperature? One might ask: What is a pound? A second? A foot? A degree of heat? At one time agreement on these concepts had to be reached. Today, we no longer question these measurement relationships, nor do we question the instruments that have been devised to measure them.

But how about less tangible, less mechanical concepts? On what basis may we believe that the Binet-Simon Test measures intelligence? That the Physical Fitness Index is a measure of physical fitness? That cardiovascular tests indicate circulatory endurance? That a ball-volleying test is a measure of general tennis ability? The relationships here are not so obvious. One wants proof that they exist.

Consequently, in constructing tests, the researcher presents evidence to support his contentions regarding the elements or traits that his tests measure. In order to do this, he establishes a criterion of the element being measured and compares the new test with this criterion measure. If the two have a high relationship—if they go together, if the test and criterion agree—the researcher may logically conclude that his test measures the same quality as does the criterion. In determining the validity of tests, therefore, the physical educator should evaluate two elements, the degree to which the criterion measure represents the quality being measured, and the amount of relationship shown between the test and the criterion.

The Criterion

Physical education researchers have used considerable ingenuity in devising criteria in the validation of tests. In general, the following five types of criteria have been utilized:

Critical Appraisal. The initial basis for the construction of many general motor ability and motor fitness tests has been critical appraisal, although usually other criteria have also been used. This process consists in analyzing the activity in terms of its fundamental elements. For example, in constructing the Youth Fitness Test for the American Association for Health, Physical Education, and Recreation, a committee of qualified professional personnel, through critical appraisal, designated the following seven components of motor fitness: arm-shoulder muscular endurance, abdominal muscular endurance, agility, speed, muscular leg power, muscular arm-shoulder power, and circulatory-respiratory endurance. Then, based on their extensive knowledge of tests, they selected one test item to represent each of the seven components. The only actual research done in developing this test consisted of

the construction of percentile norms for boys and for girls at each age 10 through 17 years for each of the seven test items.

Established Test. A simple criterion is to utilize a test of the same quality the validity of which has been established. If the relationship between the old and the new tests is close, they measure essentially the same thing. This is a practical application of the basic algebraic rule that, when two different measures agree with a third, they also agree with each other. Of course, the degree of agreement of the criterion test with the quality measured limits assurance of the validity of the new test. The new one may or may not be more valid than the criterion, but the experimenter cannot know this from his investigation. This practice of validating a new test with an established procedure has not been followed to any extent in physical education. However, several established tests have been revised or simplified in this manner, i.e., by using the original test as the criterion. Thus, we have the Iowa Revision of the Brace Test, the Methany-Johnson Test of Motor Educability, and the Oregon Simplification of the Strength Index.

Subjective Judgment. In the utilization of subjective judgment as the criterion, ratings of the relative ability of the subjects in the activity to be measured are made by experts. This criterion has been used in constructing tests in team sports, such as basketball, soccer, field hockey, volleyball, and the like. In such activities, it is otherwise difficult to isolate the quality of the individual's performance from that of his team mates.

Composite Score. The composite score is the sum of all the scores made by each individual on all the tests included in the experimental situation. These scores are usually expressed in standard score form, as, otherwise, such values as distance in the standing broad jump, number of chins, and speed in the 50-yard dash could not be added. This criterion has been in common use in the validation of motor ability and motor fitness tests.

Functional Evidence. This criterion consists of functional evidence of the element for which the test is constructed. As examples of the application of this criterion in test construction, the following may be mentioned: Dyer used round-robin play to validate her tennis test; Cureton used a manikin as a criterion of posture and a footprint in specially prepared sand as the criterion for determining the validity of footprints as a measure of the height of the longitudinal arch of the foot; Rogers used major sports letter men, captains, and "best players" as representing athletic ability.

Relationships

If the relationship between a test and its criterion measure is low, little value can be attached to the test, unless there are extenuating circumstances. One such circumstance is the use of a criterion measure that is itself inaccurate. For example, certain judgment ratings are known to be inconsistent; to use such ratings as a criterion for test results, as has been done in the construction of skill tests, would impair the value of the results. One would naturally, therefore, expect to get lower validity coefficients when such criteria are used.

Then, too, tests themselves may be somewhat inaccurate but still superior to any other available methods. To illustrate, Cureton, in constructing posture tests, obtained reliability and objectivity coefficients that were well below ordinarily accepted standards for satisfactory measurement. Yet, he was able to show that his objective procedures were much more accurate than the results of subjective inspections by experts. Therefore, the use of the objective posture scheme may be justified in lieu of a better testing instrument.

Obviously, too, not everything can be measured with the same degree of precision. Such elements as jumping distance, running speed, and muscle strength can be recorded with considerable accuracy, whereas character traits, appreciations, and attitudes still lag behind in the objectivity with which they can be determined. Consequently, these factors should be taken into account in evaluating present-day tests in physical education.

Relationship is usually shown by correlational methods, in which the proposed test is related by mathematical procedures with the criterion measure. In these instances, the most desirable standards are 0.90 and above, although correlations above 0.80 are considered significant. Validity coefficients obtained by this method in constructing certain of the tests mentioned above, for example, were as follows below:

Experimenter	Element Measured	Criterion Measure	Correlation Coefficient
F. W. Cozens	General athletic ability of college men	41 motor ability tests	0.97
T. K. Cureton	Height of arch by footprints	Height of footprints in sand	0.90
J. Dyer	General tennis ability	Round-robin play	0.92
F. R. Rogers	General athletic ability by Strength Index	Track and field events	0.81

Relationship may also be indicated by comparing the successes in the test obtained by contrasting groups: those rated as "good" and those rated as "poor." For example, the performance on the test of the upper quarter or third of the group, selected according to the criterion measure, may be compared with the performance of the lower quarter or third. Validity for the McCurdy-Larson Organic Efficiency Test was determined by this method, three contrasting groups being selected as follows: (a) good-condition group, varsity swimmers at the 440-yard distance; (b) poor-condition group, infirmary patients; and (c) average group, all Springfield College freshmen over a two-year period. The criterion for the Washburne Social Adjustment Inventory was also established by this procedure, the following four groups being utilized: (a) well-adjusted high school pupils; (b) average-adjusted high school pupils; (c) maladjusted high school pupils; and (d) second-term reform school offenders.

Validity, of course, is absolutely essential for a good test, since without it one does not know what the test measures. In fact, to use an unvalidated test is worse than useless: it is positively misleading.

ACCURACY OF TESTS

Need for Precision

The accuracy with which things are measured, or with which differences are perceived, depends first upon the precision of the measuring instruments. An alarm clock is a valid measure of time, but one would scarcely use it as a measure of speed in the 100-yard dash, because it is not precise enough. It does not register time with sufficient precision to be usable for this purpose. Neither could a wrist watch be used, even if it were equipped with a second hand. Today, in important track and swimming meets, even the stop watch is unsatisfactory, accurate timing being based upon electrical devices. In like manner, a foot long rule measures distance, but one would hesitate to use it for measuring the distance one can throw the discus or javelin. Even human ability to perceive the winner of a close race is often questioned; therefore, the photographic lens has replaced the human eye in horse-racing events, for example.

Many consider themselves able judges of weight; and, indeed, weight should be one of the easiest of the physical measurements to estimate. It is surprising, however, to note the great range of variation among any group of physical educators in estimating the weight of one of their members. To estimate the *amount* of difference in weight between two individuals when one is small and the other is large leads to even less satisfactory results. To perceive that one individual weighs more than the other is, of course, quite simple in this situation; but the more closely two individuals approach the same weight, the more difficult even this becomes.

Thus, the existence of a difference is quite easy to note when two objects are at opposite extremes, although the amount of the difference is not so simple unless *precise measuring instruments are used.* And, too, estimating the amount of an individual's change in weight after the lapse of a period of time is even more inaccurate. A set of scales, however, solves this problem simply and easily.

In measurement, we make sure rather than guess or take for granted; moreover, the more refined the testing instrument, the better the results. Of course, some individuals can attain a great degree of precision, at least of some qualities, as, for example, the "side-show" man who guesses the weight of individuals within three pounds, and the athletic coach who, with many years of experience in observing his players in a large number of situations, selects the members of his athletic teams on a judgment basis. (Incidentally, this specialist, the athletic coach, regularly and frequently corrects his mistakes in judgment by substitutions.) But a convenient index of the condition of the players on the day of a game would be a great help to any coach in selecting his starting players, and also in determining substitutions. The need for precise measuring instruments is thus readily seen. Certainly, if guessing such tangible physical factors as weight is lacking in accuracy, how much more difficult must it be to judge such intangibles as physical fitness, motor ability, and social efficiency.

Reliability

The reliability of any test may be defined as the degree of consistency with which a measuring device may be applied. A highly reliable test yields the same or approximately the same scores when administered twice to the same individuals, provided conditions and subjects are essentially the same. Unfortunately, the conditions and the subjects may not be the same each time, especially if the two tests are given with one or more days intervening. Feldt and McKee[1] have shown in skill testing that daily individual differences in skill performances occur, that skill learning results as a consequence of previous testing, and that differences in such factors as day-to-day fatigue condition, mental set, bodily health, and level of motivation may be present. The presence of any of these factors in test-retest situations can only lower test reliability. Henry[2] has discussed intra-individual variability and

other errors of measurement as related to test reliability; his reference should be consulted for a fuller understanding of this concept.

A common procedure is to repeat the full test with the same subjects and under the same conditions, and to correlate the results of the two tests. When this method is followed, test accuracy is expressed in terms of coefficients of correlation, known as reliability coefficients. It is possible, however, for this correlation to be high without the test being really reliable, which would be the case if the subjects had consistently higher scores on the second administration of the test than they had on the first. The presence of this condition may be detected by taking into account both the correlations and the difference between the average scores of the two tests.

Objectivity

Objectivity as a concept has different meanings. The common term, objective tests, usually refers to written examinations scored from a key, as for true-false and multiple-choice questions. In test construction, however, objectivity means the degree of uniformity with which various individuals score the same tests. In other words, a perfectly objective test is one in which no disagreement occurs among competent persons in scoring any given subject while using the same test. Objectivity in grading essay-type examinations has been notoriously low. Frequently great differences occur among scores assigned to the same paper by different readers. Essay examinations, however, can be scored with greater consistency if proper precautions are taken in the preparation of check lists and in the training of scorers. For example, Grant and Caplan[3] obtained correlations between two readers scoring

[1]Leonard S. Feldt and Mary Ellen McKee, "Estimation of the Reliability of Skill Tests," *Research Quarterly*, **51**, No. 2 (October 1957), 279.

[2]Franklin M. Henry and others, "Errors in Measurement," *Research Methods Applied to Health, Physical Education, and Recreation* (Washington: AAHPER, 1949), Ch. 19.

[3]D. Grant and N. Caplan, "Studies in the Reliability of Short-Answer Examinations," *Journal of Educational Research,* **51,** No. 2 (October 1957), 109.

the same short-answer examinations by college students of 0.98 when factual questions and 0.82 when comprehension questions were answered.

With the newer types of objective tests, however, acceptable consistency is possible, although their validity may be questioned as measures of, say, appreciations, ability to express oneself, and various social traits. In physical education, on the other hand, scoring is usually a fairly simple procedure, since scores are frequently recorded in units of time, distance, or height, in readings on a dynamometer dial, or in the number of times a particular exercise or skill is successfully performed.

A somewhat different concept of the meaning of the reliability and objectivity of tests is indicated in physical education performance. (This is that a measure is reliable if two or more *measurements* of the same object or function by the same device and tester yield similar scores; and that it is objective if two or more different *individuals,* using the same instrument, or procedure, secure similar results. In this case, tests with high objectivity will also have high reliability, since an individual will agree more readily with himself in administering tests than he will with others.) Frequently, therefore, in constructing tests, objectivity only is computed; the assumption is that, if this is satisfactory, reliability is automatically assured.

A test, however, can have a high degree of reliability without an appreciable degree of objectivity. For example, in establishing the footprint angle as a measure of the height of the longitudinal arch of the foot, one of the lines originally drawn was defined as a "line of best fit." Reliability for this form of the test was 0.90, no objectivity coefficient being given. Thus, the tester was able to place the line consistently in the same place, but his idea as to where it should be did not agree with the position in which it was placed by others. By defining this line precisely, the

reliability of the test was increased to 0.97 and the objectivity coefficient became 0.95. Many judgment ratings have yielded similar results. In test construction, therefore, every effort should be made to secure high objectivity, so that physical educators may compare their test scores with the test scores of other teachers or with universal norms.

The question of acceptable objectivity coefficients for health and physical education tests needs consideration. As a general rule, coefficients of 0.90 and above should be obtained before satisfactory test achievement is realized. If a lower coefficient is reported for a test, less reliance can be placed on scores when the test is used. (Rough guides for securing adequate objectivity in measurement are: (a) accurately phrased and fully detailed instructions in measuring procedures; (b) simplicity of measuring procedures; (c) the use, wherever possible, of mechanical tools of measurement; (d) reductions of results to mathematical scores; (e) selection of intelligent measurers, carefully trained; (f) maintenance of professional or scientific attitudes by testers; and (g) unremitting supervision of measuring procedures by administrative officers. Objectivity standards that have become generally accepted follow.

Objectivity
Coefficients

0.95–0.99	very high; found among the best tests
0.90–0.94	high; acceptable
0.80–0.89	fairly adequate for individual measurement
0.70–0.79	adequate for group measurement, but not satisfactory for individual measurement
0.60–0.69	useful for group averages and school surveys, but entirely inadequate for individual measurement.

It does not follow, because an objectivity coefficient of 0.90 is reported for a test, that anyone using the test will automatically achieve this degree of test precision. When tests are constructed, the testers are carefully trained in testing techniques, sufficient to achieve such accuracy. Untrained testers may not be nearly as consistent in administering the test. An essential practice is for two testers to practice with some 30 subjects, each testing them independently, until they are able to achieve an objectivity coefficient approximately as high as reported for the test.

Investigators have studied the stability of scores when multiple trials of a test are given. McCraw and McClenney[4] administered one trial each day of sit-ups, push-ups, and pull-ups for four successive days to fifth, seventh, and tenth grade boys. Even though the boys were given a week of practice on the tests prior to the experimental period and a warm-up before each testing session, push-ups continued to increase each day for all grades; pull-ups and sit-ups did not stabilize for the fifth and tenth grade boys respectively. Kane and Meredith[5] gave 12 standing broad jump trials on each of two days to elementary school children. Sixty percent of the children performed their best jumps on the second day. Kroll[6] tested college men five times a day for three successive days on the wrist flexor strength test. The strength scores were significantly higher on the third than on the first day. College students enrolled in conditioning classes were tested by Baumgartner[7] on the standing broad jump and on a side-

step test twice a week for three weeks; three trials of the jump and five trials of the side-step were given at each session. For both tests, significant variability among days was found. The reasons for the increases in scores for the various tests were not investigated. From extensive testing experiences, however, it may be speculated that some learning of testing techniques took place from test to test; and, even more important, the motivation inspired by attempting to improve previous performances could well result in improved test scores. For the sake of objectivity in testing, the tester should instruct carefully in test techniques, allow practice trials, and hold motivation as constant as possible.

NORMS AND STANDARDS

Generally, in the construction of tests, norms are prepared from testing random samples of children for whom the tests are intended. Thus, norms are based upon the status quo. For skill tests, this basis may be satisfactory, especially if the sample includes subjects ranging from poor to superior. For physical fitness testing, however, this basis is faulty inasmuch as the norms will only reflect the present condition of American youth; adequate physical fitness will not necessarily be presented. If a lack of health knowledge is normal, certainly it is not desirable. Thus, standards indicating proper levels for physical fitness components, health knowledge, and other human traits are needed; unfortunately, such standards do not exist. In this sense, *standards* differ from *norms*; a standard is the degree of attainment in a quality or characteristic held to be essential for a certain purpose or function, usually empirically determined and set for specific groups.

Yet, norms have a definite value, as will be illustrated. Is a weight of 125 pounds satisfactory? Is a Strength Index

[4]Lynn W. McCraw and Byron N. McClenney, Reliability of Fitness Strength Tests," *Research Quarterly,* **36,** No. 3 (October 1965), 289.

[5]Robert J. Kane and Howard V. Meredith,"Ability in the Standing Broad Jump of Elementary School Children 7, 9, and 11 Years of Age," *Research Quarterly,* **23,** No. 2 (May 1952), 198.

[6]Walter Kroll, "Reliability Theory and Research Decision in Selection of a Criterion Score," *Research Quarterly,* **38,** No. 3 (October 1967), 412.

[7]Ted A. Baumgartner, "Stability of Physical Performance Test Scores," *Research Quarterly,* **40,** No. 2 (May 1969), 257.

of 1500 good? How may a time of 25.5 seconds on the obstacle race in Scott's Motor Ability Test for college women be interpreted? What can be expected in athletics from an individual with a score of 190 on McCloy's General Motor Ability Test? These questions cannot be answered without additional information concerning the individuals so measured. A weight of 125 will be satisfactory for certain individuals; for others it will indicate a serious underweight condition; and for still others it may mean obesity. With norm charts based upon sex, height, and age, a satisfactory answer can readily be reached. The same is true of the Strength Index. Thus, a Strength Index of 1500 may indicate adequate strength, great strength, or general weakness, depending on the sex, age, and weight of the individual. The obstacle race time of 25.5 seconds becomes meaningful when it is discovered that it has a T-scale score of 51, representing the average performance on the test for college women. In order to understand the McCloy score of 190, one must know the norm for that individual, the norm in this case being based upon a classification index (age, height, and weight).

(Norms, therefore, are necessary in order to interpret test scores.) In physical education, norms may be based upon various combinations of age, height, and weight, as indicated above.) In this situation, average scores are usually given with other values to indicate the significance of variances from this point. For example, in the use of age-height-weight tables, usually an individual 10 percent below the average weight for his age and height is considered to be underweight, and, if 20 percent above, he is considered obese by these norms. In the case of the Strength Index, the boy or girl whose Strength Index equals the norm for his or her age and weight has a Physical Fitness Index of 100. This, then, is a median score based on sex, age, and weight. A lower score of 85 is at the first quartile according to the norms,

and a higher score of 115 is at the third quartile. Thus, these variations from average may be interpreted.

Also commonly used in physical education are scoring scales based upon absolute performances, rather than relative performances as above. One such scale is the percentile, which gives the percentage of individuals scoring below points on the scale in the sample upon which the scale was constructed. Thus, 50 percent score below the 50th percentile, 27 percent below the 27th percentile, and so on. While easily constructed and readily understood, this scale has the disadvantage of unequal values for differences in scale points. Actually, the percentile scale is crowded largely around the mean performance; approximately two-thirds of the scale is within the middle one-third of the distribution. Actually, this scale encourages mediocrity of performance, because it is easy to progress in the middle range of scores, where values are close together, and difficult to improve at the ends of the scale, where values are much farther apart.

Scales based upon standard deviation values of normal distributions[8] have been used extensively in health and physical education. Four of these are generally recognized: Z-score, T-scale, sigma-scale, and Hull-scale. For the Z-score scale, the mean is zero; the other scores are expressed in terms of plus and minus standard-deviation distances from the mean. Thus, a score of -1.5 is 1.5 standard deviations below the mean. For the other three scales, the mean is 50; they differ in the positions of 0 and 100. Zero and 100 in the T-scale are -5 and +5 standard deviations from the mean; for the sigma and Hull-scales, these distances are 3 and 3.5 standard deviations below and above the mean respectively.

Norm charts themselves must be

---

[8]The construction of these scales is presented in Appendix A.

evaluated, too, to determine their propriety. Several general evaluative factors are discussed briefly below to indicate the nature of this process.

1. Sampling procedures for the construction of norms should be based upon a wide distribution of the population. In physical education, quite frequently, such samples are definitely limited to rather small geographical areas. Typically, researchers have been restricted to their own general location in the collection of test data. To attempt a broader sampling has its difficulties. Not only is it costly; it would depend upon the utilization of many testers.

2. The testing sample should be representative of the population for which the test is intended. For example, data for skill test norms collected from athletes would be representative of athletes, but not of the population as a whole. Norms for weight charts based upon boys and girls residing in favored neighborhoods might not properly reflect the status of all classes of children.

3. Norms should be used for the specific groups for which they are prepared. As an illustration, the Dyer Tennis Test was originally constructed for college women and the norms were based upon a sampling of women in a number of colleges. To use these norms, therefore, for college men, or for any other group, would be inappropriate.

4. Norms for standard tests should be based upon a relatively large number of cases. An arbitrary assignment of a specific number for this purpose is impossible, however, as the reliability of the sample depends in part upon the variability of the test data, i.e., the range of scores for the element being tested. The greater the variability of scores, the larger the number required to reduce the standard error of estimate to a negligible quantity. To illustrate, the heights of individuals in a defined population do not vary so greatly as weight or strength for the same population, and, as a consequence, in the development of norms they will vary within narrower limits. The possibility of securing reliable norms for this trait is much better, therefore, and can be accomplished with a smaller sample of the population.

ECONOMY OF TESTS

Cut 10% of time devoted to meaningful Tests

In considering the economy of tests, two factors should be kept in mind: (1) money costs, and (2) time required of subjects and testers. Other things being equal, of course, tests requiring little in money and time should be used. Thus, the cost of apparatus may be a prohibitory factor in the use of certain tests in schools. For example, this is the chief reason why the X-ray and basal metabolism tests are not generally used. Cost, however, should not be the major consideration, but rather the value of the test in the physical education program. The cost of certain types of testing apparatus may be justified in the light of the value received.

The amount of time required for administering tests, as well as the energy and degree of effort required, is an important factor in test economy. Some authorities believe that one-tenth of program time spent in testing is justifiable. Consequently, tests that may be quickly administered are preferable. One fault of many skill tests, for example, is that they require a great deal of time to give. However, many tests that appear difficult and time-consuming can be administered economically if proper organization techniques are employed.

OBJECTIVE WRITTEN EXAMINATIONS

Objective written examinations have not been utilized in physical education as widely as in general education. However, such tests have been prepared to determine the amount of information acquired and the understanding developed in health education and in physical education. As related to sports, exercise, dance, and related activities, such tests would include historical background, terminology, rules governing the activity, equipment and facilities, techniques involved in performing the activity, strategy when appropriate as in sports, etiquette and courtesies, and values to the participant. When applied to the area of physical fitness, other factors are involved that may be considered in knowledge tests, including the importance of physical fitness, the need for exercise as a way of life, the meaning of physical fitness and its basic components, ways by which physical fitness components can be improved and maintained, and the specific and concomitant values accruing from adequate physical fitness.

The procedures for constructing tests of this sort differ somewhat from those employed with the more generally used skill and performance tests. Also, some physical educators prefer to construct locally the written tests they use; a distinct advantage of this procedure is that it permits adaptation to local needs, local course content, and specific types of teaching. A general understanding of the precautions to be taken in constructing such tests and of the techniques employed in this type of test construction should therefore be beneficial to health and physical educators.

Types of Examination Questions

Frequently in practice, objective written examinations have taken the form of true-false statements exclusively. Consequently, in the minds of many the true-false test is "the" objective test. Actually, there are several types of written objective tests. These may be classified into two general categories, (*recognition*, including such types as true-false, multiple-choice, and matching; and *recall*, including simple recall and completion.) Several of these test forms are discussed briefly below.

True-False.   In this common type of objective written test, a statement is made which the student marks as true or false; T and F or + and 0 may be used to designate true

or false as the answer. The following examples are taken from Hewitt's Comprehensive Tennis Knowledge Test, Form A, Revised:[9]

Directions: About one half of the following statements are true and about one half are false. If the statement is more true than false put a (+) sign in the space provided and an (0) if the statement is more false than true. *Answer each question as if it relates to a right-handed player.*

1. _____ A chop stroke produces a backward spin on the ball.

4. _____ If time permits, a pause at the end of the backward swing on all drives is advisable.

8. _____ Stepping on the line while in the act of serving is called a line fault.

15. _____ "Wightman Cup" play is competition for women only in England and the United States.

Unusual care must be exercised in phrasing true-false statements so that their meanings are clear without obvious clues to their answers. The following specific suggestions should be followed in constructing this type of test:

1. Avoid ambiguous statements.

2. Avoid tricky questions.

3. Do not use double negatives; in fact, avoid negative statements as much as possible.

4. Use *all* or *never* statements very cautiously.

5. Omit statements that express opinionated views, at least without definite reference to source.

6. Avoid statements that are partly true and partly false.

7. Utilize short, concise statements as much as possible.

8. Avoid trivial and meaningless items.

Scoring may be done by counting the number of statements answered correctly

[9]Jack E. Hewitt, "Hewitt's Comprehensive Tennis Knowledge Test—Form A and B Revised," *Research Quarterly,* **35,** No. 2 (May 1964), 149.

or by subtracting the number of wrong answers from the number right ("rights minus wrongs"). The latter method was devised to discourage guessing and is widely used. Actually, for college students at least, there is apparently little difference in the relative score received. Keislar[10] obtained correlations of 0.96 and 0.99 between the way the same college students answered true-false questions scored by number right and rights minus wrongs.

True-false statements can be used to test for factual information, for the application of general principles, and for reasoning. They are also well adapted to testing the persistence of popular misconceptions and superstitions.

Multiple-Choice. In the multiple-choice form, a statement or question is given with three or more responses, only one of which is correct or definitely better than the others. Examples of this type of question are taken from a health knowledge test for the seventh grade by Veenker.[11]

An answer sheet is used for this test. In the directions the mechanics of using the answer sheet are explained. The students are instructed to read each statement carefully and then to select one answer which best completes the statement.

3. To keep the hair soft and glossy (1) use a vinegar rinse after washing, (2) apply hair dressing each morning, (3) do not wear a hat or cap, (4) brush it several times daily.

15. Iron is needed in the body for the manufacture of (1) red blood cells, (2) white blood cells, (3) malaria, (4) Rocky Mountain spotted fever.

In preparing multiple-choice questions, care should be taken to avoid the inclusion of irrelevant or superficial clues and to measure other than memorized knowledge. Following are suggestions for preparing appropriate statements of this type:

1. Use at least four choices whenever possible.

2. Make all choices plausible; if obviously wrong choices are included, the real thinking situation is reduced accordingly.

3. Be sure only one of the choices is correct.

4. Keep the choices short where possible.

5. Word questions simply.

6. Scatter the position of the correct choices and avoid any set pattern.

7. Use unfamiliar phrasing rather than that from the text.

8. Avoid statements acknowledged to be disputed by authorities, or which vary from time to time, unless authority or time is stated.

9. Score by counting the number of correct responses.

The multiple-choice type of test is regarded as one of the most useful of the test forms. It is especially valuable in testing judgment, reasoning ability, and fine discrimination between various shades of meaning.

Matching. Two varieties of matching questions are as follows: (a) *sentence completion matching,* in which completion of a sentence is required by matching it with a column of items, only one being chosen as correct; and (b) *column matching,* in which words, sentences, numbers, or phrases arranged in two opposite columns are matched. In these instances, the student merely shows which items go together. Examples of matching questions from the Hewitt tennis test[12] are as follows:

1. basefault

2. volley

3. love all

4. let

5. deuce

6. overhead play

[10]Evan R. Keislar, "Test Instructions and Scoring Methods in True-False Tests," *Journal of Experimental Education,* **21,** No. 3 (March 1953), 243.

[11]C. Harold Veenker, "A Health Knowledge Test for the Seventh Grade," *Research Quarterly,* **30,** No. 3 (October 1959), 345.

[12]Hewitt, "Tennis Knowledge Test," p. 149.

direct relationship

7. thirty-all

8. end line

9. fifteen-all

10. footfault *easy to prepare*

11. baseline *difficult to grade*

12. stop-volley

13. kill *too difficult to prepare*

14. net ball

15. fifteen-love *easy to grade*

16. permissible

17. lob

18. continue play

19. pick up

20. half-volley

21. game

22. advantage receiver

23. smash

24. love-fifteen

43. _____ When each side has won two points each.

44. _____ End line of a tennis court.

45. _____ Hitting the ball overhead with an attempt to "kill."

46. _____When the receiver wins the first point.

47. _____ When serving, jumping off the ground with both feet before contacting the ball.

48. _____ Striking the ball just as it leaves the ground.

49. _____ Splitting the ball while serving.

50. _____ Winning two points in succession after deuce.

The following suggestions should prove helpful in constructing matching-type questions:

1. Include more items among the choices, so that they may act as distracters; all distracters, however, should make sense.

2. Be sure that only one word among the choices applies to each situation.

3. Have one of the lists to be matched composed of single words, numerals, or brief phrases.

4. Score by counting the number of correct answers.

The matching type of objective written examination has definite limitations. It is not well adapted to the measurement of understanding. It is likely to include irrelevant clues to the correct response, and, unless carefully made, is time-consuming in its administration. It is useful, however, in checking on precise information, such as events, places, and dates; terms, definitions, and rules; and tools, equipment, and facilities and their use.

Simple Recall.   The simple recall test is one in which the answer is not suggested but must be recalled. There are three main forms of this test, short answers, test items that require identification or specific information; and a word or phrase requiring definition. This test form permits the use of maps or diagrams with numbers to indicate the parts to be identified. The following examples of simple recall questions are again taken from the Hewitt tennis test.[13]

Directions. Enumerate the names for the following lines and spaces of a tennis court.

24. ....(1)

25. ....(2)

26. ....(3)

27. ....(4)

28. ....(5)

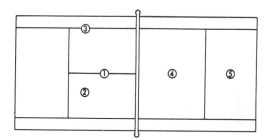

Scoring: Number right.   *Score...*

[13]Hewitt, "Tennis Knowledge Test," p. 149.

Following are suggestions to be observed in constructing simple recall questions:

1. State the test items so that the answer can be given briefly and concisely.

2. As a general rule, use direct questions rather than statements.

3. Allow, in the key, for different ways in which the question can be answered.

4. Preferably, provide numbered spaces for responses, the numbers to correspond with the recall items.

5. Make minimum use of textbook language.

6. Score by counting the number of correct answers.

The simple recall type of question is particularly valuable in the identification of various items and in problem-solving requiring computation. Many of the questions included in the essay-type examination may be broken into recall questions.

Completion. In the completion test, sentences are given in which certain important words or phrases have been omitted, the resulting blanks to be filled in by the pupils. Such sentences may be disconnected or organized into a paragraph. In these questions, recall rather than recognition is required. Hewitt's tennis test[14] supplies the questions illustrated below:

Directions. In each statement, fill in the space or spaces with the proper word:

33. Hitting a ball directly overhead with attempt "to kill" the ball is called a _____

35. All balls hitting boundary line are _____

38. Hitting a chop or cut on the ball makes the ball spin _____

42. Each side winning three points each, the score is called _____

The greatest difficulty in preparing this form is to make the sentences definite and clear. Suggestions for their construction are as follows:

[14]Hewitt, "Tennis Knowledge Test," p. 149.

1. Supply sufficient information so that the meaning of the sentence is clear to the reader.

2. Avoid phrasing the sentences so that the answer is perfectly obvious.

3. Use one to three blanks in any one sentence; avoid over-mutilated statements.

4. Make blanks call for one correct word or phrase, and not for a large number of similar words and phrases.

5. Provide blanks for all key words and omit blanks for those that are unimportant, such as *a, an,* and *the.*

6. In the key, allow for all different answers that may be used correctly, such as synonyms.

7. Compose sentences around certain key words or phrases; avoid lifting sentences from the text.

8. Arrange, if desired, spaces for pupils' answers in a column at the right of the sentence; in this case, number the blanks and the spaces to correspond.

9. Score by counting the number of correct responses.

The completion type of objective written examination is useful in determining the amount of factual information known and in problem-solving.

Evaluation of Written Tests

The requirements of a satisfactory objective written examination are the same and are fully as necessary as for other types of tests usually employed in health or physical education. Thus, the test must be valid; it must be reliable; it must be objective; it must have norms; it must be economical; and it must contribute toward the realization of health education or physical education objectives. The techniques for determining these factors, especially the validity and accuracy of such tests, however, vary somewhat.

Validity. In educational practice, the validity of written tests is determined by two well-established methods, both of which should be employed in validating tests. These methods are curricular or content validity, and statistical validity. To determine *curricular validity,* it is necessary to define carefully the extent of the test and then to insure that this range covers the course content. Sources of validity, therefore, would include courses of study, textbooks, and analyses of examination questions. If a standardized test for nation-wide use is being constructed, the sources must embrace a broader base, representing a cross section of practice in the subject throughout the country. Frequently, tests of this sort include understanding of materials only and have been based upon the memorizing of facts and familiarity with a body of knowledge. Recently constructed tests, however, have attempted to test also the mental reactions desired in the course. The evaluation of curricular validity depends upon a study of the subject matter that the test aims to cover and also the procedures followed in constructing the test. Because of this indefiniteness, such test evaluation is difficult to make.

Curricular validity can be specifically applied when a knowledge test is prepared by a health or physical educator for use in a course he teaches. For such a course, the teacher knows the stated purposes to be achieved, the attitudes and behavior pattern to be formed, the content material to be included, and the literature sources to be consulted. Questions for the test, then, can be directed toward appropriately and adequately covering these factors.

Statistical validity may be determined by relating the test to other evidence of the quality being measured, such as other valid tests, the opinions of experts in the specific field of the tests, or pupil grades in the subject. Such criteria are only fairly adequate because of their admittedly inadequate subjectivity.

Statistical validity, however, may take another form—that of determining the difficulty and discriminative value of each item in the test. This is known as *item validity.* Item validity is determined by computing the percentage of pupils passing each item; the fewer passing the item, the more difficult the question, provided, of course, that the item itself is satisfactory and correctly phrased. For item discrimination, an appreciably larger percentage of the more competent pupils than of the less competent in a grade should answer it correctly, and an appreciably larger percentage of pupils in any grade should answer it correctly than in the next lower grade. Item discrimination may also be shown by comparing the percentage of correct answers on the item given by the upper third or fourth of the group on the entire test with the percentage of correct answers given by the lowest third or fourth. In all instances, items showing little or no discrimination, or those that show a percentage of successes in favor of the poor groups or the lower grades, should be either eliminated or examined for vagueness and ambiguity and reworded.

Various *indices of discrimination* are in use. Among these is the Flanagan technique[15] based upon a discrimination of test items as shown by the variance in the scores of the upper and of the lower 27 percent from the total score made on the test.

Items which are too difficult or too easy are apt to have poor discriminatory value. When the test is intended to cover more than one school grade, a good rule to follow is to choose items that vary in difficulty rating from just above zero to close to 100 percent, with the average at approximately 50 percent. Items for a test covering a narrow range, as would be the case in many written tests on physical activities, discriminate best when their difficulty is such that each item is passed by at least 50

[15]John C. Flanagan, "General Considerations in the Selection of Test Items and a Short Method of Estimating the Product-Moment Coefficient from Data at the Tails of a Distribution," *Journal of Educational Psychology,* **30,** No. 9 (December 1939), 674.

percent of the pupils in the group.[16] In any event, questions missed by all students or answered correctly by all students are of no differentiation value and should be eliminated. It is frequently desirable to establish difficulty limits. Such limits may be set at any desired point. In health and physical education, these limits have been variously established at 10 and 90 percent (that is, by dropping those questions answered by less than 10 percent and by more than 90 percent), 7 and 93 percent, and 5 and 95 percent.

Accuracy.   The reliability of objective written tests may be determined in several different ways.

1. Correlation between equivalent forms of the test. Frequently, in constructing objective written tests, two or more equivalent forms of the test may be prepared so that the test may be administered repeatedly without duplication of the questions. If the two forms are comparable in difficulty, it is possible to give both forms to the same subjects and correlate the results. Correlational standards of reliability coefficients are the same as discussed previously in this chapter.

2. Correlation between chance halves. When only one form of the test is available, coefficients of correlation may be computed between odd- and even-numbered items on the test. The resulting correlation, however, would be for one-half of the test. Since the length of the test affects its reliability, the correlation should be corrected for the full length of the test. This is done by use of the Brown-Spearman prophecy formula.[17]

3. Correlation between repeated tests. This procedure is the one generally followed in determining the reliability of physical performance tests. It is not as satisfactory with written tests, as pupils will usually improve their scores

on the repeated test. The correlation, however, does show the degree of agreement between the two sets of scores, although the average scores of the two groups, and perhaps their variability, will differ.

Construction of Your Own Tests

The health educator or physical educator may wish to construct his own objective written tests[18] in order to focus his examination procedures around his own course of study. The following steps may be found helpful in preparing these tests:

1. The purpose of the test should be clearly in mind. Such questions as these might well be answered: To what extent do you wish to measure how well your students have learned a particular unit of study or body of material? Do you wish to evaluate their attitudes and practices, especially in health education, in relation to physical fitness, and in the use of sports skills in their daily lives?

2. Outline the scope of the proposed examination, listing the important topics and the types of thought reactions to be tested. Under each topic, list the most significant items to be included.

3. Compose test items, selecting the type of objective form best suited for each. Keep items of the same objective form together; this may be done while composing by using separate sheets of paper for each type.

4. Arrange test items in approximate order of difficulty.

5. Give clear directions for taking the various test types.

6. Specify the scoring procedure for each test type.

7. Prepare scoring key.

8. Compute the reliability of the test.

---

[16]Clay C. Ross, *Measurement in Today's Schools* (Englewood Cliffs, N.J.: Prentice-Hall, 1941), p. 87.

[17]See Appendix A, "Elementary Statistics," for an explanation of the Brown-Spearman prophecy formula.

[18]*Making the Classroom Test: A Guide for Teachers* (Princeton, N.J.: Educational Testing Service, 1959).

SELECTED REFERENCES

BARROW, HAROLD M., and ROSEMARY MCGEE, *A Practical Approach to Measurement in Physical Education,* 2nd. ed. Philadelphia: Lea & Febiger, 1971, Ch. 11.

BAUMGARTNER, TED A., "Stability of Physical Performance Test Scores," *Research Quarterly,* **40,** No. 2 (May 1969), 257.

FLANAGAN, JOHN C., "General Considerations in the Selection of Test Items and a Short Method of Estimating the Product-Moment Coefficient from Data at the Tails of a Distribution," *Journal of Educational Psychology,* **30,** No. 9 (December 1939), 674.

HENRY, FRANKLIN M., and others, "Errors in Measurement," *Research Methods Applied to Health, Physical Education, and Recreation.* Washington: American Association for Health, Physical Education, and Recreation, 1949, Ch. 19.

Making the Classroom Test: A Guide for Teachers. Princeton; N.J.: *Educational Testing Service,* 1959.

correlation
direct   negative posity
inverse

PART TWO

PHYSICAL FITNESS

In Chapter 1, physical fitness was defined as the ability to carry out daily tasks with vigor and alertness, without undue fatigue and with ample energy to enjoy leisure time pursuits and to meet emergencies. It was identified as a positive quality, extending on a scale from death to "abundant life." Thus, all living individuals have some degree of physical fitness, which is minimal in the severely ill and maximal in the highly trained athlete; it varies considerably in different people and in the same person from time to time.

Undergirding physical fitness is the organic soundness of the body. Obviously, persons with heart lesions, metabolic diseases, neurological dysfunctions, and the like are not organically sound; these individuals are at the lower levels of physical fitness. The physical educator needs to be aware of these individuals, as well as those with handicapping defects of an orthopedic nature, so that he may provide appropriate restricted or adapted activity programs for them. Other conditions of concern to the physical educator are postural defects and nutritional deficiencies. Consequently, chapters in this section are devoted to measures related to school health appraisal, to nutrition and body physique, and to posture.

Education and Fitness

Still, a great many students free of organic lesions and handicapping defects are low on the physical fitness continuum—they are deficient in basic physical fitness components. These components are the special concern of the physical educator in his efforts to improve the physical fitness of children, youth, and adults. While concensus on the components of physical fitness does not exist, there is little or no disagreement that muscular strength, muscular endurance, and circulatory-respiratory endurance are basic. Within the broader concept of motor fitness, other components are recognized, including muscular power, agility, and speed. Definitions of these components and their relationships are presented in Chapter 9.

In our sedentary society, people frequently question the need for much physical fitness, as doing one's job many times requires only a minimum of strength and endurance. The progressive mechanization of work and activities of daily living has reduced the need for cultivating physical fitness, the strength and endurance of muscles, the resistance to fatigue. However, as Missiuro[1] has demonstrated, the replacement of the motor function by the mechanical device and all kinds of labor-saving electronic instruments contains the dangers of the distintegration of the biosocial human entity. The purpose of the present chapter is to show the relationship of physical exercise—the physical educator's stock in trade—to physical fitness and to indicate the importance of physical fitness to the individual's total effectiveness.

THE PHYSICAL IN PHYSICAL EDUCATION

Little doubt exists today that the right kind and amount of exercise will develop

[1]W. Missiuro, "Biological Conflicts of Technical Civilization," *Journal of Sports Medicine and Physical Fitness,* **5,** No. 1 (March 1965), 32.

muscular strength and endurance, body flexibility, and circulatory-respiratory endurance. In fact, properly directed exercise is the only known means for acquiring the ability to engage in tasks demanding sustained physical effort. However, it is gratifying to demonstrate the presence of such benefits as a consequence of existing physical education programs.

Whittle[2] studied two groups of 81 twelve-year-old boys who were comparable in such maturity factors as chronological age, skeletal age, weight, height, and Wetzel development level. One group of these boys had participated for at least three years in good physical education programs; the other had little or no physical education in elementary school. Pronounced differences were found between the two groups in various affective factors. The means on the Rogers Physical Fitness Index (PFI) test[3] for the boys in the good and poor physical education programs were 121 and 103 respectively. The boys in the good programs also produced higher means on the Metheny-Johnson Test of Motor Educability, the Indiana Motor Fitness Test, and the vertical jump.

A further interesting disclosure of the Whittle study was that boys in each group who participated a "lot" in out-of-class physical activity showed strong superiority over those who participated a "little." Again, in terms of the PFI tests, a very high mean of 132 was scored by those participating a lot in outside activity from the good programs, while the mean for those engaging a little was 109. Of special import for those interested in the development of strong athletic programs is the comparison between the boys from both

programs who participated a lot in out-of-class activities. The PFI means were 132 and 116 for the boys in the good and poor programs respectively. Thus, athletes scored higher on physical fitness tests than did their peers. The effect of participation in good physical education programs raised the level of all boys with the athletes scoring still higher; in fact, the athletes from the poor programs were still below the average of all boys in the good programs.

Clarke and Broekhoff[4] summarized the results of Oregon studies contrasting boys and girls who participated in and did not participate in physical education. Utilizing the PFI for men and the Oregon Motor Fitness Test for women, students entering the University of Oregon with four years of high school physical education definitely had higher averages than did those with two years or less. Comparable results were obtained at Oregon State University by Koski.[5] Further, the men and women at both universities without physical education before entrance were significantly inferior to the standards presented by the norms. Drowatzky and Madary[6] demonstrated that youths without physical education in the eleventh and twelfth grades had lower average physical fitness test scores than did any other grade in the Coos Bay, Oregon school system.

Shaffer[7] reduced failures on the Kraus-Weber Test of Minimum Muscular Fitness to a marked degree in a few weeks through conditioning exercises. Forty-two percent of 2281 junior high

[2]H. Douglas Whittle, "Effects of Elementary School Physical Education upon Some Aspects of Physical, Motor, and Personality Development of Boys Twelve Years of Age," Doctoral Dissertation, University of Oregon, 1956.

[3]The Physical Fitness Index is presented in Chapter 7. A PFI of 100 is the median for the test; scores of 85 and 115 reflect the first and third quartiles respectively.

[4]H. Harrison Clarke and Jan Broekhoff, "Fitness Status of Oregon University Freshmen," Mimeographed Report.

[5]Arthur C. Koski, Department of Physical Education, Oregon State University, Corvallis, Oregon.

[6]John N. Drowatzky and Charles J. Madary, "Evaluation of the Physical and Motor Fitness of Boys and Girls in the Coos Bay, Oregon, School District," Master's Thesis, University of Oregon, 1962.

[7]Gertrude Shaffer, "Editor's Mail," *Journal of Health, Physical Education, and Recreation,* **28,** No. 2 (February 1957), 6.

school boys and girls in Johnstown, Pennsylvania, failed one or more of the six Kraus-Weber test items in September; in November, the failures dropped to eight percent. At the end of the term, only four percent failed one or more of the test items. These results have been repeated annually over a period of years.[8]

In the Medford, Oregon, public schools, Ragsdale[9] reported the differences obtained between boys who elected and did not elect physical education in the eleventh grade; for each category, differentiation was made between those who participated and did not participate in interscholastic athletics. Although the differences were not always significant, those boys who did not elect physical education and did not participate in interscholastic athletics were inferior to all other groups on 22 tests of maturity, physique, body size, muscular strength and endurance, motor performances, and scholastic achievement. The tests showing generally significant differences were 60-yard shuttle run, Rogers arm strength score, parallel bar push-ups, total-body reaction time, and amount of participation in out-of-school physical activities at the time of physical education election in the tenth grade. One year later, as seniors, these same boys had not gained as much as others in tests of muscular strength and endurance.

ORGANIC SOUNDNESS

While Kraus coined the phrase earlier, Kraus and Raab[10] extensively developed the concept of ("hypokenetic disease,"

defined as the "whole spectrum of inactivity-induced somatic and mental derangements.")Gleaned from many sources, they indicated that coronary heart disease is twice as frequent in the sedentary as in the active. Other diseases more frequent in the sedentary than in the active are diabetes, duodenal ulcer, and other internal and surgical conditions; 80 percent of low back pain is due to lack of adequate physical activity; lack of physical exercise goes parallel with emotional difficulties; the physically active show better adaptability to stress, less neuromuscular tension, and lesser fatigability; active individuals age later, do not tend toward absolute and relative overweight, have lower blood pressure, are stronger and more flexible, and have greater breathing capacity and lower pulse rate. Studies that contributed to such conclusions as these follow.

From a review of studies from many countries, the author[11] reported that the overwhelming majority supported an inverse relationship between the amount of physical activity and the incidence of coronary heart disease. The evidence indicated that regular participation in physical activity will not necessarily prevent a heart attack, but will make its occurrence less likely; also, in the event of an attack, it will tend to be less severe and the likelihood of survival will be greater.

After analytically reviewing his and other studies, Taylor[12] concluded "that men in sedentary occupations have more coronary heart disease than those in occupations requiring moderate to heavy physical activity." Hein and Ryan[13] reached a

[8]Personal correspondence.

[9]Lee V. Ragsdale, "Contrast of Maturity, Physical, and Scholastic Measures Between Boys Who Elect and Who Do Not Elect Physical Education in Grade Eleven," Doctoral Dissertation, University of Oregon, 1966.

[10]Hans Kraus and Wilhelm Raab, *Hypokenetic Disease* (Springfield, Ill.: Charles C. Thomas, Publisher, 1961).

[11]H. Harrison Clarke, "Physical Activity and Coronary Heart Disease," *Physical Fitness Research Digest*, President's Council on Physical Fitness and Sports, **2**, No. 2 (April 1972).

[12]Henry L. Taylor, "Coronary Heart Disease in Physically Active and Sedentary Populations," *Journal of Sports Medicine and Physical Fitness*, **2**, No. 2 (June 1962), 73.

[13]Fred V. Hein and Allan J. Ryan, "The Contributions of Physical Activity to Physical Health," *Research Quarterly*, **31**, No. 2, Pt. 2 (May 1960), 279.

similar conclusion when they stated: "A high level of physical activity throughout life appears to be one of those factors that inhibit the vascular degeneration characteristic of coronary heart disease, the most common cause of death among cardiovascular disorders."

In other research reviews, the author summarized the results of studies related to exercise and blood cholesterol[14] and other risk factors[15] associated with coronary heart disease. These studies generally demonstrated that dangers from these factors can be alleviated through circulatory-respiratory endurance exercise. Thus, with this type of activity, with appropriate intensity and dosage, and with regular continuance over a period of time, the following results have been achieved: reductions in serum cholesterol and triglyceride levels, development of collateral circulation around coronary artery restrictions, improvement in myocardial vascularization, increases in red blood cells and blood volume, improved fibrinolytic capability, and reduction in blood pressure.

Dudley White prescribed exercise for President Dwight D. Eisenhower following his heart attack. He has written: "Proper exercise is as essential to good health as eating and sleeping."[16] Wolffe[17] has stated: "The beneficial effect of physical activity on the cardiovascular system is becoming well recognized. This is true not only for the well but also in the sick."

Low back pain is much more prevalent in the sedentary than in the physically active. Kraus[18] reported that 80 percent of his patients with this ailment were unable to pass his test of minimum muscular fitness.

Gallagher[19] has stressed the value of athletics and other physical activities in the adolescent's development and the frequency with which strengthening activity rather than rest is the appropriate recommendation when the person is below par in health. For medical practice, he states: "The evaluation of strength, the determination of the disproportion between strength and probable stress, and the increase of strength through exercise can at times constitute better management than a regime which focuses upon the ailment, emphasizes rest, and ignores the facts regarding strength development in exercise." During World War II in the hospitals and convalescent centers of the Army, Navy, and Air Force and since the war in Veterans Administration and other hospitals, exercise was and is being used extensively in speeding the recovery of patients. Early ambulation is now a standard procedure following surgery of many kinds; even with extensive abdominal surgery, the patient is frequently out of bed within 24 hours after the operation.

The Joint Committee of the American Medical Association and the American Association for Health, Physical Education, and Recreation, has issued a pamphlet titled; "Exercise Fitness."[20] Included in this document is the following statement: "The benefits of physical exercise are more clearly observable in their relation to certain organic diseases. Regular exercise is now considered to help retard the onset or further progress of diabetes, for example, and man's most common threat to health—arteriosclerosis."

[14]H. Harrison Clarke, "Exercise and Blood Cholesterol," *Physical Fitness Research Digest*, President's Council on Physical Fitness and Sports, **2**, No. 3 (July 1972), 6.

[15]H. Harrison Clarke, "Exercise and Risk Factors Associated with Coronary Heart Disease," *Physical Fitness Research Digest*, President's Council on Physical Fitness and Sports, **2**, No. 4 (April 1972).

[16]Joseph B. Wolffe, "Cardiovascular Response to Vigorous Physical Activity," *Medicina Sportiva*, **12**, No. 1 (Gennaio), 1958.

[17]Kraus and Raab, *Hypokinetic Disease*, p. 13.

[18]Kraus and Raab, *Hypokinetic Disease*, p. 13.

[19]J. Roswell Gallagher, "Rest and Restriction," *American Journal of Public Health*, **46** (November 1956), 1424.

[20]Joint Committee of AMA and AAHPER, "Exercise Fitness," American Medical Association, 1964.

Mental alertness

Another research review by the author[21] reported the results of studies pertaining to the relationships between physical and motor traits and mental achievements. Many more studies produced positive relationships than nil or negative results. Most studies reporting little or no relationships between physical and mental measures were correlational in nature and ignored the intelligence of the subjects. By contrast, more studies showed positive relationships when only pupils who scored low on physical tests were considered or when high and low groups on physical tests were contrasted. Some correlational studies did produce positive coefficients, especially when intelligence was partialled out. Illustrated studies of these relationships follow.

The great psychologist, L. M. Terman, concluded after 25 years of studying intellectually gifted children: "The results of the physical measurements and the medical examinations provide a striking contrast to the popular stereotype of the child prodigy, so commonly predicted as a pathetic creature, over-serious, undersized, sickly, hollowchested, nervously tense, and bespectacled. There are gifted children who bear some resemblance to this stereotype, but the truth is that almost every element in the picture, except the last, is less characteristic of the gifted child than of the mentally average."[22] In Terman's initial monumental study,[23] when his gifted subjects were young, symptoms of general weakness were reported by the school nearly 30 percent less frequently for the gifted than for the control group.

Clarke and Jarman[24] investigated the academic achievement of boys nine, twelve, and fifteen years of age. At each age, high and low groups were formed separately based on Strength Indices and on Physical Fitness Indices; in each instance, the group was equated by intelligence quotients. Generally, (especially for the Physical Fitness Index) the high groups had significantly superior grade-point averages in their class work and significantly higher means on standard scholastic achievement tests.

Rogers[25] studied two group of high school boys with comparable IQ averages, but differing in muscular strength. The scholarship of the high-strength group was definitely superior to the low-strength group. Weber obtained a significant positive relationship between physical fitness test scores and grade-point averages of university men. Hart and Shay[26] found that the academic index means were grouped in descending order for Springfield College men grouped by Physical Fitness Indices. The PFI groupings and academic index means were: 115 and above, 2.01; 100 to 114, 1.94; 85 to 99, 1.85; 84 and below, 1.51. For 60 sophomore women, the following partial correlations were obtained: 0.66 between PFI and cumulative academic index with Scholastic Aptitude Test of the College Entrance Board held constant, and 0.63 between PFI and the academic index with verbal scores of the SAT held constant.

[21]H. Harrison Clarke, "The Totality of Man," *Physical Fitness Research Digest,* President's Council on Physical Fitness and Sports, **1,** No. 2 (October 1971).

[22]Lewis M. Terman, ed., *Genetic Studies of Genius. IV. The Gifted Child Grows Up* (Stanford: Stanford University Press, 1947), p. 24.

[23]Lewis M. Terman, ed., *Genetic Studies of Genius. I. Mental and Physical Traits of a Thousand Gifted Children* (Stanford: Stanford University Press, 1925), p. 211.

[24]H. Harrison Clarke and Boyd O. Jarman, "Scholastic Achievement of Boys 9, 12, and 15 Years of Age as Related to Various Strength and Growth Measures," *Research Quarterly,* **32,** No. 2 (May 1961), 155.

[25]Frederick Rand Rogers, "The Scholarship of Athletes," Master's Thesis, Stanford University, 1922.

[26]Marcia E. Hart and Clayton T. Shay, "Relationship Between Physical Fitness and Academic Success," *Research Quarterly, Springfield Studies,* **35,** No. 3, Pt. 2 (October 1964), 443.

Page[27] found that 83 percent of the freshman male students dismissed from Syracuse University because of low grades had Physical Fitness Indices below 100; 39 percent had PFI's below 85. These same students had scholastic aptitude scores well above the average; their median score was at the 72nd percentile. Coefield and McCollum[28] at the University of Oregon found that the 78 male freshmen with lowest PFI's during the 1954 fall term were definitely low in scholastic accomplishment, as compared with all freshmen at the university. As in Page's study, the low fitness students were above average in scholastic aptitude. Popp[29] conducted case studies of the highest 20 and the lowest 20 of 100 sophomore high school boys. Subsequently, he found that all but one of the high group graduated from high school, while only 60 percent of the low group graduated. Rogers and Palmer[30] presented a number of case studies of boys and girls at Nathaniel Hawthorne Junior High School, Yonkers, N.Y.; studies of "bright kids" and low PFI pupils were conducted. In many instances, improvement in physical fitness was accompanied by improved scholastic success.

Doornink[31] reported on the success of 1338 men during their four years at the University of Oregon. The PFI had been administered to these men upon entrance in the fall terms of 1953 and 1954. Two out of five of these men graduated four years later; for the lowest 7 percent on PFI, only one out of five graduated, or one-half the number for all students. One out of five of all students won a scholarship; only one in 25 in the lowest 15 percent on PFI obtained a scholarship. For all students, one in five was elected to honor societies; for the lowest 10 percent on PFI, only one in 33 was so admitted.

At the University of Illinois, Powell and Pohndorf[32] compared mental test results of older adult males who had participated in a running-type exercise regimen for more than three years with men who had exercised little or not at all during the same period. The Culture Fair Intelligence Test was administered to both groups; this test evaluates certain intelligence factors which decrease as adults get older. The regular exercisers scored higher on the mental achievement test than did the nonexercise group. In general, better fitness measures accompanied higher fluid intelligence scores.

As a consequence of this type of evidence, it may be contended that a person's *general learning potential for a given level of intelligence* is increased or decreased in accordance with his degree of physical fitness. Rogers[33] has expressed this general learning potential relationship as the product of intelligence and physical fitness squared. Thus, $GLP = if^2$. While the formula has not been scientifically validated, the concept can be supported. Basically, this concept declared that the individual is more prone to be physically and

[27]C. Getty Page, "Case Studies of College Men with Low Physical Fitness Indices," Master's Thesis, Syracuse University, 1940.

[28]John R. Coefield and Robert H. McCollum, "A Case Study Report of 78 University Freshman Men with Low Physical Fitness Indices," Master's Thesis, University of Oregon, 1955.

[29]James Popp, "Case Studies of Sophomore High School Boys with High and Low Physical Fitness Indices," Master's Thesis, University of Oregon, 1959.

[30]Frederick Rand Rogers and Fred E. Palmer, "A Notable Physical Education Demonstration," *Physical Fitness News Letter*, University of Oregon (May 20, 1955).

[31]Robert H. Doornink, "The Feasibility of Using Strength Fitness as a Predictor of Student Success at the University of Oregon," Doctoral Dissertation, University of Oregon, 1962.

[32]Richard R. Powell and Richard H. Pohndorf, "Comparison of Adult Exercisers and Nonexercisers on Fluid Intelligence and Selected Physiological Variables," *Research Quarterly*, **42,** No. 1 (March 1971), 70.

[33]Frederick Rand Rogers, "Rogers' Law of Learning Capacity," *Physical Fitness News Letter*, University of Oregon (January 31, 1955); "Revision of Rogers' Law," *Physical Fitness News Letter* (September 1955).

mentally alert, to be vigorous in his applications, and to suffer less from efficiency-destroying fatigue when he is fit.

PERSONAL-SOCIAL STATUS

In still another research review, the author[34] summarized the results of studies on the relationships of personal-social characteristics to physical and motor traits. Positive relationships were shown, as measured by psychological inventories, peer status indicators, teacher evaluations, and self-concept instruments. Generally, boys high on physical-motor tests tended to be extroverted, dominant, sociable, dependable, tolerant, active, and competitive; they were prone to be leaders and popular with their peers. Boys low on physical-motor measures showed feelings of insecurity, inferiority, and inadequacy and had difficulties in social relationships. They were also inclined to be rebellious, emotionally unstable, and defensive; and their concepts of themselves were negative, checking such adjectives applying to themselves as sissy, nervous, cry-baby, unhappy, clumsy, bossy, and careless. Illustrated studies of these relationships are indicated below.

As a part of a longitudinal study of growth in adolescence at the Institute of Child Welfare, University of California, Berkeley,[35] scores on dynamometric strength tests were related to biological, social, and psychological characteristics. Among the findings were the following.

1. As compared with "dynamic" strength (dash, jump, throw), static dynamometric strength is more closely associated with biological growth, suggesting a dependence upon

constitutional factors expressed in physical measurements and in physiological maturity.

2. Among boys, a positive relationship of strength to "prestige" traits is apparent, which is regarded as evidence of the role of physical prowess in the adolescent value system.

3. Superior strength in boys is part of a complex of physical characteristics valued highly during the adolescent period; the absence of this trait is a handicap which can be overcome only by strongly compensating personal traits in other areas also highly valued.

4. Boys high in strength tend to be well adjusted socially and psychologically; boys low in strength show a tendency toward social difficulties, feelings of inferiority, and other personal maladjustments.

In Popp's study previously mentioned in this chapter, the 20 boys with the highest PFI's and the 20 boys with the lowest PFI's were arranged in a single alphabetical list. Five judges (principal, vice-principal, dean of boys, and two physical educators) each independently selected the ten most desirable boys ("those most nearly like sons they would like to have") and the ten most undesirable boys ("those least like sons they would like to have"). Sixteen boys were named by at least one judge in the "desirable" classification. Of these, 11, or 69 percent, had high PFI's, and five, or 31 percent, had low PFI's. In selecting the "undesirable" boys, again 16 boys were chosen. Of this group, four, or 25 percent, had high PFI's and 12, or 75 percent, had low PFI's. Thus, the five judges, without knowledge of each boy's PFI, generally recognized in the boys with high scores on this test the many and varied traits they would like most to see in a son of their own.

As presented in 1949 by Appleton,[36] physical proficiency measures proved useful predictors of the nonacademic aspects of military success at the United States

---

[34]H. Harrison Clarke, "The Totality of Man Continued," *Physical Fitness Research Digest,* President's Council on Physical Fitness and Sports, **2,** No. 1 (January 1972).

[35]Harold E. Jones, *Motor Performance and Growth* (Berkeley: University of California Press, 1949).

[36]Lloyd O. Appleton, "The Relationship Between Physical Ability and Success at the United States Military Academy." Doctoral Dissertation, New York University, 1949.

Military Academy at West Point. The study of West Point cadets has continued; Kobes[37] reported on accumulated data over a period of 15 years with 9442 cadets tested. The upper 7 percent and the lower 7 percent on the West Point test were contrasted. Among the results were the following:

1. Failure to graduate: 48.3 percent in low group; 18.8 percent in high group.

2. Cadet discharge for any reason: 29.8 percent in low group; 11.3 percent in high group.

3. Cadet resignations: 18.5 percent in low group; 7.5 percent in high group.

4. Leadership ability: 6.6 percent in low group; 40.0 percent in high group.

5. Low aptitude for military service: 19.2 percent in low group; 1.2 percent in high group.

6. Academic failures: 17.2 percent in low group; 8.1 percent in high group.

Further, cadets with a history of athletic participation were better natured and cooperative, emotionally mature and realistic about life, enthusiastic and cheerful, adventurous, masculine, conservative, and willing to work with people. The attrition rate among cadets who entered the Academy with a record of athletic participation was 27 percent compared with 40 percent for those with no such record.

Results similar to those of Appleton were obtained by Doornink in his study discussed earlier in this chapter. For all men, one in seven was elected to a position of leadership in the Associated Student Body during their four years at the University of Oregon; for the lowest 10 percent on PFI, only one in 33 was so elected. Nine out of 100 students became a leader in a club or society; only one in 100 among the lowest 10 percent on PFI were elected to such offices.

In a paper before the International Symposium of the Medicine and Physiology of Sports and Athletics at Helsinki, Finland, Cureton[38] reported that personality itself is responsive to physical training in view of the changes that can be made in the autonomic nervous system and in the cardiovascular state. He concluded that men are more energetic, more buoyant and optimistic, more action-minded, more playful, more aggressive—in general, they appear more extroverted and more healthful when they are physically trained than when they are physically untrained. And, as men go through progressive training, they tend to tackle harder and harder tasks, and they are able to work relatively harder and longer.

Gottesman[39] tested men in the physical education service program at the University of Oregon with Cattell's Sixteen Personality Factor Questionnaire and related these scores to various physical traits. The physical measures with the most and best relationships with the personality factors were 160-yard shuttle run, Physical Fitness Index, pull-ups, jump and reach, Rogers' arm strength score, and bar push-ups. Cattell[40] summarized research with his test at the University of Illinois by stating: ". . . when effective personality measures are employed, indubitable relations are perceived between measures of physique and physical fitness on the one hand, and psychological measures on the other."

[37]Frank J. Kobes, "Predictive Values of Initial Physical Performance Levels of Freshmen at USMA," Paper Presented at 1965 Meeting of the American College of Sports Medicine; and materials provided by Lloyd O. Appleton.

[38]Thomas K. Cureton, "Physical Training Produces Important Changes, Psychologically and Physiologically," *Proceedings of the International Symposium of the Medicine and Physiology of Sports and Athletics at Helsinki*, 1951.

[39]Donald T. Gottesman, "Relationships Between Cattell's Sixteen Personality Factor Questionnaire and Physique, Structure, Strength, and Motor Traits of College Men," Doctoral Dissertation, University of Oregon, December 1964.

[40]Raymond B. Cattell, "Some Psychological Correlates of Physical Fitness and Physique," *Exercise and Fitness* (Chicago: The Athletic Institute, 1960), pp. 138–51.

Storey[41] rated the physiques of freshman high school boys as fat, medium, and thin by Wetzel grid procedures; each subject also indicated which of these physique categories applied to him; further, the Mooney Problem Check List was administered to the subjects. Thin boys had the poorest adjustment in the Home and Family area of the check list; fat boys had poorest adjustment on worry items. Of special significance in this study, however, was the self-concepts of the boys, whether or not they were in the physique category accorded them. Boys who perceived themselves as fat had poor adjustments in the Mooney Problem Check List categories of Health and Physical Development, Courtship, Sex and Marriage, and Morals and Religion, and in attitudes toward the Future. Boys who thought they were thin were least adjusted in the Socio-Psychological Relations and School Work categories. Boys who felt they were of medium physique had generally the best adjustments throughout.

Exercise and Fat Reduction

Excess fat on the body, commonly referred to as obesity, is a problem that concerns both children and adults. Frequently in today's society, fat reduction is undertaken for aesthetic reasons, to enhance one's appearance, by those with such excesses. However, there are many vital reasons for fat reduction; complications associated with obesity are associated with serious organic impairments and shortened life, with psychological maladjustments, with unfortunate peer relationships (especially among children); with inefficiency of physical movement, and with ineffectiveness in motor and athletic activities. Obesity is constantly en-

countered as a cause of physical unfitness among children and adults; these individuals score low on physical and motor tests, a result encountered universally by school and college physical educators.

In still another research review, the author[42] presented the value of exercise in fat reduction and indicated the forms of exercise and their applications that have been found most effective in studies of children and adults. The following are among implications that may be drawn from these studies.

1. The causes of obesity were considered as: fuel intake through diet in excess of daily needs, lack of exercise, hereditary and other familial considerations, glandular and other bodily malfunctions, and psychological, social, and emotional problems. An effective approach to fat reduction for a given individual may involve any or various combinations of these causative factors.

2. In recent years, the role of exercise in fat reduction has been ignored or minimized by health and physical educators and some physicians. A nutritionist of international repute, Jean Mayer, has effectively supported the contention that physical inactivity is the single most important factor explaining the increasing frequency of overweight people in modern western societies. He states: "Natural selection operating for hundreds of thousands of years, made men physically active, resourceful creatures, well-prepared as hunters, fishermen, and agriculturists. The regulation of food intake was never designed to adapt to the highly sedentary conditions of modern life, any more than animals were designed to be caged."[43]

3. Intensive physical conditioning causes a depletion of excess fat and an increase in lean body weight. In fact, some studies resulted in no appreciable change in body weight, but body composition did change with a decrease

[41]Stuart E. Storey, "Physique and the Self-fulfilling Prophecy," Master's Thesis, Western Kentucky University, 1968.

[42]H. Harrison Clarke, "Exercise and Fat Reduction," *Physical Fitness Research Digest*, President's Council on Physical Fitness and Sports, **5**, No. 2 (April 1975).

[43]Jean Mayer, "Exercise and Weight Control," *Exercise and Fitness* (Chicago: Athletic Institute, 1960), p. 110.

in body fat and a balancing increase in muscular tissue.

4. Fat reduction results achieved from exercise regimens not only depend on the nature of exercise but upon the manner in which a given regimen is applied. How a regimen is applied is dependent upon its frequency, duration, and intensity.

5. The most frequent physical activity utilized in studies on the effect of exercise in fat reduction is some regimen of walk-jog-run. However, special applications of weight training have proven effective.

CONCLUSIONS

In this chapter, it is not intended to present physical fitness as a panacea, as, obviously, there are many other important factors contributing to our various performances. As an example, for his level of intelligence, a physically fit person may not realize his mental potentialities due to lack of motivation, interest, time spent in study, and the like. And, a physically fit boy may devote his abundant energies toward outstanding leadership in athletics, whereby he exerts dynamic influences directly upon his teammates and upon the total school population. However, if this leadership is wrongly directed, such a physically fit person could be a dynamic influence in a gang devoted to disruptive acts.

Evidence has been provided in this chapter to show that, *other things being equal,* students will be more effective as a consequence of an adequate level of physical fitness. They should have the strength and stamina to carry out the duties of the day without undue fatigue and with an ample reserve to meet unusual situations and unforeseen emergencies; they should realize in an adequate measure their potentialities for physical activities as well as for mental accomplishments and for personal-social relations unhampered by efficiency-destroying fatigue.

Consequently, definite steps should be taken to ascertain the physical fitness of each pupil in school and to institute appropriate remedial and development programs for those who require them.[44] Individual needs cannot be known accurately, nor can the effects of individual programs be known without tests and retests of the individuals themselves. Therefore, measurement of physical fitness is essential for the physical educator in his attempt to improve the fitness of students. The teacher must try to determine their status and measure their progress.

SELECTED REFERENCES

CATTELL, RAYMOND B., "Some Psychological Correlates of Physical Fitness and Physique," *Exercise and Fitness.* Chicago: The Athletic Institute, 1960, pp. 138–51.

CLARKE, H. HARRISON, "Exercise and Blood Cholesterol," *Physical Fitness Research Digest,* **2,** No. 3 (July, 1972), 6.

CLARKE, H. HARRISON, "Exercise and Fat Reduction," *Physical Fitness Research Digest,* **5,** No. 2 (April 1975).

CLARKE, H. HARRISON, "Exercise and Risk Factors Associated with Coronary Heart Disease," *Physical Fitness Research Digest,* **2,** No. 4 (October 1972).

CLARKE, H. HARRISON, "The Totality of Man," *Physical Fitness Research Digest,* **1,** No. 2 (October 1971).

CLARKE, H. HARRISON, "The Totality of Man Continued," *Physical Fitness Research Digest,* **2,** No. 1 (January 1972).

JONES, HAROLD E., *Motor Performance and Growth.* Berkeley: University of California Press, 1949.

KRAUS, HANS, and WILHELM RAAB, *Hypokinetic Disease.* Springfield, Ill.: Charles C Thomas, Publisher, 1951.

[44]See H. Harrison Clarke and David H. Clarke, *Developmental and Adapted Physical Education* (Englewood Cliffs, N.J.: Prentice-Hall, Inc., 1963).

CHAPTER 4

The school health program has three interrelated parts: health education, healthful environment, and health services. This program is involved in evaluations of significance to the health educator and the physical educator; these evaluations include health appraisal and health knowledge and attitude. The term health appraisal is usually limited to systematic efforts to assess pupil health through use of teacher observations, health histories, medical and dental examinations, and screening tests, especially of vision, hearing, and nutritional status. In this chapter, health histories, medical examinations, and vision and hearing tests will be presented; nutrititional assessment will be found in Chapter 5 and health education tests in Chapter 15.

While primary responsibilities for the school health program are delegated to specific individuals, successful programs involve the combined efforts of many persons. Logical participants, of course, are school physicians, school dentists, nurses, and health educators; others could well be administrators, classroom teachers, physical educators, home economics teachers, and counseling personnel. This cooperative effort to improve and maintain the health of school children is essentially educational rather than medical. Basic responsibility for the health of the child belongs to the parents; the school health program should help students to develop a feeling of obligation for their own health as well as the health of others.

Historically, the school health program has been coupled with the role of the school physician. This role has changed through the years. Sellery[1] has traced this change through six "eras." The first era was his function in communicable disease control. The second, following World War I, was typified as medical inspection, during which school doctors examined children for such obvious physical defects as diseased tonsils, decayed teeth, heart abnormalities, and the like. The third era, in the 1930s, emphasized the improvement of the medical examination given in schools. In the fourth era, the school physician became a health educator by making the medical examination an educational experience for children and parents. Due to the shortage of physicians during World War II, the school physician became a medical advisor in the fifth era, during which he relied more and more on screening inspections conducted by others while he examined only those children referred by the school nurse or classroom teacher. In the sixth era, the school physician became a medical educational consultant, as related to the presence in children of physical defects, physical retardation, mental retardation, psychological maladjustments, and so on.

A booklet that provides standards for determining the health status of school children through the cooperation of parents, teachers, administrators, physicians, dentists, nurses, and others is *Health Appraisal of School Children*. This booklet was produced and has been periodically updated by the Joint Committee on Health

[1]C. Morley Sellery, "Role of the School Physician in Today's Schools," *Journal of School Health*, **22**, No. 3 (March 1952), 69.

School Health Appraisal

Problems in Education of the National Education Association and the American Medical Association.[2] Health appraisal is considered a cooperative and continuing process in which various individuals share responsibility and concern for the health evaluation of children and the subsequent management of identified health problems by appropriate methods. Ideally, each person on the health appraisal team supplements the others involved and their unified effort is child centered. Since 1947, the American Medical Association through its Bureau of Health Education has held repeated conferences to consider the functions of physicians and other medical personnel in the health appraisal and subsequent follow-up of detected health problems of individual children.[3]

In the booklet, parents are encouraged to accompany their children when given medical examinations, whether the examination is in their doctor's office or at school. Although such examinations require more time, since the physician must talk with each parent, it provides an opportunity for the parent to get a first-hand interpretation of the physician's findings. When indicated, appropriate treatment of any condition found in the examination is more apt to occur when parents are fully aware of the situation. The booklet also indicates means by which other individuals on the health team can contribute to the educational values of the health appraisal experience.

Medical examination

Representatives of education, medicine, and public health have agreed that health appraisal should be designed (a) to contribute to the maximum effectiveness of the child as an individual and a member of the community, (b) to assure the child's maximum fitness to receive an education, (c) to inform school personnel, parents, and the child regarding his health status, (d) to suggest adjustments in the school environment or instructional program based on individual needs, and (e) to serve as learning experiences for children, teachers, and parents which will be basic to lifelong programs of healthful living.

The medical examination has two very distinct values for the physical educator. *First,* pupils with serious defects, of such a nature that vigorous exercise would be harmful to them, are discovered. Such pupils should be exempted from any physical tests of a vigorous nature unless otherwise indicated, and should be placed in physical education classes in which exercise is restricted to individual capacities and modified to meet individual needs. The medical examination thus becomes a safeguard for the individual and a guide for the physical educator in prescribing physical activities for him.

Second, the medical examination is helpful in discovering physical defects that result in physiological disturbances that may be the cause of low physical fitness in those pupils so classified by other testing techniques employed by the physical educator. The school health service personnel can be of great value in discovering the cause of this condition and in suggesting remedies for its amelioration.

The school physician also has a special function in relation to teachers of physical activities: to notify them of findings and to help them conduct physical education programs in conformity with modern medical science. The school physician should be considered the physical educator's medical adviser, and should be called on repeatedly for help and guidance in classifying pupils for activity programs, in conducting individual and adapted physical education, and in handling the "excuse" problem. Informed physicians, who

[2]Joint Committee on Health Problems in Education, *Health Appraisal of School Children,* 5th ed. (Washington and Chicago: National Education Association and American Medical Association, 1970).

[3]Wallace Ann Wesley, Department of Health Education, American Medical Association, 535 North Dearborn Street, Chicago, Illinois 60610.

understand modern concepts of physical education, in general thoroughly believe in its importance for growing children and youth and give enthusiastic support to programs that are well conducted. The physical educator *should take the initiative* in developing proper and effective relationships with his school medical officer.

The frequency of medical examinations of school children is determined by law in a number of states, but there is no uniformity in these requirements. Health and physical educators, therefore, should determine whether such regulations exist and what they are for their respective states.

Differences of opinion are evident relative to the frequency medical examinations should be required; the recommendations of various groups are based on a synthesis of opinions rather than on scientific facts. However, Yankower and associates studied the need for periodic school medical examinations in the first four elementary school grades in Rochester, New York. They found that 21 percent of first grade children had an "adverse" condition, but 78 percent of these children were already under medical care, and the defects of an additional 12 percent were known by the schools. By the fourth grade, 14 percent of the children developed new defects; half of these were under care and one-fourth more were known to the schools.[4] These investigators concluded that it is more important to tailor all features of a school health program, including the frequency of periodic medical examinations, to the needs of individual schools and the communities they serve than to follow a set and standardized pattern of frequent examinations whose casefinding and educational values are dubious.[5]

The Joint Committee on Health Problems of the N.E.A. and the A.M.A. proposes that each child should be seen by a physician, preferably his family doctor, for a medical examination and review at suitable intervals during the 12-year span of the school period. Each examination should include coordination of the observations of parents, teachers, nurses, and others who have had regular contacts with the child since his previous examination. All available records pertaining in any way to his or her physical or emotional health should be assembled for use by the physician before the examination.[6]

For those who wish a more specific guide to the frequency of medical examinations, the practice preferred by some is that the most important medical examination is at entrance to school, before beginning kindergarten or the first grade. Instead of each year, other examinations are recommended at the start of the fourth and seventh grades and before graduation from high school. Under this plan, provisions should be made for special examinations when pupils are referred by teachers or school nurses. Today, too, the medical examination is usually given by the family physician; where this is not possible, the school should provide this service.

Standards for the School Medical Examination

New York State Regulations.[7] In attacking the problem of improving school medical examinations, the Bureau of Health Services, New York State Education Department, has established official regulations governing health services. The regula-

[4]Alfred Yankower and Ruth A. Lawrence, "A Study of Periodic Medical Examinations: 1. Methodology and Initial Findings," *American Journal of Public Health,* **45,** No. 1 (January 1955), 71.

[5]Alfred Yankower and others, "A Study of Periodic Medical Examinations: IV. Educational Aspects," *American Journal of Public Health,* **51,** No. 10 (October 1961), 1540.

[6]Joint Committee, *Health Appraisal of School Children.*

[7]*Regulations of the Commissioner of Education Governing Health Service,* New York State Education Department, 1970.

tions provide that the following shall be the responsibilities of all boards of education throughout the state:

1. To provide and maintain a continuous and satisfactory program of school health service.

2. To require each child enrolled in the public school to have a satisfactory health examination either by the family physician of the child or by the school physician upon the child's entrance in such school and for each child entering the first, third, seventh, and tenth grades thereof and to require such special health examinations as may be essential.

3. To require that the results of the health examination . . . shall be recorded on approved forms which shall be kept on file in the school.

4. To require the physician making the examinations to sign the health record card and make approved recommendations.

5. To advise, in writing, the parent or guardian of each child in whom any aspect of the total school health service program indicates a defect, disability, or other condition which may require professional attention with regard to health.

6. To keep the health records of individual children confidential except as such records may be necessary for the use of approved school personnel and, with the consent of the parents or guardians, for the use of appropriate health personnel of cooperating agencies.

7. Boards of education may, when the exigencies warrant, provide relief in situations wherein the child would otherwise be deprived of the full benefit of education through inability to follow instruction offered and to benefit therefrom.

8. To require adequate health inspections of pupils by teachers, school nurse-teachers and other approved school personnel.

9. To maintain a suitable program of education for the purpose of informing the school personnel, parents, nonschool health agencies, welfare agencies and the general public regarding school health conditions, services and factors relating to the health of school children.

10. To provide for adequate guidance to parents, children and teachers in procedures for preventing and correcting defects and diseases

and in the general improvement of the health of school children.

11. To furnish appropriate instruction to school personnel in procedures to follow in case of accident or illness.

12. To provide suitable inspections and supervision of the health and safety aspects of the school plant.

13. To provide adequate health examinations before participation in strenuous physical activity and periodically throughout the season for those so participating.

14. To provide health examinations necessary for the issuance of employment certificates, vacation work permits, newspaper carrier certificates, and street trades badges.

In New York State, essential data must also be carried on school medical record cards, which must first be approved by State Bureau of Health Services. An attempt is thus made to obtain a reasonable uniformity in examining and recording, and the minimum extent of the examination in all schools is defined.

Medical Record Forms

The use of proper forms on which to record the results of medical examinations is of considerable value both in defining minimum standards and in securing adequate examinations. A large number of these forms have been prepared by schools throughout the country. The most valuable and acceptable health records are those designed jointly by representatives of the persons who will use them.[8] These include teachers, health educators, physical educators, the school nurse, the school physician, and local private physicians and dentists.

School medical examinations, usually limited in scope, are planned to discover the health status of the total child and to uncover conditions that need attention. Minimum essentials are a review of the

[8]Donald A. Dukelow and Fred V. Hein, eds., *Health Appraisal of School Children*, 3rd ed. (Chicago: American Medical Association, 1961), p. 7.

health history, the results of screening tests, parent and teacher observations, and medical evaluations of the following conditions and parts of the body:[9]

Nutritional
Eyes and eyelids
Ears and eardrums
Skin and hair
Heart
Pulse: Resting
   after exercise
Lungs
Nervous system
Muscle tone
Posture
Bones and joints
Abdomen
Nose, throat, and tonsils
Thyroid gland
Lymph nodes
Teeth and gums

Numerous school systems and several states have developed medical record forms by cooperative means or through research. Certain of these projects are described below.

Oregon School Health Appraisal.[10] *Health School Services for the School-Age Child in Oregon* was first published in 1951; in revised form, the third edition was issued in 1968. This manual was developed by a committee composed of the State Board of Health, the State Education Department, and the Departments of Health Education at the University of Oregon and Oregon State University. In carrying out the recommended procedures, the State Superintendent of Public Instruction, with the advice of the State Board of Health, has the responsibility to prescribe a program of health examinations of boys and girls in the public schools. School administrators at both county and local levels are responsible for carrying out such a program.

In Oregon, health appraisals are made of all pupils entering a public school in the state for the first time. Also, every effort is made to provide such appraisals of pupils upon entrance to the ninth grade; or in junior high or three-year high schools, the examinations would be given to seventh and tenth grade pupils. In addition, pupils referred through teacher-nurse screening must be examined. All pupils taking part in interscholastic athletic contests are examined before participation in the sports program each year. The medical part of the examination is performed by a private physician, school physician, or local health officer and his assistants.

Public health departments and schools may cooperate in sending a letter to parents asking that children be examined before school opens and including the standard form, *Oregon Pupil Medical Record*. The information required for this form includes the following: history of birth and infancy; habits, personality and behavior; illnesses, immunizations, and unusual conditions; medical examination findings; height and weight, and vision testing.

When the *Oregon Pupil Medical Record* is completed and on file in the school, essential information is transferred to the *Oregon School Health Record Form*. This is a cumulative record form, designed to follow the pupil throughout his public school attendance from elementary school to his graduation from high school. The annual height, weight, vision, and hearing tests are administered by nurses or teachers; observations of the teacher relative to each pupil's eyes, ears, oral cavity, nose and throat, general condition and appearance, and behavior are recorded annually.

The Connecticut Cumulative Health Record. Byler[11] described a cumulative health record to be used in conjunction

[9]*Ibid.,* p. 37.

[10]*Health Services for the School-Age Child in Oregon,* 3rd ed. (Salem: State Department of Education; Portland: State Board of Health, 1968).

[11]Ruth V. Byler, "The Cumulative Health Record," *Journal of the Association for Health, Physical Education, and Recreation,* **20,** No. 7 (September 1949), 444.

with the school health service program in Connecticut.) In constructing this form, medical record cards in use in the local school systems of the state, plus a wide sampling of forms recommended by other states were analyzed. Regional meetings of all school health personnel concerned were held throughout the state.

This form has several unique features: (a) space is provided for recording, each September and February, the date of the pupil's last visit to a dentist; (b) a record is provided for pre-school health notes and a complete list of preventive treatments and tests; (c) both chronological age and mental age may be entered on the card; (d) considerable space is devoted both to teachers' notes on the pupil's physical, mental, and emotional health and to nurses' notes on health counseling; (e) following each examination, physicians must answer the following four questions as an aid in advising the school and parents relative to follow-up treatment: Does the pupil need medical care? Is further examination or a laboratory test recommended? Does any irremediable defect exist? Are there problems relating to growth, development, or nutrition, with which teachers and parents should be acquainted? When any of these questions are answered in the affirmative, the examining physician is asked to write his significant findings and specific recommendations in space provided for this purpose.

The Springall Cumulative Health Record.[12] Arthur N. Springall, M.D., Council on Medical Education and Hospitals, American Medical Association, studied school health record forms with the intention of suggesting such a form for common use in the elementary and secondary

[12]Arthur N. Springall, "A Suggested Cumulative Health Record Form for Use During the Elementary and Secondary School Years," Master's thesis, George Williams College, 1954.

schools of the United States. Fifty-nine forms were obtained: 36 forms from state departments, 20 from boards of education, and one each from the Y.M.C.A., the Y.W.C.A., and the Boy Scouts. After analysis, the compiled data were sent to a jury of 14 individuals designated by various health organizations as being especially well qualified in child health work. On the basis of those who voted to include the item, the values of the various items were judged as follows: 75 to 100 percent, essential; 50 to 75 percent, recommended; 25 to 50 percent, optional; 0 to 25 percent not considered for inclusion. Thus, the Springall form represents a compilation of the 59 forms analyzed, modified by the opinions of outstanding workers in the field of child health, and interpreted by the investigator.[13]

Validity and Accuracy of the Medical Examination

The validity of the medical examination as a measure of health is obvious. There is sufficient clinical evidence to support the contention that a physical defect *causing organic disturbances,* such as diseased tonsils or abscessed teeth, constitutes a drain on the individual, lowering his vitality and his capacity for physical activity, impairing the function of his vital organs, and reducing his efficiency as a total being. As previously stated, health is more than *either* being sick *or* being well; more than having a fever or not having a fever. (Health is a positive quality extending from death to abundant life.) Therefore, any defect that impairs the function of the body as a whole reduces its capacity for physical activity.

Although the validity of the medical examination is unquestioned, frequently questions may be raised concerning its

[13]Physicians' Record Company, 3000 S. Ridgeland Ave., Berwyn, Ill. 60402.

accuracy and thoroughness as conducted in public schools. The fact that this examination is, of necessity, based upon the judgments of physicians usually without the assistance of laboratory tests or other objective techniques, places it in much the same category of subjectivity as judgment in other types of observations. When subjective judgment becomes the basis for decisions, differences of opinion are apt to exist. The need for care on the part of school physicians in giving medical examinations is clearly indicated. A hurried examination actually may be worse than none at all if it fails to detect defects, thus giving pupils a false sense of security, as well as giving them an erroneous notion that medical examinations are relatively unimportant.

Examination of Athletes

The concensus overwhelmingly favors an annual pre-participation medical evaluation of athletes. The essentials of such an evaluation are provided in a pamphlet prepared in 1972 by the Committee on the Medical Aspects of Sports of the American Medical Association.[14] The aims of the examination are to: determine the health status of candidates prior to exposure to participation and competition; provide appropriate medical advice to promote optimum health and fitness; counsel atypical candidates as to the sports or modification of sports which would provide suitable activity for them; restrict from participation those whose physical limitations present undue risks. The pamphlet presents a number of suggestions of value to the examining physician, including a Sports Candidates' Questionnaire, a Health Examination Form, a Return to Play Form, and a list of Disqualifying Conditions for Sports Participation.

[14]Obtained through the American Medical Association, 535 N. Dearborn Street, Chicago, Illinois 60610.

VISION SCREENING TESTS

Visual defects, if not discovered and compensated for, impair pupils' general physical fitness. Physical ailments, such as headaches, indigestion, and neuromuscular hypertension, are often traceable to eyestrain caused by noncompensated visual defects. Such defects also affect children's school achievement. Stump[15] in 1952 compared the visual performance of "best" and "fair" students in 11 school subjects; the average scholastic advantage in visual performance for the best students ranged from 11 to 35 percent for the various subjects. Kephart[16] demonstrated that a significant relationship exists between the visual status of school children and their academic success and that improvement of visual skills through professional attention leads to more rapid progress in school achievements.

Visual demands made on school children are very great. It has been estimated that 80 to 85 percent of the learning process is done via the visual pathway.[17] The prevalence of visual defects has been checked through surveys of school children in Denver, St. Louis, and Detroit. The percentages of children referred to opthalmologists as a consequence ranged between 20 and 30 percent. As an example of these surveys, Cromwell[18] studied the cumulative records of 996 children in grades one through twelve. Each of these children had received ten or more visual

[15]N. Franklin Stump, "Visual Performance and Educational Success," *The Optometric Weekly* (September 4, 1952).

[16]Newell C. Kephart, "Visual Skills and Their Relation to School Achievement," *American Journal of Ophthalmology*, **30** (June 1953).

[17]Otto Lippman, "Eye Screening," *Archives of Ophthalmology*, **68** (November 1962), 690.

[18]Gertrude E. Cromwell, "A Study of Visual Screening and Referrals on 996 Pupils During Their 12 Years School Experience," *Journal of School Health*, **22**, No. 8 (October 1952), 229.

screening tests utilizing the Snellen eye chart. Among her findings were the following: 24.6 percent were referred for visual evaluation by a specialist; of those children referred to an eye specialist, 64 percent were in kindergarten and elementary school; and of those children referred to a specialist, no visual corrections were made for 17 percent.

Blackhurst and Radke[19] have indicated that one-third of the school population will need treatment for a significant vision defect before completing high school. Such evidence points to the need for annual vision screening tests in the schools, both to discover new defects and to indicate additional corrections of previously determined deficiencies in vision.

Symptoms of Visual Disorders

Classroom and health education teachers, especially, and physical educators, to some extent, should be alert to detect signs of visual discomfort in the appearance and behavior of children. The Joint Committee on Health Problems in Education of the National Education Association and the American Medical Association[20] presented the following manifestation of eye difficulties to be observed:

Before a Child Begins to Read

1. Attempts to brush away blur.
2. Blinking more than usual.
3. Frequent rubbing of the eyes.
4. Squinting when looking at distant objects.
5. Frequent or continuous frowning.
6. Stumbling over objects.
7. Undue sensitivity to light.
8. Red, encrusted, or swollen eyelids.
9. Recurring styes.

10. Inflamed or watery eyes.
11. Crossed eyes, "wall" eye, or "wandering" eye (regardless of degree).

Other Signs After Reading Begins

12. Holding a book too far away or too close to the face when reading.
13. Inattention during reading periods, chalkboard, chart, or map work.
14. Difficulty in reading or in other work requiring accurate use of the eyes.
15. Inability or lack of desire to participate in games requiring accurate distance vision.
16. Frequent complaints of headaches associated with close work.
17. Poor alignment in written work.
18. Tilting head to one side or thrusting head forward when looking at near or distant objects.
19. Irritability when doing close work.
20. Shutting or covering one eye when reading.

In view of the great importance of vision, it would be ideally desirable for every child to have a periodic examination by an eye specialist. Since the expense of such a practice is prohibitive for most schools, however, it becomes necessary to utilize tests that will select or screen out those who require careful examinations. Screening tests are not diagnostic; they are intended to identify those with potential vision problems for referral to an opthalmologist for a complete eye examination. Parents should be informed of this distinction and should not assume that a screened child has an eye defect in need of correction until a complete examination is given by a specialist. Screening tests may be given appropriately by properly instructed non-medical personnel; in fact, the use of such persons is considered desirable in order to avoid the impression that diagnostic eye examinations are being given. Classroom teachers, health educators, nurses, physical educators, volunteers, and part-time employed technicians

[19]Robert T. Blackhurst and Edmund Radke, "Is Snellen Screening Enough?" *E.E.N.T. Digest,* **28** (July 1966), 57.

[20]Charles C. Wilson, ed., *School Health Services* (Washington: National Education Association; Chicago: American Medical Association, 1964), p. 76.

are logical individuals who may develop competency in using one or more of the vision tests currently available.[21]

In evaluating vision tests for screening purposes, Hitz[22] proposes the following four criteria:

1. The test should pick up most errors without finding minor transient psychic effects.

2. The test should be easy to operate without the need for specialized training or technical knowledge.

3. The test should not be more discriminating than the accepted thorough examination utilized by the majority of competent well-trained ophthalmic physicians.

4. If the principles upon which the test is based are different from those accepted by competent ophthalmologists, then at least the findings must agree fairly accurately with the findings of a thorough ophthalmic test.

The Snellen Letter Chart

In 1862, Professor H. Snellen of Utrecht presented a practical method of determining visual acuity. Since that time the Snellen Letter Chart has become a common method of testing vision in schools. This chart consists of several rows of letters, each succeeding row from top to bottom being reduced in size, thereby requiring a consecutively greater amount of visual acuity in order to read them.

The E Chart, or Snellen Egyptian block letter chart, is similar to the Snellen letter test and is of particular value in testing the vision of young children, although it may also be considered for general use. On this chart only the letter E is used, facing in different directions. The procedures for administering and scoring this test are the same as for the Snellen test, except that a single symbol is shown at a time, seen through a hole in a card held by an assistant. The subject by pointing indicates the direction of the "E", whether up, down, to the right, or to the left. This chart may, therefore, be used with young children who do not know the alphabet, and it eliminates with older subjects the possibility of memorizing a sequence of letters on the chart.

Frequently, local or state health departments, local or county school systems, or state departments of education can supply Snellen eye charts.[23] Techniques for testing follow.

1. The vision testing room should be quiet and the atmosphere friendly for best results. Only one subject should be in the room at a time in order to eliminate any opportunity for memorizing the letter sequences prior to testing. If the tester suspects subjects of such memorizing, he may ask the person being tested to read lines right to left instead of left to right.

2. The person being tested should stand or sit 20 feet from the chart, with the "20-foot line" on the chart approximately level with the eyes. If standing, the heels should touch a line drawn on the floor 20 feet from the chart; if seated, the back legs of the chair should touch this line, with the person sitting erect in taking the test.

3. The chart should be illuminated with approximately 20 foot-candles of light, evenly diffused over the chart with no glare. This amount of illumination should be checked through use of a light meter. General illumination in the vision-testing room should not be less than one-fifth of the chart illumination and should not be more than the illumination on the chart. There should be no bright light in the child's field of vision.

4. Each eye should be tested separately, the other being covered with a square of cardboard

[21]Joint Committee, *Health Appraisal of School Children,* p. 10.

[22]H. B. Hitz, "An Evaluation of Vision Testing Methods in Schools," *American Journal of Ophthalmology,* **21,** No. 9 (September 1938), 1024.

[23]If not available at one of these sources, they may be obtained from the National Society for the Prevention of Blindness, 79 Madison Ave., New York City 10016. A Snellen chart with built-in illumination is available from Good Lite Company, 7426 Madison Street, Forest Park, Illinois 60130.

held obliquely against the nose to cover the eye completely, avoiding any pressure on the eyeball. Both eyes should be kept open. If the person wears glasses, a test with the glasses only is necessary. Test the right eye first, then the left eye, then both eyes.

5. In testing, begin with the 30-foot line on the chart and follow with the 20-foot line. It is not necessary to test below the 20-foot line since visual acuity is considered satisfactory at this point. If the person fails the 30-foot line, move up to the 40-foot line and above until a line that can be seen is located. Actually, testing at the 20- and 30-foot lines is adequate, as referrals would be made for pupils failing the 30-foot line. Vision at a given test line is considered satisfactory if three out of four letters are correctly read.

6. The scoring is in fractions, the numerator being the distance the subject is from the chart (20 feet, usually), and the denominator the number on the chart which indicates the distance that would be read by the normal eye. If the subject's vision is just normal, then his acuteness of vision will equal 20/20. A score of 20/30, 20/40, or 20/50 indicates that the child can just see at 20 feet letters large enough for the normal eye to see at 30, 40, or 50 feet, respectively.

7. According to the 1972 edition of *Health Appraisal of School Children*,[24] parents should be urged to secure professional eye examinations for children who are in the following categories: (a) those who consistently exhibit symptoms of visual disturbance, regardless of the results of the Snellen test; (b) children eight years of age or older who have visual acuity of 20/30 or less in either eye, with or without symptoms; (c) children seven years of age or less who have visual acuity of 20/40 or less in either eye, with or without symptoms. It is recommended that children failing the screening test be retested before referrals to an eye specialist are made.

The Snellen test has several distinct advantages for use in schools. It is inexpensive, requires no special electrical apparatus (although the amount of light on the chart should be controlled), is easy to administer, and takes an average of only about one minute per child. In the Michigan survey, over 90 percent of the children who failed the test received treatment.[25] Evidence is not presented on the number of children with visual defects who might have been missed by the Snellen test.

As useful as the Snellen test has proven, however, it has received criticism. The major criticism is that it primarily identifies the myopic, or nearsighted, child, who would probably be functioning well academically since he has good vision for reading and other desk work. Obviously, at 20 feet, the hyperopic, or farsighted, child will pass the test easily. Therefore, a test of visual acuity at reading distance, 10 to 16 inches, is needed. Other deficiencies of the Snellen Test are that it does not detect eye muscle imbalance or astigmatism. Some individuals can with conscious effort force their eyes to read small enough to pass the test even though their refractive errors are such as to make sustained reading difficult and uncomfortable.

A handy practical device for shielding the eye not being tested is the occluder, proposed by the Army-Navy-NRC Visual Committee. Specifications for this instrument are given in Figure 4.1. It should be constructed from rigid material, such as wood, translucent plastic, or metal.

Commercial Screening Devices

Attempts to incorporate tests of several visual functions into a standardized form resulted in fixed batteries of tests contained in sterioscopic testing devices. The early instruments contained such ocular tests as monocular and binocular vision at both near and far distances, color vision, muscle balance, fusion, and depth perception. The devices contained test plates

---

[24]Joint Committee, *Health Appraisal of School Children*, p. 11.

[25]Blackhurst and Radke, "Is Snellen Screening Enough?" p. 57.

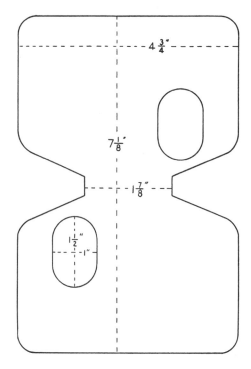

$4\frac{3}{4}''$

$7\frac{1}{8}''$

$1\frac{7}{8}''$

$1\frac{1}{2}''$

$1''$

FIGURE 4.1. *The Occluder*

used at a linear distance of one foot, but provided an "optical" distance of 20 feet by use of lenses and reduction in the size of test letters.[26] Advantages of these instruments were standard illumination without interference from room lighting, small space for testing, exact definition of tests, and provision for more visual characteristics than just visual acuity at 20 feet as in the Snellen test.

The original devices were found to yield too many referrals that were subsequently found by specialists' examinations not in need of visual corrections. Over the years, manufacturers strove to improve their effectiveness as visual screening devices. A noteworthy development was the Massa-

chusetts Vision Test, designed by the Division of Maternal and Child Health, Massachusetts Department of Public Health. The kit for this test consisted of an improved form of the Snellen E chart; a house card mounted on a frame with an electrical unit and light source; a near phoria tester; and spectacles, some with plus sphere lenses and others with Maddox rods. This kit is no longer available commercially, but its principles have been incorporated in other stereoscopic testing devices. Several of the visual screening instruments presently available are described below. These devices are used in business and industry and for traffic testing safety, as well as by schools.

Denver Eye Screening Test.[27] The Denver Eye Screening Test was developed in the B. F. Stolinsky Laboratories, Department of Pediatrics, University of Colorado Medical Center. The test has four parts: a vision screening test, responses to questions, a cover test, and a pupillary light reflex test.[28] Only the screening test will be described here (any E or a picture card test may be given for this purpose). The E test is given to children three years of age and older; the picture card test is intended for younger children.

The materials needed for the E test are an E card, an occluder, and a 15-foot string, used to measure the distance for the test. The card has a small E on one side and a large E on the other. The large E is utilized to instruct the child in responding to the direction the E is pointing; at 15 feet, this E indicates 20/40 vision or better.

When the child understands the test, he is shown the small E at the 15-foot distance with one eye at a time occluded by using the occluder. The position of the E is ro-

[26]Renee A. Sherman, "The First Thirty Years of Stereoscopic Visual Training," *American Journal of Optometry*, March 1964. (Reprinted by Titmus Optical Company, Inc., Petersburg, Virginia.)

[27]John Barker, Arnold Goldstein, and William K. Frankenburg, *Denver Eye Screening Test*, Rev. Ed. (Denver: Project and Publishing Foundation), 1972.

[28]Manual and test items may be purchased from Project and Publishing Foundation Inc., E. 51st Ave. and Lincoln St., Denver, Colorado 80216.

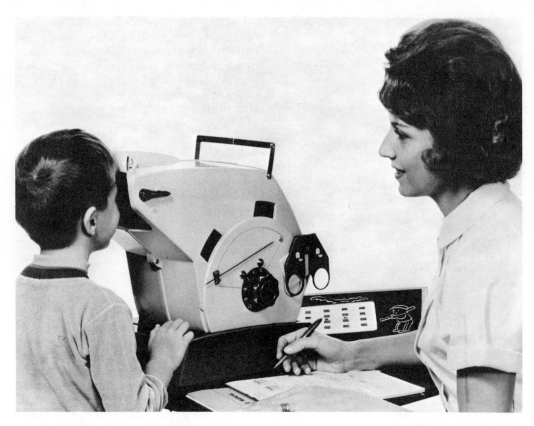

FIGURE 4.2. *Titmus Vision Tester*

tated several times at random; the tester should cover the card with his hand each time so that the pupil cannot see the direction the card is being turned. The rotations for each eye are repeated until the child has either three correct responses or three failures, whichever is first. If he gives three correct responses first, he passes the vision screening test; if three incorrect responses are given first, he fails the test.

Titmus Vision Tester.[29]   The Titmus Vision Tester, portrayed in Figure 4.2, is a compact, portable instrument developed after 30 years of laboratory research and field studies. This tester has slides and acces-

sories for many uses. For pediatric, school, and general use, three groups of slides are available: pre-school children, primary grade children, and older children and adults. The primary age series conforms to the Massachusetts Vision Test; the older children and adult series has been approved by the Federal Aviation Agency for aeromedical use. The school visual screening tests include acuity of right and left eyes separately and both eyes together at far and near distances and vertical and lateral balance tests at far and near distances. Other slides may be obtained for special purposes. Among the desirable features of the Titmus tester are: easy height adjustment to the eye level of the short child or the tall adult; occlusion of the non-tested eye by touch of a switch without the subject closing his eye;

[29]Titmus Optical Company, Petersburg, Virginia 23803.

observation window, which permits the tester to see the slide being viewed by the subject and to point to a specific test symbol; and easy "far-near" change by use of a switch.

Keystone Ophthalmic Telebinocular.[30] (The Telebinocular is a modification of the Brewster stereoscope with stand, attached movable slide holder, and light.) The construction of the instrument separates the fields of vision and permits each eye to see only its half of the slide.(The vision of both eyes may be tested together or either eye may be tested separately.) A special arrangement whereby measurements can be made at reading-distance equivalents ranging from 12 inches to infinity is also provided (ordinarily, infinity is considered 20 feet and beyond).

The *Keystone Visual Survey Tests* consist of stereographic cards, which provide information on the pupil's visual efficiency covering a wide field of functional aspects of vision. Instead of testing visual acuity by occlusion, the usable vision of each eye is tested with the other eye open and seeing; stress is placed on binocularity, with the two eyes working together. The fourteen tests included are for the following: simultaneous perception, vertical posture, lateral posture at far point, fusion at far point, usable vision of the right eye at far point, usable vision of the left eye at far point, depth perception (stereopsis), color perception (two cards), lateral posture at near point, fusion at near point, usable vision of the right eye at near point, usable vision of the left eye at near point. If this test indicates vision is not up to normal, before referral to an eye specialist it is urged that pupils be re-tested with great care.

School Vision Tester.[31] As for the telebinocular described above, this vision tester,

developed by Bausch and Lomb, employs the stereoscopic principle with optical equivalents for far and near distances. Six visual performance tests may be given from slides, as follows: monocular acuity of each eye, farsightedness of each eye, simultaneous testing of vertical and lateral muscle balance at far distance, and gross muscular imbalances at near point. In 1973, a new model of the School Vision Tester was introduced, which utilizes molded plastic to provide a more compact, lighter, and easier to operate instrument. The three slides, which contain the six tests, however, remain the same.

Sight Screener.[32] Again, this instrument employs the stereoscopic principle at the optical equivalent of distance; near vision is tested without the interposition of lenses. The targets for right and left eyes are superimposed on Polaroid vectograph film. The visual functions tested are: simultaneous binocular vision, visual acuities of right eye, left eye, and both eyes, stereopsis, and vertical and lateral phorias.

Studies Pertaining to Visual Screening

Many studies have been made pertaining to methods and instruments utilized in the visual screening of school children. Certain of these are summarized below.

In 1962, Lippman[33] reviewed research pertaining to the referral rates of children from school visual screening procedures. The studies showed that the Massachusetts Vision Test compared favorably with clinical examination results and that tests of hyperopic are fairly reliable. General agreement was indicated for a referral rate of 20 to 30 percent. Under-referrals usually escape detection; however, in one study, it was reported that only three in 1000 non-referred children from a screen-

---

[30]Keystone View Company, 2112 E. 12th St., Davenport, Iowa 52803.

[31]Bausch & Lomb, Ophthalmic Division, 635 St. Paul Street, Rochester, N.Y. 14602.

[32]American Optical Corporation, Southbridge, Massachusetts 01550.

[33]Lippman, "Eye Screening," p. 69.

ing process were in need of visual attention. Of course, the referral cut-off point makes a difference: if over 30 percent are referred, an excess of over-referrals and few underreferrals will result; the reverse will happen if the cut-off is below 20 percent. This situation is further confused due to some disagreement among eye doctors as to the degree of visual acuity requiring visual attention.

The reliability and validity of scores obtained on the Telebinocular, the Ortho-Rater, and the Sight Screener were studied at the U.S. Submarine Base, Groton, Connecticut.[34] Reliability coefficients by the test-re-test method compared well for the three instruments, ranging from 0.81 to 0.84. In checking far and near vision against visual targets developed by the investigators, an early model Telebinocular proved inferior to the other devices. Hitz[35] found that the old-model Telebinocular was more discriminatory in detecting visual defects than is the ophthalmic examination; the tests with this instrument produced 20 percent more visual cases than did the specialist's examination. Similar results were obtained by Oak and Sloane,[36] utilizing 200 boys and girls ranging in age from 6 to 15 years. Gates and Bond[37] found that Telebinocular tests sometimes give inconsistent results when used with young children. These investigators concluded, however, that this situation may be due to fluctuations in attention and distractibility in young children rather than to any fundamental defects of the tests. (In evaluating these findings, it should be recognized that early-model Telebinoculars were used in the studies, so

it does not follow that similar results would be obtained with current improved instruments).

Gutman[38] compared the Massachusetts Vision Test and the Snellen Test as school vision screening devices. 6500 school children in three Oregon counties were screened with one or both methods; 1533 children were tested by both methods. The author concluded that both tests coupled with observation will, when given by a trained operator, yield an equivalent number of referrals for professional eye examinations. One component common to both tests, the Snellen Test, had a high degree of efficiency with but one "over-referral" in seven when failure to read 20/30 with either eye was used as the criterion for referral; it disclosed from two-thirds to three-fourths of all cases meriting professional care. The subsidiary tests of the Massachusetts Vision Test produced an additional small group of cases, but did so with a higher ratio of over-referrals.

A comprehensive study of visual screening procedures was conducted in the St. Louis schools with the joint support of the National Society for the Prevention of Blindness, the Children's Bureau of the Federal Security Agency, the Division of Health of the State of Missouri, the St. Louis Board of Education, the Department of Ophthalmology of Washington University School of Medicine, and the Bureau of Naval Research.[39] The children tested were 606 first-grade and 609 sixth-grade pupils; all subjects were given a complete ophthalmological examination, along with a number of screening tests, including the Snellen, the Massachusetts, the Telebinocular, the Ortho-Rater, and the Sight-Screener. The

[34]John H. Sulzman, Ellsworth B. Cook, and Neil R. Bartlett, 1948.

[35]Hitz, "Vision Testing Methods," p. 1024.

[36]Lura Oak and Albert E. Sloane, "The Betts Visual Sensation and Perception Tests," *Archives of Ophthalmology,* **22** (November 1939), 832.

[37]Arthur I. Gates and Guy L. Bond, "Reliability of Telebinocular Tests of Beginning Pupils," *Journal of Educational Psychology,* **28,** No. 1 (January 1937), 31.

[38]Eleanor B. Gutman, "School Vision Screening: A Comparison of Two Methods," *Sight-Saving Review,* **26** (1956), 212.

[39]Marian M. Crane and others, "Study of Procedures Used for Screening Elementary School Children for Visual Defects: Referrals by Screening Procedures vs. Ophthalmological Findings," *The Sight-Saving Review,* **22,** No. 3 (1952).

Ortho-Rater, Sight-Screener, and the Telebinocular correctly referred about 75 percent of the pupils referred by the ophthalmologist; however, these screening tests referred incorrectly an even larger number of pupils. The Massachusetts Vision Test and a combination of high standard Snellen with teacher judgment, both correctly referred about two-thirds of the students who need care. While this proportion is not quite as high as obtained with the other screening procedures, there were fewer incorrect referrals. This was particularly true of the Massachusetts Vision Test's incorrect referrals, which, for sixth grade students, were between half and two-thirds of the number of correct referrals, while for the first grade students correct and incorrect referrals were in about equal proportion. The investigators concluded that none of the vision-testing methods provides more than a rough screening procedure.

In 1962, the Department of Health in Detroit, Michigan, conducted a pilot school vision screening investigation. Using stereoscopic instruments, trained vision technicians screened a total of 36,554 children in grades one, seven, and ten. Referrals on the tests were those with poorer visual acuity than 20/30 without and 20/20 with a 1.75 diopter plus sphere lens and phoria tests at 20 feet and reading distance in either eye. Nearly 17 percent of the children failed the initial screening test and a retest. Of the referrals, 71 percent failed the visual acuity test; these children would have been identified had the screening been limited to a Snellen Test. The remaining 29 percent, however, would have remained unidentified. A followup study of the latter group revealed that 90 percent had a significant vision defect in need of treatment.[40]

Hearing tests

Auditory defects are serious handicaps in all phases of individual growth. It has been shown that even slight losses of hearing in school children cause speech defects, retardation, inferiority complexes, and unsocial behavior. Hearing losses are also an important cause of reading difficulties, frequently resulting in inability to distinguish between words that sound alike: if the child does not hear the difference between two words, he may have difficulty in distinguishing between their printed symbols.

In 1958, Newby[41] reported estimates of hearing loss in from 5 to 10 percent of the school population. Many of these, he stated, will respond to medical treatment or will spontaneously regain normal hearing at a later date; however, about 1 percent will have irremediable hearing loss of a handicapping nature. Cameron[42] found that a newly discovered hearing loss has more than a 50–50 chance of regaining average hearing with medical attention. If the child becomes an "old case," because of delayed medical attention, his chance of regaining average hearing with medical attention drops to about one in eight. Thus, the need for *early* detection and treatment of defective hearing is essential.

Symptoms of Ear Disorders

In addition to testing hearing acuity periodically, all teaching personnel should be alert to signs of hearing loss and ear diseases and disorders. Such signs are as follows.

1. Complaints of earaches or pain in the area around the ear; drainage from the ears.

[40]Robert T. Blackhurst and Edmund Radke, "School Vision Testing in The State of Michigan," *The Sight-Saving Review,* **34,** No. 1 (Spring 1964), 8.

[41]H. A. Newby, "School Hearing Conservation Programs," *Hearing News* (September 1958).

[42]Robert M. Cameron, "An Audiologist Looks at Hearing in the High School," *Journal of Health, Physical Education, and Recreation,* **29,** No. 2 (February 1958), 45.

2. Frequent complaints of the ear being "stopped up," or of noises in the ears, such as ringing, buzzing, or roaring.

3. Constant mouth breathing.

4. Frequent failure to respond when called upon or to locate properly the source or direction of a sound; frequent requests for repetition of words or phrases.

5. Inattention, interrupting conversations of others, being unaware that others are talking, leaning forward to hear, or cocking the head in an effort to hear better; unusual dependence upon visual cues.

6. Distortion of speech out of proportion to age; poor or defective articulation of speech sounds.

7. Poor balance in walking, running, leaping, and other similar activities, especially in dark places.

Many or all of the above manifestations of hearing impairment can represent other kinds of problems, so such observations should merely arouse suspicion concerning pupil's hearing. They indicate a need for further consideration.

Simple Hearing Tests

Two simple tests of hearing have been used in the schools for the purpose of screening out those in need of further examinations by otologists. These are the *watch-tick* test and the *voice* test.

Watch-Tick Test. The watch is a convenient instrument for roughly testing hearing. Directions for giving this test are as follows:

1. Stand behind the child seated in a chair. With one hand, hold a postal-size card at the side of the head, which will serve as a "blinder" to keep him from seeing the watch. The palm of the subject's hand should be held over the ear not being tested.

2. With the other hand, hold the watch toward one of the child's ears and on a level with it. Start testing by holding the watch one foot

from the ear; if the child can hear it, move it back one foot at a time until the tick is no longer discernible. Test the other ear in the same manner.

3. Hearing by this test can be scored by use of a fraction. In this instance, the denominator is the longest distance at which most children can hear the tick; the numerator is the longest distance at which it is heard by the child being tested. The score for each ear should be recorded.

An obvious problem encountered in the use of this test is differences that exist between the tick sounds from different watches, as, obviously, some watch ticks are lower than others. As a consequence, a sample of children should be tried with a given watch to determine the distance at which most can hear it; this distance can then be used as a guide for detecting those with hearing difficulties.

Voice Test. The voice test is another crude hearing screening procedure, given as follows:

1. The pupil is placed 20 feet from and with his back to the tester. He covers the ear not being tested with his hand.

2. In a conversational voice, the tester pronounces disconnected numbers, such as 2–4–7–8–1–9, and so forth, or words or short sentences. The child repeats what the tester says. If he cannot hear at 20 feet, the tester moves up to 15 feet, and further if necessary. Test the other ear in the same way.

The pupil who cannot hear with either the watch-tick or the voice test at two-thirds the distance established may be in need of medical attention. Both of these hearing screening tests, as has been mentioned, are but crude measures of auditory acuity, as the testing conditions are not sufficiently standardized. While they may serve to disclose marked hearing losses, they are unsatisfactory when compared with more adequate testing methods.

Audiometry[43]

The Audiometer. By far the most satisfactory way of measuring hearing in the schools is to use the audiometer. This instrument has raised hearing tests to the level of an effective and objective measure. The audiometer selected should meet the specifications established by the American Standards Association. Specifications may be obtained from the U.S. Bureau of Standards or the American Speech and Hearing Society, both in Washington, D.C. Audiometers, especially those in constant use, should be returned to the factory or designated center for calibration check at least once each calendar year. In using the audiometer, the testing room *must* be quiet, free from interruptions and removed from the sounds of music rooms, gymnasiums, typewriters, telephones, student traffic, and outside noises. Preferably, testing should be done in a sound-proof room.

The audiometer produces tones of various frequencies (pitches) over a wide range of intensities (loudness). The intensities range from a sound that is barely perceptible to the keenest ear to a sound at a very loud level. Frequency is measured in units of cycles per minute (cps); the range is from 125 to 8000 cps. Intensity is measured in decibels (db); the range is from −10 db to 100 db. Zero db intensity at each frequency represents the intensity required for the average ear to detect the presence of a tone. The pupil being tested hears the tone presented through an earphone.

Screening Test. The audiometer may be used either as a screening device or as an instrument for measuring the threshold of

[43]The information on the use of audiometry in the schools given here was checked against proposals contained in *Health Appraisal of School Children,* 1972 edition, prepared by the Joint Committee on Health Problems of the National Education Association and the American Medical Association.

hearing. The Joint Committee on Health Problems recommends that screening be done at the 10 db level, with reference to the present American Standard Audiometric zero for the frequencies of 1000, 2000, and 6000 cps, and at the 20 db level for the frequency of 4000 cps. Because the tester can "sweep" through all the frequencies in rapid order, this procedure is often called a sweep test. A child who hears each tone under these conditions is considered to have normal hearing. Those children who fail to hear one or more frequencies in either ear should be given a threshold test; that is, their thresholds at each of the test frequencies should be charted on an audiogram.

In administering pure-tone audiometer tests, the tester should explain to the children the purposes of the test and the procedures to be followed. The child should be seated so that he cannot see the dials of the audiometer. He is asked to nod or give a hand signal when he hears each new tone. The tester should be seated in order to watch carefully the child's face; he should use the interrupter switch at intervals as a check on the subject's responses.

Group Audiometry. Although not considered as desirable as individual testing, group audiometry is possible. The group audiometer is similar to a phonograph, and is equipped with earphones for the testing of as many as 40 subjects at one time. An instrument for testing one individual at a time is also available, and is superior for use when careful examining is required. The test consists in playing a record on which are recorded the voices of a man and a women speaking a series of numbers in a lower and lower tone. Each subject, listening through the earphones, writes down the numbers he hears on a special form provided for this purpose. Each ear is tested separately. One side of the disk is for the right ear, the other for the left.

Normal hearing is represented by a

zero-line on the typical record form. Hearing loss is recorded in decibels. A loss of six decibels is considered within the normal hearing range; pupils with a loss of nine decibels or more should be referred to a specialist for further examination.

Evaluation of Audiometer Testing

The desired screening program for the detection of children with hearing losses would select from a group of individuals with apparently normal hearing the maximum number with a significant or potentially significant disability and the minimum number without such disability. In most school surveys, between 5 and 10 percent of the children have failed the screening hearing test. If more than 10 percent fail in a given school situation, the tester should re-examine his technique, check the accuracy of calibration of the audiometer, and evaluate the possible effect of environment noise on his test results.

Yankower and associates[44] compared the case-finding effectiveness of the group phonograph fading numbers test, the group pure tone test, and the individual pure tone check test. The subjects were 2404 pupils in the third through seventh grades of the Rochester, N.Y., public schools. Approximately 5 percent of these children were found to have a verified hearing loss by otological examination. Not one of the three screening devices was able to select all of these cases: 33 percent were selected by the group phonograph screening procedure, 69 percent by the group pure tone method, and 95 percent by the individual sweep check process. Although the individual pure tone sweep check was the best case finder, it also se-

lected more children with no hearing loss than did either of the two group tests.

In the Cleveland public schools, Kinney[45] found that the percentage of suspected cases selected by the sweep check method was very little higher than by the group phonograph screening process. Both methods were used to screen 2068 children; each child was tested by both methods on the same day. There were 118 suspected cases (5.75 percent) by the phonograph method; the sweep check method identified the same 118 cases plus five additional ones.

The time required to administer the various hearing screening tests may frequently be a factor in selecting the device to use. Obviously, the group methods require much less time per pupil than do the individual methods. Also, the skill required of the tester is less for the group phonograph process than for the pure tone procedures.

EVALUATING HEALTH SERVICE PROGRAMS

Kirk[46] developed an instrument for evaluating college and university health service programs. From the literature on the subject and with the assistance of several health service directors, 764 standards were obtained. An analysis of these standards resulted in 291 for inclusion in a preliminary instrument. The preliminary instrument was rated by a jury of 40 authorities; 247 of the standards were considered acceptable and were arranged as a revised instrument. The revised instrument was weighted by 48 health ser-

[44]A. Yankower, M. L. Geyer, and H. C. Chase, "Comparative Evaluation of Three Screening Methods for Detection of Hearing Loss in Children," *American Journal of Public Health*, **44**, No. 1 (January 1954), 77.

[45]Charles E. Kinney, "Cleveland Hearing Conservation Program," *Transactions of American Academy of Ophthalmology and Otolaryngology*, **50** (November-December 1945), 94.

[46]Robert H. Kirk, "An Instrument for Evaluating College and University Health Service Programs," *Research Quarterly*, **35**, No. 3, Pt. 1 (October 1964), 307.

vice directors representing all types and sizes of colleges and universities throughout the United States. The final instrument was administered by visitation to 12 Indiana colleges and universities.

The Kirk Health Service Standards contain eight divisions: organization and administration; health advisory, counseling, and educational services; finance; health appraisal; medical care; sanitation; records and reports; and plant, facilities, and equipment. The instrument is well constructed and should be suitable for evaluating health service programs in practically all types and sizes of colleges and universities.

Selected references

Dukelow, Donald A., and Fred V. Hein, eds., *Health Appraisal of School Children,* 3rd. ed. Chicago: American Medical Association, 1961.

Joint Committee on Health Problems in Education, *Health Appraisal of School Children,* 5th ed. Washington: National Education Association; Chicago: American Medical Association, 1972.

Joint Committee on Health Problems in Education, School Health Services, 2nd. ed. American Medical Association, 1964. Washington: National Education Association.

CHAPTER 5

The effectiveness of many physical performances are related to various basic traits found in boys and girls, including their maturation, body size, and physique type. Some of these traits are related to heredity; others, such as body weight, have hereditary implications, but may also be affected by environmental influences, including the nature and amount of exercise, nutritional practices, and health habits.

Students differ dramatically in these basic traits.[1] Changes in some of these traits may be possible, at least to a limited degree. Logically, physique type, or body form, may be changed somewhat through diet and exercise. Yet, changes in maturity and the height and breadth of the skeleton do not seem possible through exercise. However, individual differences in maturity, body size, and physique type will definitely influence physical performances. Thus, they should be considered in judging the potentialities of students for participation in physical activities of many kinds. For example, those with a high de-

---

[1]H. Harrison Clarke, "Individual Differences, Their Nature, Extent, and Significance," *Physical Fitness Research Digest,* President's Council on Physical Fitness and Sports, Series 3, No. 4 (October 1973).

Maturity, Nutrition, Body Size, and Form

gree of mesomorphy are generally favored in many sports; the endomorph, on the other hand, is definitely handicapped. Mature and large students have great advantages over immature and small students, although compensations are possible through various developmental traits.

Maturity

According to Greulich,[2] the chronological age of a child is often little more than an indication of the length of time he or she has lived; it does not necessarily bear a close relationship to the amount of progress the child has made toward maturity. Tanner[3] has stated " . . . the bald statement that a boy is aged 14 is in most contexts hopelessly vague."

Great differences exist in the physiological maturity of boys and girls of the same chronological age. Utilizing skeletal age[4] as the maturity indicator in the Medford Boys' Growth Study,[5] boys were tested within two months of their birthdays at each age from seven through 17 years. The standard deviations fluctuated between 11.9 and 15.1 months. The ranges varied from a low of 58 months (about five years) at age 17 to a high of 85 months at age 13 (about seven years); the median range was 71 months, nearly six years. To illustrate the magnitude of these differences at age 14 years, approximately two-thirds of 168 boys tested had skeletal ages between 14 and 16 years—a span of two

---

[2]W. W. Greulich, "Skeletal Status and Physical Growth," *Dynamics of the Growth Process* (Princeton, N.J.: Princeton University Press, 1950).

[3]J. M. Tanner, *Growth at Adolescence,* 2nd ed. (Springfield, Ill.: Charles C Thomas, 1962), p. 55.

[4]Skeletal age is a measure of how far the ossification of the bones has progressed in their course of development from birth to maturity. This ossification is usually revealed from an X-ray of the wrist and hand.

[5]H. Harrison Clarke, *Physical and Motor Tests in the Medford Boys' Growth Study* (Englewood Cliffs, N.J.: Prentice-Hall, Inc., 1971), Ch. 2.

years; yet, these same boys were tested within two months of their birthdays, so they could not vary chronologically by more than four months. The skeletal range, of course, was much greater, between 10.3 and 16.9 years.

From studies of the significance of individual differences in maturity in the Medford series, the following generalizations may be made: the more mature boys were taller, heavier, stronger, and had a greater potential for success in interscholastic athletics; they were prone to higher levels of aspiration and better psychological adjustment. Significant relationships were not found between skeletal age and relative physical measures, such as the Physical Fitness Index, pull-ups, push-ups, and standing broad jump distance, since, for these measures, the effect of body weight on their performances has been neutralized.

The best method of evaluating the maturity of growing children is by determination of skeletal age. However, as this method involves an X-ray, usually of the wrist and hand, it is not considered practical for routine school use. Other methods of maturational assessment are limited and crude, but do have value as rough classifiers.

Dental Age

A general indicator of the maturational level of pre-pubescent boys and girls is related to the eruption of the permanent teeth. In general, those who have advanced dental development during childhood are larger and enter adolescence earlier than those who have retarded dental development.

(Dental age is obtained by counting the number of permanent teeth erupted at any age and relating this number to norms for each age.) These teeth erupt from about 6 to 13 years, which covers the elementary school and early junior high school ages, reaching at least to the start of

TABLE 5.1 *Dental Age Based on Number of Permanent Teeth Erupted*

Dental Age	Boys	Girls
6	2–3	2–3
7	6	7
8	9	10
9	12	13
10	15	17
11	19	21
12	23	25
13	26	27

pubescence. As adapted from Shuttleworth, the average number of permanent teeth erupted at each age is given in Table 5.1.[6] A tooth is considered to be erupted upon the first appearance of the crown or a part of it through the gum.

After counting the number of permanent teeth that have erupted, obtain the child's dental age from the table. For example, if a girl has 17 erupted teeth, her dental age is 10 years. If her chronological age is also 10 years, her maturity level is normal. However, if her chronological age is 11 years, then she is retarded by one year. Interpolations on the scale will be necessary unless maturation determinations are made on or near birthdays.

In a review of the literature, Schwartz[7] found conflicting correlations, as low as 0.29 and as high as 0.94, between skeletal age and the number of erupted permanent teeth. In his own dissertation (completed in 1960), type 3 dental examinations, using mouth mirror and explorer instrument, were performed by a dentist on 171 boys 7 to 12.5 years of age. He reported the following correlations with

[6]Frank K. Shuttleworth, "The Physical and Mental Growth of Girls and Boys Ages Six to Nineteen in Relation to Age at Maximum Growth," *Monograph of the Society for Research in Child Development,* **4,** No. 3, Serial No. 22 (1939).

[7]Samual Schwartz, "The Validity of the Human Dentition as an Indicator of Physical Maturity of Boys ranging from Seven Years to Twelve Years Six Months of Age," Doctoral Dissertation, Temple University, 1966.

the number of erupted permanent teeth: 0.81 for dental development status; 0.76 for chronological age; 0.71 for skeletal age; 0.65 for standing height; 0.62 for body weight; and 0.59 for grip strength.

Pubescent Assessment

Once boys and girls enter adolescence, pubescent assessment may be utilized to evaluate their maturity. For girls, the age at menarche (the time of first menstruation), is a simple and effective means of maturity classification. A correlation of -0.85 between the age at menarche and skeletal age at the chronological age of 13 years was obtained by Simmons and Greulich.[8] Thus, girls who are skeletally advanced at the time of adolescence also menstruate early. Deming[9] reported a correlation of 0.93 between age at menarche and the peak height velocity in girls.

The maturity of adolescent boys may be evaluated by assessment of their secondary sex characteristics. In this method, pubescent status is described in terms of five categories which represent successive stages in the development of the genitals and the pubic hair. Group 1 represents the sexual development of prepubescent boys; group 5 has reached the external sexual characteristics of adults. Illustrated descriptions of the five stages of pubescent development for both boys and girls have been provided by Greulich and associates,[10] Tanner,[11] and others. If longitu-

dinal observations are established, a simple maturity evaluation could be the beginning of penis growth. Stoltz and Stoltz[12] obtained a correlation of 0.87 between the beginning of the adolescent height spurt and the beginning of penis growth.

Clarke and Degutis[13] compared the skeletal ages and various body size, strength, and motor tests with the pubescent development of 10-, 13-, and 16-year-old boys. Physical maturation was differentiated most effectively at 13 years of age, although it was not as sensitive to maturational changes as skeletal age. At 16 years, maturational differentiation by pubescent assessment was much more limited; at 10 years of age, little or no value could be attributed to this method. With few exceptions, the 13- and 16-year-old boys who were advanced in pubescent development had higher mean scores on the body size, strength, and motor tests included in the study. Generally, the differences between means were significant.

Nutrition

The use of tests to measure the nutritional status of children in school has been common for many years. The purpose of this measurement is primarily to discover those who are undernourished and those who are obese so that appropriate remedial procedures may be applied. Efforts in this direction should continue, constituting an essential phase of measurement in health and physical education.

Undernourishment is particularly serious and a threat to health among children and young adults; it is most apt to develop dur-

[8]K. Simmons and W. W. Greulich, "Menarcheal Age and the Height, Weight, and Skeletal Age of Girls Age 7 to 17 Years," *Journal of Pediatrics,* **22** (1943), 518.

[9]J. Deming, "Application of the Gompertz Curve to the Observed Pattern of Growth in Length of 48 Individual Boys and Girls During the Adolescent Cycle of Growth," *Human Biology,* **29,** No. 1 (February 1957), 88.

[10]W. W. Greulich and others, "Somatic and Endocrine Studies of Puberal and Adolescent Boys," *Monograph of the Society for Research in Child Development,* **7,** No. 3, Serial No. 33 (1942).

[11]Tanner, *Growth at Adolescence,* 32–37.

[12]H. R. Stoltz and L. M. Stoltz, *Somatic Development of Adolescent Boys* (New York: The Macmillan Company, 1951), p. 332.

[13]H. Harrison Clarke and Ernest W. Degutis, "Comparison of Skeletal Age and Various Physical and Motor Factors with the Pubescent Development of 10, 13, and 16 Year Old Boys," *Research Quarterly,* **33,** No. 3 (October 1962), 356.

ing the period of rapid growth in children's lives. A normal amount of fat is desirable to the body: to act as reserve fuel, to furnish padding about the nerve endings, and to buoy up the visceral organs. Undernourishment may be due to insufficient food, to food lacking in essential nutrients, or to inability of the body processes to utilize properly the food intake. The undernourished child is apt to be high-strung and nervous; the abdominal organs commonly sag out of normal position; and the poorly nourished muscle tissues, including the muscles of the abdominal wall and the muscle layers of the intestines, become relaxed and flabby. Such persons suffer from nervous indigestion, constipation, and a wide variety of ill-defined ailments. Furthermore, undernourished individuals are usually listless and fatigue easily, or else keep going under strain, which results in a dangerous accumulation of fatigue products. They also show diminished resistance to fatigue and general lowered vitality. Various respiratory infections are especially apt to develop in young people if they are undernourished.

Obesity is a problem that chiefly concerns adults, although many obese children are found in school. Although a well-filled body and a moderate store of fat are advantageous for children and young adults, nevertheless, definite obesity is disadvantageous. It results in disfigurement and inefficiency of physical movement. It also increases risks in operations. Moreover, resistance to infectious disease is lowered, and excessive weight places an additional burden upon the circulatory system and the kidneys, so that obese persons are prone to develop functional disorders of the heart, high blood pressure, nephritis, and so forth.

Armstrong and associates[14] contrasted the mortality rate of overweight persons, limited to substandard life insurance, with persons accepted for standard insurance. The mortality rates were 79 percent for men markedly overweight and 42 percent for men moderately overweight above the standard risk group; comparable percentages for women were 61 and 42 percent respectively. The excess mortality rate was due to the greater number of deaths from degenerative diseases. Joslin and associates[15] found from an analysis of 3000 clinical records that 63 percent of males and 67 percent of females showed evidence of overweight at the outset of diabetes. From a survey of 74,000 industrial workers, Master and associates[16] found at every age and for both sexes that average blood pressure increased with body weight for a given height.

In making judgments of the nutritional status of school-age children, it should be recognized that they have a high degree of subjectivity. Consequently, they are open to the inaccuracies and differences of opinion between judges which are typical of other ratings of this sort. In a study by Franzen,[17] children in five different groups were examined by a number of physicians, using an adaptation of the Dunfermline Scale, and their judgments of the same children were intercorrelated. The median correlation between any two physicians was 0.60; correlations between pairs of physicians occurred as low as 0.18 and as high as 0.82. When the physicians used 46 items, each of which was credited as satisfactory or debited as unsatisfactory for each child, the median correlation between pairs of physicians was raised to 0.65. Although the agreement between physicians' ratings of nutritional status was fairly low, the reliability of an analytic rating scheme for 46 nutritional items was

[14]D. B. Armstrong and others, "Obesity and Its Relation to Health and Disease," *Journal of American Medical Association*, **147** (1951), 1007.

[15]E. P. Joslin and others, *Treatment of Diabetes Mellitus* (Philadelphia: Lea and Febiger, 1952).

[16]A. M. Master and others, "The Normal Blood Pressure Range and Its Clinical Implications," *Journal of American Medical Association*, **143** (1950), 1464.

[17]Raymond Franzen, *Physical Measures of Growth and Nutrition* (New York: American Child Health Association, 1929).

high. Correlations by the split-half method, 23 odd-numbered correlated with 23-even. numbered items, using 61 subjects, were 0.99, 0.97, 0.96, 0.95, and 0.90. These correlations mean that when a physician judges a child to be mal-nourished, he is consistent in rating the child high or low on most items.

EVALUATING NUTRITION

In order to eliminate the judgment errors in the subjective evaluation of nutritional status, various objective tests have been proposed and widely used, not only for children but for adults as well. Frequently, these are used in conjunction with physician's health appraisals, as considered in Chapter 4. Several of these measures will be described next.

Age-Height-Weight Tables

For many years, "standard" age-height-weight tables have been used in this country. As early as 1900, life insurance companies prepared such tables to determine the weights of men and women who were acceptable for life insurance. The schools used the tables as indices of nutritional status, and monthly weighing of children and the plotting of their individual weight curves became fairly common practice.[18] The best known tables of this type used for school children are the Wood-Baldwin Age-Height-Weight Tables. The usual policy has been to consider as undernourished all children who were 10 percent below the average for their sex, age, and height; as obese, those who were 15 to 20 percent above the average. The advantages of this practice are the universal appeal and understanding of weight, the simplicity and economy of the measurement, and the opportunity to center health lessons in the classroom around the numerous and varied reasons for losing and gaining weight. Excellent health programs have been developed in this way, the periodic weighing effectively motivating the child.

Recent research has cast considerable doubt on the reliance that can be placed upon age-height-weight tables as a measure of nutritional status. A number of conflicting statements have been made. Certain authorities on nutrition maintain that the use of these table results largely in omissions rather than commissions. Children who are from 7 to 10 percent below average weight are definitely malnourished and exhibit signs of lowered vitality and lowered physical efficiency, while to be more than 10 percent underweight usually means a dangerous reduction in fitness and stamina. Also, malnourished children are not necessarily underweight, since frequently individuals may be up to or may exceed the average weight for their type and yet have low vitality or be in poor health, with soft, flabby flesh, poor color, and often poor bones and teeth.

The most serious faults in applying age-height-weight tables to determine nutritional status are the complete neglect of body build, or skeletal dimensions, and of the gross proportion of bone, muscle, and fat in considering the standard weight that one should equal. For example, two individuals may be of the same age, height, and weight, and yet be totally different in their nutritional status. One may be of tall, slender build with good muscle development and adequate subcutaneous flesh; the other may be tall, big-boned, of stocky build, with poor muscle development and little subcutaneous flesh. Furthermore, two individuals may be of the same skeletal size, may weigh the same, and still be vastly different in the proportions of muscle and fat, as well as the size and

---

[18] The following reference contains several age-height-weight charts for both sexes at all ages: L. Jean Bogert, *Nutrition and Physical Fitness*, 9th ed. (Philadelphia: W. B. Saunders Company, 1973), pp. 578–79.

density of the internal organs. Yet, in both of these situations, the individuals are classified alike. Actually, one's weight cannot be completely understood unless differentiated according to body build and the components of the various tissue types.

Behnke and Wilmore[19] have discussed overweight when related primarily to well developed musculatures. They show that the average weight of a lean, muscular athlete may well exceed 30 percent of average weight for stature in standard tables. Excess muscle is primarily responsible for the greater lean bulk, but bone may also be ancillary, as revealed by the thickened cortex of long bones in radiography. Weight lifters show some remarkable examples of muscular hypertrophy. Wilhelm and Behnke[20] dramatized this situation during World War II when they showed that "according to height-weight tables, the majority of football players could be unclassified for military service and as not qualified for first class insurance by reason of overweight." Obviously, overweight in these men is due largely to non-fat components of the body.

Meredith Height-Weight Chart

A method of using age, height, and weight in the appraisal of pupil growth, which avoids some of the weaknesses of the age-height-weight tables, was developed by Meredith. Charts representing growth curves of height and weight for boys and girls four to eighteen years of age are available; each chart has five zones for height and five zones for weight, as seen in Figure 5.1 for boys and Figure 5.2 for

girls. The height and weight measurements for constructing the charts were collected on boys and girls attending public and private schools in Iowa City, Iowa. To obtain the channels, age distributions for height and weight were subdivided as follows: Upper 10 percent, tall-heavy; next 20 percent and middle 40 percent, average; lowest 30 percent, short-light. The original and revised forms were prepared for the Joint Committee on Health Problems of the NEA and the AMA by Howard V. Meredith and Virginia B. Knott.[21]

Before using the Meredith charts, of course, the height and weight of each child must be tested. These tests should be given as follows:

Height.   A height scale in inches may be fastened to an upright board or wall without wainscoting. After removing shoes, the child stands erect with his heels, buttocks, and upper back contacting the scale; the arms should hang naturally at the side; the chin should be lifted but not tilted. Height should be taken by placing some flat object, such as a chalk box, with one of the ends against the scale, and the long side resting on the highest point of the head. The height should be recorded to the nearest one-fourth inch.

Weight.   Weighing scales should be checked annually for dependability, and they should be adjusted for proper balance on each occasion of use. The pupils should be weighed wearing as little clothing as practicable, which will minimize the influence of seasonal and daily variation in the weight of school clothing; shoes, of course, should always be removed. Record the weight to the nearest one-half pound.

The height and weight scores are then plotted on the chart in accordance with the sex and age of the child. Normally, the

---

[19]Albert R. Behnke and Jack H. Wilmore, *Evaluation and Regulation of Body Build and Composition* (Englewood Cliffs, N.J.: Prentice-Hall, Inc., 1974), p. 130.

[20]W. C. Welhelm and A. R. Behnke, "The Specific Gravity of Healthy Men," *Journal of American Medical Association,* **118** (1942), 498.

[21]Copies may be secured through the American Medical Association, 535 N. Dearborn Street, Chicago, Illinois 60610.

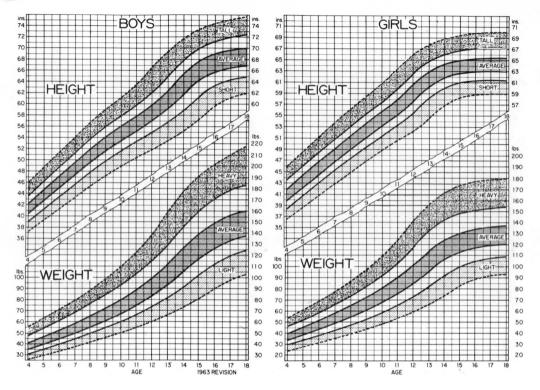

FIGURE 5.1 *Meredith Height-Weight Chart for Boys. Reproduced with permission of Joint Committee on Health Problems in Education of the National Education Association and the American Medical Association.*

FIGURE 5.2. *Meredith Height-Weight Chart for Girls, 1967 Revision. Reproduced with permission of Joint Committee on Health Problems in Education of the National Education Association and the American Medical Association.*

pupil's height and weight points fall in like zones, such as tall and heavy or average and average. When a boy's or girl's height and weight points do not lie in corresponding channels, the discrepancy may denote natural slenderness or stockiness of build, or it may reflect an undesirable state of health. For example, if a boy's scores fall in average height and moderately heavy weight zones, the dissimilarity may indicate stockiness of build or it may be related to obesity. Generally, the child's height and weight curves should follow the same zones as he is re-tested from time to time; this procedure gives some idea as to whether he is growing satisfactorily. If either of the child's curves moves into an-

other zone, the reason for such a change should be examined.

Wetzel Grid

The Wetzel Grid[22] was devised as a direct reading control chart on the quality of growth and development in individual boys and girls. It is divided into nine physique channels, designated as follows: A_4, obese; A_3 and A_2, stocky; A_1 M, and B_1 good; B_2, fair; B_3 borderline; and B_4 poor. The child's position on the grid is plotted

[22]Norman C. Wetzel, *The Treatment of Growth Failures in Children* (Cleveland: NEA Service, Inc., 1948). Grids may be obtained from the NEA Service.

from his age, height, and weight. From this plotting, his developmental level and his age schedule of development are determined; repeated plottings indicate the direction of his growth and development. If the child's growth is "normal," he will stay in the same channel as time goes on, moving progressively upward. But, if malnutrition, fatigue, or illness hampers growth, the child's growth changes channels.

A copy of the Wetzel Grid appears in Figure 5.3. Directions for its use follow with an illustration for a boy 10 years of age with a weight of 55¼ pounds and a height of 50 inches at the time of initial testing.

1. Plot the pupil's height and weight on the physique channels. For this boy, the plot fell in channel M; from the Clinical Ratings, lower left corner of the grid, he is classified as "good." The subject's developmental level is 66, as shown by the diagonal lines crossing the channels. At each subsequent testing, this plot is made again; this indicates his growth pattern.

2. The pupil's Age Schedule of Development (Auxodrome) is plotted next; the panel for this purpose is at the right side of the grid. Thus, for the developmental level of 66, the 10-year-old boy's age schedule falls between the 82 and 98 percent lines, about 90 percent. The auxodrome is a curve representing the age at which a child arrives at any developmental level in the channel. Five such time tables of development are included in the panel; these have been standardized to give the percentage of children on or ahead of these respective schedules. Thus, for the illustration, 90 percent of boys have reached the 66th level in the channel as early as 10 years. The 67 percent auxodrome is taken as the standard of reference for determining whether the child's growth is advanced, normal, or retarded.

3. Methods employed to determine a child's physical advancement from the auxodrome are as follows. (a) *Position of auxodrome relative to the standard.* This position was explained above with the subject falling on the 90 percent line. Thus, the boy's growth would be considered retarded, since he is below the 67 percent line. (b) *Developmental age.* This is determined by read-

ing the age at which the 67 percent line crosses a given developmental level. For the 10-year-old boy, his level of 66 crosses the 67 percent line at age 8⅓ years, which, thus, becomes his developmental age. (c) *Developmental ratio.* This ratio is as follows, illustrated for the boy in question:

$$\text{Developmental ratio} = \frac{\text{Developmental age}}{\text{actual age}}$$

$$= \frac{8.33}{10} = 0.833$$

In his original work, Wetzel compared Grid ratings of 2093 school children, kindergarten through the twelfth grade, with physicians' estimates. Agreement was reported for 94 percent, except for those children rated as fair, and upon whom physicians themselves had difficulty in agreeing. Moreover, the Grid caught 95 percent of those children classified as poor or borderline by the doctors. Kahn and associates[23] found growth failures by Wetzel Grid methods in 157 children with acute rheumatic fever; the followup position determination of 130 of the children revealed a shift toward marked improvement in growth and development. Bruch[24] confirmed the usefulness of the Grid technique in the early recognition of abnormal changes in the height-weight relationship. However, he obtained no agreement between developmental age, as assessed by the grid, and skeletal age, as appraised from hand and wrist x-rays.

In the Medford Boys' Growth Study, Weinberg[25] investigated the structural, strength, and maturity characteristics, as related to various aspects of the Wetzel

[23]Lawrence Kahn, George Brown, and David Goldring, "Wetzel Grid Analysis of Rheumatic Children," *Journal of Pediatrics,* **41,** No. 1 (July 1952), 47.

[24]Hilde Bruch, "The Grid for Evaluating Physical Fitness (Wetzel)," *Journal of American Medical Association,* **118,** No. 15 (April 11, 1942), 1289.

[25]Herbert A. Weinberg, "Structural, Strength and Maturity Characteristics as Related to Aspects of the Wetzel Grid for Boys Nine Through Fifteen Years of Age," Doctoral Dissertation, University of Oregon, December 1964.

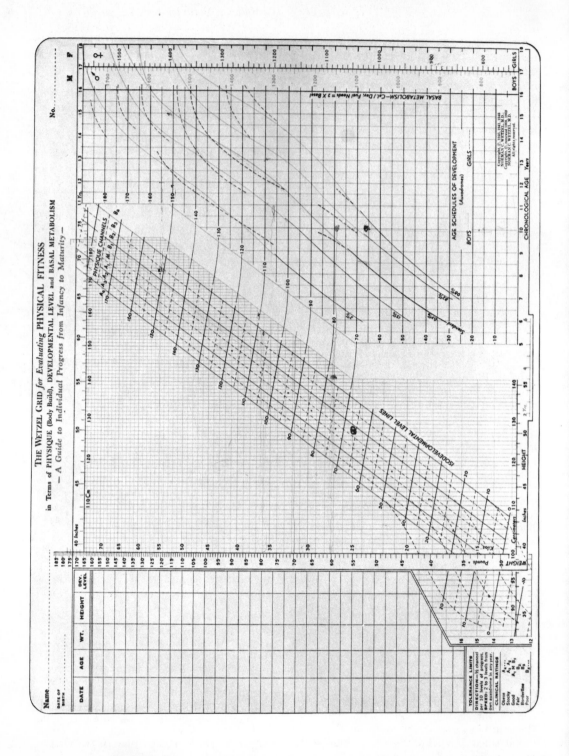

THE WETZEL GRID for Evaluating PHYSICAL FITNESS
in Terms of PHYSIQUE (Body Build), DEVELOPMENTAL LEVEL and BASAL METABOLISM
— A Guide to Individual Progress from Infancy to Maturity —

Grid, of boys 9 through 16 years of age. Among his findings were the following: (a) Low but significant correlations were obtained between the physique channels[26] and anthropometric and strength tests; the highest correlations were 0.519, 0.453, and 0.449 with upper arm, chest, and calf girths respectively. (b) A multiple correlation of 0.901 was found between the channels and upper arm girth, standing height, and body weight; this correlation was increased to 0.962 with the addition of sitting height and leg length. (c) The correlation between Wetzel's developmental level and body weight was 0.984. (d) The highest correlations with Wetzel's developmental ratios were 0.552 for calf girth, 0.506 for chest girth, 0.505 for weight, and 0.480 for upper arm girth. For 15-year-old boys, Jarman[27] reported the following relation with Wetzel physique channels: 0.88 for ectomorphy, 0.71 for endomorphy, 0.64 for arm girth, and 0.52 for body weight.

The Wetzel Grid has been studied by several investigators for application to performances in physical education activities. With 1977 elementary school boys, Bookwalter and associates[28] found that large boys, classified as thin to medium by grid channels, performed equally well on the Indiana Motor Fitness Test; for average size, thin boys performed better than medium physique boys; the very obese were the poorest physical performers. Wear and Miller[29] found that junior high school boys medium in physique and normal in development were superior in pull-ups, 50-yard dash, standing broad jump, and softball distance throw; boys with heavy physiques (many overweight) were the most inferior.

Rousey[30] obtained a critical ratio of 7.05 when the mean performance on the Indiana Motor Fitness Test of 429 secondary school boys classified on the Grid as growth successes was compared with 233 boys who were classified as growth failures. His correlations between fitness items and physique channels, however, were low (0.29 to 0.47). According to Rains,[31] outstanding secondary school athletes are classified in physique channels M through A5, with channel A2 as the most satisfactory; over 75 percent of the athletes had developmental levels over 150, while less than 50 percent of the non-athletes exceed this level. In contrasting the characteristics of boys 10 to 15 years of age in elementary and junior high schools, Clarke and Petersen[32] found no significant differences between the means of athletes and non-athletes for Wetzel's physique channel ratings.

It appears that the Wetzel Grid has

---

[26]In scoring the Wetzel physique channels for statistical purposes, numerical values were assigned the channels, starting with 1 for channel B4 and ending with 9 for channel A4.

[27]Boyd O. Jarman, "Interrelationships Between Academic Achievement and Selected Maturity, Physique, Strength, and Motor Measures of Fifteen Year Old Boys," Doctoral Dissertation, University of Oregon, 1965.

[28]Karl W. Bookwalter and others, "The Relationship of Body Size and Shape to Physical Performance," *Research Quarterly*, **33,** No. 3 (October 1952), 271.

[29]C. L. Wear and Kenneth Miller, "Relationship of Physique and Developmental Level to Physical Performance," *Research Quarterly*, **33,** No. 2 (December 1962), 616.

[30]Merle A. Rousey, "The Physical Performance of Secondary School Boys Classified by the Grid Technique," Doctoral Dissertation, Indiana University, 1949.

[31]David D. Rains, "Growth of Athletes and Non-Athletes in Selected Secondary Schools as Assessed by the Grid Technique," Doctoral Dissertation, Indiana University, 1951.

[32]H. Harrison Clarke and Kay H. Petersen, "Contrast of Maturational, Structural, and Strength Characteristics of Athletes and Nonathletes 10 to 15 Years of Age," *Research Quarterly*, **32,** No. 2 (May 1961), 163.

FIGURE 5.3. *Wetzel Grid for Evaluating Physical Fitness*

possibilities for use in detecting nutritional and growth disturbances in children. A weakness of the grid technique is in the degree of assurance that the child is actually placed in the appropriate channel at the time his initial measurements are made. If the child is wrongly placed at this time, the health or physical educator may help perpetuate an improper growth pattern. Solley[33] demonstrated, too, that many changes occur in the physiques of children, as plotted with the grid over a five-year period, and that physique has a definite tendency to be more variable as grade level increases. Of pupils classified as extreme physiques in his study, about half showed physique shifts from the preceding measurement; the shifts tended strongly toward increased obesity or thinness. Some doubt is expressed as to the effectiveness of any of the grid measures in classifying children for physical education activities.

Wellesley Weight Prediction Method

In studying methods of weight prediction for college women, Ludlum and Powell found that height, chest depth, and chest width were the most effective of the items studied. The following regression equation was between these tests and the weights of 1580 women from 19 colleges throughout the United States:

$$\text{weight} = 2.6(\text{sum of measurements}) - 154.3$$

The coefficient of correlation between actual and the predicted weights was 0.71, with a predictive index of 0.30. Height correlated with actual weights was 0.57, with a predictive index of 0.17. Thus, the new formula is approximately twice as effective in predicting weight as is height alone.

Measurements for the Wellesley weight prediction[34] method are taken in the following manner:

1. *Height:* standing; readings taken to the nearest ½ inch.
2. *Chest depth:* horizontal distance between the midsternal and midspinal lines at the level of the lower end of sternum; readings taken to the nearest ½ centimeter.
3. *Chest width:* horizontal midaxillary distance at the same level as for chest depth; readings taken to the nearest ½ centimeter.

In measuring chest depth and chest width, readings are taken at the end of a normal expiration. A straight arm sliding caliper, calibrated in centimeters, is used for measuring these chest diameters. Appendix Table B.1 is provided, from which weight in pounds may be read directly from the sum of the three measurements.

Other Evaluative Methods

ACH Index. In an analysis of various combinations of anthropometric measures made on over 10,000 children in 75 cities of the United States, Franzen and Palmer[35] proposed the ACH Index as a means of determining the nutritional status of children seven to 12 years of age. The index is based upon three measurements: arm girth (A), chest depth (C), and hip width (H). The selection of boys and girls may be done by using the scoring standards to select either a fourth or a tenth of the children measured. Children thus selected should then be given the full

---

[33]William H. Solley, "Status of Physique, Changes in Physique, and Speed in the Growth Patterns of School Children, Grades 1–8," *Research Quarterly,* **30,** No. 4 (December 1959), 465.

[34]F. E. Ludlum and Elizabeth Powell, "Chest-Height-Weight Tables for College Women," *Research Quarterly,* **11,** No. 3 (October 1940), 55.

[35]Raymond Franzen and George Palmer, *The ACH Index of Nutritional Status.* (New York: American Child Health Association, 1934).

test proposed by the authors, which consists of seven rather than three anthropometric measures, before being referred to a physician or nutrition specialist.

Sheldon's Age-Height-Weight Tables. Sheldon's *Atlas of Men*[36] contains an age-height-weight table for each of his 88 basic somatotypes; ages are from 18 to 63 years. When somatotyping is done, these tables may be used as the norms for weight.

Cureton's Tissue Symmetry Analysis. Cureton[37] has presented four indices for use in making a tissue symmetry analysis. The four indices are for skeletal growth, muscle girth, adipose tissue, and weight prediction. Weight prediction is based upon the other three indices. Complete directions for giving the tests involved, together with photographs of the testing techniques appear in the reference.

Nutrition Test Evaluation

The evaluation of nutritional status, which is usually related to the prediction of the individual's desirable weight, has taken many directions. The simplest forms utilize age and height only as the components. Thus, age-height-weight tables were used early and extensively. Their most serious faults are that they do not provide for individual differences in body build and in proportions of bone, muscle, and fat in establishing weight standards. The Meredith height-weight charts and the Wetzel Grid avoid some of these weaknesses, although they, too, are limited to age, height, and weight as measures.

In Pryor's width-weight tables (now out of print), and in Wellesley's weight prediction method, indices of body build have been utilized to predict weight. Both of these processes include height and chest width; also, the Pryor test includes hip width and the Wellesley method includes chest depth.

While indices of body build are superior to height alone as a basis for evaluating nutritional status, they still indicate only the percentage by which an individual is inadequate, as it does not show the direct body condition causing malnutrition. For example, it is quite possible for two individuals to weigh the same and have comparable skeletal proportions, but have greatly different proportions of fat and muscle: one individual may have a large amount of fat and poor musculature; the other may have little subcutaneous tissue but be well developed physically.

Both a normal amount of fat and good musculature are necessary. The amount of fat just under the skin, especially in certain select body areas, such as the upper arm, chest, abdomen, back, and side, bears a high relationship to the total amount of fat on the body, and the total amount of fat on the body is closely related to the general nutritive condition of the individual.[38] From measures of subcutaneous tissue, therefore, one may determine to what extent underweight may be due to undernutrition. Likewise, the development of the muscular system varies with different skeletal proportions, and should be considered if underweight or poor nutrition is due to poor muscular development. Nutritional tests utilizing this consideration are the ACH Index and the Cureton tissue symmetry analysis. These tests, although complicated and difficult to administer, are superior to other measures of this sort.

A number of studies have compared various tests for identifying the nutritional status of individuals. The results have shown that fairly extensive disagreements exist.

[36]William H. Sheldon, C. W. Dupertuis, and Eugene McDermott, *Atlas of Men* (New York: Harper & Row, 1954).

[37]Thomas K. Cureton, *Physical Fitness Appraisal and Guidance* (St. Louis: C. V. Mosby, 1947), Ch. 5.

[38]C. H. McCloy, "Anthropometry in the Service of the Individual," *Journal of Health and Physical Education,* **5,** No. 7 (September 1934), 7.

Marshall,[39] using a group of 77 boys aged 7 to 12 years, compared four methods of appraising physical status: the Baldwin-Wood age-height-weight tables, the Pryor-Stolz age-height-hip-weight standards, the Franzen-Palmer ACH Index, and the McCloy age-height-weight-chest-knee-weight tables. The frequencies of underweight for the four methods presented marked disagreement, varying from 72 percent by Pryor-Stolz, through 23 percent by Baldwin-Wood and McCloy, to 5 percent by Franzen-Palmer. A study by Allman[40] in which the Baldwin-Wood age-height-weight tables, the Pelidisi Formula and the ACH Index were related to an experienced physician's estimates of nutritional status, resulted in similar disagreement among the tests. In the case of girls, the Baldwin-Wood Tables agreed very closely with the physician's ratings; in the case of boys, the Pelidisi more nearly approximated the doctor's ratings.

Craig[41] determined the expected weight of 101 Wellesley College women between the ages of 17 and 22 by the Medico-Actuarial Mortality Investigation age-height-weight tables, the revised Pryor width-weight tables, the Boillin weight expectancy regression equation, the McCloy method for appraising physical status, and the Ludlum (Wellesley) method of weight prediction for college women. The five methods were found to disagree on the classification of college women as underweight, normal weight, or overweight to such an extent that the methods should not be used interchangeably. The Ludlum method was recommended for use with college women.

SKINFOLD

The direct measurement of fat deposits on various parts of the body by use of skinfold calipers has not been a common practice in physical education, but could well be useful in determining the effectiveness of weight reduction programs. A number of skinfold calipers are available commercially, although the better ones are expensive. The recommended amount of pressure to be applied to the skinfold is 10 grams per square millimeter; the size of the contact surface of the caliper may vary from 20 to 40 square millimeters, depending in part on the shape of the contact surface.[42] Three calipers that meet these specifications are the Vernier, the Harpenden, and the Lange.

Skinfold measures are considered to be a superior indicator of obesity than is overweight as determined from weight tables. Skinfold thickness gives an estimation of total body fat, inasmuch as 50 percent of total fat lies immediately under the skin.[43] The skinfold sites generally accepted for determination of body fat are at the back of the arm and at the subscapular position on the back; a third site is suggested on the mid-axillary line at the level of the umbilicus.

Directions for testing skinfolds are as follows: grasp the skinfold between the thumb and index finger about one centimeter from the site at which the calipers are to be applied. The amount of the skinfold should be great enough to include two thicknesses of skin with intervening fat, but not enough to involve muscle or fascia. To insure against including these latter structures, when in doubt, the tester should instruct the subject to tense the underlying muscles. The caliper is applied above the fingers holding the skinfold; all

[39]Everett L. Marshall, "Comparison of Four Current Methods of Estimating Physical Status," *Child Development,* **8** (1937), 89.

[40]Delmar I. Allman, "A Comparison of Nutritional Indices," *Research Quarterly,* **8,** No. 2 (May 1937), 79.

[41]Margaret B. Craig, "A Comparison of Five Methods Designed to Predict the 'Normal' Weight of College Women," *Research Quarterly,* **15,** No. 1 (March 1944), 64.

[42]Josef Brozek, ed., *Body Measurements and Human Nutrition* (Detroit: Wayne State University Press, 1956), p. 10.

[43]Jean Mayer, *Overweight: Causes, Cost, and Control* (Englewood Cliffs, N.J.: Prentice-Hall, 1968), p. 31.

measurements are made to the nearest millimeter. Instructions for giving the three recommended skinfold tests follow and are illustrated in Figure 5.4.[44]

Back of Arm. The skinfold is taken over the triceps muscle at a point halfway between the tip of the shoulder (acromial process) and the tip of the elbow (alecranon process). The point is located with forearm flexed to 90 degrees; in making the measurement, however, the arm should hang free. The fold is lifted parallel to the long axis of the arm.

Subscapular. The skinfold is taken at the tip of the scapula (inferior angle) with the subject in a relaxed standing position. The fold is lifted in the diagonal plane at about 45 degrees from the vertical and horizontal planes.

Lateral Abdomen. The skinfold is taken on the side of the abdomen at the mid-axillary line at the level of the umbilicus. The fold is lifted parallel to the long axis of the body.

The three skinfold measures described were included in the Medford Boys' Growth Study,[45] with all the skinfold tests made on the left side. In this project, Geser[46] found that the intercorrelations among these measures for 12-year-old boys clustered between 0.797 and 0.810.

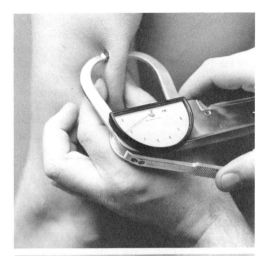

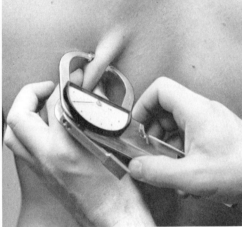

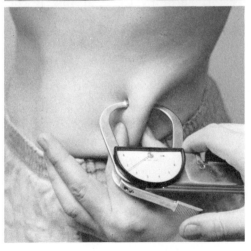

[44]The instrument used in the illustrations is the Lange Skinfold Calipers; it may be obtained from J. A. Preston Corporation, 71 Fifth Avenue, New York, N.Y. 10003.

[45]Clarke, *Medford Boys' Growth Study,* pp. 142–47.

[46]L. Richard Geser, "Skinfold Measures of Twelve-year-old Boys as Related to Various Maturity, Physique, Strength, and Motor Measures," Doctoral Dissertation, University of Oregon, 1965.

FIGURE 5.4. *Skinfold Tests.* Top: *Back of arm.* Middle: *Subscapular.* Bottom: *Lateral abdomen.*

The correlations between each of the skin-fold measures and the composite of all three tests were 0.908 for subscapular, 0.912 for arm, and 0.963 for lateral abdomen. Clarke, Geser and Hunsdon[47] obtained a correlation of 0.79 between caliper and x-ray measures of adipose tissue over the biceps muscle. Garn and Gorman[48] obtained a higher correlation (0.88) between these measures at the same site.

Through his research and that of others, Mayer[49] indicated that triceps (back of arm) skinfold is most representative of the total body fat of obese individuals. Based on this belief, he and Selzer[50] developed minimum triceps skinfold thicknesses indicating obesity for males and females of different ages. These thicknesses appear in Appendix Table B.2. Minimum thickness was placed at one standard deviation above the mean; thus 16 percent of the population would be designated as obese. The standard for obesity over age 30 was taken at 30 years on the assumption that weight gain after adult size has been reached is excess fat.

BODY DIMENSIONS

The type of an individual's physical structure is an essential factor in his motor performance. Evidence of this is commonplace: observe the well-proportioned physiques of boxers and gymnasts, the superstructure of great basketball competitors, the solidarity of top-flight football players, the wiriness of champion distance runners, and the massive builds of great shot putters and discus throwers.

Anthropometry is the oldest type of body measurement used, dating back to the beginning of recorded history. The concepts of the ideal proportion varied over periods of time. For example, Polycletus fashioned Doryphorus, the Spear Thrower, as a fighter and an athlete, broad shouldered, thick set, and square chested—the perfect man. As the arts of civilization became more gentle, however, grace rather than ruggedness appealed to the Athenians; the ideal man then became slender, graceful, and skillful, albeit also well proportioned.

In the United States, anthropometric measurement was the first type of measurement to be used generally in physical education. On the theory that exercise should be prescribed to affect muscle size, emphasis was placed upon body symmetry and proportion. In 1861, Hitchcock, and later Sargent, produced profile charts to reveal how individuals compared with their standards. Sargent's chart required 44 anthropometric measurements, as well as a number of strength tests. Fifty measurements of this sort were recommended by the American Association for the Advancement of Physical Education.

As seen earlier in this chapter, anthropometric tests have been utilized as a basis for evaluating nutritional status. They have also been used extensively in determining growth changes of children. Many studies have related measures of body dimensions to physical and motor performances. In this section, four anthropometric measures found to be significantly related to various physical education activities will be presented.

The materials utilized below for these tests were obtained from the Medford boys' growth study; the reference contains much more detail related to these and other anthropometric measures and indices of body proportion obtained from

[47]H. Harrison Clarke, L. Richard Geser, and Stanley B. Hunsdon, "Comparison of Upper Arm Measurements by Use of Roentgenogram and Anthropometric Techniques," *Research Quarterly,* **27,** No. 4 (December 1956), 379.

[48]Stanley M. Garn and E. L. Gorman, "Comparison of Pinch Caliper and Teleroentgenogrammetric Measurements of Subcutaneous Fat," *Human Biology,* **28,** No. 4 (December 1956), 407.

[49]Mayer, *Overweight,* p. 32.

[50]C. C. Selzer, and J. Mayer, "A Simplified Criterion of Obesity," *Postgraduate Medicine,* **38,** 2 (1965), A–101. Also Mayer, *Overweight,* p. 34.

them.[51] It should be observed that the Medford study correlations are generally lower than for studies by others, due to the fact that, when testing was done, age was limited to a single age and to within two months of each boy's birthday. For the measures considered here, scores increase with age, which permit higher correlations when age is not controlled.

Body Weight

Without doubt, body weight has been utilized more extensively than any other anthropometric test in physical education. It has formed the basis for arm strength formulae; it has been a basic factor in constructing strength norms. With age and height, it has been used in classification indices and athletic exponent plans. It has frequently been the criterion measure in nutrition-type tests. Directions for obtaining body weight were given earlier in this chapter.

The individual differences for body weight are great for boys of the same chronological age; these tested boys were within two months of their birthdays, which makes these differences more significant than the usual span of one year. For boys tested at each age, seven through 18 years, the standard deviations increased steadily from 6.3 pounds at age seven to 21.3 pounds at age 14. Thereafter, the deviations were fairly consistent, ranging between 19.2 and 22.6 pounds. The ranges varied with the presence of extreme scores at some of the ages; the lowest range was 33 pounds at seven years, and the highest was 141 pounds at 17 years. At all but one age, the heaviest boy was at least twice as heavy as the lightest; at some ages, this differential was nearly three times as great.

Generally, in regard to the significance of these individual differences, weight was positively related to gross strength and negatively related to relative strength and muscular endurance (in tests where body weight was lifted or its effects eliminated in scoring). Weight, within limits, was an advantage in making and being successful on interscholastic athletic teams at all school levels. Heavier boys generally, except for the obese, enjoyed greater peer status and had higher levels of aspiration.

Chest Girth

For this test, the subject was in a normal standing position; a tape was brought around his chest at the level of the nipples, as shown in Figure 5.5. The score recorded was the average of the girth measurements taken on full inhalation and full exhalation.

In the Medford analyses, chest girth was found to correlate between 0.92 and 0.93 with body weight for upper ele-

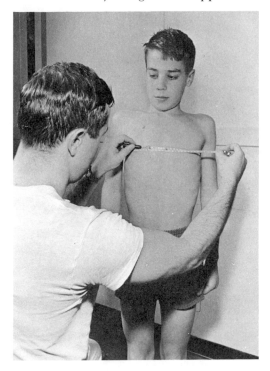

FIGURE 5.5. *Chest Girth Measurement*

---

[51]Clarke, *Medford Boys' Growth Study*, Ch. 4.

mentary, junior high, and senior high school boys. As would be expected, therefore, the correlations of these two variables followed a comparable pattern.

Arm Girth

For this test, the girth of the left flexed-tensed upper arm was taken. The subject sat in a chair, feet flat on the floor. The arm was flexed at the shoulder to about 90 degrees and the forearm in supine position was flexed at the elbow; the muscles of the upper arm were contracted to form as "large a muscle" as possible. The girth was measured around the most prominent part of the upper arm, as shown in Figure 5.6. A Gulick tape was used for this test, as well as the one for chest girth. This tape has a spring encased in a handle which facilitates the application of a consistent

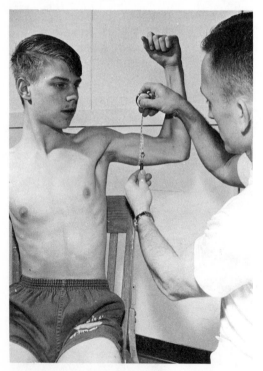

FIGURE 5.6. *Arm Girth Measurement*

pressure in making girth measures over soft tissue.[52]

In the Medford boys' growth study, the correlations of arm girth with weight and other girth measures were mostly in the 0.80's for each age 7 through 18 years. For these same ages, the correlations of this measure with gross strength batteries, such as the Strength Index and the average of 11 cable-tension strength tests, varied between 0.35 and 0.65. Further, boys with the highest arm girths were 50 to 100 percent greater than for boys with the smallest girths at the different ages.

Lung Capacity ~~strength~~

Lung capacity has been a controversial item in physical education testing, especially since Rogers included it in his Strength Index battery. In the Medford series, the test was administered with a wet spirometer, as described in Chapter 7.

In an early study, Cureton[53] concluded that lung capacity was largely a measure of body size. In the Medford study, lung capacity correlated higher with various anthropometric tests at the junior high school ages, 13 through 15 years. For these ages, the correlations with arm, chest, and buttocks girths ranged between 0.39 and 0.55. Higher correlations were obtained with the linear tests of standing height, sitting height, and leg length; over half of the correlations for these ages were in the 0.70's. For gross strength measures, the correlational ranges for boys from 7 through 18 years were 0.42 to 0.67 for Strength Index and 0.32 to 0.60 for the average of 11 cable-tension strength tests; again, the highest correlations were at the ages 13, 14, and 15 years. Boys with highest lung capacities were two to three times

[52]Gulick tapes may be obtained from J. A. Preston Corporation, 71 Fifth Ave., New York, N.Y. 10003.

[53]Thomas K. Cureton, "Vital Capacity as a Test of Condition for High School Boys," *Research Quarterly,* **7,** No. 4 (December 1936), 80.

greater than for boys with the smallest capacities at all ages 7 through 18 years. For college men, Davis[54] obtained a correlation of −0.59 between lung capacity and time in the 200-yard freestyle swim. Only one other test in Davis' study (−0.61 for shoulder flexion strength) exceeded the lung capacity-swimming time correlation; tests with lower correlations included the Rogers' Strength and Physical Fitness Indices and the Navy Physical Fitness Test, and the test items composing these batteries.

BODY COMPOSITION

In evaluating the body in relation to its structure and nutritional status, health and physical educators are generally limited to external measures of body bulk, linearity, and skinfold thickness. These measures do not permit an adequate differentiation between lean and fat body tissues. A number of sophisticated laboratory methods have been developed for making this as well as other differentiations. Behnke and Wilmore[55] have discussed such methods, including hydrostatic weighing, radiographic analysis, and biochemical approaches.

While still largely a laboratory method, the simplest approach to the determination of lean body weight by employing the Archimedian principle that a body immersed in fluid is acted upon by a buoyancy force, which is evidenced by a loss of weight equal to the weight of the displaced fluid. Thus, when as individual is weighed underwater, while totally submerged, his total body volume is equal to his loss of weight in water. Specific gravity, which reflects body density, may be obtained by dividing the body weight in air by the body weight displaced in water. Behnke and Wilmore[56] have proposed several regression equations based upon anthropometric measures for predicting lean body weight (*LBW*). Two of these equations with the multiple correlations upon which they are based follow.

$$R = 0.931 \ LBW = 10.260 + 0.793 \text{ (weight)} - 0.367 \text{(abdominal skinfold)}$$
$$R = 0.938 \ LBW = 44.636 + 1.082 \text{ (weight)} - 0.740 \text{(abdomen circumference)}$$

The anthropometric tests required for these equations are given as follows:

Abdominal skinfold: horizontal fold adjacent to umbilicus.
Abdominal girth: laterally at level of iliac crests and anteriorly at umbilicus.

SOMATOTYPES

The concept that an individual's body type is related to his health, immunity from disease, physical performance, and personality characteristics has developed from ancient times.[57] Hippocrates designated two fundamental physical types, the *phthisic habitus* and the *apopletic habitus*. The *phthisic* had a long, thin body, which was considered particularly subject to tuberculosis. The *apoplectic* was a short, thick individual with a predisposition toward diseases of the vascular system leading to apoplexy. Rostan defined three essentially different types: the *type digestif, type mus-*

---

[54]Jack F. Davis, "Effects of Training and Conditioning for Middle Distance Swimming upon Measures of Cardiovascular Condition, General Physical Fitness, Gross Strength, Motor Fitness, and Strength of Involved Muscles," Doctoral Dissertation, University of Oregon, 1955.

[55]Behnke and Wilmore, *Body Build and Composition*, p. 130.

[56]Behnke and Wilmore, *Body Build and Composition*, p. 99.

[57]W. B. Tucker and W. A. Lessa, "Man: A Constitutional Investigation," *Quarterly Review of Biology*, **15**, (September 1940), 265, 411.

culaire, and *type cérébral.* Kretschmer's three types, *pyknic, athletic,* and *asthenic,* received considerable attention. The concept of body types, as shown in numerous studies, proved inadequate, in many respects. However, there remained considerable evidence that the physique pattern is significant and is related to an understanding of the individual, physically, mentally, emotionally, and socially.

Primary Components

Sheldon, assisted by Stevens and Tucker,[58] after extensive research came to the belief that human beings could not be classified into just three physique types, but that nearly all individuals were mixtures. However, they did designate three primary components of body build that provide first-order criteria for differentiating among individuals. The names of the three components were derived from the three layers of the embryo, as follows: (a) First component, *endomorph,* named after the endoderm from which the functional elements of the digestive system emanate; (b) second component, *mesomorph,* named after the mesoderm from which come the muscles and bones; (c) third component, *ectomorph,* named after the ectoderm from which develops the sensory organs. Brief descriptions of these components follow.

In *endomorphy,* the digestive viscera dominate the body economy. A predominance of soft roundness throughout the various regions of the body is evident, with mass concentration in the center. Other characteristics are: large, round head; short, thick neck; broad, thick chest, with fatty breasts; short arms, with "hammy" appearance, large abdomen, full above the navel and pendulous; heavy buttocks; and short, heavy legs.

In *mesomorphy,* muscle, bone, and connective tissue are dominant. The mesomorphic physique is heavy, hard, and rectangular in outline, with rugged, massive muscles and large, prominent bones. Other characteristics are: prominent facial bones; fairly long, strong neck; thoracic trunk dominant over abdominal volume; broad shoulders, with heavy, prominent clavicles; muscular upperarm and massive forearms, wrists, hands, and fingers; large, heavily muscled abdomen; slender, low waist; heavy buttocks; and massive forelegs.

Linearity and fragility predominate in the *ectomorph.* The dominant ectomorph has a frail, delicate body structure, with thin segments, anteroposteriorly. Other characteristics are: relatively large cranium, with bulbous forehead; small face, pointed chin, and sharp nose; long slender neck; long narrow thorax; winged scapula and forward shoulders; long arms, muscles not marked; flat abdomen, with hollow above navel; inconspicuous buttocks; and long, thin legs.

Determination of Somatotypes

Each of the three components is rated on a 7-point scale to indicate its relative contribution to the total physique; the scale may be recorded in half units for finer differentiation. In each instance, the first numeral in the sequence refers to endomorphy; the second, to mesomorphy; the third, to ectomorphy. The entire somatotype process is described in Sheldon's *Atlas of Men.*[59] These materials include specifications of the camera needed in photographing the subjects, the type of film and its developing and printing, posing of the subject in three planes (front, side, and rear), and various aids in making assessments.

While Sheldon's *Atlas* is restricted to

[58]W. H. Sheldon, S. S. Stevens, and W. B. Tucker, *The Varieties of Human Physique* (New York: Harper & Row, 1940).

[59]Sheldon, Dupertuis, and McDermott, *Atlas of Men.*

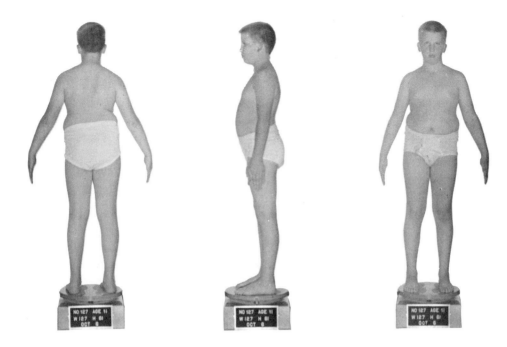

FIGURE 5.7. *Dominant Endomorph Somatotype*

somatotyping of men, 18 to 65 years of age, it has been utilized by Sheldon and others at younger ages. The somatotype was included as a basic measure of physique type in the Medford Boys' Growth Study.[60] Description of the many somatotypes found among human beings goes beyond the scope of this text. However, the following four examples may aid the physical educator in forming a concept of this form of body assessment.

Dominant Endomorph (Figure 5.7). This boy is 11 years of age; his somatotype designation is 6–3–2. Note the overall endomorphic characteristics, especially the high waist and the double chin.

[60]Clarke, *Medford Boys' Growth Study*, Ch. 3.

Dominant Mesomorph (Figure 5.8). This boy is 14 years of age and is an outstanding junior high school athlete. His somatotype is 2–6–3. He has an excellent muscular physique.

Dominent Ectomorph (Figure 5.9). This boy's somatotype designation is 2–2–7. He is 15 years of age. The linearity of this physique type is obvious.

Mid-Type. (Figure 5.10). The somatotype of this boy is quite evenly divided among the three components; the designation is 4–4–4. He is 14 years of age.

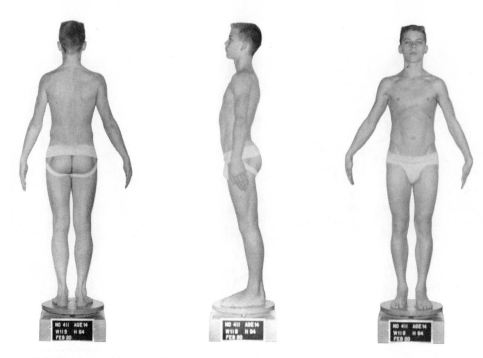

FigURE 5.8. *Dominant Mesomorph Somatotype*

In studying the consistency of the somatotype process, Tanner[61] reported objectivity coefficients among three well-trained somatotype evaluators from 0.82 to 0.93 for the three components. He indicated further that trained observers agree to within half a rating on a 7-point scale in 90 percent of the instances. Hawthorne reported similar objectivity coefficients; his coefficients ranged from 0.87 to 0.91.

Female Somatotypes

Although Sheldon's *Atlas of Men* describes the male somatotype only, he has also studied the female somatotype, although a published atlas has not appeared. Instead of developing distinctive physique criteria for women, Sheldon decided to use his original somatotype system for both sexes. However, he recognized that the distribution of female physique types differs from the men's distribution. For example, women at all ages are much more endomorphic than men and are heavier in proportion to stature. Further, women do not possess the same degree of mesomorphy as do the men; Sheldon has rarely found a woman with a rating as high as 6 in this component. The commonest male somatotypes are found in the area between the 3–4–4 and 3–4–3; the commonest female somatotypes are around 5–3–3.[62] Thus, the somatotyping process for women parallels the process described above for men.

[61]J. M. Tanner, "Reliability of Anthroposcopic Somatotyping," *American Journal of Physical Anthropology,* **12** n.s., No. 2 (June 1954), 257.

[62]Sheldon, *Atlas of Men,* p. 14.

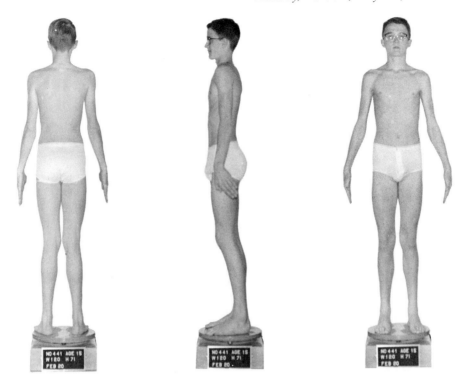

FIGURE 5.9. *Dominant Ectomorph Somatotype*

Children's Somatotypes

Although Sheldon has studied children, he has not yet provided an atlas of their somatotypes, so his somatotype descriptions of 18-year-old men must be adapted to younger boys and girls. Clarke, Heath, and Irving[63] found that a distribution of the somatotypes of 259 boys, ages 9 to 15 years, did not vary significantly from Sheldon's distribution based on 46,000 adult American males; many of the adult somatotypes were not encountered, naturally, in the much smaller boys' sample. In this study, too, the differences between ponderal indices were small for the

seven ages; they ranged from 12.99 at 9 years of age to 13.38 at 15 years of age; the median ponderal index reported by Sheldon for 18-year-old males is 13.20. For the younger boys, the progression in ponderal index continued steadily downward from those established by Sheldon for men.

In the Medford series, Sinclair longitudinally studied the somatotype consistency of boys 9 to 12[64] and 12 to 17 years of age.[65] The highest inter-age correlations of somatotype components were obtained for adjacent years; the ranges of these

[63]H. Harrison Clarke, Robert N. Irving, and Barbara H. Heath, "Relation of Maturity, Structural, and Strength Measures to the Somatotypes of Boys 9 Through 15 Years of Age," *Research Quarterly,* **32,** No. 4 (December 1961), 449.

[64]Gary D. Sinclair, "Stability of Physique Types of Boys Nine Through Twelve Years of Age," Master's Thesis, University of Oregon, 1966.

[65]Gary D. Sinclair, "Stability of Somatotype Components of Boys Twelve Through Seventeen Years of Age and Their Relationships to Selected Physical and Motor Factors," Doctoral Dissertation, University of Oregon, 1969.

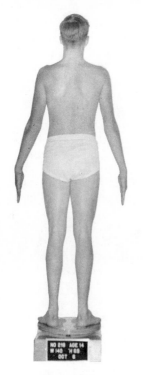 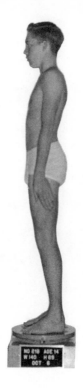 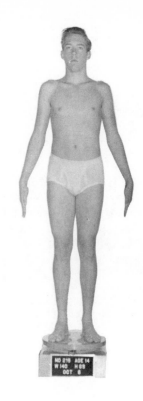

FIGURE 5.10. *Mid-Type Somatotype*

correlations were 0.75 to 0.85 for endo-morphy, 0.83 to 0.93 for mesomorphy, and 0.85 to 0.90 for ectomorphy. The lowest such correlations were for the five-year gap, 12 to 17; these were 0.50, 0.60, and 0.67 respectively. Inspection of somatotype assessments also revealed considerable instability of somatotype components. The numbers of changes for 100 boys ages 9 through 12 and 106 boys ages 12 through 15 were 94 for endomorphy, 42 for mesomorphy, and 91 for ectomorphy. Kurimoto[66] found that mean meso-morphy rose from 4.12 to 4.65 and mean ectomorphy decreased from 3.71 to 3.18 during the age span 15 through 18 years.

Modifications

Various modifications of Sheldon's somatotyping process have been proposed, some to simplify for practical use by physical educators and reduce the cost by avoidance of photography. Certain of these modifications will be presented here.

Heath Modification.[67] Heath proposed some slight modifications for Sheldon's somatotype procedures, as follows: (a) the rating scale was opened at both ends; thus, component values less than 1 and more than 7 were possible; and (b) the tables of possible somatotypes for various intervals of height divided by cube root of weight

[66]Etsuo Kurimoto, "Longitudinal Analysis of Maturity, Structural, Strength, and Motor Development of Boys Fifteen Through Eighteen Years of Age," Doctoral Dissertation, University of Oregon, 1963.

[67]Barbara Honeyman Heath, "Need for Modification of Somatotype Methodology," *American Journal of Physical Anthropology,* **21** n.s. (June 1963), 227.

were revised to provide a more linear relationship between changes in component ratings and this ratio. These modifications were employed by Heath in the somatotype assessments in the Medford Boys' Growth Study.

Sheldon's Trunk Index.[68] Sheldon's investigations led to an objective differentiation between *phenotype* and *genotype*. The phenotype refers to the individual's physique type at the time his somatotype picture is taken—the phenotype may change during growth and thereafter. The genotype refers to the individual's hereditary physique, and is not affected by nutritional conditions, developmental activities, the ravages of disease, and the like. Unfortunately, the determination of the genotype is impossible for school use, as its assessment requires semi-annual tests throughout the growth period. These tests are the trunk index, minimum ponderal index (height divided by cube root of weight) during growth, and adult height. However, in the Medford series, Morton[69] found that the phenotype had greater significance in physical and motor performances than does the genotype for boys at each age from 9 through 16 years.

Parnell's M.4 Deviation Chart.[70] Parnell proposed the use of anthropometric measures and somatotype photography to assess Sheldon's physique components. The anthropometric measures are: height and weight; skinfold measures over triceps,

subscapular, and suprailiac; diameters of humerus and femur; girths of biceps and calf. An M.4 standard deviation chart is provided for component determinations, so called because it is based on the assumption that a rating of 4 in "Muscularity" (mesomorphy) bears a constant proportional relationship to stature. When applied to the chart, the skinfold measures determine endomorphy; the bone and girth measures determine mesomorphy; and height divided by cube root of weight determine ectomorphy. The method can be applied without photography, although Parnell recommends its use to permit a preliminary estimate of somatotype components, to provide a permanent portrayal of physique type, and to disclose indications of displasia (Sheldon's concept of possible different somatotype designations for five body regions).

Heath-Carter Somatotype Rating Method.[71] Heath and Carter proposed a modification of the Parnell method of rating somatotype components by anthropometric tests. The anthropometric tests were the same in both rating methods, except Heath and Carter included calf skinfold in the assessment of mesomorphy. Further, the scoring methods were changed for the determination of mesomorphy, and the scales were revised. The Heath modification mentioned above was also employed.

Cureton's Simplified Physique Rating.[72] Subjective criteria for rating physique types were proposed by Cureton based upon three gross aspects: external fat, muscular development and condition, and skeletal development. His descriptive scales follow.

[68]William H. Sheldon, "Brief Communication on Somatotyping and Psychiatyping and Other Sheldonian Delinquencies," Maudsley Bequest Lecture, Royal Society of Medicine, London, England, May 13, 1965.

[69]Alan R. Morton, "Comparison of Sheldon's Trunk Index and Anthroposcopic Method of Somatotyping and Their Relationships to the Maturity, Structure, and Motor Ability of the Same Boys Nine Through Sixteen Years of Age," Doctoral Dissertation, University of Oregon, 1967.

[70]R. W. Parnell, *Behavior and Physique* (London: Edward Arnold, Ltd., 1958).

[71]Barbara Honeyman Heath and J. E. Lindsay Carter, "A Modified Somatotype Method," *American Journal of Physical Anthropology,* **27** m.s. (July 1967), 57.

[72]From Cureton, *Physical Fitness Appraisal and Guidance* (St. Louis: The C. V. Mosby Company, 1947) p. 120.

A. Scale for Rating Endomorphic Characteristics

1   2

Extremely low in adipose tissue and relatively small anterior-posterior dimensions of lower trunk

3   4   5

Average tissue, and physical build of lower trunk

6   7

Extremely obese with large quantities of adipose tissue and an unproportionately thick abdominal region

B. Scale for Rating Muscular Development and Condition

1   2

Extremely underdeveloped and poorly conditioned muscles squeezed or pushed in contracted state (biceps, abdominals, thighs, calves)

3   4   5

Average in skeletal muscular development and condition

6   7

Extremely developed with large and hard muscles in the contracted state, firm under forceful squeezing

C. Scale for Rating Skeletal Development

1   2

Extremely thick and heavy bones, short and ponderous skeleton with relatively great cross-section of ankle, knee, and elbow joints

3   4   5

Average size bones and joints in cross-section and length

6   7

Extremely thin, frail bones, tall, linear skeleton with relatively small cross-section of ankle, knee, and elbow joints

Willgoose's Rating.[73]   Willgoose suggested a subjective rating procedure, which he has used successfully in instructing some 1200 elementary school teachers-in-training in estimating somatotype designations. This process consists of the following steps:

1. Study the physical characteristics of the three somatotype components.

2. Inspect subjects in gymnasium or swim suits.

3. For each subject, decide on the primary component present, unless the subject is a mid-type.

4. Rate the primary component on the 1-to-7 scale; then, rate the other two components in turn.

5. Compute the ponderal index (height divided by cube root of weight) and relate it to possible somatotypes, as shown in Figure 5.11. Make rating adjustments considered appropriate.

6. Consult the *Atlas of Men* before deciding on the final somatotype assessment.

Willgoose has indicated that somatotype estimates can be made close enough for teacher use with school children and college students without the ponderal index or the *Atlas of Men*. However, if the height and weight of the subjects are available, the ponderal index can easily be obtained by use of the nomograph in the *Atlas*.

Medford Somatotype Prediction Formulae.[74] With 207 12-year-old boys in the Medford Boys' Growth Study, Monroe obtained the following multiple correlations and prediction equations with the somatotype components:

[73]Carl E. Willgoose, *Evaluation in Health Education and Physical Education* (New York: McGraw-Hill Book Company, 1961), p. 303.

[74]Richard A. Munroe, "Relationships Between Somatotype Components and Maturity, Structural, Strength, Muscular Endurance, and Motor Ability Measures of Twelve Year Old Boys," Doctoral Dissertation, University of Oregon, December 1964.

Component	R		Prediction Formulae	Standard Error Estimate
Endomorphy	0.887		− 1.85 (Ponderal Index) + 0.17 (Leg Length) + 23.08	0.48
Mesomorphy	0.900		− 2.15 (Ponderal Index) − 0.68 (Endomorphy) + 34.66	0.28
Ectomorphy	0.964		2.30 (Ponderal Index) − 27.02	0.31

[handwritten: correlation]

[handwritten: known]

The somatotypes of 40 subjects were predicted by the formulae; those predicted ratings were then correlated with the actual ratings assessed by the Sheldon method. The resultant correlations were 0.944 for endomorphy, 0.789 for mesomorphy, and 0.981 for ectomorphy. When rated endomorphy, rather than predicted endomorphy, was placed in the formula for mesomorphy, the correlation between the predicted and actual mesomorphic scores was 0.967. As can be seen, the only measures required for use with the prediction formulae are standing height, weight, and leg length. In this study, leg length was determined as the difference between standing and sitting heights.

The equations given above were for 12-year-old boys. Differences in the equations occur with age, as revealed in the Sinclair studies of boys at each age from 9 through 17 years. All of the latter equations appear in his theses and in the Medford monograph by the writer.[75]

Inasmuch as the ponderal index has been mentioned several times in connection with the assessment of somatotype components, a nomograph for its computation appears in Figure 5.11. The formula for ponderal index is:

[handwritten: know]

$$\frac{\text{height}}{\sqrt[3]{\text{weight}}}$$

To use the nomograph, place a ruler between the individual's height in inches in the left column and his weight in pounds in the right column; read his ponderal index at the point where the ruler crosses the center column.

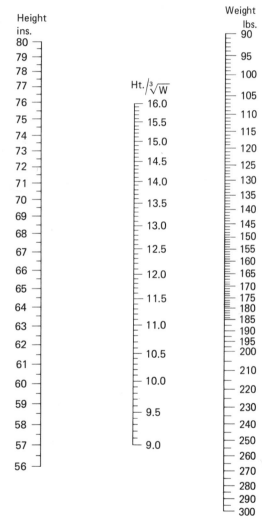

[75]See footnotes 65 and 66 this chapter; see also Clarke, *Medford Boys' Growth Study*, pp. 91–93.

FIGURE 5.11. *Ponderal Index:* $\dfrac{\text{Ht}}{\sqrt[3]{\text{W}}}$

Implications

The individual's physique type has considerable importance for health and physical education. In the realm of measurement, it should be considered in the establishment of norms for many types of physical education tests, if the results of tests are to be properly interpreted. This is true, for example, with the determination of nutritional status previously discussed in this chapter, a problem that has already become an area of study for recent experimenters in this field. In considering somatotypes as related to age-height-weight tables, the endomorph is normally overweight, the mesomorph is nearer average, and the ectomorph is well below these standards. Yet, if based upon weight tables alone, they are all judged alike. In Sheldon's *Atlas,* however, as previously mentioned an age-height-weight table for adult males is presented for each of his 88 somatotype designations. Likewise, tests of posture, strength, flexibility, endurance, or circulatory-respiratory functions may be understood more clearly in terms of their biological and social significance when reviewed against the general background of constitutional potentialities and limitations.

The somatotype is not subject to the size of the individual; thus small and large boys may have the same somatotype designation. To study component relationships when the effects of body size were eliminated, Munroe[76] found that the correlations between somatotype components and measures of body structure were markedly greater than corresponding zero-order correlations when contrasting structural measures were partialed out. Endomorphy was highly related to body bulk when linear measures were partialed; ectomorphy was highly related to linearity when body bulk measures were

partialed; and mesomorphy seemed to relate to a combination of these factors, especially a large trunk and short legs. Illustrations are as follows. The correlation between endomorphy and standing height was 0.187; with weight held constant, the partial correlation was −0.709. The correlation between ectomorphy and standing height was insignificant; with weight held constant, the partial correlation rose to a high 0.926.

From many analyses in the Medford boys' growth study, the following brief generalizations may be made. High endomorphic boys were handicapped by excessive bulk, by low strength relative to size, by inability to perform muscular endurance tests involving moving the body, and inability to make and be successful on athletic teams. They had negative self-images but seemed fairly well adjusted psychologically. High mesomorphic boys had advantages related to greater gross and relative muscular strength, muscular endurance, successful athletic participation, peer status, and psychological adjustments. Ectomorphic boys had disadvantages related to less body bulk and gross strength, but they had advantages in relation to relative strength and muscular endurance. They demonstrated some lack of peer status and psychological adjustments and some favorable self-image characteristics.

Certain somatotypes are also related to specific types of athletic performance. Findings by Cureton[77] after experimenting with a group of Springfield College men made up largely of athletes and with practically no endomorphs in the group were as follows: (a) mesomorphs received the highest scores in athletic performance involving strength and power; (b) ectomorphs were favored in the Brace test, a

---

[76]Munroe, "Somatotype Components and Maturity."

[77]Thomas K. Cureton, "Body Build as a Framework of Reference for Interpreting Physical Fitness and Athletic Performance," *Supplement to the Research Quarterly,* **12,** No. 2 (May 1941), 301.

test which requires body balance, flexibility, and agility; (c) mesomorphs and meso-endomorphs did better in aquatic events; (d) ectomorphs received the lowest scores in the McCurdy-Larson Organic Efficiency Test.

Cureton[78] made extensive studies of the body build of Olympic men and women athletes of the 1932, 1936, and 1948 Olympiads. The results of these and other analyses of athletic groups are as follows: heavy athletes are relatively more mesomorphic (solid, dense muscle) types; track athletes run to slim body build with considerable ectomorphy (frail, linear) types but with well developed musculature; swimmers are more frequently meso-endomorphic (muscular and fat) types; weight lifters and weight throwers are frequently meso-endomorphics; and gymnasts, tumblers, and agile athletes are often meso-ectomorphic. Very seldom do men and women low in mesomorphy succeed in athletics. The dynamic athlete type has an above-average component of muscular fitness. Tanner[79] contrasted Olympic athletes in different sports and events. Some of the characteristics found were: sprinters were short and muscular, throwers were tall and heavy, and hurdlers had long legs. He suggested a relationship between mechanical and physiological requirements of a particular event and the physique of successful participants.

Clarke and Petersen[80] contrasted the somatotypes of boys in grades five through nine who were participants in inter-school athletics. The somatotype distribution of junior high school boys differed from the elementary school boys in the following respects: a greater percentage of mesomorphs was found among three classifica-

tions of athletes; a much greater percentage of mid-types was present among nonparticipants and a much smaller percentage from this category was found among outstanding athletes; a greater percentage of endo-mesomorphs was evident among the outstanding athletes and regular players. At both school levels, rarely was a boy classified as an endomorph found on an inter-school athletic squad. With a small sample of outstanding athletes in upper elementary and junior high schools, Clarke and Shelley[81] tentatively characterized the somatotypes of boys in various sports as follows: track and basketball, ectomorphs; football, wrestling, and baseball, mesomorphs and midtypes. In these studies, physique type and body size were more significant factors in athletic success for junior high than for elementary school athletes.

In addition, Sheldon has shown that body build is related to endocrine function. From somatotyping several groups of clinical patients on whom endocrine data were available, it was found that mesomorphic endomorphs have sluggish thyroids, that in acromegalics and other mesomorphs there is relatively active secretion by the anterior lobe of the pituitary and by the adrenal cortex, and that the ectomorphic endomorphs and the endomorphic ectomorphs tend to lack secretions from the posterior lobe of the pituitary, and the males lack gonadal secretion. It appears from these studies, that different standards of normality are needed for the interpretation of basal metabolic rates. Normal persons who are mesomorphic ectomorphs show an average BMR reading at least 20 points higher than normal individuals of the same age who are predominantly mesomorphic endomorphs.

The rate of physiological sexual matura-

[78]Cureton, *Physical Fitness Appraisal and Guidance*, p. 108.

[79]James M. Tanner, *The Physique of Olympic Athletes* (London: George Allen and Unwin, Ltd., 1964).

[80]Clarke and Petersen, "Maturational, Structural, and Strength Characteristics," p. 163.

[81]H. Harrison Clarke and Morgan E. Shelley, "Maturity, Structure, Strength, Motor Ability and Intelligence Test Profiles of Outstanding Elementary and Junior High School Athletes," *Physical Educator*, **18**, No. 4 (December 1961), 132.

tion, at least in females, can be better understood in relation to the individual's somatotype. From studies so far conducted, it seems apparent that dominance of the ectomorphic component tends to postpone sexual maturation, as indicated by appearance of the menses, and a modest predominance of either of the endomorphic or mesomorphic conponents tends to hasten it. On the other hand, a strong predominance of either of the latter components alone tends, in the female, to suppress sexual development.

For boys 12 years of age in the Medford Boys' Growth Study, skeletal age was not highly related to somatotype components, but the direction of the correlations indicated that endomorphy and, to a lesser extent, mesomorphy were associated with advanced skeletal age; ectomorphy was associated with somewhat retarded skeletal development. With boys 9 through 15 years, Clarke, Irving, and Heath[82] found a significantly greater percentage of boys classified as endo-mesomorphs were advanced than were retarded in maturity; the reverse was true for boys classified as mid-types.

[82]Clarke, Irving, and Heath, "Relation of Maturity, Structural, and Strength Measures to Somatotypes," p. 449.

SELECTED REFERENCES

BEHNKE, ALBERT R., and JACK H. WILMORE, *Evaluation and Regulation of Body Build and Composition.* Englewood Cliffs, N.J.: Prentice-Hall, Inc., 1974.

BROJEK, JOSEF, ed., *Body Measurements and Human Nutrition.* Detroit: Wayne State University Press, 1956.

CLARKE, H. HARRISON, "Individual Differences, Their Nature, Extent, and Significance," *Physical Fitness Research Digest,* President's Council on Physical Fitness and Sports, Series 3, No. 4 (October 1973).

CLARKE, H. HARRISON, *Physical and Motor Tests in the Medford Boys' Growth Study.* Englewood Cliffs, N.J.: Prentice-Hall, Inc., 1971.

CURETON, THOMAS K., *Physical Fitness Appraisal and Guidance.* St. Louis: The C. V. Mosby Co., 1947.

MAYER, JEAN, *Overweight: Causes, Cost, and Control.* Englewood Cliffs, N.J.: Prentice-Hall, Inc., 1968.

McCLOY, C. H., "Anthropometry in the Service of the Individual, *Journal of Health and Physical Education,* **5,** No. 7 (September 1934), 7.

SHELDON, WILLIAM H., C. W. DUPERTIUS, and EUGENE McDERMOTT, *Atlas of Men.* New York: Harper & Row, 1954.

TANNER, J. M., *Growth at Adolescence.* Springfield, Ill.: Charles C Thomas, 1962.

CHAPTER 6

In this chapter, tests especially related to remedial physical education will be considered. Remedial programs have been instituted in many schools and colleges throughout the country in the belief that the correction of certain types of defects and deficiencies is conducive to the well-being of the individual. Thus, tests designed to evaluate the following conditions will be presented: anteroposterior posture, lateral spinal deviations, foot condition, bodily flexibility, strength of individual muscle groups, and muscular fatigue.

POSTURE VALUES

Studies on the values of posture were much more prevalent some 40 years ago than is true in recent years. In substantiation of this statement, Fox[1] reported that 33 articles were published in the *Research Quarterly* under the heading of posture during 1930–1939. From 1940–1949, only

[1]Margaret Fox, "Body Mechanics," *Research Methods in Health, Physical Education, Recreation,* 2nd. ed., M. Gladys Scott, Ed. (Washington: American Association for Health, Physical Education, and Recreation, 1959), p. 315.

Measurement in Remedial Work

four more additions were made on this subject in the *Research Quarterly;* the numbers during other decades were six during 1950–1959 and five during 1960–1969. A survey of medical journals by Fox also indicated little interest in this area, except in foreign literature.

The lack of current studies related to posture should not infer that problems in this area have mostly been solved—far from it, as much work needs to be done. Although published data on the prevalence of postural defects are sparse, studies that are available point to the general presence of such defects among students. For example, Alderman[2] reported that 93 percent of the sophomore girls at Belair High School, Houston, Texas, had postural faults. The most frequent faults were: forward head, 62 percent; round shoulders, 36 percent; lateral asymmetry of shoulders, 31 percent; hollow back, 29 percent; pelvic tilt, 21 percent. Thus, physical educators have problems to solve, if the value of good posture is accepted.

Posture involves the mechanical coordination of the various systems of the body with reference to the skeletal and muscular systems and their neurological associations. From a theoretical standpoint, therefore, it seems reasonable to believe that poor posture, with the resulting pressure upon and displacement of visceral and other internal organs, nerves, and blood vessels, must impair their functioning, thus reducing the physical fitness of the individual. Many critical thinkers have carefully considered this relationship, although many of the data are based on extreme case studies. Adequate proof of the relationship itself does not exist. A brief summary of present information on the subject follows.

[2]Melba K. Alderman, "An Investigation of the Need for Posture Education Among High School Girls and a Suggested Plan of Instruction to Meet These Needs," Master's Thesis, University of Texas, 1966.

Goldthwaite[3] suggests a strong relationship between posture and circulation, and indicates that good circulation in the vital organs is impossible with a slumped chest because of resultant poor breathing and mechanical blockage. He maintains further that ulcered stomach, postural diabetes, gasteroptosis and enteroptosis are traceable to poor posture. Many researchers of this problem describe the harmful effects on health of visceroptosis, the abnormal falling downward of the abdominal viscera. Extreme cases of this sort show lack of endurance and are usually afflicted with constipation, headaches, and offensive breath. Karpovich[4] indicated that lordosis may be associated with orthostatic albuminaria, but maintains there is no scientific proof that improvements of "slight" irregularities in posture leads to "definite" improvement in the physical functions of the body. He explained that the lordosis-albuminaria relationship was due to veinous congestion in the kidneys resulting from lordosis.

Fox[5] reports that dysmenorrhea occurs with greater severity among college women with a sway-back postural condition. Ringo[6] obtained a low but definite relationship among college women between posture and trunk strength imbalance. Flint[7] found significant relationships between trunk strength and anteroposterior alignment of elementary school girls. In a later study, however, Flint and Diehl[8] reported that hip and trunk flexibility and back and abdominal muscular strength are not related to lumbar lordosis. Moriarity and Irwin[9] concluded from a study of school children that there is a significant association between poor posture and physical and emotional factors, including disease, fatigue, self-consciousness, fidgeting, hearing defects, restlessness, timidity, underweight, and asthma.

Experiments conducted on the relationship between posture and physical and mental efficiency, reveal very little or no relationship. Deaver[10] reported a slight tendency for physical fitness, motor ability, and health to be related to posture, but no relationship so far as vital capacity, intelligence, scholarship, personality integration, or leadership is concerned. Alden and Top[11] found practically no relationship between posture and weight, vital capacity, and intelligence. DiGiovanna[12] concluded that there seems to be a fairly definite tendency for posture to be positively related to athletic achievement only. Dunbar[13] found a positive correlation between posture and athletic ability, but it

[3]J. E. Goldthwaite, *Body Mechanics*, 5th ed. (Philadelphia: J. B. Lippincott Company, 1952), Ch. 6.

[4]Peter V. Karpovich, *Physiology of Physical Activity*, 5th ed. (Philadelphia: W. B. Saunders Company, 1959), pp. 297–98.

[5]Margaret G. Fox, "The Relationship of Abdominal Strength to Selected Postural Faults," *Research Quarterly*, **22**, No. 2 (May 1951), 141.

[6]Mildred B. Ringo, "An Investigation of Some Aspects of Abdominal Strength, Trunk Extensor Strength, and Anteroposterior Erectness in College Women," Doctoral Dissertation, University of Oregon, 1956.

[7]M. Marilyn Flint, "Lumbar Posture: A Study of Roentgenographic Measurement and the Influence of Flexibility and Strength," *Research Quarterly*, **34**, No. 1 (March 1963), 15.

[8]M. Marilyn Flint and Bobbie Diehl, "Influence of Abdominal Strength, Back-Extensor Strength, and Trunk Strength Balance upon Antero-Posterior Alignment of Elementary School Girls," *Research Quarterly*, **32**, No. 4 (December 1961), 490.

[9]Mary J. Moriarity and Leslie W. Irwin, "A Study of the Relationship of Certain Physical and Emotional Factors to Habitual Poor Posture Among School Children," *Research Quarterly*, **23**, No. 2 (May 1952), 221.

[10]George D. Deaver, "Posture and Its Relation to Mental and Physical Health," *Research Quarterly*, **4**, No. 1 (March 1933), 221.

[11]Florence D. Alden and Hilda Top, "Experiment on the Relation of Posture to Weight, Vital Capacity, and Intelligence," *Research Quarterly*, **2**, No. 3 (October 1931), 38.

[12]Vincent G. DiGiovanna, "A Study of the Relation of Athletic Skills and Strength to Those of Posture," *Research Quarterly*, **2**, No. 2 (May 1931), 67.

[13]Ruth O. Dunbar, "A Study of Posture and Its Relationship," *American Physical Education Review*, **32**, No. 2 (February 1927), 75.

was not high. Rawles[14] concluded, after experimenting with 300 young adult women, that "it appears there is much current exaggeration of the connection in the adult between posture and performance efficiency, physical or intellectual." With college women as subjects, Davies[15] found very little, if any, relationship between postural divergencies and performance on Scott's motor ability test.

Klein and Thomas,[16] on the other hand, reported that improvement in nutritional condition was more frequent among children who received posture training than among those who did not (*especially among those who actually improved their posture*). The rate of absence due to sickness for those receiving posture training was 38 percent lower in the spring quarter than it had been in the fall, while, for those not receiving posture training, the rate for the spring quarter showed an increase of 2 percent over the rate in the fall. The unique feature of this study was that a fairly well controlled experiment was conducted over a period of two years; thus, the effects of posture training over a period of time were evaluated.

Aside from potential physical fitness values, it should be stressed that good posture has strong aesthetic values. Good posture contributes positively to a pleasing appearance. No one would judge a person with sagging abdomen, rounded shoulders, and protruding head as being physically attractive. Certainly, art forms portraying the human body to best advantage show well-proportioned figures with grace and poise, which all add to a pleasing posture.

Lack of Posture Standards

A common handicap faced by most of the experimenters investigating the benefits of posture is that they have lacked precise testing instruments and methods for measuring posture, all these investigators having used either the silhouette or some form of general inspection. Deaver took silhouettes of his subjects and judged them according to the Harvard Posture Charts. Alden and Top used Bancroft's "Straight Line Test" as applied to silhouettes. DiGiovanna gave each individual a segmental posture examination and a final check-up of general posture by a process of careful inspection, a mental comparison being made between the findings in the examination and the standards illustrated in the posture charts of the Children's Bureau, United States Department of Labor. Klein and Thomas compared silhouettes with the posture charts of the Children's Bureau. Dunbar used the Bancroft Triple Posture Test. Davies used subjective postural screening by three judges.

There is ample proof to substantiate the statement that posture standards based upon the measures mentioned are lacking in precision and accuracy, a condition that lowers greatly the validity of the experiments conducted on the relationship between posture and the mental and physical traits of individuals. Cureton[17] faulted the profile silhouette alone *for quantitative measurement or evaluation,* as it is misleading and does not represent accurately the true spinal curvatures, showing instead the muscular contours of the back, the scapulae, and frequently the elbows. Other errors found in the silhouette-ograph method were: difficulty in measuring the silhouettes exactly due to lack of sharply defined edges, caused by improper adjustment of the camera lens or

[14]H. P. Rawles, "Objective Evaluation of Standards and Types of Posture." Master's Thesis, Wellesley College, Wellesley, Mass., 1925.

[15]Evelyn A. Davies, "Relationship Between Selected Postural Divergencies and Motor Ability," *Research Quarterly,* **28,** No. 1 (March 1957), 1.

[16]Armin Klein and Leah C. Thomas, *Posture and Physical Fitness* (Washington: U.S. Department of Labor, Children's Bureau, 1931).

[17]Thomas K. Cureton, "Bodily Posture as an Indicator of Fitness," *Supplement to the Research Quarterly,* **12,** No. 2 (May 1941), 348.

improper lighting; the smallness of the silhouette, causing likelihood of an error in determining the multiplier for the particular picture to enlarge the measurement to full size; and the photographic errors due to improper adjustment of the lens or improper location of the subject.

The unreliability of the subjective judgment of certain physical and mental traits is a well-established fact. In a subsequent study, Cureton and associates[18] found that the subjective inspectional scheme for measuring posture, as carried out by three trained and experienced examiners, who had worked intimately with each other for at least three years, gave results only 13.4 percent better than chance guesses as an average in ranking pupils, the mean correlation being 0.51.

Phelps and Kiphuth[19] question the "Straight Line Test" as proposed by Bancroft, when they state that "the position of the mastoid with regard to the acromion of the shoulder is valueless because of the mobility of the shoulders."

The problem of establishing posture standards is further complicated by other factors, as follows: (a) posture evaluation should not be confined to the standing stance, as is the situation in most of the studies mentioned above; other positions, such as lying, sitting, walking, and the like, should be considered; (b) appropriate individual differences should be recognized in determining proper posture standards. Kelly[20] has indicated that stocky individuals are less likely to show posture faults, because their massive bone structure provides greater stability, and that fat deposits, especially below the umbilicus, may mistakenly be considered posture faults. With high school girls, Alderman[21] found the following: a higher percentage of tall girls had forward head and round shoulders than did medium and short girls; a higher percent of heavy girls had round shoulders than did medium and light weight groups, slender girls were prone to forward heads and pelvic tilt. Posture as related to somatotype components is discussed by Clarke and Clarke.[22]

Thus the inability of previous experimenters to measure posture adequately is a fundamental reason why most attempts to correlate posture with health, scholarship, intelligence, athletic activity, organic condition, and similar criteria have failed. When measures of any one of these are correlated with posture, the result will not be higher than the reliability of the posture test. Therefore, until the value or lack of value of posture can be definitely established, the conscientious physical educator must decide for himself whether the results derived from good posture are beneficial to the physical well-being of the individual and whether or not he will continue with posture training.

TESTS OF ANTEROPOSTERIOR POSTURE

Posture measurement has attracted the attention of physical educators for many years. A number of special instruments were brought forward in the 1890s to measure anatomical and physiological relationships. These included devices for measuring the amount of the pelvic tilt, for showing the exact contour of the chest, for tracing the anteroposterior depth at all

[18]T. K. Cureton, J. S. Wickens, and H. P. Elder, "Reliability and Objectivity of the Springfield Postural Measurements," *Supplement to the Research Quarterly,* **6,** No. 2 (May 1935), 81.

[19]W. W. Phelps, R. J. H. Kiphuth, and C. W. Goff, *The Diagnosis and Treatment of Postural Defects,* 2nd ed. (Springfield, Mass.: Charles C Thomas, 1956).

[20]Ellen D. Kelly, *Adapted and Corrective Physical Education,* 4th ed. (New York: Ronald Press Company, 1965), p. 82.

[21]Alderman, "Need for Posture Education."

[22]H. Harrison Clarke and David H. Clarke, *Developmental and Adapted Physical Education* (Englewood Cliffs, N.J.: Prentice-Hall, Inc., 1963), p. 194.

points of the trunk, and for recording outlines of the body and abnormalities of spinal curvature. Other approximate schemes for measuring posture have considerable value as motivating devices in teaching posture, such as Bancroft's Triple Posture Test, Denniston's Double-Pole Posture Test, and Crampton's Work-a-Day Tests. There are also a number of postural scales based largely upon the opinions of experts in the field, such as the Brownell scale of silhouettes for ninth-grade boys, and a similar scale by Crook for measuring the anteroposterior posture of preschool children. Buhl has presented a "posture-meter" which is based upon the principle that, as the posture of the thoracic region improves, the chest moves forward and upward and the head moves backward, thus improving the general posture of the individual.

All of the tests so far mentioned consist of "over-all" postural measurement; that is, a general posture grade is assigned. In these instances no attempt has been made to break up posture into its component parts. Thus, it is not possible to tell from a posture score what parts of the body are faulty or the exact areas wherein the individual is defective. No basis is presented upon which specific postural exercises may be prescribed. Posture tests constructed recently break with this procedure and consider each of the parts of posture separately, such as the position of the head, the shoulders, the abdomen and so on. This is a step in the right direction, since "composite" posture scores are usually misleading and do not give an adequate description of the individual situation.

Subjective Posture Appraisals

Phelps, Kiphuth, and Goff Appraisal.[23] Phelps, Kiphuth, and Goff, in their subjective examination procedures for mea-

suring posture, painstakingly and effectively describe, with excellent illustrations, each of the various aspects of a complete posture appraisal, including the position or alignment of the neck, shoulders, thoracic spine, lumbar spine, pelvic tilt, overcarriage, chest, abdomen, lateral spinal deviation, knees, and feet. This system is subject to the errors common to other types of subjective measurement, as shown by the results of Cureton's experiments given below.

Iowa Posture Test.[24]   The posture and body mechanics test developed by the Women's Department of the Division of Physical Education, State University of Iowa, has been used with considerable success. This test provides a three-point rating scale for each of the following functional conditions: foot mechanics, standing position, walking, sitting, stooping to pick up a light object, and ascending and descending stairs. Foot mechanics appraisal will be described later in this chapter; criteria for evaluating the other postural conditions are presented here.

General Procedure.   While this test was developed for evaluating the body mechanics of college women, it can readily be adapted for others. The class is divided into groups of ten or twelve. Each group sits in a row of chairs or stools about two feet apart, facing forward or each chair turned at a 45-degree angle to facilitate rising and walking away from the chair. Ratings may be made more satisfactorily if the students wear bathing suits or leotards; they should also be barefooted.

Standing Position.   Students stand at the sides of their chairs; the examiner passes down the line checking correct alignment of body segments. The scoring:

3 points   axis through head, neck, trunk and legs approximately a straight line

[23]Phelps, Kiphuth, and Goff, *Postural Defects*, Ch. 6.

[24]*Posture and Body Mechanics*, rev. ed. (Iowa City: State University of Iowa Extension Bulletin, No. 792, July 1, 1962).

2 points   slight general deviation or moderate deviation of one part

1 point   marked general deviation

Walking.   Half of each group at a time walks around the row of chairs, some five or six feet between each person. The examiner studies the side view of the group and checks for correct alignment of body segments and lack of stiffness. The scoring:

3, 2, or 1 point(s)   rate as for standing, checking particularly for any change from the standing position; record stiffness, if present.

Sitting.   With the group sitting on the chairs or stools, the examiner checks the sitting position of the first person. Then, the subject rises and walks forward a few steps, turns, returns to the chair, and sits down. The examiner then proceeds to the next person and the others in turn. The scoring:

3 points   upper trunk well balanced over pelvis, head erect, chest high, shoulders back (not stiff), abdomen controlled, normal upperback curve

2 points   slight to moderate deviation from above sitting standard

1 point   marked deviation from correct standard

Stooping to Pick up Light Object.   Each person in turn stands and picks up a small object from the floor, walks a few steps, and places it on the floor again. The scoring:

3 points   one foot slightly ahead of the other, feet and hips well under body; bend at knees, slight bend at hips; relatively straight line of trunk, back controlled; arms relaxed, smooth movement, balance maintained throughout; object picked up slightly ahead of foot

2 points   very slight deviation from good standard in several items listed or moderate deviation in no more than three

1 point   markedly incorrect performance, especially bending from hips with knees straight

Ascending and Descending Stairs.   Each person is checked while ascending and descending some eight to ten stairs. The construction of a portable set of stairs would be a convenience in administering this test. Score each subject separately on ascending and on descending the stairs. The criteria for scoring 3, 2, or 1 point(s):

Ascending   weight only slightly forward from ankles (not hips); straight push up from ankle and knee, avoiding sideward sway of hips

Descending   controlled lowering of weight onto forward foot (not a relaxed drop; smoothness (avoid bobbing)

This test is inexpensive, easy to administer, its functional application is not limited to the static standing posture, and individual testing requires about five minutes. Lee and Wagner[25] claim that 40 children have been examined in as many minutes through group testing methods. A reliability coefficient of 0.97 for this posture scoring scheme was obtained by Moriarity.[26]

New York State Posture Rating Test.[27]   The New York State Physical Fitness Test manual includes a posture assessment method. A series of profiles illustrating 13 posture areas is presented; these profiles appear in Figure 6.1. For each area, three profiles

[25]Mabel Lee and Miriam M. Wagner, *Fundamental Body Mechanics and Conditioning* (Philadelphia: W. B. Saunders Company, 1949), p. 283.

[26]Moriarity and Irwin, "Physical and Emotional Factors and Habitual Poor Posture," p. 221.

[27]*The New York State Physical Fitness Test: For Boys and Girls Grades 4–12*, rev. ed. (Albany, N.Y.: State Education Department, 1966).

POSTURE RATING CHART

Grade 4 5 6 7 8 9 10 11 12

Rater's Initials

Date of Test

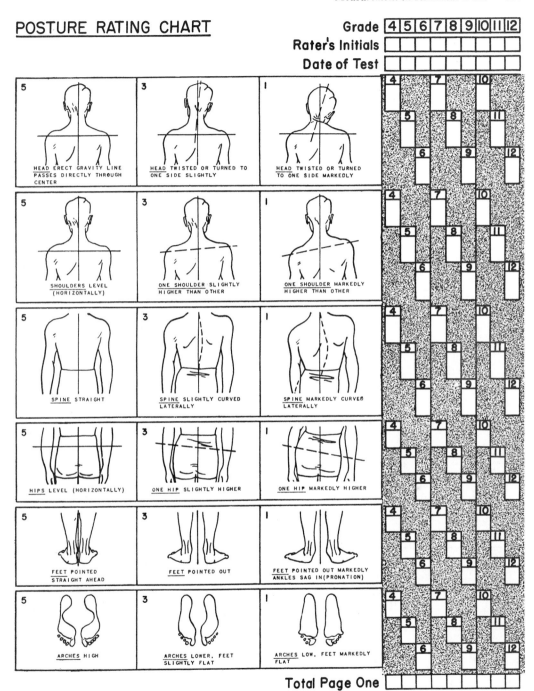

FIGURE 6.1. *New York State Posture Rating Chart*

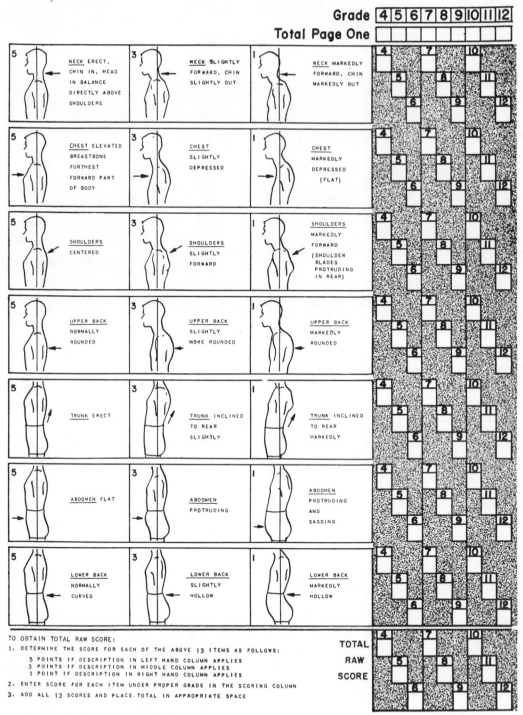

FIGURE 6.1. *(continued)*

are provided for good, fair, and poor posture; these are scored 5, 3, and 1 respectively, although the intervening numerals of 2 and 4 may be used. The 13 scores are totaled to obtain a subject's posture grade. Provisions are made to record annual posture scores under grade in school each year from the fourth grade through high school. Norms for this posture rating test follow.

Achievement Level	Percentile Rank	Posture Score
10	99	—
9	98	65
8	93	63
7	84	61
6	69	59
5	50	55–57
4	31	49–53
3	16	45–47
2	7	39–43
1	2	35–37
0	1	0–33

The following instructions are given for this posture rating process.

Test area: Suspend a heavy, clearly visible plumb line from a stationary support in front of an appropriate screen so that the bob almost touches the floor. Directly under the bob, provide a straight line using one-inch masking tape. This line should begin at a point on the floor three feet from the bob toward the screen, pass directly under the bob, and extend ten feet on the examiner's side of the bob.

Testing procedure: The pupil being examined first assumes a comfortable and natural standing position between the plumb bob and the screen, straddling the floor line and facing the screen, as shown in Figure 6.2A. After the pupil's lateral posture and feet have been rated, he then turns left, sideward to the examiner, and stands with his feet at right angles to the floor line; his left malleolus must be in line with the plumb bob (Figure 6.2B).

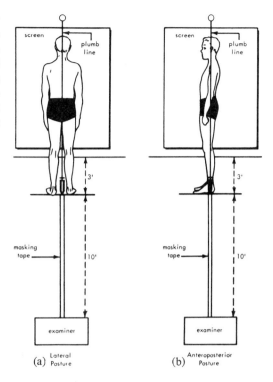

FIGURE 6.2. *New York State Posture Rating Positions*

Woodruff Body Alignment Posture Test.[28] A body alignment frame was designed by Woodruff to avoid the time consuming and expensive photographic techniques of posture examination while providing a more reliable procedure than subjective appraisal alone. The construction of this frame is shown in Figure 6.3. The nine strings running lengthwise of the frame are three-fourths of an inch apart. The center string is a different color for easy identification.

In using the frame, a base line six feet long is drawn on the floor at right angles to a wall; the frame is centered at the end of this line and at right angles to it.

[28]Janet Woodruff, School of Health, Physical Education, and Recreation, University of Oregon, Eugene, Oregon.

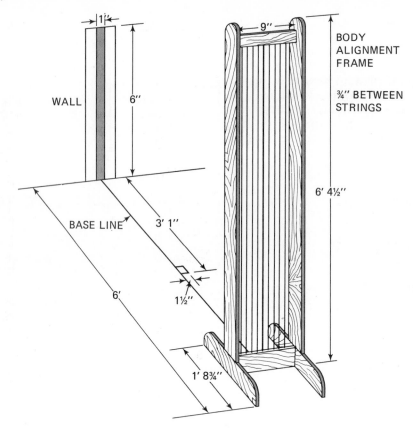

FIGURE 6.3. *Woodruff Posture Frame. Courtesy of Janet Woodruff, School of Health and Physical Education, University of Oregon.*

Another line, one inch wide, is drawn on the wall perpendicular to the floor and intersecting the line on the floor. A one and one-half inch line is drawn perpendicular to the base line, three feet one inch (inclusive of the line) from the wall.

The subject stands between the body alignment frame and the wall with the left side toward the tester. The left foot is placed in such a position that the ankle bone is opposite the free end of the one and one-half inch line; the right foot is placed parallel to the left foot. The subject should then adjust the foot position so that the base line runs under the top of the instep. A natural standing position, looking straight ahead, is assumed by the subject.

The examiner takes a position ten feet in front of the frame.

In giving the test, the examiner looks through the frame and lines the center string of the frame with the wall line. For perfectly balanced posture, the "plumbline" test applies, in which the center string, if the posture is "perfect," passes in front of the ankle joint, just in front of the dimple behind the knee cap, through the center of the hip and shoulder joints, and through the mastoid process. Posture scoring is accomplished by judging the deviation, either forward or backward, for the number of strings for each of the following segments from the one directly below (therefore, not necessarily the deviation from the center string each time): ankle, knee, hip, shoulder, head. A score of 25 shows no deviations from this line; one point is deducted for each string deviation. For the first test given college women, the mean posture score was around 20; the range of scores was from 16 to 25.

By the test-retest method, 80 percent agreement was obtained in scoring "overhang," which denotes the distance the shoulders are carried posterior to the center of the hip joint.

Objective Posture Tests

A number of objective posture tests have been proposed, most of which require either special apparatus or some form of photography or both.

Cureton's Posture Measurement. One of the first thorough analyses of objective posture measurement was made by Cureton, who studied the validity of various posture-testing devices and attempted to measure objectively many of the separate items included in the Phelps and Kiphuth posture appraisal, mentioned above.

Cureton's first task was to determine the validity of various instruments proposed for posture measurement, including the conformateur, the spinograph (a spine-tracing device), and the silhouetteograph.[29] Preliminary measurements utilizing all three devices were taken on 15 subjects, the conformateur and spinograph giving comparable results, but the silhouetteograph being greatly in error. A manikin was next measured with the various devices, in order to eliminate the errors resulting from the inconstancy of the subject in assuming the same position exactly in a series of trials. A metal conformateur with measurements taken directly from the rods was found to be superior to other measurements taken separately in order to record conveniently the posture picture. A recommended procedure, proposed after additional research, called for a combination of the conformateur, as perfected by Cureton and Gunby, and the silhouetteograph. Details for the improvement of the conformateur will be found in the reference. This conformateur lends itself readily to use in combination with the silhouetteograph, allowing a double check upon gross errors and the opportunity of obtaining quantitative results. It also provides a personal picture, which may have value in motivating the subject to improve his posture.

In a subsequent study, Cureton, Wickens and Elder[30] studied the reliability and objectivity of the postural appraisals by the Cureton method. They found that the objective measurement scheme was 2 to 5 times as reliable as subjective inspection, depending on the part measured, and from 3 to 15 times as objective.

Cureton did not attempt to define either good or bad posture, nor did he present norms for evaluating postural status. In a subsequent study, however, he stated that postural measurements do not correlate highly with each other, most of the relations of distinctly different items being below 0.30, a fact that supports the belief that each aspect of posture is due to specific mechanical forces and neural learnings, and that each must therefore be dealt with specifically.[31]

Wellesley Posture Measurements. In studying the posture of girls and women, MacEwan and Howe[32] recognized what Cureton subsequently proved, that in photographs and silhouettes the profile pic-

[29]Thomas K. Cureton, "The Validity of Antero-Posterior Spinal Measurements," *Research Quarterly,* **2,** No. 3 (October 1931), 101.

[30]Cureton, Wickens, and Elder, "Springfield Postural Measurements," p. 81.

[31]Thomas K. Cureton, "Bodily Posture as an Indicator of Fitness," *Supplement to the Research Quarterly,* **12,** No. 2 (May 1941), 348.

[32]C. G. MacEwan and E. C. Howe, "An Objective Method of Grading Posture," *Research Quarterly,* **3,** No. 3 (October 1932), 144.

ture alone does not accurately represent the true spinal curvatures. In an attempt to locate the actual position of the spine from a photograph of the subject, aluminum pointers, 9 cm. long by 4 mm. wide and ¼ gm. in weight, were attached at the end of the sternum, on the prominence of the first piece of the sacrum, and on the spinous processes of every second vertebra beginning with the seventh cervical. By measuring inward the proper distance from the tips of the pointers, the real position of the chest and spine is located and drawn on the picture regardless of the musculature of the back or projecting scapulae, arms, or other protuberances. The following postural measurements may be made by the Wellesley technique: (a) the amount of anteroposterior curvature in the dorsal and lumbar areas of the spine; (b) the amount of segmental angulation and body tilt; and (c) the position of the head and neck.

Validity for this posture test was claimed on the grounds that the battery of measurements was in "reasonable agreement" with the composite judgment of a group of physical educators who were authorities on the posture of girls and women. With 243 subjects, the correlation between the criterion posture grade (five judges) and thoracic depth was 0.47; and between the criterion posture grade and lumbar depth, 0.56.

Wickens and Kiphuth Posture Test.   Wickens and Kiphuth[33] designed a posture test for use with men at Yale University. This test utilized certain of the Cureton measurement procedures; instead of the conformateur, the Wellesley aluminum pointers were employed to locate the actual position of the spine; photography was used to record the image. Before the student was photographed the following

points on the left side of the body were marked with a black flesh pencil to serve as landmarks for determining segmental alignment on the picture: tragus of the ear, front tip of the shoulder, acromion, greater trochanter of the femur, styloid process of the fibula, and center of the external malleolus. In order to determine the amount of anteroposterior spinal curvature, five aluminum pointers were attached to the back, located at the spinous process of the seventh cervical vertebra, the greatest convexity backward of the dorsal curve, the point of inflection between dorsal and lumbar curves (the point where the curve reverses its direction), the greatest convexity backward of the lumbar curve, and the most prominent part of the sacrum. One pointer was placed at the lower end of the sternum to determine the carriage of the chest. The feet were adjusted so that a plumb bob fell through the external malleolus, and the anteroposterior photograph was taken.

After the picture had been printed, small perforations were made at the proximal ends of each of the pointers, through the flesh pencil marks, and at the flesh line of the most protuberant part of the abdomen. The glossy side of the picture was placed face down on the frosted-glass surface of a mimeoscope illuminated from underneath, thus making the picture transparent; measurements were made on the back of the photograph. The following measurements were taken, as illustrated in Figure 6.4:

1. Head and Trunk: The position of the head and neck was determined by scaling the angle made by a horizontal line through the seventh cervical and a line from the seventh cervical through the tragus of the ear. (Angle E.)

2. Kyphosis: The amount of kyphosis was determined by scaling the angle made by a line from the greatest convexity backward of the dorsal curve through the seventh cervical and a line from the greatest convexity backward through the inflection point. (Angle H.)

[33]Stuart Wickens and Oscar W. Kiphuth, "Body Mechanics Analysis of Yale University Freshmen," *Research Quarterly,* **8,** No. 4 (December 1937), 38.

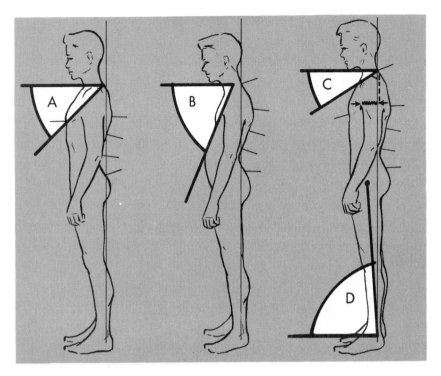

FIGURE 6.4. *Wickens-Kiphuth Posture Test*

3. Lordosis: The lordosis angle was formed by a line from the greatest concavity backward of the lumbar curve through the inflection point and a line from the greatest concavity backward through the most prominent part of the sacrum. (Angle J.)

4. Chest: The angle formed by a horizontal line through the seventh cervical and a line from the seventh cervical through the end of the sternum gave a measure of the carriage of the chest. Men carrying their chests in an elevated position show a smaller angle than those having a flat chest. (Angle A.)

5. Abdomen: If the abdominal line is straight and does not extend beyond the sternum, then the angle formed by a line from the most prominent part of the abdomen through the end of the sternum and a horizontal line through the seventh cervical will be 90 degrees or greater. On the other hand, if the abdomen extends beyond the sternum, the angle will read less than 90 degrees. (Angle B.)

6. Shoulders: The shoulder angle was determined by scaling the angle made by a horizontal line through the seventh cervical and a line from the seventh cervical through the front tip of the shoulder. (Angle C.) Measuring with vernier calipers the horizontal distance between two vertical lines erected through these points gives a linear rating of the shoulder's position.

7. Trunk: An important item in segmental alignment is the amount of lean of the trunk forward or backward as it is balanced on the hip joint. The term *overcarriage* is applied to faulty carriage of the trunk where its weight is carried backward so that a vertical through the seventh cervical falls outside the most prominent part of the sacrum. This may be objectively measured by using the angle formed by a horizontal line through the sacral point and a line from the sacral point to the seventh cervical. As the trunk leans forward, the angle becomes less than 90 degrees, while in overcarriage it increases beyond 90 degrees. (Angle F.)

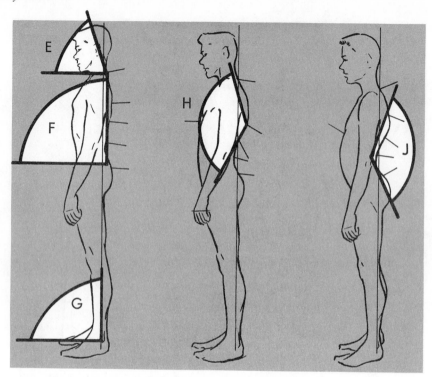

FIGURE 6.4. *(continued)*

8. Hips: The position of the hips was measured by the degree that the greater trochanter of the femur was carried forward or backward relative to the external malleolus. (Angle D.)

9. Knees: Although "bow-legs" or "knock-knees" cannot be determined from a picture taken in the anteroposterior plane, an idea of knee posture with regard to "flexed knees" or "hyper-extended knees" may be obtained by scaling the angle formed by a horizontal line through the external malleolus and a line from the external malleolus through the styloid process of the fibula. In case of flexed or "easy" knees, the angle will be less than 90 degrees; with hyper-extended knees, greater than 90 degrees. (Angle G.)

Objectivity coefficients were determined for the different measurements by photographing and rephotographing 30 subjects after the points were affixed by two different examiners independent of each other. The following coefficients show the precision of affixing the pointers and scaling the pictures: 0.72 for head and neck, 0.85 for kyphosis, and 0.73 for lordosis. Duplicate sets of 100 pictures were graded by two different examiners with correlations of 0.96 and 0.97 for the same three measurements. Thus, the application of the measurement procedures to the photographs has a high degree of consistency. When the whole process of preparing and photographing the subject is repeated, the objectivity coefficients are only slightly better than those obtained by Cureton with his conformateur procedure.

Subsequently, a method of taking PhotoMetric posture pictures for use with the Wickens and Kiphuth posture measurements was developed at Yale University.[34] By a system of mirrors placed in

[34]Phelps, Kiphuth, and Goff, *Postural Defects,* Ch. 6.

specific positions, four images of the individual from the following four angles are produced in a single exposure: left side, front, rear, and overhead. Before taking the picture, the subject is prepared with aluminum pointers and body markings, as for the Wickens and Kiphuth method. From slides of the photographs, images of half life size are projected on a screen, from which measurements within a tolerance of $^1/_{16}$th inch in 72 inches may be made. In addition to the Wickens and Kiphuth posture measurements, the PhotoMetric picture permits an assessment of shoulder displacement.

A distinct advantage of the Wickens and Kiphuth technique is that it can be applied without the use of a conformateur. Silhouettes could be used instead of photographs by utilizing Cureton's scheme of lights over essential points on the body, such as the tragus of the ear, the acromion, and so forth.

Alderman's Adaptation.[35] Alderman successfully adapted a photographic method of taking posture pictures proposed by Fishman[36] in the detection of various posture faults. A grid was constructed from a peg board three feet by six feet with string interwoven through the holes to form a grid of two-inch squares, which was placed against a wall to form the background for the picture. A plumb line was suspended in the front-center of the grid, allowing enough room for the subject to stand between the board and the line. The lighting consisted of two photoflood lamps with built-in reflectors screwed into small table lamp bases. The lamp to the right of the grid was placed four feet from the subject at an angle of 45 degrees, approximately shoulder height; the lamp to the left was at the same distance and angle but at waist height. A 100-watt bulb

[35]Alderman, "Need for Posture Education."

[36]Harry R. Fishman, "One-Minute Posture Pictures," *Journal of Health, Physical Education, and Recreation,* **29,** No. 1 (January 1958), 72.

was suspended one foot above the grid to put more light on the subject's face. Each subject had a number on a tag, which was placed on a nail in the grid for identification purposes. The subjects wore swim suits.

Three photographs were taken of each subject, back, right and left sides. Posing directions for the side views were: stand between the plumb line and the grid, place hands on front of thighs, and align the front of the ankle joint with the plumb line. The plumb line was applied; thus, if the body segments were correctly balanced, the line passed through the lobe of the ear, the center of the shoulder, the greater trochanter of the hip, just behind the knee cap, and front of the ankle joint. To assist in subject placement for the rear view, two marks were drawn on the floor two inches apart, bisected by the plumb bob. When the subject's feet were on these marks, the plumb line fell between the heels and, when correctly aligned, continued through the cleft of the buttocks and along the spinal cord. The subject's arms hung naturally at the sides of the body.

The following antero-posterior postural faults were identified: (a) forward head, when plumb line passed behind lobe of ear; (b) round shoulders, when line passed behind tip of shoulders; and (c) pelvic tilt, when line passed behind center of hip joint. The position of the knees helped to determine pelvic tilt; if the knees were hyperextended, the line passed more to the front of the patella. In addition, protruding abdomen, round back, and increased dorsal curve can be seen from the side views.

Lateral asymmetries of the hips and shoulders were detected from the rear view photograph. This detection was more accurate when a thin ruler was placed on the horizontal line nearest to the upper positions of the hips and shoulders. A severe lateral deviation of the spine can also be seen from this view, but is difficult to detect unless the vertebrae column is marked with a flesh pencil. In addition to lateral deviations, pronation of the ankles can be seen from the back view; and, round shoulders can be detected, since drooping of the shoulders can be seen.

Alderman's postural photographic procedures were confined to the detection of postural faults; evaluations of their severity were not included. She concluded that her photographic method was more effective in detecting postural deviations than was visual screening. Posture photographs were also found to be an important motivational factor in a subsequent posture improvement program.

Massey's Posture Technique.[37]   In selecting the combination of body adjustments which best reflect the total posture of the body, Massey developed a criterion composed of the combined ratings of three qualified judges. The Cureton-Gunby conformateur technique was utilized to record posture, with small angle-iron pointers instead of lights being used to designate such landmarks as would be invisible in the silhouette. From the resultant silhouette, 30 angles and seven linear deviations, representing segmental alignments were made. The following angles proved to be of greatest significance in over-all posture evaluated: Angle I, head and neck-trunk alignment; Angle II, trunk-hip alignment; Angle III, hip-thigh alignment; and Angle IV, thigh-leg alignment. This combination of angles resulted in a multiple correlation of 0.985 with the criterion.

Howland Alignometer.[38]   In studying various posture relationships, Howland

found that when the structural alignment of the trunk approximates the line of gravity, the tilt of the pelvis and the upper trunk are aligned vertically. To measure this relationship as a posture test, she designed an alignometer. This device consists of a vertical rod secured to a portable base, to which two adjustable and calibrated pointers are attached. In use, these point to the center of the sternum and the superior border of the symphysis pubis. If the subject has proper alignment, the two pointers will be the same distance from the vertical rod. Objectivity for this test is approximately 0.90.

Conclusion

Good work has been done in the development of postural measurements. Certain of these measures, however, have objectivity coefficients which, while much superior to subjective judgment, are still below the accepted standard of 0.80, and all are below the preferred standard of 0.90. This seeming lack of precision is due not entirely to the measurement itself, but to the inability of the subject to assume exactly the same position on each repetition of the test.

Another weakness of posture tests is that norms have not been developed, except for the Wellesley and the New York state evaluations. Such scales, as well as the ideal toward which physical educators should work in their posture instruction, are needed.

The question of practicability may also be raised in connection with the posture measures, as the administration of any one of the objective tests requires special equipment and necessitates the expenditure of considerable time. This drawback is also true of other good tests in physical education and is not an insurmountable obstacle. Physical educators should give careful consideration to the values to be obtained from the subsequent program. If major emphasis on posture training is to

[37]Wayne W. Massey, "A Critical Study of Objective Methods for Measuring Anterior Posterior Posture with a Simplified Technique," *Research Quarterly*, **14**, No. 1 (March 1943), 3.

[38]Ivaldare Sprow Howland, *Body Alignment in Fundamental Motor Skills* (New York: Exposition Press, 1953), p. 78.

be a part of the physical education program, then the expenditure of time and money will be justified.

CENTER OF GRAVITY TEST

The center of gravity is the weight center of the body, the point around which it balances in all directions. Its determination and significance have been of interest to body mechanics investigators since the turn of the century. Tests of this trait have utilized body weight, either in the lying or standing position. Cureton and Wickens[39] proposed one such test, which is effective and simple to administer. Their test indicates the distance the individual's center of gravity is in front of his internal malleoli. The equipment consists of a balance board supported at the ends on blocks located in the center of two weight scales, such as the Toledo dial scale or the lever-arm type, with a vertical pin located in the exact center of the board. A variation of the test permits its administration from a single weight scale, as described in the reference.

In administering the test, the subject stands on the balance board in a normal postural position, facing in the direction of the length of board and with his internal malleoli lined up even with the vertical pin. The examiner balances the scales, first the forward one and then the rear scale, until both scales have their lever arms swinging freely between the guide stops, or reads the weights directly, if the Toledo dial scales are used. The scales are read and both readings recorded. Half of the weight of the board is deducted from each reading. The individual's score from the weights, showing how far the center of gravity is being balanced in front of the internal malleoli, may be read directly from a prepared table, and the percentile score determined from a percentile rating scale, both given in the reference.

The reliability and objectivity coefficients for this test were approximately 0.90. Correlations of center of gravity and other measures were: 0.86 with body lean, 0.75 with Physical Fitness Index, 0.50 with Strength Index, and 0.49 with vertical jump.

LATERAL DEVIATION OF THE SPINE

Fitz[40] described a "scoliometer" for measuring and graphically plotting lateral curvatures of the spine, which consisted of transparent celluloid, $^2/_{100}$ in. in thickness, 52 cm. in length, and 16 cm. in width, ruled with longitudinal gradations 1 cm. apart and horizontal gradations 4 cm. apart. Two small level glasses, the tubes of which were bent to the curve of a circle of 12-inch radius, were attached to the celluloid; one of these was fastened at a right angle to the longitudinal lines and the other was fastened at a right angle to the horizontal lines. The subject was prepared by marking with a skin pencil the tops of the spinous processes of the vertebrae, the posterior-superior spines, and the spines and lower angles of the scapulae. The major purposes of this device were to determine lateral curvature of the spine, lateral tilt of the spine, lateral tilt of the pelvis, and level of the shoulders.

Believing that the scoliometer had definite possibilities for objective measurement of lateral deviations of the spine, Clarke and Shay conducted a study of its use as a precision instrument.[41] A scoliom-

[39]T. K. Cureton and J. Stuart Wickens, "The Center of Gravity Test of the Human Body in the Antero-Posterior Plane and Its Relation to Posture, Physical Fitness and Athletic Ability," *Supplement to the Research Quarterly,* **6,** No. 2 (May 1935), 93.

[40]George W. Fitz, "A Simple Method of Measuring and Graphically Plotting Spinal Curvature and Other Assymetrics by Means of a New Direct Reading Scoliometer," *American Physical Education Review,* **11,** No. 1 (March 1906), 18.

[41]H. Harrison Clarke and Clayton T. Shay, "Measurement of Lateral Spinal Deviations," *Black and Gold of Phi Epsilon Kappa,* **17,** No. 2 (March 1940), 38.

eter was constructed after the manner described by Fitz, except that the prescribed levels were omitted. Thus, the experiment was limited to the measurement of lateral curvatures only. The use of this scoliometer is shown in Figure 6.5.

An objectivity coefficient of 0.89 was obtained for the scoliometer test, when successive measurements were taken within a short time (the back markings not being repeated). It was not entirely satisfactory when the measurements were made after the lapse of several days, the correlations being approximately 0.60 for both reliability and objectivity. Considerable doubt, however, exists concerning the subject's ability to assume the same position each time he is measured. Marking the entire back proved most exact.

The following criticisms may be made of the scoliometer as a precision instrument in measuring lateral curvatures of the spine.

1. The main difficulty encountered in the use of the scoliometer is in keeping the celluloid from twisting, especially when projecting scapulae tend to displace it.

2. The scoliometer is too short for taller individuals.

3. If only lateral deviations are measured, the scoliometer may advantageously be made smaller, reducing its width by half.

Another method of objectively measuring lateral curvatures, the taut-string test, was also tried. This test consists of stretching a string from the seventh cervical to the fifth lumbar vertebrae, and noting the amount of lateral deviation from the string. Inside calipers were used for measuring the curvature and a steel metric rule for determining the amount of deviation.

The taut-string test as administered was found to be slightly superior to the scoliometer. Criticisms concerning its use are as follows.

1. Difficulty is encountered in keeping the string straight between the seventh cervical and the fifth lumbar vertebrae, especially when a pronounced kyphosis is present and bows the string posteriorly, and when the lateral curvature is of such a nature that the erector spinae muscles of the back tend to deflect the string sideward.

2. Difficulty is also encountered in measuring the deviation when the convexity is in the lumbar area and the individual has a pronounced lordosis. The string is then two to three inches from the back, and sighting the calipers through this distance is not easy.

3. The point of greatest convexity of the curvature is occasionally found to be in error when only one mark on the back is used, as contrasted with measures where the entire back is marked.

4. An assistant is required in giving the test in order to hold the string while the calipers are being applied.

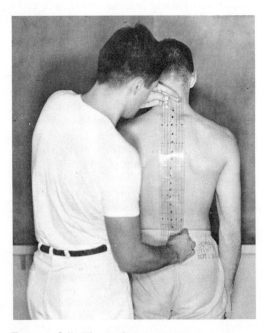

FIGURE 6.5. *The Scoliometer in Use*

FOOT MEASUREMENT

Examinations of the feet have generally consisted of subjective checkings of certain foot characteristics considered indicative of the status of the foot. (Among these characteristics are the following: angle of stance, ankle overhang, height of the longitudinal arch, bowing of the Achilles tendon, pronation or supination, foot flexibility, presence of callouses on bottom of foot, and the like.) Pronation, or inward rolling of the ankles with resulting disalignment of the feet and legs, has been a widely accepted criterion of foot weakness and strain. Kelly[42] reported that 50 to 60 percent of the child population shows pronation to a greater or lesser degree. However, she points out, functional foot complaints are relatively uncommon among children and very common among adults. To identify and correct potential foot disturbances is a logical purpose of remedial physical education.

Pain on Pressure

Kelly[43] studied 35 anthropometric and x-ray variables with three groups of children, 8 to 14 years of age, to determine their relative effectiveness in identifying criteria of potentially painful feet. The three groups of children were as follows: (a) 75 children judged to have symptomless, normal, or well aligned feet and legs; (b) 52 children were symptomless, but with markedly weak or pronated alignment; (c) 51 children reported persistent symptoms typical of functional foot strain. Both pronated and painful groups showed greater flexibility than the normal group with regard to the arch, the ankle, and the trunk and hamstrings, and similar but less significant greater flexibility in 10 of 11 additional variables studied. Pain on pressure to the sole of the foot differentiated the normal from the painful feet, and the pronated from the painful feet.

The following three pressure points were used to determine the presence of pain in the foot: (a) under the junction of the first and second metatarsal with the first cuneiform bone, (b) under the insertion of the tibialis anterior muscle, and (c) under the posterior insertion of the plantarcalcaneo-navicular ligament into the calcaneus bone. As shown in Figure 6.6, the subject lowers the weight of the leg and foot onto a half-inch diameter padded nailhead inserted into a block, which is resting on the platform of a bathroom-type scale. With the foot relaxed, the minimum pounds pressure required to elicit a pain response is the score used. If no pain is recorded at 12 pounds, the pressure is stopped.

Iowa Foot-Mechanics Test[44]

As indicated above, a foot mechanics test is included in the Iowa Posture Test for college women, and is administered from the same seating arrangement described. In this instance, the examiner takes a position at the side of the row of subjects; each girl in turn walks out toward her and returns, while she is checked on toeing straight ahead and the presence or absence of pronation. The scoring:

A. Weight Distribution

3 points	no bony bulge in front of and below medial malleolus; no marked inward protrusion of navicular bone; no inward bowing of heel cord
2 points	some pronation
1 point	marked pronation

[42]Ellen D. Kelly, "A Comparative Study of Structure and Function of Normal, Pronated, and Painful Feet Among Children," *Research Quarterly*, **18,** No. 4 (December 1947), 291.

[43]Ibid.

[44]State University of Iowa, *Posture and Body Mechanics.*

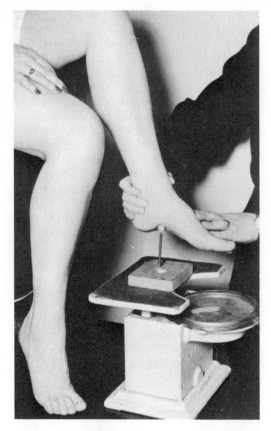

FIGURE 6.6. *Kelly Test for Foot Pain Symptoms. Courtesy of Ellen Kelly.*

B. Direction of Feet

3 points   feet parallel; a very slight angle of
               toeing out is allowed
2 points   moderate toeing out
1 point   marked toeing out

Height of Longitudinal Arch

Footprint Angle. The use of footprints as measures of foot condition, especially of the height of the arch, has been the subject of several studies. Footprints are easily taken and yield pictures easily comprehended by the subject. They also lend themselves to objective measurement.

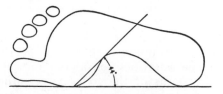

FIGURE 6.7. *The Footprint Angle*

Footprints may be made with a pedograph or with homemade devices. One homemade device for taking footprints consists of an ordinary picture frame across which is stretched light rubber sheeting. Fingerprint ink is rolled on the underside of this sheeting and the print taken on ordinary paper. This device is inexpensive, takes an excellent footprint, and in addition shows the callouses and other growths on the underside of the foot. Its main disadvantage is the necessity of constantly re-applying the fingerprint ink to the rubber sheeting.

Schwartz, Britton, and Thompson[45] proposed the footprint angle as a measure of the height of the longitudinal arch, based on the observation that, as arches become higher, the angles increase steadily. He obtained high reliability coefficients but failed to indicate objectivity for this test. By refining the method of determining the arch angle, Clarke[46] obtained a reliability coefficient of 0.97 and an objectivity coefficient of 0.95.

The procedures used in scoring the footprints, as illustrated in Figure 6.7, follow.

1. Draw a line to represent the medial border of the foot between the points of the imprint at the base of the first metatarsal bone (base of the big toe) and the calcaneus or heel bone.

[45]L. Schwartz, R. H. Britton, and J. R. Thompson, *Studies in Physical Development and Posture,* U.S. Public Health Bulletin No. 179 (Washington: Government Printing Office, 1928).

[46]H. Harrison Clarke, "An Objective Method of Measuring the Height of the Longitudinal Arch of the Foot," *Research Quarterly,* **4,** No. 3 (October 1933), 99.

2. Locate the point where this line first touches the inner side of the imprint at the base of the first metatarsal bone.

3. Then, with a ruler held on this point, swing it down from the toe until it just touches the edge of the print on the inside of the arch, and draw a line from the point across the print. No white paper should show between this line and the print.

4. Measure the angle at the junction of the two lines with a protractor.

The average footprint angle for adult males is placed at about 42 degrees. Some question has been raised, however, as to whether the footprint angle actually measures the height of the arch. Cureton[47] pointed out that the footprint shows the fleshy pads and musculature of the plantar surface of the foot rather than the bony alignment of the arch. He did, however, show that the footprint angle does measure the external height of the arch, when he obtained a correlation of 0.96 between it and the height of imprints made in moist sand (sandbox method).

Cureton further found that the height of the arch, as measured by either the footprint or the sandbox method, was not a significant factor in the functional efficiency of the foot. These data explode the popular theory that a measure of the external height of the arch may be used as a diagnostic device in the selection of individuals needing foot correction. Apparently, therefore, the principal value of the footprint angle is to measure the increase in arch height in those cases selected by other means for treatment, and then only where arch height is one of the factors involved. The footprint, however, is a motivating device, which, like the silhouette in posture training, portrays to the individual obvious facts concerning the condition of his feet, thus emphasizing in his mind the need for correction.

Navicular Drop. DePiero[48] proposed the navicular drop as a test of essential foot function. This test determines the depression of the longitudinal arch which occurs when a person stands or supports a weight. In a study of college men by Thompson,[49] the test was administered in the following manner.

1. The subject, barefooted, sat in a chair with the feet resting on the floor, legs perpendicular to the floor.

2. With a felt pen, the tester marked the most prominent part of the navicular bone; the distance of this mark to the floor was measured to the nearest millimeter.

3. The subject stood and the distance from the mark to the floor was again measured. The difference between the two distances is the amount of the navicular drop.

Thompson related the amount of the drop to a number of structural aspects and functional performances of the feet by comparing two groups of college men, an experimental and a control group. The experimental group was composed of subjects who had observed and measured deviations of the structure and posture of their feet, while the feet of the control group were essentially without such variations. Among his findings were the following: (a) the strength of the muscles activating ankle movements were weaker for men with a navicular drop; (b) men with a navicular drop of 5.5 mm. or more in both feet recorded plantar-flexion, dorsiflexion, pronation, and supination muscular strengths which were at least 28.7 percent below the control group; and (c) the

[47]Thomas K. Cureton, "The Validity of Footprints as a Measure of Vertical Height of the Arch and Functional Efficiency of the Foot," *Research Quarterly,* **6,** No. 2 (May 1935), 70.

[48]H. H. DePiero, "A Device for Measuring Foot Deviation," *Journal of American Podiatry Association,* **31** (March 1961), 203.

[49]Cameron Thompson, "Relationships Between Deviations of Human Feet and Their Strength and Flexibility," Doctoral Dissertation, University of Oregon, 1969.

feet of those with navicular drop were more flexible than were the feet of those in the control group.

Pedorule. The pedorule was proposed by Danforth[50] to measure the amount of deflection of the Achilles tendon from the perpendicular. In the normal foot, this tendon forms a straight line up the back of the leg from the heel. The pedorule consists of a rectangle of heavy plate glass, seven inches wide and nine inches high; the surface is marked in parallel lines one-tenth inch apart, the center line being colored for convenience in use.

Before testing, two ink dots are placed on the subject's tendon: midpoint as high on leg toward calf as possible and midpoint on back of heel. The center line of the pedorule should bisect the two ink dots on a normal foot. Two methods of using the pedorule were tried, with the following found to be most satisfactory.

1. Place the center line on the pedorule directly behind the center of the tendon at the point where it is bowed inward the farthest.

2. Count the number of lines from this point to the tips of the malleoli and subtract the distance from the tendon to the internal malleolus from the distance from the center of the bowed-in tendon to the external malleolus.

3. The score for correct position is zero, thus showing that the Achilles tendon is equidistant between the malleoli.

The reliability coefficient for this test was reported as 0.94. The correlations with the arch angle and the judgments of examiners were low, around 0.30 to 0.38.

FLEXIBILITY TESTS

The term *flexibility* is commonly defined as the range of possible movement about a joint or a sequence of joints. Range of motion tests have been in use for 75 years by orthopedists, physiatrists, and physical therapists in the treatment of orthopedic conditions that have temporarily restricted joint movement. These tests have mostly been confined to single joints. Special attention to overall trunk-hip flexibility came into prominence in physical education when the floor-touch test (contained in the Kraus-Weber Test of Minimum Muscular Fitness) received attention in the mid-fifties. Consideration is given below to both types of flexibility tests.

Single Joints

The Goniometer. In a literature review, Moore[51] showed that instruments for measuring the range of motion in joints of the body have been discussed since the turn of the century. The medical needs of both World Wars intensified its use in evaluating the rate of improvement of patients recovering from orthopedic disabilities. Many types of goniometers have been devised. Generally, measurement is based on degrees of a circle.

One form of the goniometer is illustrated in Figure 6.8. This device consists of a 180-degree protractor with extended arms, constructed from plexiglas. The two arms are 15 inches long; the one at the zero line is fixed, the other movable. A winged nut at the center point where the two arms meet may be tightened to hold the movable arm in position once the measurement is made.

The application of the goniometer is simple. For example, if the range of motion of the elbow joint is to be tested, the arms of the goniometer are placed parallel with the upper and lower arms of the body, with the center of motion at the elbow joint; readings are taken with the

[50]Harold R. Danford, "A Comparative Study of Three Methods of Measuring Flat and Weak Feet," *Supplement to the Research Quarterly,* **6,** No. 1 (March 1935), 43.

[51]Margaret L. Moore, "The Measurement of Joint Motion: Introductory Review of the Literature," *Physical Therapy Review,* **39,** No. 1 (January 1959), 1.

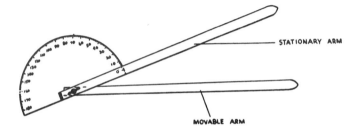

FIGURE 6.8. *The Goniometer*

elbow flexed as fully as the disability permits, and again with as full extension as possible; the difference between the two readings represents the range of motion.

Leighton Flexometer. Another device for measuring the range of motion of various joints is the flexometer, developed by Leighton,[52,53] illustrated in Figure 6.9. This instrument consists of a weighted 360-degree dial and a weighted pointer,

[52]Jack R. Leighton, "An Instrument and Technique for the Measurement of Range of Joint Motion," *Archives of Physical Medicine and Rehabilitation*, **36,** No. 9 (September 1955), 571.

[53]The Flexometer may be obtained from Leighton Flexometer, E. 1321 Fifty-fifth Avenue, Spokane, Washington 99203.

both moving freely and independently as affected by gravity. When the instrument is ready for use, the dial and the pointer point upward and coincide. A locking device is provided for the dial and another for the pointer. In use, the instrument is strapped on the moving part being tested. The dial is locked at one extreme position (that is, full flexion of the elbow); the movement is made and the pointer is locked at the other extreme position (that is, full extension of the elbow). Thus, the direct reading of the pointer on the dial is the range of motion which takes place. Thirty flexibility tests have been devised, involving movements of both trunk and extremities. Reliability coefficients for the various tests range from 0.889 to 0.997. Average range of motion for the tests are given in the reference.

Elgon. Karpovich and associates[54] have developed an electrogoniometer, called an elgon. In the elgon, a potentiometer is substituted for the protractor customarily used in goniometers; the potentiometer was designed originally for hearing-aid and transistor radio volume control. While a manual goniometer can only measure joint angles in stationary positions, the elgon can record continuously the changes in degrees of joint angles during motion.

[54]P. V. Karpovich and G. P. Karpovich, "Electrogoniometer: A New Device for Study of Joints in Action," *Federation Proceedings*, **18** (1959), 79.

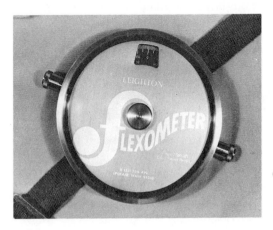

FIGURE 6.9. *Leighton Flexometer. Courtesy of Dr. J. R. Leighton.*

Trunk-Hip Flexibility Tests

General body flexibility, represented by hip and back flexion, has long been of interest to physical educators, as body suppleness has been considered advantageous in physical performances. A number of tests have been proposed to test this trait.

Scott and French Test.[55]   A 20-inch scale, marked in halfinch units, is attached to a stable bench or chair, so that half the scale is above and half below the level of the bench. An alternative method is to arrange the scale so that the bench level is zero with half-inch deviations progressing upward and downward from that point. The scale should not be more than three inches wide.

In taking this test, the subject stands with toes even with the front edge of the bench and against the sides of the scale. The trunk is bent forward, fingers in front of the scale. The subject then reaches slowly downward as far as possible, the finger tips of both hands moving parallel and equally down the scale. The knees must be kept straight. The score is the distance on the scale at the lowest point reached by the finger tips in the downward stretch. The authors advocate easy warm-up bobbings before taking the test.

Wells and Dillon Sit and Reach Test.[56]   The equipment for this test consists of a platform scale, two gymnasium (stall-bar) benches, and a piece of rubber matting about four feet square. The platform scale consists of a scale similar to that used by Scott and French, described above, with a center line marked zero, and with plus and minus scales on either side of the zero line. The support for this scale is in the form of

an elongated plus sign made of 11-inch boards resting on their edges. For convenience, these are referred to as the cross board and the stem board. Footprints are outlined on the cross board, one on either side of the stem board. The scale is attached to the upper edges of the support in such a way that when the subject is seated on the floor with the feet against the footprints, the zero line coincides with the near surface of the cross board and the minus values are toward the subject.

The equipment is placed near a wall. The two benches are placed side by side on their sides about 12 inches apart, with their legs against a wall. The scale is placed between the benches with the cross board braced against the benches. The rubber matting is spread on the floor in front of and partially under the scale.

In taking the test, the subject sits on the rubber matting, legs separated just enough to straddle the stem board, with the feet placed on the footprints and pressed firmly against the cross board. The arms are extended forward with the hands placed palms down on the upper surface of the scale. In this position, the subject bobs forward four times and holds the position of maximum reach on the fourth count. The knees must remain straight. If the hands reach unevenly, the hand reaching the shorter distance determines the score. The score is taken to the nearest half inch.

Kraus-Weber Floor-Touch Test.   This test will be described in Chapter 7 as an item in the Kraus-Weber Test of Minimum Muscular Fitness. It consists of the ability to touch the floor from a standing position, keeping the knees straight.

Evaluation

Considerable research has been done on the interrelationships among flexibility tests and their relationships with anthropometric and performance variables. Such results as the following may be cited.

[55]M. Gladys Scott and Esther French, *Measurement and Evaluation in Physical Education* (Dubuque, Iowa: Wm. C. Brown Company, 1959), p. 311.

[56]Katharine Wells and Evelyn Dillon, "The Sit and Reach: A Test of Back and Leg Flexibility," *Research Quarterly*, **23**, No. 1 (March 1952), 115.

1. The various flexibility tests presented are valid and reliable. The goniometer tests have a long history in orthopedics. The newer measures show face validity by measuring the range of motion in the joints specified. Reliability coefficients for these tests are consistently in the 0.90's.

2. Harris[57] factor analyzed the flexometer and several trunk-hip flexibility tests with 147 college women as subjects. Many of the correlations between the flexibility tests had zero or near zero values. The factor clusters were restricted to a very few variables and the clusters were essentially uncorrelated. The major conclusion stated by the investigator was that flexibility does not exist as a general characteristic of the human body; no one test gives a satisfactory indication of the flexibility characteristics of the individual. The same conclusion was reached by Holland[58] in a review of studies on the physiology of flexibility. However, Mathews, Shaw, and Bollen[59] obtained the following intercorrelations between trunk-hip flexibility tests for college women: 0.95, Kraus-Weber versus Wells-Dillon tests; 0.80, Kraus-Weber versus Leighton tests; and 0.74 Leighton versus Wells-Dillon tests.

3. Downie[60,61] studied the age differences in the flexibility of girls from 6 through 14 years, utilizing 19 flexometer tests. Generally, flexibility increased by age until 12 years and then declined. Odgers[62] obtained similar results with 160 boys ages 6 through 13 years.

4. Leighton[63] reviewed five of his articles containing studies with the flexometer. Among his findings were: (a) flexibility varies with habitual physical activity patterns; (b) flexibility patterns differ for different sports, paralleling skills and habits of basic movements peculiar to the skills involved; and (c) extending flexibility of some joints may detract from a given skill, and limiting range of movement in some joints may enhance some skills, such as those in track, basketball, and baseball. McCue[64] found that college women who had a past history of greater physical activity tended to be more flexible than did those who were less active.

5. Ferris[65] obtained low, mostly insignificant, correlations between trunk flexibility and measures of abdominal isometric and isotonic strength and endurance. For the most part, Odgers[66] found that boys 6 through 13 years of age with high and low scores on motor ability items did not differ significantly on flexometer tests. The significant differences obtained were: the more skilled boys in the standing broad jump, 30-yard dash, and softball distance throw were more flexible in trunk-extension-flexion; those with greatest distances in the softball throw had greater neck rotation and trunk lateral flexion flexibility.

6. Correlations are low between flexibility and such anthropometric measures as height, leg length, arm length, and trunk length.

CABLE-TENSION STRENGTH TESTS

In medicine, physical therapists have used "manual" tests to measure the strength of muscle groups weakened or impaired as a result of disease or injury. These tests have been used to determine the strength status of affected muscle groups at the beginning

[57]Margaret L. Harris, "A Factor Analytic Study of Flexibility," *Research Quarterly,* **40,** No. 1 (March 1969), 62.

[58]George J. Holland, "The Physiology of Flexibility," *Kinesiology Reviews,* 1968, p. 49.

[59]Donald K. Mathews, Virginia Shaw, and Merla Bollen, "Hip Flexibility of College Women as Related to Length of Body Segments," *Research Quarterly,* **28,** No. 4 (December 1957), 352.

[60]Patricia D. Downie, "A Study of the Relationship Between Flexibility Measures and Chronological Ages of Six to Ten Year Old Girls," Master's Thesis, University of Oregon, 1965.

[61]Patricia D. Downie, "A Study of the Flexibility Characteristics of Ten, Eleven, Twelve, Thirteen, and Fourteen Year Old Girls," Doctoral Dissertation, University of Oregon, 1970.

[62]Thomas W. Odgers, "A Study of the Relationships Between Flexibility Measures, Skill Performances, and Chronological Ages of Six to Thirteen Year Old Boys," Master's Thesis, University of Oregon, 1969.

[63]Jack R. Leighton, "On the Significance of Flexibility for the Physical Educator, *Journal of Health, Physical Education, and Recreation,* **31,** No. 8 (November 1960), 27.

[64]Betty F. McCue, "Flexibility Measures of College Women," *Research Quarterly,* **24,** No. 3 (October 1953), 316.

[65]Blake F. Ferris, "The Relationship Between Spinal Flexibility and Selected Measures of Abdominal Strength and Endurance," Master's Thesis, University of Oregon, 1966.

[66]Odgers, "Flexibility Measures, Skill Performances, and Chronological Ages."

of therapeutic exercise and, periodically, during the period of treatment in order to follow their improvement. In applying these tests, the examiner subjectively estimates the ability of muscles to overcome gravity and resistance applied manually. Williams[67] has presented the development and use of this form of testing. Daniels, Williams, and Worthingham[68] have carefully described the techniques involved in the administration of these tests. An early objective-type test for measuring the strength of muscles activating various joint movements was devised by Martin,[69] in which a spring balance was used for measuring the strength of 22 muscle groups. In this test a sling was fastened to the extremity with the pull at right angles to the long axis of the limb. An assistant held the spring balance, fastened to the other end of the sling. The subject contracted the muscle being tested and held it against the pull of the spring balance.

More recently, Clarke adapted the tensiometer,[70] an instrument designed to measure the tension of aircraft control cable, for testing the strength of individual muscle groups. Cable tension is determined from the force needed to create offset on a riser in a cable stretched between two set points, or sectors. This tension can be converted into pounds on a calibration chart. Thirty-eight strength tests were subsequently devised to measure the strength of muscles activating the following joints: fingers, thumb, wrist, forearm, elbow, shoulder, neck, trunk,

hip, knee, and ankle. Descriptions of the equipment needed for these tests and the testing techniques for the 38 strength movements are presented by Clarke and Clarke.[71] Illustrations of four of these tests appear in Chapter 7.

Research in the construction of these tests included: determination of body position which permitted greatest application of strength for each joint movement, selection of the joint angle which resulted in the strongest movement, and the study of such factors as the position of the pulling strap and the effect of gravity upon the test scores. The effectiveness of the following four instruments for recording muscle strength was studied: cable tensiometer, Wakim-Porter strain gauge, spring scale, and Newman myometer.[72] As reflected by objectivity coefficients, the tensiometer has greatest precision for strength testing (0.90 and above). It was the most stable and generally useful of the instruments.

Selected references

CLARKE, H. HARRISON, and DAVID H. CLARKE, *Developmental and Adapted Physical Education.* Englewood Cliffs, N.J.: Prentice-Hall, Inc., 1963, Chapter 4.

CURETON, THOMAS K., "Bodily Posture as an Indicator of Fitness," *Supplement to the Research Quarterly,* **11,** No. 2 (May 1941), 348.

HARRIS, MARGARET L., "A Factor Analytic Study of Flexibility," *Research Quarterly,* **40,** No. 1 (March 1969), 62.

KELLY, ELLEN D., *Adapted and Corrective Physical Education,* 4th ed. New York: Ronald Press Company, 1965.

[67]Marian Williams, "Manual Muscle Testing: Development and Current Use," *Second Congress Proceedings,* World Confederation for Physical Therapy, 1956, p. 115.

[68]Lucile Daniels, Marian Williams, and Catherine Worthingham, *Muscle Testing* (Philadelphia: W. B. Saunders Company, 1947).

[69]E. G. Martin, "Tests of Muscular Efficiency," *Physiological Review,* **1** (1921), 454.

[70]Manufactured by the Pacific Scientific Company, 6280 Chalet Drive, City of Commerce, California 90022.

[71]H. Harrison Clarke and David H. Clarke, *Developmental and Adapted Physical Education* (Englewood Cliffs, N.J.: Prentice-Hall, Inc., 1963), pp. 73–96.

[72]H. Harrison Clarke, "Comparison of Instruments for Recording Muscle Strength," *Research Quarterly,* **25,** No. 4 (December 1954), 398.

LEIGHTON, JACK R., "An Instrument and Technique for the Measurement of Range of Joint Motion," *Archives of Physical Medicine and Rehabilitation,* **36,** No. 9 (September 1955), 571.

LEIGHTON, JACK R., "On the Significance of Flexibility for the Physical Educator," *Jour-nal of Health, Physical Education, and Recreation,* **31,** No. 8 (November 1960), 27.

PHELPS, W. W., R. J. H. KIPHUTH, and C. W. GOFF, *The Diagnosis and Treatment of Postural Defects,* 2nd ed. Springfield Ill.: Charles C Thomas, 1956.

CHAPTER 7

The consensus of knowledgeable physical educators accepts strength as a primary component of physical fitness. While freedom from disease, organic soundness, and proper nutrition are essential elements for physical fitness, they are not alone sufficient to satisfy the definition of physical fitness proposed in Chapter 1; they do not by themselves provide "the ability to carry out daily tasks with vigor and alertness, without undue fatigue, and with ample energy to enjoy leisuretime pursuits and to meet unforeseen emergencies." The positive qualities of muscular strength, muscular endurance, and circulatory endurance are also needed. It is these elements that the physical educator is trained to understand, interpret, and use in developing the physical fitness of all.

Strength tests, although they do not measure all aspects of physical fitness as the physical educator views the problem, do deal with a basic element of the individual's general physical status. They have been used successfully in practical field sitautions, both as a means of selecting students for developmental classes, and for general classification in physical activities. The former use will be discussed in this chapter; the latter, in Chapter 12.

Strength Tests

The idea of using strength tests as a measure of physical condition is not new. Feats of strength and trials of endurance, practiced by savage tribes as well as by civilized man, have come down through the ages. Nor is the idea of combining strength tests into a formal battery for the purpose of measuring athletic ability a new one. Dudley A. Sargent, M.D., in 1880 proposed such a battery in which the individual elements were measured by calibrated mechanical instruments. It was not until 1925, however, when Dr. Frederick Rand Rogers standardized testing procedures and developed norm tables for their interpretation, that the relationships among physical condition, athletic performance, and muscular strength were demonstrated.[1]

The January 1973 issue of the *Physical Fitness Research Digest* was devoted to "a better understanding of muscular strength."[2] It was shown that strength is highly specific to various muscle groups of the body rather than general to all muscle groups. However, the overall strength of the musculature does not require testing of a large number of muscle groups, but can be accomplished from small batteries of three or four tests. The battery tests are typically selected by multiple correlation procedures with the composite of a larger number of similar tests serving as the criterion measure.

ROGERS PHYSICAL FITNESS INDEX

In selecting the individual elements composing the PFI battery, Rogers included only tests that would measure most of the

---

[1]Frederick Rand Rogers, *Physical Capacity Tests in the Administration of Physical Education* (New York: Bureau of Publications, Teachers College, Columbia University, 1926).

[2]H. Harrison Clarke, "Toward a Better Understanding of Muscular Strength," *Physical Fitness Research Digest*, President's Council on Physical Fitness and Sports, Series 3, No. 1 (January 1973).

large muscles of the body. As a result, the complete test involves the following muscle groups: forearms, upper arms, shoulder girdle, back, and legs. Most of the large muscles not tested are antagonistic to those tested—Rogers' composite test of seven elements is a reduction from ten tests given by Sargent.

With the construction of norm tables for many combinations of sex, age, and weight, two major scores are possible—the Strength Index and the Physical Fitness Index—each of which has a distinctly different purpose. By the construction of these norm tables, Rogers created the PFI.

The Strength Index. The Strength Index is the gross score obtained from the six strength tests plus lung capacity. It is proposed as a measure of *general athletic ability* and should be conceived neither as a measure of skill in any particular sport nor as a measure of physical fitness. It is with this measure, scored in kilograms and points rather than pounds and points, that Sargent was familiar. The old Sargent test was an athletic ability test only.

The Physical Fitness Index. The Physical Fitness Index is a score derived from comparing an achieved Strength Index with a norm based upon the individual's sex, weight, and age. It is a measure of basic physical fitness elements, including both muscular strength and muscular endurance.

ADMINISTRATION OF THE PFI TESTS

The Physical Fitness Index Test may be used for both boys and girls, the elements being the same for both sexes; however, the pull-up and push-up test for girls are less strenuous than those for boys. The various parts of the test, in the order in which they are usually administered, are described in detail here. In all tests, the subject should be encouraged to do his best *but should not strain.* "Normal strains of effort" should be encouraged; "extreme strains" should be avoided.

Age, Height, Weight

The age, height, and weight of the individual should be recorded, according to the following instructions:

1. Age should be taken in years and months, as 15 years, 7 months.

2. Height and weight should be taken in gymnasium uniforms, and recorded at the nearest half-inch and half-pound.

Lung Capacity

Lung capacity is measured in cubic inches with a *wet spirometer* (Figure 7.1).

1. The spirometer should be equipped with an extra-length rubber hose (36 to 42 inches), filled with water to within one inch of the top, and placed at such a height that all subjects can stand erect when beginning the test. A good arrangement for the majority of students is to place the base from four to four and one-half feet from the floor.

2. An individual wooden mouthpiece, the most hygienic, is used for each subject. The mouthpieces should not be handled by the tester, but should be inserted into the tube by the subject being tested. The wooden mouthpiece may be used repeatedly if thoroughly sterilized by boiling, steaming, or soaking for half an hour in an antiseptic solution, such as zephiran aqueous solution, $1/1000$. A glass mouthpiece is not recommended unless some method can be devised for instantaneous sterilization.

3. The subject should take one or two deep breaths before the test. Then, after the fullest possible inhalation, he should exhale slowly and steadily while bending forward over the hose until all the air within his control is expelled. Care should be taken to prevent air from escaping either through the nose or around the edges of the mouthpiece, and to see that a second breath is not taken by the subject during the test. If the test is improperly performed, or if, in the opinion of the tester,

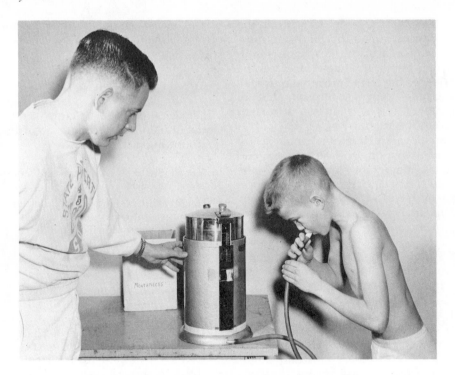

FIGURE 7.1. *Test of Lung Capacity with Wet Spirometer*

the pupil did not do his best, it should be repeated after an explanation of the precautions necessary to make the test a successful one.

4. The tester should watch the indicator closely to note when it reaches the highest point.

5. The rubber plug at the base of the spirometer should be removed when lowering the inner can after a test has been administered. (Some spirometers, as in the illustration, have an air-release valve on the top of the inner can rather than a plug at the base.) Care should be taken in lowering this can so that the water is not spilled. If at any time the inner can should "bobble" and refuse to rise higher with continued blowing into the hose, additional water is required. This situation will occur if there is an insufficient amount of water in the can, which may happen if the water level has been lowered through spilling.

Grip Strength

A *manuometer,* or *hand dynamometer,* of the rectangular type, is used to measure grip strength, both right and left hands being tested (Figure 7.2).

1. The tester should take the right corner of the manuometer between the thumb and forefinger of his right hand and place it in the palm of the subject's hand while holding the hand to be tested with his left hand in such a manner that the convex edge of the manuometer is between the first and second joints of the fingers and the rounded edge is against the base of the hand. The thumb should touch, or overlap, the first finger. The dial of the manuometer should be placed face down in the hand.

2. In taking the test, the subject's elbow should be slightly bent and his hand should describe a

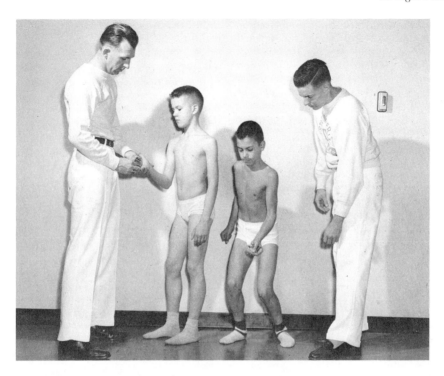

FIGURE 7.2. *Testing Grip Strength with Manuometer*

sweeping arc downward as he squeezes the manuometer. The hands should not be allowed to touch the body, or any object, while the test is being administered. If they do, the score should not be read at all, and retest should be given after a short rest period of 30 seconds.

3. The right hand should be tested first and then the left. Scores should be read to the nearest pound.

4. A cake of magnesium carbonate should be available for dusting the hands if they should become moist and slippery.

5. The indicator should be returned to zero after each test.

Back and Leg Dynamometer

The back and leg dynamometer is the instrument used in measuring the strength of both back and leg muscles.

1. Several back and leg dynamometers are on the market, the better ones being rather expensive. The instrument selected should be easy to read, should be calibrated in pounds, and should be capable of measuring a lift of at least 2500 pounds. The chain purchased with the dynamometer should be at least 24 inches in length, and the handle should be from 20 to 22 inches long.

2. Certain dynamometers are equipped to measure compression, or crushing strength. In testing for back and leg strength, the handles supplied for this purpose should be removed. The outer edge of the dynamometer carries the scale for measuring the lifting strength, while the inner scale is for crushing power.

3. Small pointers of white adhesive with the weight indicated on the broad ends may be placed at each hundred-pound interval on the dial to facilitate reading the lifts.

4. The dynamometer base should be placed on a small elevated platform, such as a stall bar bench. It is very important that this base be solid and steady so that the subject will have a feeling of security throughout the test. Stall-bar type benches may be purchased with the instrument. A runner should be attached to the supports of the bench platform, (as shown in Figure 7.4), for maximal stability.

5. The handle or cross-bar should be taped to facilitate firm handling by the subject; a block of magnesium carbonate or chalk should also be supplied with which to dust the hands if they are moist and slippery. Hinojosa and Berger[3] studied the use of a bare handle, a taped handle, and a strap to secure the hands to the lifting bar in performing the back lift. They

[3]Ralph Hinojosa and Richard A. Berger, "Effect of Variations in Hand Grip on Recorded Dynamometer Back Strength," *Research Quarterly,* **36,** No. 3 (October 1965), 366.

found that a taped bar was essential for maximal lifts.

6. In all lifting tests, the feet should be placed parallel, about six inches apart, with the center of the foot opposite the chain. To save the tester's time and energy, foot outlines should be painted on the base to indicate the position of the feet.

7. In back and leg lifts, the tester should guard against any snap resulting from a kink in the chain, which might jar the indicator beyond the true lift made by the subject.

Back Lift

1. With the feet in the proper position on the base of the dynamometer (see Figure 7.3), the subject should stand erect with the hands on the front of the thighs, fingers extended downward. The tester should then hook the chain so that the bar level is just below the finger tips. The subject should grasp the

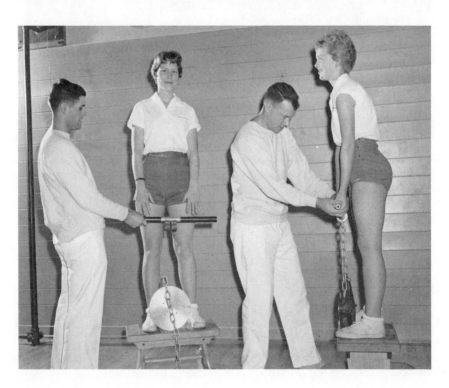

FIGURE 7.3. *Back Lift with Dynamometer*

handle firmly at the ends of the bar, with thumb clenching fingers and *with one palm forward and one palm backward.* When the subject is in position to lift, the back should be slightly bent at the hips, so that he will not completely straighten when lifting, but the legs should be straight with no bend at the knees. The head should be up and eyes directed straight ahead.

It is highly important not to bend the back too much, as the resultant poor leverage is conducive to a poor lift as well as to the possibility of strain. With the back properly bent, however, there is very little likelihood of injury from lifting.

2. The tester should grasp the subject's hands firmly during the lift. Hinojosa and Berger found that grasping of the hands actually did not make a difference in back lift scores of college men. The practice is recommended, however, if for no other reason than to give added stability of the subject and to enhance his confidence in making a maximal lift.

3. The subject should lift steadily. Care should be taken to keep the knees straight. The feet should be flat on the platform. It is necessary to retest after shortening the chain, if attempts to lift result in rising on the toes. Any initial lateral sway should be immediately checked.

4. At the end of lifting effort, the back should be almost straight. If not, repeat the test. Singh and Ashton[4] found that the best back lift scores were obtained with back angles of 163 to 170 degrees, which verifies the usual practice for this test.

Leg Lift

Two methods have been proposed for administering the leg lift on the back and leg dynamometer (see Figure 7.4). These methods may be characterized as "without the belt" and "with the belt." Everts and Hathaway[5] perfected the belt technique in order to obtain more objective results and to improve the validity of the PFI battery itself. The belt technique is now advocated and has been generally adopted by physical educators as the standard technique in the administration of the test. Consequently, the leg lift with the belt only is described below.

A belt may be purchased or may be made from pliable, tightly woven canvas belting, 5 feet 8 inches long, 4 inches wide, and about ⅛ inch thick. A loop is formed at one end of a size to fit snugly over one end of the lifting bar. This loop is formed by doubling back the last four inches of the belt and sewing firmly with double cross and diagonal stitching.

1. The subject should hold the bar with both hands together in the center, both palms down, so that it rests at the junction of thighs and

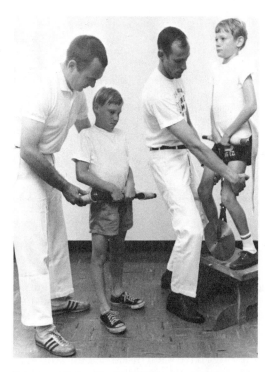

FIGURE 7.4. *Use of Belt in Testing Leg Strength*

[4]Mohan Singh and T. Edwin J. Ashton, "A Study of Back Lift Strength with Electrogoniometric Analysis of Hip Angle," *Research Quarterly,* **41,** No. 4 (December 1970), 562.

[5]Edgar W. Everts and Gordon J. Hathaway, "The Use of the Belt to Measure Leg Strength Improves the Administration of Physical Tests," *Research Quarterly,* **9,** No. 3 (October 1938), 62.

trunk. Care should be taken to maintain this position after the belt has been put in place and during the lift.

2. The loop end of the belt is slipped over one end of the handle or crossbar: the free end of the belt should be looped around the other end of the bar, tucking it in under so that it rests next to the body. In this position, the pressure of the belt against the body and the resultant friction of the free end against the standing part holds the bar securely. The belt should be placed as low as possible over the hips and gluteal muscles.

3. The subject should stand with his feet in the same position as for the back lift. The knees should be slightly bent. Maximum lifts occur when the subject's legs are nearly straight at the end of the lifting effort. Experienced testers become adept at estimating the potential lift by noting the degree of muscularity of the subject's legs. As a consequence, they will start the stronger subjects at a lower chain link, to allow for the extra distention in the dynamometer. If too high a link is used, the subject's knees may snap into hyperextension during the lift, although an alert tester can always anticipate such an occurrence and interrupt the performance.

4. Before the subject is instructed to lift, the tester should be sure that the arms and back are straight, the head erect, and the chest up. These details are of great importance to accurate testing. Beginners will err in results by from 100 to 300 or more pounds if the single detail of leg-angle is wrong. Therefore, even experienced testers repeat leg-lift tests for most subjects immediately, changing slightly the length of chain—*even by twisting, if a link seems too great.*

Pull-up Tests

In Rogers' construction of his strength battery, he administered the pull-up tests for boys and girls from rings attached loosely to a bar in order to allow the wrists to twist naturally as the subject performed the test. However, generally in practice, the rings have been discarded and the tests are given with hands grasping the chinning bar.

Boys' Pull-up Test. (The bar (see Figure 7.5) should be located high enough so that the feet of the tallest boy do not touch the floor when performing the test.)

1. In taking the pull-up test, the subject hangs from the bar by his hands with forward hand grip and chins himself as many times as he can. In executing the movement, he should pull himself up until his chin is even with his hands, then lower himself until his arms are straight. He should not be permitted to kick, jerk, or use a kip motion.

2. Half-counts are recorded if the subject does not pull all the way up, if he does not straighten his arms completely when lowering the body, or if he kicks, jerks, or kips in performing the movement. Only four half-counts are permitted.

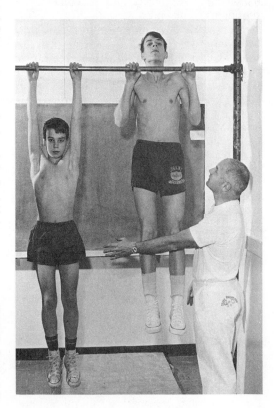

FIGURE 7.5. *Pull-up Test for Boys*

Girls' Pull-up Test. For the girls' pull-up test, Figure 7.6, use either an adjustable horizontal bar or one bar of the parallel bars, which permits convenient raising and lowering. A mat should be laid on the floor to prevent the feet from slipping.

1. The bar should be adjusted to approximately the height of the apex of the sternum, thus requiring each girl to pull approximately the same proportion of her weight. Time may be saved in adjusting the bar if the girls are arranged by heights at the beginning of the test.

2. The girl should grasp the bar with palms outward and should slide her feet under the bar until the body and arms form approximately a right angle when the body is held straight. The weight should rest on the heels.

3. The test is to pull up to the bar with the body held perfectly straight as many times as possible. The girls should pull a dead weight, the exercise being performed by the muscles of the arms and shoulder girdle only.

4. If the body sags, if the hips rise, or if the knees bend in a kip motion, or if the subject does not pull completely up or go completely down, half-credit only is given up to four half-credits.

A. E. Gay, formerly of the Lockport, New York, Public Schools, perfected a device that improves the procedure for administering the girls' pull-up test. This device consists of a platform with an adjustable heel rest which may be raised or lowered depending upon the height of the girl being tested, the bar remaining at a fixed height.

Push-up Tests

Boys' Push-up Test. The push-up test for boys (Figure 7.7) may be administered either on the regular gymnasium parallel bars or on wall parallels (or "dipping

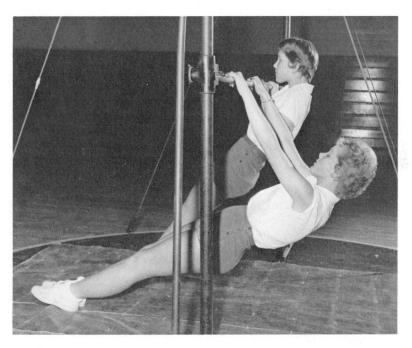

FIGURE 7.6. *Pull-up Test for Girls*

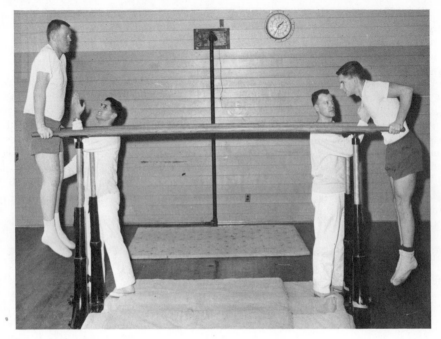

FIGURE 7.7. *Push-up Test, or Bar Dips, for Boys*

bars"). The regulation parallel bars are preferred, since their width and height may be adjusted to the height of the subject.

1. The bars should be adjusted at approximately shoulder height.

2. The subject should stand at the end of the parallel bars, grasping one bar in each hand. He jumps to the front support with arms straight (this counts *one*). He lowers his body until the angle of the upper arm and forearm is less than a right angle, then pushes up to the straight-arm position (this counts *two*). This movement is repeated as many times as possible. The subject should not be permitted to jerk or kick or stop and rest when executing push-ups.

3. At the first dip for each subject, the tester should gauge the proper distance the body should be lowered by observing the elbow angle. He should then hold his fist or fingers so that the subject's shoulder just touches it on repeated movements.

4. If the subject does not go down to the proper bent-arm angle or all the way up to a straight-arm position, half-credit only is given, up to four half-credits.

Push-Up Test for Girls. The push-up test for girls (Figure 7.8) is executed from a stall bar bench, or a stool, 13 inches high by 20 inches long by 14 inches wide. It should be placed on a mat about six inches from a wall so that subjects will not take a position too far forward.

1. The girl should grasp the outer edges of the bench or stool at the nearest corners and assume the front-leaning rest position, with the balls of her feet resting on the mat and with her body and arms forming a right angle.

2. The test is to lower the body so that the upper chest touches the near edge of the stall bar bench, then raise it to a straight-arm position as many times as possible. In performing the test, the girl's body should be held straight throughout.

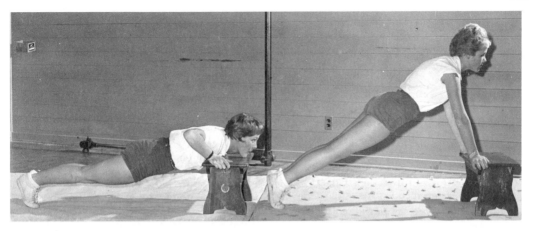

FIGURE 7.8. *Push-up Test for Girls*

3. If the body sways or arches, or if the subject does not go completely down or does not push completely up, half-credit is given, up to four half-credits.

General Instructions for Pull-up and Push-up Tests.   General instructions in administering pull-ups and push-ups tests follow.

1. After four half-credits have been recorded in the push-up and pull-up tests for both boys and girls, no more should be allowed for partial performance. The tester should give reasons for half counts scores as they occur.

2. At the fifth incomplete exercise, it is advisable to stop the test and repeat after a rest period.

3. Counting should be audible to the subject, the count being made sharply at the end of each evolution.

4. The subject should rest five minutes between the pull-up and push-up tests unless fewer than three counts have been made. No rest periods are necessary between the other parts of the test.

Scoring

Scoring of the Physical Fitness Index tests is accomplished in the following manner.

Arm Strength: Arm strength is scored according to the following formula:

$$(\text{pull-ups} + \text{push-ups})\left(\frac{W}{10} + H - 60\right),$$

in which W represents the weight in pounds, and H the height in inches. Fractions are corrected to nearest whole numbers.

For example, a boy pulls up 7 and pushes up 8 times. His weight is 155 pounds and his height 68 inches.

$$(7 + 8)\left(\frac{155}{10} + 68 - 60\right),$$
$$\text{or}$$
$$(15)(16 + 8)$$

which gives an arm strength of 360 pounds. If the subject is below 61 inches in height, height should be disregarded in the formula.

Strength Index: The Strength Index, or SI, is the total score determined by adding together the scores made on each test item: lung capacity, right grip, left grip, back strength, leg strength, and arm strength.

The Norm: The norm charts are based upon sex, weight, and age, the normal score being changed for each two-pound increase in weight and for each half-year increase in age. Instead of interpolating to determine the *norm* for those individuals between points on the norm chart, the weight above and the age below should be taken. For example, if an individual weighs 151 pounds, the norm at 152 should be taken; if he is 16 years and 5 months of age, the norm at 16 years should be taken.

As norm charts have been prepared for PFI tests both when the belt is used in the leg lift and when it is not used, care should be taken to use the proper chart in scoring the tests. Norm charts (with belt) appear in Appendix Table B.2.

Physical Fitness Index: The Physical Fitness Index is computed from the following formula:

$$ \text{PFI} = \frac{\text{achieved SI}}{\text{normal SI}} \times 100. $$

SUGGESTIONS FOR ADMINISTERING PFI TESTS

Many problems are encountered in administering the Physical Fitness Index tests efficiently and accurately.[6] Several suggestions that may prove helpful are given below; others that apply to testing in general will be found in Chapter 16.

1. Accurate instruments: The accuracy of testing instruments should be checked at least once a year. A rough check on the back and leg dynamometer may be made by suspending several known weights from it and reading the scores on the dial. In a study by Clarke and Geser,[7] the mean right grip strength scores for 34 col-

lege men obtained with three manuometers purchased from two manufacturing concerns were as follows: 136 pounds, 124 pounds, and 103 pounds. Murray[8] describes a number of ways for the physical educator to check the accuracy of this and other testing instruments.

2. Trained testers: Trained testers are essential. Unless tests are given properly and accurately, the results will be misleading and, thus, the time spent in giving them worse than wasted. Mathews[9] demonstrated pronounced differences between skilled and unskilled testers in results obtained in administering the PFI test. For all test items, the skilled testers obtained significantly higher mean scores than did the unskilled testers. For example, the skilled testers obtained a mean PFI of 107; for the unskilled testers, the mean was 90.[10] Hubbard and Mathews[11] found that, when testing for leg lift strength, higher scores were achieved when the subjects attained a maximum lift and then lunged backward (a practice which is not a permissible PFI testing technique).

Van Dalen and Peterson[12] and Wear[13] obtained significantly higher grip strength scores when the manuometer was placed with the dial toward the palm than when placed with the dial turned outward.

Thus, careful attention to the prescribed detail of administering these strength tests is

[6]Strength testing instruments may be obtained from such concerns as the following: Narragansett Gymnasium Equipment Corp., 110 West Carpenter St., Moberly, Mo. 65270; Nissen Corp., 930 27th Ave., S. W. Cedar Rapids, Iowa 52406; J. A. Preston Corp. 71 Fifth Ave., New York, N.Y. 10003.

[7]H. Harrison Clarke and L. Richard Geser, "Comparison of Three Manuometers," *Research Quarterly,* **28,** No. 2 (May 1957), 173.

[8]Kenneth Murray, "Calibration and Uses of Fitness Tests in Westmount High School, Quebec," *Supplement to the Research Quarterly,* **6,** No. 1 (March 1935), 12.

[9]Donald K. Mathews, "Comparison of Testers and Subjects in Administering Physical Fitness Index—Tests," *Research Quarterly,* **24,** No. 4 (December 1953), 442.

[10]Some, but by no means all, of this difference may be due to the skilled testers giving the second test to all subjects; the subjects, therefore, had the benefit of some experience in taking the test, which may logically have increased their scores.

[11]Alfred W. Hubbard and Donald K. Mathews, "Leg Lift Strength: A Comparison of Measurement Methods," *Research Quarterly,* **24,** No. 1 (March 1953), 33.

[12]D. B. Van Dalen and C. A. Peterson, "A Comparative Study of the Administration of the Manuometer," *Physical Educator,* **7,** No. 2 (May 1950), 52.

[13]C. L. Wear, "Further Study of the Administration of the Manuometer," *Physical Educator,* **9,** No. 3 (October 1952), 82.

imperative for the proper results. The back and leg strength tests are the most difficult to administer and require not only proper instruction and supervision but considerable practice.

3. Organization for testing: With a sufficient number of trained testers available, the next problem is to organize procedures so that a maximum number of pupils are tested during each hour or day of testing. Economy in testing time requires that pupils be made available in a continuous, unbroken procession. The method of testing pupils during their physical education class period results in tremendous loss of time, conservatively estimated at from 30 to 40 percent, as the testing line must be started and stopped each period.

With pupils readily available, testing stations should be set up in such a manner that pupils can pass from one to another in a continuous line. Student lines should not cross when passing from station to station. The stations should be as follows:

Station 1: Age, height, and weight: record cards, scales, stadiometer.

Station 2: Lung capacity: wet spirometer.

Station 3: Grip strength: manuometer.

Station 4: Back and leg strength: preferably two back and leg dynamometers, two belts, and three dynamometer handles.

Station 5: Pull-ups (boys): Horizontal bar (or substitute). Pull-ups (girls): Adjustable horizontal bar (or one bar of the parallel bars, Gay's apparatus, or substitute) and floor mat.

Station 6: Push-ups (boys): Parallel bars or wall parallels (or substitute). Push-ups (girls): Stall bar bench and mat.

Station 7: *Scoring Method A:* four scorers, each of whom makes one of the following calculations: (a) arm strength, (b) strength index, (c) normal-strength index, and (d) physical fitness index (an adding machine is very helpful in scoring). *Scoring Method B:* an electrical calculator (one operator and an assistant to look up norms). By either method, A or B, PFI's can be computed as fast as the tests are given.

Special mention should be made of organization procedures that may be followed in administering back and leg lifts rapidly. Owing to the extra operation of placing the belt on the subject, more time is necessary for administering the leg lift than for any other single test in the PFI battery. Two methods may be followed to reduce the time necessary for the test, as follows:

a. If two back and leg dynamometers are available, one may be used for the back lift and the other for the leg lift. With an extra tester and two handles and two belts for the latter instrument, the belt can be adjusted to one subject while the subject preceding him is taking the lift. The subject is thus ready for the lift as soon as he takes his place for the test.

b. If only one back and leg dynamometer is available, the order of the tests may be reversed, giving the leg lift first and the back lift last. With an extra tester and a second handle, the belt can be adjusted to one subject while the subject preceding him is taking the back lift. Obviously, back and leg lifts cannot be given as rapidly with one instrument as with two, but the procedure described will reduce considerably the testing time from what otherwise would be required for these tests.

With a sufficient number of trained testers, therefore, with pupils available in a continuous procession, and with the testing apparatus arranged on the gymnasium floor as indicated above, pupils can be tested at the rate of one a minute, or 60 per hour.

4. Order of tests: Rogers originally contended that the order of administering his strength test items should be maintained in the following order: lung capacity, grip tests, back lift, leg lift, pull-ups, and push-ups. However, Allen[14] found that the order in which test items were administered did not influence the results obtained with the MacCurdy Force Index. The MacCurdy index contains the same test items as the PFI, except pulls and pushes on a dynamometer are substituted for pull-ups and push-ups. Thus, the exact order of PFI test

[14]James H. Allen, "Influence of Order upon the MacCurdy Force Index," Doctoral Dissertation, Indiana University, 1956.

administration is not essential, except the pull-ups and push-ups should be last to avoid possible carry over of fatigue effects to the other strength efforts. In this situation, however, some time can be saved, without adverse effect, by testing lung capacity during the rest period between pull-ups and push-ups.

5. Practice tests: It is essential that physical fitness tests be administered accurately, and that the derived PFI of a pupil be his true score. If the testing period is preceded by class sessions during which the tests have been taught and practiced, he may be reasonably sure of his results. If, however, this has not been possible, it is advisable to retest low students before studying their individual cases or starting developmental programs. This procedure is especially important if pupils have not been previously tested. Retests are advisable, also, if the situation at the time of the annual tests does not approximate normal conditions. For example, the initial tests in one school system were conducted at a time when many pupils had been absent from school because of measles and many others had just been vaccinated. The retests in this situation, quite naturally, showed many significant increases. In addition, pupils who feel they can "do better" on the test should be allowed to repeat it. Fundamentally, the physical educator should be sure that the score assigned to a low-fitness pupil is an accurate one. A little extra time spent at this point will be well worthwhile in the saving of pupil- and teacher-time later on.

6. Warm-up period: A few light calisthenic exercises are advisable before students take the Physical Fitness Tests. Better results are achieved through this brief warm-up period, and there is less likelihood of sore muscles following the completion of the test.

THE PFI AS A MEASURE
OF PHYSICAL FITNESS

The reliability and objectivity of the Physical Fitness index tests, when administered by competent testers, were established by Rogers[15] and have since been verified by other investigators working independently. With tests taken four months apart, the test-retest correlations ranged from 0.86 for leg lift to 0.97 for lung capacity; the correlation for the Strength Index was 0.94.

Physical Fitness Elements

The Physical Fitness Index battery contains test items for two basic elements of physical fitness, muscular strength and muscular endurance. It does not contain items which measure the circulatory-respiratory type of endurance, so essential in sustained running, swimming, and the like. Thus, the PFI does not measure all aspects of fitness, as the physical educator views the problem.

Muscular strength and muscular endurance are not the same, although they are related. Individuals with greatest muscular strength have greatest absolute endurance; however, stronger muscles tend to maintain a smaller proportion of maximum strength than do weaker muscles. Tuttle and associates[16] obtained a correlation of 0.90 between the maximum strength of the back and leg muscles and their absolute endurance; the correlation between the strength and relative endurance (average strength maintained) was −0.40 and −0.48 for back and leg muscles respectively. Clarke[17] verified these results, and, further, showed a number of other muscular strength-endurance relationships resulting from his studies with the tensiometer and the ergograph. As a consequence, the need for including both strength and endurance elements in physical fitness testing was demonstrated.

In order to understand the PFI better and to evaluate its significance, two impor-

---

[15]Rogers, *Physical Capacity Tests,* p. 32.

[16]W. W. Tuttle, C. D. Janney, and J. V. Salzano, "Relation of Maximum Back and Leg Strength to Back and Leg Strength Endurance," *Research Quarterly,* **26,** No. 1 (March 1955), 96.

[17]H. Harrison Clarke, *Muscular Strength and Endurance in Man* (Englewood Cliffs, N.J.: Prentice-Hall, Inc., 1966), p. 184.

tant concepts should be made clear. First, in order for a condition to affect strength, it must have systemic implications, that is, be total-body in its reaction. For example, if one has a sore toe, it might be an inconvenience and an annoyance, but it would not affect one's strength or lower the PFI. When, however, that same toe becomes infected, a systemic condition is established, muscles weaken, and the PFI drops. If, therefore, such conditions as body fatigue, lack of exercise, improper diet, diseased tonsils, abscessed teeth, ulcers, cancers, and the like, have total-body reactions, the strength of the muscles is affected—and the PFI declines.

The second important concept is that the PFI is a generalized index, as the name implies—not a diagnosis. It may be compared to the use of a clinical thermometer by a physician. If the thermometer reading indicates that the individual has a temperature above normal, it tells the physician that something is wrong, not what that something is. In like manner, a low PFI indicates a lack of physical condition, a lowered body vitality, but not what the cause might be. Like the patient with a fever, the individual with a low PFI should be studied in order to determine the cause of this condition. The analogy may be carried further. Individuals with high or rapidly changing temperatures almost always need a physician's care. Individuals with low, high, or rapidly changing PFI's need the physical educator's care, and they may or may not also need the attention of physicians.

Validity of the Physical Fitness Index

Physicians' Estimates of Health Status. In studying the validity of the PFI as an indicator of physical fitness, Chamberlain and Smiley[18] gave Rogers' original form of the

test to 65 university men. These men were also given physical examinations by university physicians upon which estimates of health status were made. Fifty-two, or 80 percent, of the subjects fell into the same fitness classification by both physicians' judgments and PFI scores.

Significance of a Change in Strength. A number of studies have been conducted showing the significance of a change in strength to a change in physical fitness. The effects of illness, fatigue, and organic drains upon the strength of the body are shown, for example, by experiments with grip strength. In these studies, the manuometer was used to make a daily record of grip strength, and any changes that occurred were noted.

Only the original investigation by Rogers[19] will be reported here as an illustration of the use of grip strength as a *measure* of changing body condition. This experiment was performed on an adult male subject who, after being trained in grip-test technique, tested himself daily or oftener. Following are several of his observations: (a) his grip strength dropped 30 points (from 170 to 140) before he was aware of approaching influenza; (b) an unusually fatiguing day (90 holes of golf and a square dance) resulted in no change in grip strength at bed time, but a drop of 30 points was recorded the next morning; (c) severe fatigue of the forearms caused drops of 35 to 60 points, depending upon the degree of exhaustion induced, with corresponding delay in return to normal.

Representative Case Studies. The mass of material contained in case studies of pupils with low Physical Fitness Indices gives considerable evidence of the significance of the PFI in revealing physical condition. Many cases are on record in which low or

[18]C. C. Chamberlain and D. F. Smiley, "Functional Health and the Physical Fitness Index," *Research Quarterly,* **2,** No. 1 (March 1931), 193.

[19]F. R. Rogers, "The Significance of Strength Tests in Revealing Physical Condition," *Research Quarterly,* **5,** No. 3 (October 1934), 43.

declining PFI's have indicated the presence of organic drains within the individual. The number of such cases, however, is relatively small. The majority of low-fitness students require mostly the proper amount and kind of exercise, the modification of health habits, relaxation programs, and the like. However, over many years, physicians who have examined referrals of pupils with low PFI scores by physical educators have often found such causes of low relative strength: thyroid deficiency, spinal meningitis, encephalitis, anemia, post-malarial condition, ulcer, cancer, syringomyelia, tuberculosis, and emotional strain. Subsequent improvement in strength scores following effective treatment is a typical experience in following such cases.

After studying carefully the case studies of 50 college freshmen and sophomores with low PFI's, Page[20] described the average college "low PFI student" as follows: John Doe, 20 percent overweight, high scholastic aptitude (although doing poor scholastic work), below normal in social adjustment, lives at home or commutes, is employed, did not participate actively in the high-school physical education program, is not (at first) particularly interested in physical activity, is lacking in physical skills, and has such faulty health habits as smoking, insufficient sleep, and incorrect diet. Similar results were obtained from case studies of 78 low PFI college students by Coefield and McCollum.[21,22]

Athletic Abilities.   While the PFI is not intended as an athletic ability test, studies have shown that this measure of relative (to age and weight) strength does contribute to success in sports participation. In the 12-year longitudinal growth study in the Medford, Oregon public schools,[23] boys playing on interschool teams were classified by their coaches as outstanding (3), regular players (2), and substitutes (1). The following tabulation shows the PFI means of nonparticipants (NP) and athletes in the various classifications at the upper elementary and junior high school levels:

	Coaches Ratings			
	NP	1	2	3
Upper elementary school	108	113	121	123
Junior high school	114	122	126	131

The average PFI's of the nonparticipants was high, appreciably exceeding the normal PFI of 100 and, for the junior high school boys, nearly equalling the normal third quartile of 115. Still, the athletes at both school levels were higher, with the means increasing with athletic classifications. These results were substantiated in Whittle's study[24] of 12-year-old sixth grade boys from poor and good elementary school physical education programs who participated "a lot" in out-of-class physical activities.

Limitation of Norms

Before pupils can be properly selected for individual attention in physical fitness programs, the limitations of norms should be understood. Norms are derived from testing many representative subjects and

[20]C. Getty Page, "Case Studies of College Men with Low Physical Fitness Indices." Master's Thesis, Syracuse University, 1940.

[21]John R. Coefield and Robert H. McCollum, "A Case Study Report of 78 University Freshman Men with Low Physical Fitness Indices," Master's Thesis, University of Oregon, 1955.

[22]See Chapter 6, "The Case Study Approach," in H. Harrison Clarke and David H. Clarke, *Developmental and Adapted Physical Education* (Englewood Cliffs, N.J.: Prentice-Hall, Inc., 1963).

[23]H. Harrison Clarke, "Characteristics of Young Athletes," *Physical Fitness Research Digest*, President's Council on Physical Fitness and Sports, Series 3, No. 2 (April 1973).

[24]Presented in Ch. 3.

determining averages and distributions from these data. Thus, norms present the status quo, which may not and probably do not reflect desirable standards. Factors that might be considered by the physical educator in applying norms follow.

1. As applied to developmental traits, such as muscular strength, the norms may not coincide with local situations. For example, in the presence of little or no physical education, the normal PFI pattern of 85–100–115 for the first quartile, median, and third quartile fits well. However, in schools with strong physical fitness programs, a much higher pattern exists as has been shown in the Medford, Oregon and Ellensburg, Washington schools, at LaSierra High School in California, and elsewhere. What is said of the PFI can also be said of motor fitness tests, as many physical educators have experienced with the AAHPER Youth Fitness Test.

2. The establishment and application of norms for all subjects in a particular designation do not allow for factors that make individuals "normally" different. An obvious example, as related to strength, is the person's somatotype. In the Medford Boys' Growth Study,[25] the PFI's of endomorphs were much lower than were the PFI's of mesomorphs, ectomorphs, and mid-types; all boys classified as primary endomorphs were unable to perform a single pull-up. Attempts to improve the endomorphic boy or girl should surely be made through weight reduction and strength improvement, but limited initial performances in physical activities should be expected.

Often norms do not fit extreme cases. In establishing norm tables, a sufficiently large number of cases usually is not available to describe adequately individuals at the upper and lower ends of the scale so that typical performances can be determined. In terms of the Physical Fitness Tests, this exception means the very large and the very small individuals.

THE SELECTION OF PFI CASES FOR FOLLOW-UP ATTENTION

The High PFI

Another factor that further complicates the selection of pupils in need of fitness programs is the high PFI individual, as there is evidence to support the contention that his condition *may* be dangerous. Individuals with such scores may be "on edge," "keyed up," about to "go stale," or even in danger of a nervous breakdown.

A median PFI of 150, with but six cases below 95, was recorded in testing 116 boys and girls from 10 to 16 years of age in a Massachusetts state rest camp for children with tubercular tendencies. The most noticeable condition of these children on entering camp was an extreme nervousness, characterized by inability to relax, to sleep during rest periods, and to get to sleep at night. Elizabeth Zimmerli[26] has reported several cases of extremely high PFI's running from 156 to 202. These individuals were variously described by the following characteristics: over-trained, overactive, high-strung, overstimulated, overanxious, overambitious, overdeveloped. The late Ellis H. Champlin summed up this condition when he called these individuals "activity drunkards."

Selection of PFI Cases for Study

It is apparent from the above that the selection of PFI cases for study and treatment is not so simple as many believe. The designation of "all below" an arbitrary PFI point, such as 85, as "needing individual care" is inadequate, since by so doing many cases in need of special developmental programs are missed. Actually, there are at least three groups needing special consideration:

---

[25]H. Harrison Clarke, *Physical and Motor Tests in the Medford Boys' Growth Study* (Englewood Cliffs, N.J.: Prentice-Hall, Inc., 1971), p. 81.

[26]Elizabeth Zimmerli, "Case Studies of Unusual Physical Fitness Indices," *Supplement to the Research Quarterly,* **6,** No. 1 (March 1935), 246.

1. Individuals with PFI's in the lower ranges. The abnormally weak obviously need attention. The physical educator should decide upon the number of pupils for whom he can provide individual programs and select a large portion of these from the low PFI scores.

2. Individuals whose PFI's decline on repeated tests, regardless of their PFI level. Such drops are usually definite danger signs, indicating changes in physical condition which need to be checked. It is essential, after each general testing period, to examine all record cards to discover those whose PFI's are dropping. A drop of from five to ten points is significant.

3. Individuals with PFI's in the upper ranges. An extremely high PFI may indicate that the individual is over-trained, overactive, high-strung, overstimulated, overdeveloped. A PFI of 150 is considered sufficiently high to warrant investigation for factors that may cause this condition, and to provide a program of rest and relaxation if indicated. It should be recognized, of course, that high PFI's may be due to the development of excellent physiques through participation in such activities as weight lifting, gymnastics, modern and ballet dance, and the like, and are proper for those individuals.

SUGGESTED CHANGES IN PFI TESTS

Since its origin, the Physical Fitness Index battery has been repeatedly changed in procedures, norms, and interpretations. While the PFI test remains as described above, there have been a number of modifications proposed.

Oregon Simplification

While the Physical Fitness Index and the Strength Index have been used effectively in school and college physical education programs, many users readily acknowledge that the following extraneous factors prevent their more general use: cost of testing equipment, time required for giving the test to many students, and necessity for well-trained testers. As a con-

sequence, several investigators at the University of Oregon undertook the simplification of the battery for both boys and girls from the fourth grade through college. Multiple correlations between 0.977 and 0.998 were obtained between the Strength Index and various test items composing the SI battery for the different studies.

Regression equations for each of the multiple correlations were computed. By use of the appropriate equation, the physical educator is able to estimate approximately the SI each boy or girl would have achieved had he or she taken the full test. Thus, the regular SI norms may be used to estimate Physical Fitness Indices. For some groups, two equations were computed; as will be seen, the B equation requires one more test than the A equation. The B equations approximate actual Strength Indices with greater accuracy than the A equations. The various regression equations appear on page 143.

The physical educator using one or more of these equations may easily prepare tables for their ready computation. At the top of page 144 is an illustration based on 1.35 (back lift) appearing in the equation for upper elementary school boys.

Following is an illustration of computing the PFI by use of a regression equation. The subject is a junior high school boy, 14 years 5 months of age and 149 pounds in weight (equation A): 1.33 (leg lift) + 1.2 (arm strength) + 286.

Test Item	Score	Repression Weighting
Leg lift	1260	1676
Arm strength	480	576
Constant		286
Predicted Strength Index		2538

From the norm chart, Appendix Table B.2, this boy's norm for age and weight is 1878. Thus, his predicted PFI is 135.

Upper Elementary School Boys[27]

$$SI = 1.05 \text{ (leg lift)} + 1.35 \text{ (back lift)} + 10.92 \text{ (push ups)} + 133$$

Upper Elementary School Girls[28]

A: $SI = 1.25 \text{ (leg lift)} + 1.01 \text{ (arm strength)} + 254$
B: $SI = 1.16 \text{ (leg lift)} + 1.07 \text{ (arm strength)} + 1.06 \text{ (lung capacity)} + 164$

Junior High School Boys[29]

A: $SI = 1.33 \text{ (leg lift)} + 1.20 \text{ (arm strength)} + 286$
B: $SI = 1.12 \text{ (leg lift)} + .99 \text{ (arm strength)} + 5.19 \text{ (right grip)} + 129$

Junior High School Girls[30]

A: $SI = 1.19 \text{ (leg lift)} + 1.06 \text{ (arm strength)} + 442$
B: $SI = 1.04 \text{ (leg lift)} + 1.03 \text{ (arm strength)} + 1.37 \text{ (back lift)} + 175$

Senior High School Boys[31]

A: $SI = 1.22 \text{ (leg lift)} + 1.23 \text{ (arm strength)} + 499$
B: $SI = 1.07 \text{ (leg lift)} + 1.06 \text{ (arm strength)} + 1.42 \text{ (back lift)} + 194$

Senior High School Girls[32]

A: $SI = 1.19 \text{ (leg lift)} + 1.15 \text{ (arm strength)} + 408$
B: $SI = 1.04 \text{ (leg lift)} + 1.08 \text{ (arm strength)} + 1.46 \text{ (back lift)} + 125$

College Men[33]

A: $SI = 1.27 \text{ (leg lift)} + 1.19 \text{ (arm strength)} + 544$
B: $SI = 1.54 \text{ (leg lift)} + 1.06 \text{ (arm strength)} + 1.13 \text{ (back lift)} - 357$

College Women[34]

A: $SI = 1.18 \text{ (leg lift)} + 1.10 \text{ (arm strength)} + 468$
B: $SI = 1.26 \text{ (leg lift)} + \text{ (arm strength)} + 1.37 \text{ (back lift)} + 68$

[27]H. Harrison Clarke and Gavin H. Carter, "Oregon Simplification of the Strength and Physical Fitness Indices for Upper Elementary, Junior High, and Senior High School Boys," *Research Quarterly*, **30,** No. 1 (March 1959), 3.

[28]Marilyn R. Parrish, "Simplification of Rogers' Strength and Physical Fitness Indices for Upper Elementary School Girls," Master's Thesis, University of Oregon, 1965.

[29]Clarke and Carter, "Strength and Physical Fitness Indices," p. 3.

[30]Joanne Widness, "Simplification of the Rogers' Strength and Physical Fitness Indices for Junior and Senior High School Girls," Master's Thesis, University of Oregon, 1964.

[31]Clarke and Carter, "Strength and Physical Fitness Indices," p. 3.

[32]Widness, "Rogers' Strength and Physical Fitness Indices."

[33]Calvin K. Yasumiishi, "Simplification of the Rogers' Strength and Physical Fitness Index for College Men," Master's Thesis, University of Oregon, 1960.

[34]Judith B. Hall, "Simplification of the Rogers' Strength and Physical Fitness Index for College Women," Master's Thesis, University of Oregon, 1964.

1.35 (Back Lift)

	0	10	20	30	40	50	60	70	80	90
		14	27	41	54	68	81	95	108	122
100	135	149	162	176	189	203	216	230	243	257
200	270	284	297	311	324	338	351	365	378	392
300	405	419	432	446	459	473	486	500	513	527

Use of Tensiometer

The most expensive instrument necessary for administering the PFI test is the back and leg dynamometer. Also, the two tests given with this instrument are the most difficult to administer in the battery. This is especially true for the leg lift, where considerable judgment is necessary in placing the subject at the start of the test so that his knees will be nearly straight at the end, as the dynamometer spring elongates somewhat as pressure is applied. As a consequence, Kennedy[35] sought to substitute the tensiometer for the dynamometer in back and leg lift testing; this instrument is much cheaper than the dynamometer and the pull is against a cable which does not stretch.

The capacity of the tensiometer used was 800 pounds, which was sufficient to measure back lifts directly. However, for the leg lift test, a lever system was devised, which permitted lifts up to 2400 pounds. The correlations between strength scores obtained with the dynamometer and tensiometer were 0.92 and 0.95 for the back and leg lifts respectively. The means and standard deviations obtained with the two instruments for these tests were comparable. Thus, it was demonstrated that the tensiometer could be substituted for the dynamometer in back and leg strength testing without essential loss of validity for these tests.

[35]Frank T. Kennedy, "Substitution of the Tensiometer for the Dynamometer in Back and Leg Lift Testing," *Research Quarterly,* **30,** No. 2 (May 1959), 179.

McCloy's Revisions

McCloy proposed three changes in the PFI battery: one known as his Strength Index Revision; a second, as the Athletic Strength Index; the third, as the Pure Strength Index.

1. Strength Index Revision.[36] Two changes in the PFI battery are suggested: a different formula for computing arm strength, and the elimination of lung capacity. Otherwise, the test items remain the same, except that the old method of testing leg strength (without belt) is followed.

In discussing arm strength determined from push-ups and pull-ups, McCloy states that the formula used by Rogers unduly penalizes the individual who is small and unduly rewards the person whose dipping and chinning are above the average. He experimentally developed the following formula for the computation of chinning and dipping strength.

Boys: Chinning *or* dipping strength = 1.77 (weight) + 3.42 (chins or dips) − 46.
Chinning *and* dipping strength = 3.54 (weight) + 3.42 (pull-up + push-ups) − 92.

Girls: Chinning strength = .67 (weight) + 1.2 (chins) + 52.
Dipping strength = .78 (weight) + 1.1 (dips) + 74.

In subsequent studies, correlations of the magnitude of 0.95 were obtained between McCloy's arm strength scores and body weight for both college men and junior high school boys. These results are supported logically when it is realized that weight is nearly doubled

[36]C. H. McCloy and Norma D. Young, *Tests and Measurements in Health and Physical Education,* 3rd ed. (New York: Appleton-Century-Crofts, 1954), p. 129.

(1.77 weight) in the equation and the constant deducted (-46) usually equals or is more than the amount included for chinning or dipping (3.42 chins or dips).

McCloy advocated the elimination of lung capacity from the PFI battery since it is not a test of strength. In Chapter 5, lung capacity was shown to be well correlated with linear measures of body size, in the 0.70's for boys 13, 14, and 15 years of age. For these same ages, the correlations with gross strength measures were nearly as high.

For his Strength Index revision, McCloy reported a correlation of 0.77 with a battery of four track and field events. Norms based upon sex, age, and weight are available in the McCloy and Young reference when the battery is given with and without lung capacity for boys, ages 11 to 18, and for girls, ages 11 to 17. When the belt is used in the leg lift, these norms are inappropriate.

2. Athletic Strength Index.[37] In constructing an Athletic Strength Index (boys only), McCloy weighted the test items in his revision of the strength Index to give the total amount of strength usable in athletic events. Two formulas are given, as follows:

Long form: Right grip + left grip + 0.1 (back lift) + 0.1 (leg lift) + 2 (chinning strength) + dipping strength $-$ 3 (weight).

Short form: Same, except omit back and leg lifts.

The two forms of the test were correlated with a criterion composed of six track and field events. The coefficients of correlation were the same, 0.91. Norms for boys based on weight and age, for ages 11 to 18, are available in the reference.

3. Pure Strength Index.[38] Through factor analysis, McCloy found that two elements emerge from strength tests: one of these is "pure" strength or force; the other is dependent on body size. To predict "pure" strength, he gave the following weighting: $0.5(R + L \text{ grips}) + 0.1(\text{leg lift}) + \text{chinning strength} + \text{dipping strength}$. The test items were administered and scored in accordance with his revision of the Strength Index. No

norms have been published, which makes this revision the only one of the three proposed by McCloy without a means of obtaining from the index a score comparable to the PFI.

STRENGTH TESTS FOR GIRLS

Many of the strength batteries presented above are as applicable for girls as for boys, especially the Rogers Strength Index and Physical Fitness Index, and McCloy's Strength Index and PFI norms. Several investigations in this field, however, have been directed toward the construction of tests to measure the general athletic ability of girls, rather than toward measures of relative strength. Criteria have generally been athletic events. Norm charts are based on the standard-score technique, rather than on weight and age or some other such relative measure. As a result, these tests are comparable *in purpose* to the Strength Index, but not to the Physical Fitness Index. Presentation of these tests, therefore, will be found in Chapter 12.

The appropriateness of strength tests for girls rests on a fuller understanding of the need for strength in the realization of values of importance to girls, especially body grace and poise. Yet these qualities cannot be developed in girls without adequate body strength. Further, sufficient strength and vitality to meet the demands of everyday life and with sufficient reserve to enjoy leisure and enough reserve to meet emergencies are essential to everyone.

OREGON CABLE-TENSION STRENGTH TESTS

The origin and development of cable-tension strength tests were described in Chapter 6. The original purpose of these tests was to measure the strength of muscles involved in orthopedic disabilities. However, they have subsequently been

[37]McCloy and Young, *Tests and Measurements*, p. 25.
[38]Ibid., p. 26.

used for other purposes, especially in research. A large project was undertaken at the University of Oregon to study the strength of boys and girls from fourth grade through college. The ultimate goal achieved was the construction of cable-tension strength test batteries with norms for each sex at the upper elementary, junior high, senior high school and college levels. A manual is available describing and illustrating the test batteries and presenting norms for them.[39]

In the Oregon project, 25 cable-tension strength tests were administered to 72 boys and 72 girls at each of the four school levels; the respective averages of these tests served as a criterion of total strength for the various school levels. In each instance, three tests were selected by multiple correlation procedures; the correlations ranged between 0.928 and 0.965. The test batteries follow.

Boys,   all school levels: shoulder extension, knee extension, ankle plantar flexion

Girls,   upper elementary school: shoulder extension, hip extension, trunk flexion

Girls,   junior high school: shoulder extension, hip extension, trunk extension

Girls,   senior high school and college: shoulder flexion, hip flexion, ankle plantar flexion

In order to show the testing procedures for the cable-tension strength tests, the three tests in the boys' battery are described and illustrated.

Shoulder Extension

Starting Position.   (Figure 7.9A) Subject in supine lying position, hips and knees flexed comfortably; arm on side being tested close to side, shoulder flexed to 90 degrees, elbow in 90 degrees flexion; free hand resting on chest.

[39]H. Harrison Clarke and Richard A. Munroe, *Test Manual: Oregon Cable-Tension Strength Batteries for Boys and Girls from Fourth Grade Through College* (Eugene, Oregon: Microform Publications in Health, Physical Education, and Recreation, University of Oregon, 1970).

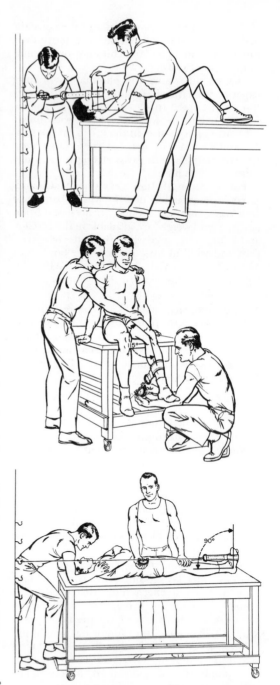

FIGURE 7.9. *Oregon Cable-Tension Strength Tests for Boys.* Top: *Shoulder extension.* Middle: *Knee extension.* Bottom: *Ankle plantar flexion*

Attachments. Strap around upper arm midway between elbow and shoulder joints; pulling assembly attached to wall behind subject's head.

Bracing. Brace subject's shoulder from behind, although shoulder braces are preferred; prevent shoulder elevation and keep elbow in line with pull (prevent adduction).

Knee Extension

Starting Position. (Figure 7.9B) Subject sitting on end of testing table with hands grasping table sides at hips, knee on side being tested in 115 degrees extension.

Attachments. Regulation strap around right leg midway between knee and ankle joints; pulling assembly attached to hook under table.

Bracing. Brace subject's shoulders to prevent backward lean, and brace across thigh to prevent lifting buttocks.

Ankle Plantar Flexion

Starting Position. (Figure 7.9C) Subject in supine lying position with legs fully extended; arms folded on chest; ankle on side being tested in 90 degrees flexion.

Attachments. Strap with stirrup around ball of foot; pulling assembly attached to wall behind subject's head.

Bracing. Use shoulder brace to prevent body movement; prevent eversion, knee flexion, and hip abduction by holding leg against table.

In an effort to determine desirable bases for cable-tension strength test norms, 12 anthropometric tests were administered to all subjects; in addition, 24 indices or ratios were derived from the anthropometric tests. For each sex at each school level, multiple correlations were computed with the average of the 25 strength tests as criterion and the 36 anthropometric tests and indices as experimental variables. On this basis, age and weight were selected for public school boys and girls. The multiple correlations were low for college men and women, so two sets of norms were constructed for each sex: a T-scale for both men and women and double entry tables based on arm and abdominal girths for men and arm girth and sitting height for women.

The process adopted by Rogers[40] in the construction of Strength Index norms to obtain the Physical Fitness Index was followed. The essential norm construction problem for public school boys and girls separately, therefore, was the determination of the increase in strength associated with an increase in weight for a given age; a double-entry table containing amounts of strength for the various categories was the final result. For college men and women, the double-entry tables were based on their respective anthropometric tests. Two battery scores were obtained for the two sexes at the various school levels:

Strength Composite (SC): A gross strength score, obtained by adding the three strength tests in each battery.

Strength Quotient (SQ): A relative strength score, derived from the following formula (except for the T-scores for college men and women):

$$SQ = \frac{\text{achieved SC}}{\text{normal SC}} \times 100$$

KRAUS-WEBER MUSCULAR TESTS

Emerging from their clinical practice in physical medicine and rehabilitation, Kraus and associates[41] presented tests of

[40]Frederick Rand Rogers, *Physical Capacity Tests*, p. 32.

[41]Hans Kraus and Ruth P. Hirschland, "Minimum Muscular Fitness Tests in School Children," *Research Quarterly*, **25**, No. 2 (May 1954), 178.

"minimum muscular fitness," commonly known as the Kraus-Weber tests. Originating in a posture clinic, the tests were further developed as a basic means of measurement in the treatment of low back pain; 80 percent of a total of over 4000 patients, free from organic disease, were unable to pass one or more of the test items. When treated with therapeutic exercise, their test results improved as they improved. In an eight-year follow-up, it was found that as the patients stopped exercising, they again failed the tests as their back complaints reappeared.

The Kraus-Weber (K-W) Tests of Minimum Muscular Fitness consist of six items. They are proposed as tests which indicate the level of strength and flexibility for certain key muscle groups below which the functioning of the whole body as a healthy organism seems to be endangered. As commonly given, the tests are graded on a pass-fail basis. However, partial movements on each test can be scored from 0 to 10. These tests are described below and are illustrated in Figure 7.10; tests are administered in the order given.

Test 1, Abdominal Plus: strength of the abdominal plus psoas muscles. Subject in supine lying position, hands behind neck; examiner holds feet down. *Pass:* perform one sit-up. *Scoring:* 0, cannot raise shoulders from table; 10, full sit-up.

Test 2, Abdominal Minus: strength of the abdominal minus psoas muscles. Subject in same position as Test 1, except knees are bent. *Pass:* perform one sit-up. *Scoring:* 0, cannot raise shoulders from table; 10, full sit-up.

Test 3, Psoas and Lower Abdomen: strength of psoas and lower abdominal muscles. Subject in supine lying position, hands behind neck; raise feet 10 inches with knees straight, while examiner counts to 10 seconds. *Pass:* position held for 10 seconds.

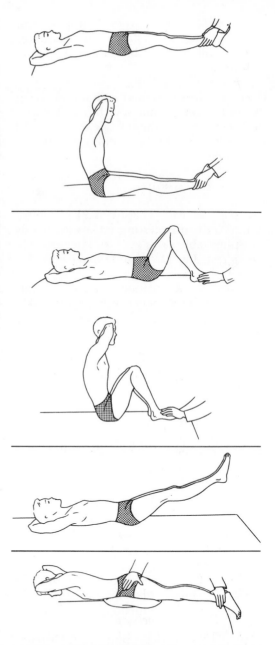

FIGURE 7.10. *Kraus-Weber Test of Minimum Muscular Fitness.* Left column, from top: *Abdominal plus; Abdominal minus; Psoas (lower abdomen); Upper back.* Right column, from top: *Lower back; Length of back and hamstring muscles*

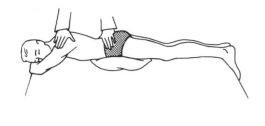

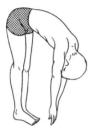

Scoring: 0–10, depending on number of seconds position is held.

Test 4, Upper Back: strength of upper back muscles. Subject in prone lying position with pillow under hips and lower abdomen, hands behind neck; examiner holds feet down; raise chest, head, and shoulders, while examiner counts to 10 seconds. *Pass:* position held for 10 seconds. *Scoring:* 0–10, depending on number of seconds position is held.

Test 5, Lower Back: strength of lower back muscles. Subject is in same position as Test 4, except feet are raised with knees straight. *Pass:* position held for 10 seconds; *Scoring:* 0–10, depending on number of seconds position is held.

Test 6, Length of Back and Hamstring Muscles: trunk flexibility, or floor-touch test. Subject stands erect in stocking or bare feet, hands at sides, feet together; lean down slowly and touch floor with fingertips, hold for three seconds (bouncing is not permitted); examiner holds knees in order to prevent any bend and to detect a

slight bend if it occurs. *Pass:* floor touch held for three seconds. *Scoring:* 10, reaches floor and holds for three seconds; 0, distance reached 10 or more inches from floor.

With these tests, Kraus and Hirschland examined 4458 eastern United States school children from both urban and rural communities, and compared their achievement with 3156 Swiss, Austrian, and Italian children. The results of this testing revealed that 57.9 percent of the United States children and only 8.7 percent of the European children failed one or more of the tests. Ample verification of the failure rate of United States children on K-W tests has been provided by surveys in Indiana,[42] Iowa,[43] Oregon[44] cities and elsewhere; the percentages of failures from these states were 45.1, 66.1, and 38.1 respectively.

As experience with K-W testing has been gained, several characteristics of the tests as applied to United States children have become obvious. Among these are the following.

1. The flexibility test (length of back and hamstring muscles) has produced by far the greatest number of failures. Nearly twice as many boys as girls fail this test; in the Eugene sample, of those failing at least one test, the percentages were 59.4 for boys and 33.0 for girls.

2. For the abdominal minus psoas test, the opposite was the case. Again, in the Eugene survey, 35.2 percent of the girls and 18.8 percent of the boys who failed one or more of the tests, failed this one.

[42]Marjorie Phillips and others, "Analysis of Results from the Kraus-Weber Test of Minimum Muscular Fitness in Children," *Research Quarterly,* **26,** No. 3 (October 1955), 314.

[43]Margaret Fox and Janet Atwood, "Results of Testing Iowa School Children for Health and Fitness," *Journal of Health, Physical Education, and Recreation,* **26,** No. 7 (September 1955), 20.

[44]Glenn Kirchner and Don Glines, "Comparative Analysis of Eugene, Oregon, Elementary School Children Using the Kraus-Weber Test of Minimum Muscular Fitness," *Research Quarterly,* **28,** No. 1 (March 1957), 16.

3. Very few children fail the two back strength tests; of nearly 1200 children in the Eugene group, only three failed the upper back test and 11 failed the lower back test. Almost identical situations occurred in the Indiana and Iowa studies.

4. Girls have a lower failure rate than boys on the entire K-W test, but this is due to their much lower failure rate on the flexibility test. When the strength tests only are considered, the boys show a slight superiority.

5. For both sexes, there is a definite decrease in strength failures as children become older; however, the opposite is true for the flexibility test, as these failures increase with age.

6. In the presentation of flexibility tests in Chapter 6, low correlations were reported between trunk-hip flexibility tests and such anthropometric measures as height, leg length, and trunk length, and muscular strength tests.

7. Brault[45] found that elementary school boys and girls who passed all K-W tests performed better than those who did not pass the tests on motor fitness tests of throwing for distance, standing broad jump, one-minute sit-ups, pull-ups, thrust and pull strengths, and trunk forward and backward flexion.

8. The percentage of K-W failures is much lower in schools where strong physical education programs exist. Furthermore, participation in vigorous body-building activities will rapidly reduce the failure rate in any school. Shaffer[46] demonstrated that K-W failures of junior high school girls can be reduced to less than 5 percent as a result of conditioning exercises "requiring less time than it is necessary for the classes to take showers, done twice each week for part of two semesters."

9. In a second study, Shaffer[47] reported a significant relationship between intelligence

quotient and K-W test failures; the trend line showed that as intelligence increased, K-W failures decreased. Age, height, and weight also influenced failures on this test; interestingly, weight had a greater effect than did height.

Many questions have been raised relative to the validity of the K-W tests in evaluating the muscular fitness of school children. It should be remembered that they are proposed by the originators as minimum fitness tests. It is surprising that so many United States boys and girls fail such simple tests; actions to correct this situation can certainly be justified. However, they should be supplemented or replaced by more complete tests, which extend through all levels of fitness, as soon as time and resources permit.

BERGER'S 1-RM

Berger[48] developed the use of 1-RM as a method for evaluating strength improvement. The 1-RM test consists of determining the maximum amount of weight a person can raise only once for a given movement. As an example, for the bench press, the subject lies supine on a bench; a barbell is placed across chest with hands grasping bar shoulder width apart, palms facing upward; bar is raised vertically until the arms are straight. Maximum weight for one lift is determined by trial. This procedure can be applied to other lifts, including curls, upright rowing, deep knee bends, military press, and back hyperextension.

In a subsequent study, Berger[49] formed a criterion of total strength by summing the 1-RM loads for six weight-lifting

[45]Donald A. Brault, "A Comparison of the Performance of Elementary School Children on the Kraus-Weber Test of Minimum Muscular Fitness with Achievement on Selected Motor Fitness Measures," Master's Thesis, University of Wisconsin, 1964.

[46]Gertrude Shaffer, "Why the American Children are Physically Unfit," *Physical Educator,* **17,** No. 2 (May 1960), 60.

[47]Gertrude Shaffer, "Variables Affecting Kraus-Weber Failures Among Junior High School Girls," *Research Quarterly,* **30,** No. 1 (March 1959), 75.

[48]Richard A. Berger, "Determination of the Resistance Load for 1-RM and 10-RM," *Journal of Association for Physical and Mental Rehabilitation,* **15,** No. 4 (July-August 1961), 108.

[49]Richard A. Berger, "Classification of Students on the Basis of Strength," *Research Quarterly,* **34,** No. 3 (December 1963), 514.

movements. The highest correlation was 0.87 for the military press. With the addition of back hyperextension, a multiple correlation of 0.92 was obtained.

SELECTED REFERENCES

CLARKE, H. HARRISON, *Muscular Strength and Endurance in Man.* Englewood Cliffs, N.J.: Prentice-Hall, Inc., 1966.

CLARKE, H. HARRISON, "Toward a Better Understanding of Strength," *Physical Fitness Research Digest,* President's Council on Physical Fitness and Sports, Series 3, No. 1 (January 1973).

CLARKE, H. HARRISON, and DAVID H. CLARKE, *Developmental and Adapted Physical Education.* Englewood Cliffs, N.J.: Prentice-Hall, Inc., 1963, Ch. 6.

KRAUS, HANS, and RUTH P. HIRSCHLAND, "Minimum Muscular Fitness Tests in School Children," *Research Quarterly,* **25,** No. 2 (May 1954), 178.

ROGERS, FREDERICK RAND, "PFI Questions and Answers," *Journal of Health and Physical Education,* **11,** No. 6 (June 1940), 352.

ZIMMERLI, ELIZABETH, "Case Studies of Unusual Physical Fitness Indices," *Supplement to the Research Quarterly,* **6,** No. 1 (June 1935), 246.

CHAPTER 8

As is well recognized, circulatory-respiratory (C-R) endurance is a basic component of physical fitness. This form of endurance is characterized by moderate contractions of large-muscle groups for relatively long periods of time, during which maximum adjustments of the circulatory-respiratory system are necessary, as in sustained running, swimming, climbing, bicycling, and the like. This physical fitness component is very complex. The elements of the C-R system affected include the heart and lungs, the vessels supplying blood to all parts of the body, the oxygen-carrying capacity of that blood, and the capillary network receiving the blood. Other body systems are also affected by endurance exercise, including the muscles, the digestion-absorption-elimination processes, the various internal secretion glands, the bones, the bone marrow's production of red blood corpuscles, and the brain.

Several investigators have studied the measureable elements involved in C-R endurance through factor analysis procedures. Such factors as the following have been identified: blood ejection velocity, oxygen requirement, pulse pressure after work, pulse recovery after easy work, vagus tone, splanchnic tone, and aerobic

Circulatory-Respiratory Endurance

capacity. The factor analyses rendered sharper meaning to several elements in the complex of C-R endurance. The many tests administered for these analyses, 101 by Cureton,[1] grouped into clusters according to their similarities. The intercorrelations between factors were low and mostly insignificant. A review of factor analysis studies was recently presented by the writer.[2] Included in this statement is an evaluation of some of the tests currently in use, especially maximum oxygen uptake and various measures taken from the brachial pulse wave obtained from heartometer tracings.

Physical educators have long been concerned with the measurement of circulatory-respiratory endurance. The early approaches were made by medical pioneers in physical activity as preventive medicine; these approaches were through responses of the cardiovascular system to exercise. Currently, interest is high on the use of circulatory-respiratory elements in the evaluation of C-R endurance. Many physical education scientists are well qualified in exercise physiology and are capable of performing and interpreting sophisticated evaluation processes. They have cooperated effectively with exercise specialists in physiology and medicine in the American College of Sports Medicine. The stature of their combined researches is well shown in the quarterly journal of the College, *Medicine and Science in Sports*.

Another approach to the evaluation of C-R endurance is through its functional manifestations in performances demonstrating such endurance, especially in prolonged running, although swimming and other activities have been employed. Both forms of evaluation, circulatory-

[1]Thomas K. Cureton and L. F. Sterling, "Factor Analyses of Cardiovascular Tests," *Journal of Sports Medicine and Physical Fitness,* **4,** No. 1 (March 1964), 1.

[2]H. Harrison Clarke, *Physical Fitness Research Digest,* President's Council on Physical Fitness and Sports: "Circulatory-Respiratory Endurance," **3,** No. 3 (July 1973); "Circulatory-Respiratory Endurance Improvement," **4,** No. 3 (July 1974).

respiratory responses to exercise and functional manifestations to sustained activity, are considered in this chapter.

CRAMPTON BLOOD-PTOSIS TEST

The Crampton Blood-Ptosis Test[3] was one of the earliest of the cardiovascular tests proposed to evaluate the general condition of the individual. The principle of the test is based on changes in heart rate and systolic blood pressure upon standing from a reclining position. Directions for administering this test are as follows.

1. The subject reclines until his pulse rate reaches a steady rate. A constant rate is reached when two repeated 15-second counts are the same.

2. While still in the reclining position, his heart rate is taken for one minute; then, his systolic blood pressure is taken.

3. The subject stands. When his pulse rate has reached a steady state, and while standing, heart rate and systolic blood pressure tests are again taken.

A norm chart for this test, which may be used for both men and women, appears in Appendix Table B.4. This is a double-entry table, which must be entered with the differences between the reclining and standing heart rates and systolic blood pressures. Thus, if a person's increase in heart rate is five and his systolic pressure increases 8 mm. Hg., his cardiovascular rating is 90. The individual who has a heart rate increase of 20 and a systolic blood pressure decrease of 6 mm. Hg. has a cardiovascular rating of 40. Crampton maintains that most people in good to fair condition will score between 60 and 100; scores below zero are evidence of impaired circulation, a toxic state, or acute severe physical disturbance.

McCloy[4] has pointed out that the Crampton Test seems to reflect changes in relative sickness, but does not reflect adequately the more positive changes in health. Furthermore, it does not appear to differentiate differences in athletic condition. The test, therefore, may have special value to determine the readiness of patients for bed exercises in convalescent care.

Hyman[5] proposed a "posture mean blood pressure index," which also records standing and recumbent blood pressures. However, the derivation of this index is much more complicated than the Crampton Blood-Ptosis Test. Systolic and diastolic pressures must be taken with the subject in a standing position for at least one minute, after he has been in a recumbent position for three minutes, immediately after he stands up quickly, and after he has been standing for one minute.

BARACH ENERGY INDEX

Another early cardiovascular test is the Barach Energy Index.[6] This test purports to measure the energy expended by the heart in blood output: the systole gives the energy factor in the work of the heart itself; the diastole provides the energy factor in the peripheral resistance; the pulse rate indicates the number of systoles and diastoles occurring in a minute. The test items utilized, then, are systolic and diastolic blood pressures and pulse rate per minute. All measures are obtained with the subject in a sitting position. Before tak-

[3]C. Ward Crampton, "A Test of Condition: Preliminary Report," *Medical News,* **87** (September 1905), 529.

[4]Charles H. McCloy and Norma D. Young, *Tests and Measurements in Health and Physical Education,* 3rd ed. (New York: Appleton-Century-Crofts, 1954), p. 291.

[5]Albert S. Hyman, "The Postural Mean Blood Pressure Index," *Journal of Sports Medicine and Physical Fitness,* **4,** No. 2 (December 1962), 218.

[6]J. H. Barach, "The Energy Index," *Journal of American Medical Association,* **62** (February 14, 1914), 525.

ing the tests, a constant pulse rate should be reached.

Scoring for the Barach Index is as follows:

$$\text{Energy Index} = \frac{\text{pulse rate} \left(\begin{array}{c} \text{systolic pressure} + \\ \text{diastolic pressure} \end{array} \right)}{100}$$

Thus, if an individual has a systolic blood pressure of 120, a diastolic pressure of 82, and a pulse rate of 70:

$$\text{Energy Index} = \frac{70(120 + 80)}{100} = 140$$

According to Barach's early studies, a robust person will have an Energy Index varying from 110 to 160. The upper normal limit is considered to be 200; the lower limit, 90. Those scoring above 200 may be hypertensed; those below 90 may be hypotensed. With 200 University of Illinois men, Cureton[7] obtained a mean Energy Index of 141; the range was 70 to 220.

In a validation of cardiovascular tests, Hunsicker[8] utilized a criterion of cardiac output, consisting of heart stroke volume for an all-out treadmill run divided by body surface area. The Barach Energy Index correlated −0.50 with this criterion. This correlation exceeded those with such other cardiovascular tests as the Harvard Step Test and the Schneider Test.

SCHNEIDER TEST

The Schneider Test[9] was the earliest of the more comprehensive cardiovascular tests. It was devised during World War I to test whether or not aviators were functionally

fit to fly. The six items comprising the test, with directions for their administration, are as follows.

1. Reclining pulse rate: After the subject has reclined quietly for five minutes, count his heart rate for 20 seconds every 20 seconds until two consecutive counts are the same; multiply this count by three to obtain the rate for one minute, and record.

2. Resting systolic pressure: Before the subject stands, take the systolic pressure. This reading should be checked two or three times before recording.

3. Standing pulse rate: After the subject has stood for two minutes to allow the pulse to reach its normal rate, count the heart rate until two 15-second counts agree; multiply this count by four, and record.

4. Increase in pulse rate on standing: Calculate the difference between the standing and reclining pulse rate, and record.

5. Increase in systolic blood pressure standing compared with reclining: Take the systolic pressure; calculate the difference between standing and reclining, and record.

6. Pulse rate increase immediately after exercise: Timing him with a stop watch, have the subject step up on a chair 18½ inches high five times in 15 seconds; count the pulse for 15 seconds immediately at the cessation of exercise; multiply this count by four; record. In the stepping procedure, the subject should stand with one foot on the chair at the first count; keeping his foot on the chair, he should continue to step up and down with the other foot; both feet should be on the floor at the end of the 15 seconds.

7. Return of pulse rate to standing normal after exercise: Continue taking the pulse in 15-second counts until the rate has returned to the normal standing rate; record the number of seconds it takes for this return. This time is taken from the end of the exercise bout to the beginning of the first normal 15-second pulse count. If the pulse has not returned to normal at the end of two minutes, record the number of beats above normal.

Norm charts for this test appear in Appendix Table B.5. The scores for each test

[7]Thomas K. Cureton, *Physical Fitness Appraisal and Guidance* (St. Louis: The C. V. Mosby Co., 1947), 285.

[8]Paul A. Hunsicker, "A Validation of Cardiovascular Tests by Cardiac Output Measurements," Doctoral Dissertation, University of Illinois, 1950.

[9]E. C. Schneider, "A Cardiovascular Rating as a Measure of Physical Fitness and Efficiency," *Journal of the American Medical Association,* **74,** No. 5 (May 29, 1920), 1507.

item range between $+3$ and -3. A perfect record, the sum of the values for all six tests, is a score of $+18$; deficiency is rated as 9 or less. In using the scoring table, parts A and B and parts C and D must be used together. For example, if an individual's pulse increase on standing is 13 (see part B) and his reclining rate is 75 (see part A), he is graded 2 on his standing increase.

Reliability for the Schneider Test by the test-re-test method is variously reported, but, when the test is given with extreme care, it is as high as 0.86 and 0.89. Recent research indicates that the test is related to endurance criteria; however, there are conflicting reports of the degree of this relationship. McCloy[10] obtained a correlation of 0.43 between the Schneider Test and a measure of the present status of the health of his subjects. Using this test with college men, Cureton[11] obtained the following correlations: mile run, -0.65; two-mile run, -0.63; three and one-half mile steeplechase, -0.50; composite of four endurance runs, -0.81. In Cureton's study, however, the subjects were highly selected. Taylor and Howe[12] reported a correlation of 0.68 between Schneider's scores and instructor's ratings of "physical fitness" of 60 college women. Henry and Herbig[13] obtained a correlation of 0.44 between scores on this test and improvement in time on the 800-yard run.

The evidence pertaining to this test is conflicting. One variable that may account for these differences is the degree of care required to obtain proper test scores on the test. Also, there is evidence that a revised weighting of the items may result in an improvement in the predictive value of the index. The test has value as one physiological fitness item to supplement the findings on the medical examination.

McCURDY-LARSON TEST OF ORGANIC EFFICIENCY

McCurdy and Larson constructed an Organic Efficiency Test[14] consisting of five items: (1) sitting diastolic pressure, (2) breath-holding 20 seconds after standard stair-climbing exercise, (3) difference between standing normal pulse rate and pulse rate two minutes after exercise, (4) sitting pulse pressure, and (5) standing pulse pressure. As a result of further research, Larson[15] devised a short test consisting of three items, numbers 1, 2, and 5 as listed above.

McCurdy and Larson maintain that endurance is basic in measuring organic capacity, believing that, if one is able to run or swim more than a normal distance without undue fatigue, he is in good physical condition. The criteria used for the validation of their Organic Efficiency Test were: the "good" physiological group, represented by 60 Springfield College varsity swimmers in mid-season condition and 40 American Olympic swimmers in the peak of condition before the start of the Olympic games in 1936; and the "poor" physiological group, represented by 138 infirmary patients examined immediately after confinement in the infirmary for two or more days with respiratory infections. The bi-serial correlation obtained between

[10]C. H. McCloy and Norma D. Young, *Tests and Measurements in Health and Physical Education*, 3rd ed. (New York: Appleton-Century-Crofts, 1954), p. 292.

[11]Thomas K. Cureton and others, *Endurance of Young Men* (Washington: Society for Research in Child Development, 10, No. 1, Serial No. 40, 1945), 214.

[12]M. W. Taylor and E. C. Howe, "Alkali Reserve and Physical Fitness," *American Physical Education Review*, **34** (1929), 570.

[13]Franklin Henry and W. Herbig, "The Correlation of Various Functional Tests of Cardio-circulatory System with Changes in Athletic Condition of Distance Runners." Mimeographed report presented at Research Section, A.A.H.P.E.R., San Francisco, 1939.

[14]J. H. McCurdy and L. A. Larson, "Measurement of Organic Efficiency for the Prediction of Physical Condition," *Supplement to the Research Quarterly*, **6**, No. 2 (May 1935), 11.

[15]Leonard A. Larson, "A Study of the Validity of Some Cardiovascular Tests," *Journal of Experimental Education*, **3**, No. 3 (March 1939), 214.

the test and the criterion groups was 0.70, and between the test items and "time" for the 440-yard swim was 0.68.[16]

HEARTOMETER

Cureton and his associates[17] have reported considerable research with the heartometer and have used the instrument extensively as a means of evaluating the functional capacity of the heart. The Heartometer provides a heartograph, a tracing made by a pen activated by the pulsation of the brachial artery transmitted by blood pressure apparatus of the sphygmomanometer type. The writing pen is activated by air pressure and a leverage system. The energy of the pulse wave is shown vertically and time pulse is shown horizontally. The tracing is somewhat comparable to the electrocardiogram; the main difference is that the heartometer registers variations in air pressure rather than electrical patterns.

Measures from the brachial pulse wave have been shown to relate to the cardiovascular fitness of the individual; trained athletes show more vigorous brachial pulse wave tracings than do nonathletes; the wave is improvable through rigorous, regularly practiced circulatory-respiratory endurance fitness programs; and deterioration of the wave occurs during prolonged physically sedentary periods.[18] The parts of the pulse wave that have greatest significance in reflecting the individual's cardiovascular fitness are the area under the curve and systolic, diastolic, and diastolic surge amplitudes. Diastolic and systolic blood pressures and heart rate may also be obtained from the heartograph.

While the heartometer has had limited use in school and college physical fitness programs, it is utilized by some YMCA physical educators, due to the literally hundreds of physical fitness clinics conducted by Cureton across the country and throughout the world; many of these clinics were held in YMCAs.

MAXIMUM OXYGEN UPTAKE

Maximum oxygen uptake (maxVO$_2$) is commonly used to evaluate the oxygen transport system of the body for various workloads; workloads may be applied by use of a treadmill, a bicycle ergometer, or a step bench. When expressed as liters per minute (l/m), absolute maxVO$_2$, it is highly related to such physique and body size measures as ectomorphy, height, weight, and especially lean body weight. As a consequence, maximum oxygen uptake relative to body weight (ml/kg/min) has come into general use in order to minimize the effect of body bulk on the uptake measure. In evaluating this measure, it is essential to differentiate between these two maxVO$_2$ tests, as the results in their use are quite different depending on the one utilized. They will be known here as absolute and relative maxVO$_2$, respectively.

In considering the maxVO$_2$ test, the following evaluation[19] seems pertinent.

1. The mean maxVO$_2$ is greater in all-out performances on the treadmill than on the bicycle ergometer, although maximum heart rates obtained are approximately the same.

2. Some investigators have questioned the use of submaximal workloads in determining maxVO$_2$ on the basis that only crude extrapolations from submaximal to maximal tests can be made. Generally, submaximal tests to predict maxVO$_2$ have been based on the concept that a task requiring a submaximal heart rate of 180 beats per minute can be used to evaluate circulatory-respiratory endurance.

[16]J. H. McCurdy and L. A. Larson, "The Validity of Circulatory-Respiratory Measures as an Index of Endurance Condition in Swimming," *Research Quarterly,* **11,** No. 3 (October 1940), 3.

[17]Thomas K. Cureton, *Physical Fitness Appraisal and Guidance* (St. Louis: C. V. Mosby Company, 1947), Ch. 8.

[18]Clarke, *Physical Fitness Research Digest.*

[19]Ibid.

3. The relationships between maxVO₂ tests and cardiovascular measures are only moderate, the highest reported being with heart rate (−0.57).

4. The correlation between relative maxVO₂ and time for the 600-yard run has been as high as −0.66, although lower and even nonsignificant correlations have been reported.

5. The highest correlations obtained between relative maxVO₂ and other motor fitness items are 0.58 for pullups and 0.45 for medicine ball throw for distance.

6. The comparison of the aerobic capacity of males and females indicates that males have higher oxygen uptake; the difference is attributed to females having smaller organs, including heart and lungs, and muscles.

7. Physical fitness programs that stress the improvement of circulatory-respiratory endurance improve the individual's maxVO₂; this is true at all ages, although, generally, the older the subject, the slower is the progress.

Although, as indicated above, the validity of using submaximal work to predict maxVO₂ has been questioned, submaximal tests do provide a rough estimate of the effectiveness of the oxygen-transport system. The full test is not feasible in school and college physical fitness programs since it requires intricate laboratory equipment, needs considerable expertise by the tester, and is time consuming to administer. Also, the subjects must perform to an exhaustive state, which involves strong motivation, extreme discomfort, and possible hazard for the unfit and sedentary. Consequently, submaximal VO₂ testing has come into use.

Astrand and Ryhming[20] proposed a step test utilizing submaximal efforts in the prediction of maxVO₂, which has become widely known. Work loads may be applied by use of a treadmill, a bicycle ergometer, or a step bench; the use of the step bench

puts this test within the purview of school and college physical education programs. Further, the measurement of oxygen uptake is not necessary for this test, as this measure may be obtained from a nomograph based on pulse rate and body weight. In addition to the Astrand-Ryhming article, this test is described and the nomograph presented by Clarke and Clarke.[21]

TUTTLE PULSE-RATIO TEST

The fact has been demonstrated that the physical condition of an individual has a definite effect upon both the rate of the heart beat and the time required for the rate to return to normal after the cessation of exercise. It has also been shown that the individual who is physically conditioned will be less affected by a given amount of exercise than when in poor condition. It is on the basis of these factors that pulse-ratio tests have been mostly justified. These tests are based on the ability of the heart to compensate for exercise. The first pulse-ratio test was developed in the physiology laboratory of Guy's Hospital, London, England.[22] Subsequently several tests of this sort were reported in this country, particularly the Tuttle Pulse-Ratio Test and the Harvard Step Test.

Tuttle's Pulse-Ratio Test[23] was announced in 1931; for a few years thereafter, considerable research related to the test was conducted. The pulse ratio is the ratio between resting pulse and pulse rate after exercise. A score on the Tuttle test is the amount of exercise required to increase the pulse rate 2.5 times above the resting pulse. In order to make this de-

[20]P. O. Astrand and Irma Ryhming, "A Nomograph for Calculation of Aerobic Capacity (Physical Fitness) from Pulse Rate during Submaximal Work," *Journal of Applied Physiology,* **7**, No. 2 (September 1954), 218.

[21]H. Harrison Clarke and David H. Clarke, *Developmental and Adapted Physical Education* (Englewood Cliffs, N.J.: Prentice-Hall, Inc., 1963), p. 68.

[22]G. H. Hunt and M. S. Pembrey, "Tests of Physical Efficiency," *Guy's Hospital Reports,* **71** (1921), 415.

[23]W. W. Tuttle, "The Use of the Pulse-Ratio Test for Rating Physical Efficiency," *Research Quarterly,* **2**, No. 2 (May 1931), 5.

termination, two step tests of contrasting efforts are performed for one minute each from a bench 13 inches high, as follows: Test 1, 20 steps for males and 15 steps for females; test 2, 40 steps for males and 35 steps for females. Pulse ratios are computed for each test, based on pulse rates two minutes after stepping: PR two minutes/PR resting. From these two ratios, the number of steps needed for a ratio of 2.5 is computed by formula. The means for the test are: 33 steps for boys 10 to 12 years of age; 30 steps for boys over 12 and adult men; 25 steps for adult women. An "efficiency rating" is also provided, which places results on a percentage basis; the percentages are based on 50 steps per minute, which was the number found to produce a ratio of 2.5 in well-conditioned athletes.

Subsequently, Tuttle and Dickinson[24] found that the ratio from a single stepping performance of 30 to 40 steps of exercise is nearly as satisfactory as the ratio obtained from the two stepping exercises. A correlation of 0.957 was obtained between the original test and the single pulse with 40 steps per minute; with 30 steps per minute, this correlation was 0.930.

Some evidence exists which relates Tuttle pulse ratios with physical condition. Three investigators have shown that the ratio agrees with the findings of physicians concerning the status of the cardiovascular system.

HARVARD STEP TEST

The Harvard Step Test[25,26] was originally constructed for college men. Following are instructions for its administration.

[24]W. W. Tuttle and R. E. Dickinson, "A Simplification of the Pulse-Ratio Technique for Rating Physical Efficiency and Present Condition," *Research Quarterly,* **2,** No. 2 (May 1931), 5.

[25]Lucien Brouha, "The Step Test: A Simple Method of Measuring Physical Fitness for Muscular Work in Young Men," *Research Quarterly,* **14,** No. 1 (March 1943), 31.

[26]Lucien Brouha, Norman W. Fradd, and Beatrice M. Savage, "Studies in Physical Efficiency of College Students," *Research Quarterly,* **15,** No. 3 (October 1944), 211.

1. The subject steps up and down 30 times a minute on a bench 20 inches high. Each time the subject should step all the way up on the bench with the body erect. The stepping process is performed in four counts, as follows: 1, one foot is placed on bench; 2, other foot is placed on bench; 3, one foot is placed on floor; 4, other foot is placed on floor. The testee may lead off with the same foot each time or may change feet as he desires, so long as the four-count step is maintained. The steps may be timed with a metronome. If a metronome is not available, count the cadence as "up, up, down, down."

2. The stepping exercise continues for exactly five minutes, unless the subject is forced to stop sooner due to exhaustion. In either case, the duration of the exercise in seconds is recorded; the maximum number of seconds is 300 for the full five-minute period.

3. Immediately after completing the exercise, the subject sits on a chair. The pulse is counted 1 to 1½, 2 to 2½, and 3 to 3½ minutes after the stepping ceases.

4. A Physical Efficiency Index (PEI) is computed, utilizing the following formula:

$$PEI = \frac{\text{duration of exercise in seconds} \times 100}{2 \times \text{sum of pulse counts in recovery}}$$

To illustrate: The subject completed the exercise period, 300 seconds; his recovery-period pulse counts were: 75 for 1–1½ minutes, 50 for 2–2½ minutes, and 35 for 3–3½ minutes (the sum is 160). Substituting in the formula,

$$PEI = \frac{30,000}{2 \times 160} = 94$$

Based on about 8000 tests of college men, the following norms were prepared:

Physical Condition	PEI
Excellent	90 and above
Good	80 to 89
High Average	65 to 79
Low Average	55 to 64
Poor	54 and below

[handwritten: Got spewts win from real extreme weakness - negative p135 how do you give test?]

In the validation of the Harvard Step Test, Brouha tested 2200 Harvard male students. The following means were obtained: 75 for all students, 93 for all athletes, 88 for the freshman track team, 90 for the varsity baseball team, 95 for the varsity track team, and 109 for the varsity crew. The freshman class before training averaged 69; after training, their average was 76. Using the short form, Taddonio and Karpovich[27] obtained the following means: 62, sedentary individuals; 86, sprinters and hurdlers; 99, marathon runners; 105, freshman cross-country runners; and 111, varsity cross-country runners.

In general, correlations between scores on the Harvard Step Test and various measures of physical strength and endurance have been low; this may be due to the fact that, while the step performance is rigorous, the score is based entirely on a pulse rate evaluation. With 117 male students, Cureton and his associates,[28] using a 15-inch bench, obtained correlations between 0.002 and 0.31 with 27 different tests of muscular strength, muscular endurance, and running endurance. Bookwalter,[29] utilizing 1269 college-age men as subjects, reported no relationship between this test and the Army Physical Fitness Test, nor between it and age, height, weight, 100-yard pick-a-back, and 300-yard run criteria. Neff and Steitz[30] also obtained low correlations between the test and strength and endurance items and batteries. On the positive side, Taddonio

and Karpovich[31] obtained a rank-difference correlation of 0.63 between the short form of the Harvard test and the order in which Springfield College men finished an intramural cross-country race.

Rapid Form. A "rapid" form of the Harvard Step Test was proposed by Johnson and Robinson.[32] The exercise phase is the same as for the regular test; however, the pulse is counted once from one minute to one minute thirty seconds. The single post-exercise pulse count is justified because of a high correlation between the first and the sum of the three pulse counts of the original test. The score is obtained from the formula:

$$\times \quad PEI = \frac{\text{duration of exercise in seconds} \times 100}{5.5 \times \text{pulse count}}$$

[handwritten: 300 sec.] *[handwritten: pulse count 1 once / min - 1:30]*

The norms for the short form are: below 50, poor; 50–80, average; above 80, good.

Carter and Winsman[33] maintain that the Harvard Step Test scoring formula is inadequate when individuals do not complete the prescribed stepping duration of five minutes. They proposed a variation of the rapid form, which renders PEI scores independent of the duration of stepping, as follows:

$$\times \quad PEI = \left(\frac{D \times 100}{5.5 \times P} \right) + \left(0.22 \, (300 - D) \right)$$

[handwritten: duration of ex.] *[handwritten: pulse]*

in which D = duration of stepping in seconds and P = 1 to 1½ minute pulse count, after stepping.

[27]Dominik A. Taddonio and Peter V. Karpovich, "The Harvard Step Test as a Measure of Endurance in Running," *Research Quarterly*, **22**, No. 3 (October 1951), 381.

[28]Cureton and others, *Endurance of Young Men*, Ch. 7.

[29]Karl W. Bookwalter, "A Study of the Brouha Step Test," *The Physical Educator*, **5**, No. 3 (May 1948), 55.

[30]Charles B. Neff and Edward S. Steitz, "A Study to Determine Physical Fitness Test Items against Criteria of Composite Scores of PFI, Army, and Harvard Step-Up Tests." Master's thesis, Springfield College, Springfield, Mass., 1948.

[31]Taddonio and Karpovich, "Harvard Step Test," p. 381.

[32]Peter V. Karpovich, *Physiology of Muscular Activity*, 4th ed. (Philadelphia: W. B. Saunders Company, 1953), p. 270.

[33]R. P. Carter, and F. R. Winsmann, "Study of Measurement and Experimental Design Problems Associated with the Step-Test," *Journal of Sports Medicine and Physical Fitness*, **10**, No. 2 (June 1970), 104.

MODIFICATIONS OF THE HARVARD STEP TEST

A number of modifications of the Harvard Step Test have been proposed to adapt the test to groups other than college men.

Girls and Women

Skubic and Hodgkins[34] proposed a three-minute step test for girls and women. The rate of stepping is 24 steps per minute; the height of the bench is 18 inches. Following exercise, the subjects rested for one minute in a sitting position; the pulse was then counted for 30 seconds at the carotid artery by palpation. For those who were unable to complete three minutes of stepping, the total time was recorded and their recovery pulse was counted after one minute for the usual 30 seconds. These investigators found that the test differentiated between trained, active, and sedentary subjects. The reliability coefficient for the test was reported as 0.82.

In subsequent studies, Skubic and Hodgkins,[35,36] developed national norms for their Cardiovascular Efficiency Test. Norms were prepared separately for junior high school girls, senior high school girls, and college women in accordance with six ratings: excellent, very good, good, fair, poor, and very poor. The samples upon which the norms are based were 2360 women from 66 colleges, 1362 senior high school and 686 junior high school girls from 55 secondary schools throughout the country. A Cardiovascular Effi-

ciency Score (CES) is computed in a manner similar to the Short Form of the Harvard Step Test. The formula is as follows:

$$CES = \frac{\text{number of seconds completed} \times 100}{5.6 \times \text{pulse count}}$$

The ratings and cardiovascular test scores comprising the norms appear in Appendix Table B.6. For subjects who complete the full three minutes of stepping, the table may be entered with the 30-second recovery pulse rate; the CES formula must be used for those who did not step for three minutes. These investigators found that 13.3 percent of girls and women tested did not complete the three-minute test.

College Women

The Queens College Step Test for college women was presented by McArdle and associates.[37] For this test, the woman steps up and down on a bleacher step for three minutes at a cadence of 22 steps per minute. At the end of the stepping, the subject remains standing while a partner counts her pulse rate by palpation of the carotid artery for 15 seconds, from 5 to 20 seconds after exercise. Subsequently, percentile norms for post-exercise 15-second pulse rates were presented,[38] as provided in Appendix Table B.7. Relative maxVO$_2$ correlated -0.75 and -0.64 with this test and with the Skubic-Hodgkin step test, respectively. The correlation with the Skubic-Hodgkins test was 0.87.

Harvey and Scott[39] proposed the Kent

---

[34]Vera Skubic and Jean Hodgkins, "Cardiovascular Efficiency Test for Girls and Women," *Research Quarterly,* **34,** No. 2 (May 1963), 191.

[35]Jean Hodgkins and Vera Skubic, "Cardiovascular Efficiency Test Scores for College Women in the United States," *Research Quarterly,* **34,** No. 4 (December 1963), 454.

[36]Vera Skubic and Jean Hodgkins, "Cardiovascular Efficiency Test Scores for Junior and Senior High School Girls in the United States," *Research Quarterly,* **35,** No. 2 (May 1964), 184.

[37]William D. McArdle and others, "Reliability and Interrelationships Between Maximum Oxygen Intake, Work Capacity, and Step-Test Scores in College Women," *Medicine and Science in Sports,* **4,** No. 4 (Winter 1972), 182.

[38]William D. McArdle and others, "Percentile Norms for a Valid Step Test in College Women," *Research Quarterly,* **44** (December 1973), 498.

[39]Virginia P. Harvey and Gwendolyn D. Scott, "The Validity and Reliability of a One-Minute Step

State University Step Test for college women. This test consists of stepping on a bench 18 inches high at a cadence of 30 steps per minute for one minute; pulse rate is counted for 30 seconds, from 1 to 1½ minutes after stepping. A correlation of 0.71 between this and the Skubic-Hodgkins tests was reported. Further, women athletes obtained significantly better scores on the test than did nonathletes.

Clarke[40] studied the use of the step test with Radcliffe College women as subjects. She used a bench 18 inches high; the exercise consisted of 30 steps per minute for four minutes. The pulse counts and scoring was the same as for the Harvard Step Test. Based on the Harvard men's norms, the distribution of scores for these women was as follows: excellent, 20 percent; good, 15 percent; high average, 31 percent; low average, 9 percent; poor, 43 percent. Scores on this test improved significantly from participation in six weeks of physical education.

High School Girls

Brouha and Gallagher[41] adapted their Harvard Step Test for girls of high school ages. The testing technique is the same as for the Harvard test, except the bench is 16 inches high and the duration of stepping is four minutes; the scoring is also the same, that is, sum of the three 30-second post-exercise pulse counts. In order to facilitate the calculation of the Physical Efficiency Index, Table 8.1 was provided for girls who continued stepping for four minutes. Enter this table with the sum of

the three 30-second pulse counts and read the PEI directly. For example, a girl has the following post-exercise pulse counts: 1–1½ min., 60; 2–2½ min., 55; 3–3½ min., 50. The total of the three counts is 165. Enter the table with 165; the PEI is 73.

Girls who stop stepping before the end of the four minutes may be scored by use of the usual formula, or, for the sake of simplicity, may be assigned an arbitrary score, as follows: 25, 2 minutes; 30, 2½ minutes; 35, 3 minutes; and 45, 3½ minutes. A score of 45 is also assigned to all girls who finish 4 minutes but who lag behind in the cadence, crouch, or show other evidence of doing less work than is demanded by the test.

TABLE 8.1 *Calculation of Girls' Physical Efficiency Index: Modified Harvard Step Test*

Pulse Score	Pulse Score	Pulse Score	Pulse Score
105-114	133-90	163-74	193-62
106-113	134-90	164-73	194-62
107-112	135-89	165-73	195-61
108-111	136-88	166-72	196-61
109-110	137-88	167-72	197-61
110-109	138-87	168-71	198-61
111-108	139-86	169-71	199-60
112-107	140-86	170-71	200-60
113-106	141-85	171-70	201-60
114-105	142-85	172-70	203-59
115-104	143-84	173-70	208-58
116-103	144-83	174-69	210-57
117-102	145-83	175-69	214-56
118-102	146-82	176-68	218-55
119-101	147-82	177-68	222-54
120-100	148-81	178-67	226-53
121- 99	149-81	179-67	230-52
122- 98	150-80	180-67	235-51
123- 98	151-80	181-66	240-50
124- 97	152-79	182-66	
125- 96	153-78	183-66	
126- 95	154-78	184-65	
127- 95	155-77	185-65	
128- 94	156-77	186-65	
129- 93	158-76	189-64	
130- 92	160-75	190-63	
131- 92	161-75	191-63	
132- 92	162-74	192-63	

Note: If pulse total is beyond limits of this table divide 120 by the pulse total to obtain the score.

Test for College Women, *Journal of Sports Medicine and Physical Fitness*, **10**, No. 3 (September 1970), 185.

[40]Harriet L. Clarke, "A Functional Physical Fitness Test for College Women," *Journal of Health and Physical Education*, **14**, No. 7 (September 1943), 358.

[41]Lucien Brouha and J. Roswell Gallagher, "A Functional Fitness Test for High School Girls," *Journal of Health and Physical Education*, **15**, No. 10 (December 1943), 517.

Secondary School Boys

In preliminary trials of the step test, Gallagher and Brouha[42] found a wide range of size in boys between the ages of 12 and 18 years. As a consequence, two heights of benches were used for the small and large boys. The division of the boys was made on the basis of body surface area, as follows:

Less than 1.85 square meters: 18-inch bench

1.85 square meters and above: 20-inch bench

Surface area may be easily determined from the nomographic chart in Figure 8.1. Place a straightedge between the boy's height on the left scale and his weight on the right scale; his surface area is read at the point where the straightedge crosses the center scale.

The rate is the same for four minutes; otherwise the test and scoring are the same as for the Harvard Step Test. Inasmuch as the duration of this test is for four minutes, the same as for the girls' test, Table 8.1 may be used to obtain the Physical Efficiency Index. The investigators presented the following distribution of scores after testing 600 private school boys:

50 or less: very poor physical condition	2 percent
51–60: poor physical condition	18 percent
61–70: fair physical condition	50 percent
71–80: good physical condition	25 percent
81–90: excellent physical condition	4 percent
91 or more: superior physical condition	1 percent

Elementary School Children

Brouha and Ball[43] made a further modification of the Harvard Step Test for use with elementary school boys and girls. The bench was lowered in height to 14 inches. The stepping times were changed

by ages: two minutes at 7 years and three minutes from 8–12 years. Scoring and classification are the same as for college men in the original test.

PCPFS Test

The President's Council on Physical Fitness and Sports proposes the use of a Recovery Index Test,[44] which is a modification of the Harvard Step Test. The differences in procedures are that the duration of stepping is four minutes and the height of the bench varies from 14 to 16 to 20 inches depending on the height of the subjects, although no height designations are given. To determine the recovery index, three post-exercise heart rates are taken and summed: $1–1\frac{1}{2}$, $2–2\frac{1}{2}$, and $3–3\frac{1}{2}$ minutes. Reference is then made to the norms as follows:

When the Three 30-second Pulse Counts Total:	The Recovery Index Is:	Then the Response to This Test Is:
199 or more	60 or less	poor
171–198	61–70	fair
150–170	71–80	good
133–149	81–90	very good
132 or less	91 or more	excellent

The PCPFS suggests that when a youth fails to complete the test or makes a score of 60 or less according to the norms, medical referral may be desireable. Those who do poorly on the test may be unfit to engage immediately in a strenuous exercise program.

Convalescent Patients

Karpovich, Starr, and Weiss[45] used the 20-inch bench and a cadence of 24 steps per minute over a period of 30 seconds for evaluating the condition of patients in army hospitals for participation in mild

[42]J. Roswell Gallagher and Lucien Brouha, "A Simple Method of Testing the Physical Fitness of Boys," *Research Quarterly*, **14**, No. 1 (March 1943), 23.

[43]Lucien Brouha and M. V. Ball, *Canadian Red Cross Society's School Meal Study* (Toronto: University of Toronto Press, 1952), p. 55.

[44]*Youth Physical Fitness*, rev. ed. (Washington: Government Printing Office, 1973), p. 9.

[45]Peter V. Karpovich, Merritt P. Starr, and Raymond A. Weiss, "Physical Fitness Test for Convalescents," *Journal of the American Medical Association*, **126** (December 2, 1944), 873.

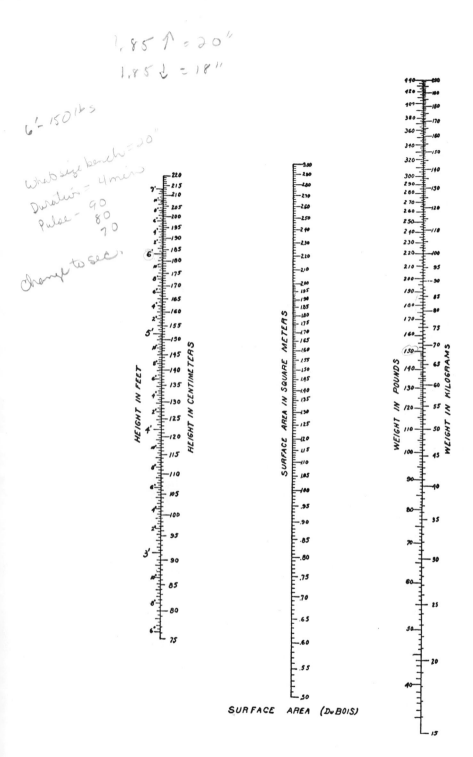

FIGURE 8.1. *DuBois Body Surface Chart: Nomograph. Copyright 1920, by W. M. Boothby and R. B. Sandiford, Mayo Clinic, Rochester, Minn.*

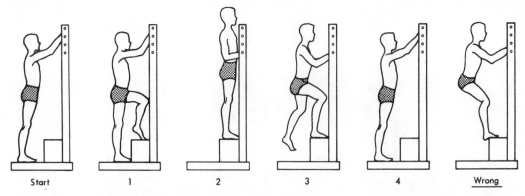

| Start | 1 | 2 | 3 | 4 | Wrong |

FIGURE 8.2. *Modified Step Test with Handholds*

physical activity. As the condition of the patient improved at the direction of the ward medical officer, his readiness for more strenuous exercise was measured by his ability to perform the same exercise for longer periods, until he reached five minutes. His physical condition was evaluated both by the pulse response and by ability to endure exercise. In addition to the reference, the scoring table for this test appears in Clarke and Clarke.[46]

MODIFIED STEP TEST APPARATUS

The step apparatus for the Harvard Step Test was modified by Patterson and associates[47] by including horizontal bars for handholds and for steadying purposes. Several horizontal bars are arranged so that subjects of different heights can select one which is above shoulder level and in a vertical plane with the back of the step. The step is a 20-inch bench and the cadence is 30 steps per minute, as for the Harvard test. The modified step test apparatus in use is shown in Figure 8.2.

[46]H. Harrison Clarke and David H. Clarke, *Developmental and Adapted Physical Education* (Englewood Cliffs, N.J.: Prentice-Hall, Inc., 1963), p. 67.

[47]John L. Patterson and others, "Evaluation and Prediction of Physical Fitness, Utilizing Modified Apparatus of the Harvard Step Test," *American Journal of Cardiology*, **14**, No. 6 (December 1964), 811.

Two maximal tests, termed the capacity step test and the capacity pack test, are similar in technique, except for the use in the pack test of a back pack loaded to one-third of the subject's body weight. The endpoint of these maximal tests is the inability of the subject to continue stepping at the prescribed rate. The test was scored by the length of time stepping could be continued.

In validating the capacity tests, U.S. Navy military and civilian men 18 to 45 years of age at the Naval Air Stations, Pensacola and Corpus Christi, were classified on the basis of previous athletic training into five groups: excellent, good, average, fair, and poor. Only athletes in finest training were graded as "excellent." The means and standard deviations of these groups for the two maximal tests appear in Table 8.2.

TABLE 8.2 *Capacity Step-Test Performances (Minutes)*

	Step Test		Pack Test	
Training Level	Mean	S.D.	Mean	S.D.
Excellent	27.2	10.5	5.9	2.3
Good	11.4	6.9	3.1	1.9
Average	6.8	4.3	3.0	1.3
Fair	4.9	3.0	2.9	1.3
Poor	4.1	2.0	2.7	1.3

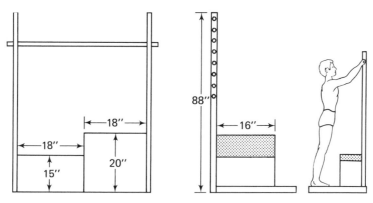

FIGURE 8.3. *Ohio State University Step Test. Redrawn from Mathews, Kurucz, and Fox, Research Quarterly, March 1969.*

The capacity step test was found to differentiate significantly among all training level groups. However, the capacity pack test was found more suitable for the excellent group of well-trained athletes.

With horizontal bars for handholds, the subjects in the study could usually exercise considerably longer on the 20-inch step test. The authors maintained that an advantage was gained from using the muscles of the arms, shoulder girdles, and upper back to assist in mounting the step, thereby reducing muscle fatigue in the legs as a limiting factor in the exercise; skill required in performing the step test was also reduced.

OHIO STATE UNIVERSITY STEP TEST

The Ohio State University Step Test was developed by Kurucz, Fox, and Mathews,[48] as a submaximal test of cardiovascular fitness for men aged 18 years and over. The test is based on the concept that the time required to reach a heart rate of

150 beats per minute is a valid indicator of the subject's capacity for more strenuous work. A split-level bench, 15 inches high at one end and 20 inches high at the other, with a hand bar adjustable at 3-inch intervals, that the subject grasps in performing the test, is needed, as shown in Figure 8.3. A metronome, or other device for indicating cadence, and a stop watch are also necessary.

Before taking the test, the hand bar is adjusted to the level closest to the top of the subject's head; the bar is grasped with both hands throughout the test in order to balance the subject and to assist him in the stepping movements. Instructions and a demonstration of the test are given before each subject is tested.

The OSU step test comprises 18 innings of bench stepping, each of 50 seconds duration. In each inning, the subject steps for 30 seconds and rests for 20 seconds; during each rest period, he counts his own pulse for 10 seconds, between 5 and 15 seconds. The test is terminated when the pulse rate reaches 25 beats (150 beats per minute) or when the subject completes the entire 18 innings. The individual's score is the number of innings completed. The stepping consists of three consecutive phases, as follows:

[48]Robert S. Kurucz, Edward L. Fox, and Donald K. Mathews, "Construction of a Submaximal Cardiovascular Step Test," *Research Quarterly,* **40,** No. 1 (March 1969), 115.

Phase I: six innings; 15-inch bench;
             24 steps per minute
Phase II: six innings; 15-inch bench;
             30 steps per minute
Phase III: six innings; 20-inch bench;
             30 steps per minute

Mean scores on the test clustered between 11.8 and 13.0 innings for men ranging in age from 19 to 56 years. The standard deviations decreased with age, as follows: 4.7 innings, 19 to 29 years; 4 innings, 30 to 40 years; and 3.4 innings, 41 to 56 years. Test-retest reliability coefficient was 0.94. The same correlation of 0.94 was obtained between the OSU and the Balke treadmill test.[49] In a study by Williams,[50] the OSU test correlation with Cooper's 12-minute run test was 0.54.

Witten[51] modified the OSU step test for college women. Three bench heights were used, 14, 17, and 20 inches. The distribution of innings was as follows:

Phase I: five innings, 14-inch bench,
             24 steps per minute
Phase II: five innings, 14-inch bench,
             30 steps per minute
Phase III: five innings, 17-inch bench,
             30 steps per minute
Phase IV: five innings, 20-inch bench,
             30 steps per minute

The test-retest reliability coefficient reported for this modification was 0.90. Correlations between the modification and the Balke treadmill test for the subjects reaching the same heart rate per minute on both tests was highest, 0.85, for the rate of 168 beats per minute.

A modification of the OSU step test for boys in grades four through six was developed by Callon.[52] The following changes were made: (a) depth of the bench reduced to to 13½ inches (instead of 16 inches); (b) pulse rate taken by examiner using a stethoscope; (c) test terminated when pulse rate reached 29 beats for 10 seconds (174 beats per minute); (d) subjects completed 18 innings given a score of 19; (e) bench height for third phase of stepping lowered to 18 inches; (f) hand bar adjusted to eye level. Test-retest reliability coefficient was 0.96. Mean performance for boys in the three grades was 13.5 innings; the standard deviation was 4.0 innings.

COMMENTS ON CARDIOVASCULAR TESTS

Accuracy of Cardiovascular Tests

The elements most frequently measured in cardiovascular testing include pulse rate at rest, after exercise, and after rest following exercise, systolic and diastolic blood pressures, and venous pressures. These may be taken reclining, sitting, or standing, and the changes that take place after activity or after various shifts of position may be recorded, as well as the direct readings themselves.

Great care must be exercised in the administration of circulatory-respiratory measures in order to obtain reliable results. It is generally agreed by experimenters that many factors influence the elements included in the cardiovascular-type test. In an early review of the cardiovascular-respiratory function, Larson[53] pointed out that both heart rate and blood pressure are affected by the following:

[49]The Balke treadmill test consists of walking at a speed of 3.5 miles per hour on a motor driven treadmill, the slope of which increases each minute; the score is the length of time a subject walks to reach a heart rate of 180 beats per minute.

[50]Melvin H. Williams, "Comparison of Submaximal Cardiovascular Step Test to a Maximum Aerobic Performance Task," *American Corrective Therapy Journal,* **24,** No. 5 (September-October 1970), 127.

[51]Chet Witten, "Construction of a Submaximal Cardiovascular Step Test for College Females," *Research Quarterly,* **44,** No. 1 (March 1973), 46.

[52]Donald E. Callon, "A Submaximal Cardiovascular Fitness Test for Fourth, Fifth, and Sixth Grade Boys," Doctoral Dissertation, Ohio State University, 1968.

[53]Leonard A. Larson, "Cardiovascular-Respiratory Function," *Supplement to the Research Quarterly,* **12,** No. 2 (May 1941), 456.

exercise, age, sex, diurnal changes, season and climate, altitude, changes in body posture, digestion, air and water movements, loss of sleep, respiration, metabolism, and emotional and nervous conditions. These factors increase considerably the complexity of cardiovascular measurement. Emotional and nervous states, such as worry, fear, and anger, are particularly difficult to control, as is the amount of physical exercise engaged in by the subject immediately preceding the taking of such tests. Even slight nervousness or muscular tension will increase the individual's score.

McCurdy and Larson[54] studied the reliability and objectivity of blood-pressure measurement under controlled experimental conditions. The reliabilities for systolic, diastolic, and pulse pressures ranged from 0.72 to 0.91 indicating that high reliability and objectivity for after-exercise tests of these measures are difficult to achieve; thus, special care is necessary in making the observations.

Evaluation

Considerable clarification on the application of cardiovascular tests in health and physical education has occurred in recent years. The factor analyses mentioned earlier in this chapter have contributed to this clarification—several factors have emerged, which have low and mostly insignificant correlations with each other. Thus, low correlations between tests representing these factors would be expected; no one test would necessarily be adequate to evaluate the totality of circulatory-respiratory endurance.

Research generally supports these observations, except when like test items or conditions appear in correlated batteries. Some examples follow. Sambolin[55] obtained low intercorrelations between several cardiovascular tests, with one exception, a correlation of 0.68 between McCloy's Efficiency Index and Schneider's Physical Efficiency Index. For the exception, however, the test items were comparable, both being based upon changes in heart rate and blood pressure from reclining to standing and following a standard amount of exercise. Correlations between step tests are reasonably high, as shown for women: 0.87 and 0.71 between the Skubic-Hodgkins test and the Queens College and Kent State University tests. The Ohio State University Step Test correlated 0.94 and 0.85 with the Balke Treadmill Test for men and women respectively. These tests have a common element, inasmuch as the subjects continue to perform until a set heart rate is attained.

Generally, cardiovascular tests have shown positive relationships, sometimes conflicting, with functional manifestations of circulatory-respiratory endurance, as indicated in this chapter. Athletes scored higher than nonathletes on such tests as the brachial pulse wave and several of the step tests for both men and women. A correlation of 0.63 was obtained between the rapid form of the Harvard Step Test and the order of finish in a college intramural cross-country race. The Ohio State University Step Test correlated 0.54 with distance run in 12 minutes. Relative maxVO₂ correlated as high as -0.66 with time for the mile run, although lower and even insignificant correlations have been reported. A correlation of 0.68 was obtained between the McCurdy-Larson Test of Organic Efficiency and time for the 440-yard swim.

Conflicting reports have been made on the relationships between cardiovascular tests and muscular strength and muscular endurance. Rifenberick[56] obtained correlations between 0.80 and 0.94 between the Tuttle Pulse-Ratio Test and Rogers' Physi-

[54]J. H. McCurdy and L. A. Larson, "The Reliability and Objectivity of Blood-Pressure Measurements," *Supplement to the Research Quarterly,* **6,** No. 2 (May 1935), 3.

[55]Luis F. Sambolin, "Extent of Relationship Between Several Strength and Cardiovascular Tests," Master's Thesis, Syracuse University, 1943.

[56]Robert F. Rifenberick, "A Comparison of Physical Fitness Ratings as Determined by the Pulse-Ratio and Rogers' Test of Physical Fitness," *Research Quarterly,* **13,** No. 1 (March 1942), 95.

cal Fitness Index (PFI) for seventh and eighth grade boys. Contrarily, with college men, Neff and Steitz[57] obtained an insignificant correlation between the PFI and the Harvard Step Test; Sambolin did likewise with the Schneider, Crampton, and McCloy cardiovascular-type tests. Relative maxVO₂ has correlated 0.58 and 0.45 respectively with the number of chins and the medicine ball throw for distance.

Certain studies point to possible modifications or substitutes for the present forms of the step tests. Russell[58] experimented with the length of time college men could continue stepping up and down on a 17-inch bench at a rate of 40 steps per minute; each subject continued stepping until unable to do so because of exhaustion. He obtained the following correlations between the length of time this all-out step test was performed, and various motor fitness tests: 0.70 with the Illinois test, 0.64 with the Army Air Forces test, 0.64 with the Navy test, and 0.61 with the Indiana test. He also obtained the high correlation of 0.85 between the length of time the step test was continued and the gross oxygen intake on a treadmill run to exhaustion.

Cardiovascular testing aids

In this section, a number of aids for those who wish to use cardiovascular testing in their physical education programs will be presented.

Benches for Step Tests

Several heights of benches have been utilized for the various step tests described in this chapter. Such benches can easily be constructed; they should be sturdy and the

surface of ample size so that the subject will feel secure in mounting them. Where it is desirable to test a number of subjects simultaneously, a long bench can be used so that several boys or girls can mount it at the same time. A number of assistants will be needed, each to count the pulse rate of a single subject. These assistants should be well trained so that they perform the pulse counts correctly and alike. The tester can then supervise the entire operation, count the cadence, signal the end of the test (preceded by a warning signal), and indicate the start and stop of pulse-count periods. The timer needs to call out the elapsed time for any subject who quits before the termination of the stepping time. Gallagher and Brouha[59] have reported that 600 boys have been given this test in a little more than three hours with the assistance of 30 helpers.

In the Schneider and Tuttle Pulse-Ratio tests, the pulse counts must start immediately upon the cessation of exercise. The timer should give a warning signal 15 seconds before the end of testing time. The pulse counter should grasp the subject's wrist, being careful not to interfere with his stepping, and find his pulse before the exercise is completed in order to start the count promptly.

Where individual testing is done and where the physical educator is using more than one test with different bench heights, a combination bench may be constructed. Such a bench is illustrated in Figure 8.4. The step heights of this bench are 13, 18, and 20 inches. The surface area for each bench is 18 by 18 inches.

Cadence and Pulse Count

Stepping counts may best be regulated by a metronome, which may be set for the proper cadence for the test to be administered. As stepping is a four-count movement, the metronome may be set for any

[57]Neff and Steitz, "Physical Fitness Test Items."

[58]Walter L. Russell, "A Study of the Relationship of Performance in Certain Generally Accepted Tests of Physical Fitness to Circulatory-Respiratory Capacity of Normal College Men," Doctoral Dissertation, Louisiana State University, 1948.

[59]Gallagher and Brouha, "Testing Physical Fitness," p. 23.

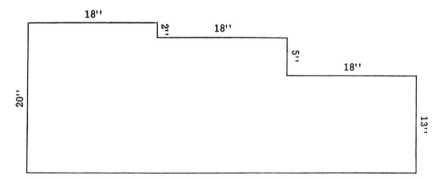

FIGURE 8.4. *Combination Step-up Bench*

one of these movements. For example, in the 30-step-per-minute Harvard Step Test, the metronome may be set at "30," in which case the subject completes the four-count step each time; or, the metronome may be set at "60," in which case the subject mounts the bench on one beat and returns to the floor on the next; or the metronome may be set at "120," in which case the subject completes each part of the step at each beat. The first situation is a bit too slow to follow smoothly; the latter situation is too fast and may result in some confusion. Thus, the 60 cadence is recommended. The tester also helps as needed by calling out the cadence.

If several subjects are taking the test simultaneously, it may be difficult for all to hear the count. The tester may help by calling out the count: "up, up, down, down." It is also possible to connect the metronome to an amplifier; the amplifier can then be adjusted to a degree of sound which can be clearly heard by all. Another device which has proven effective is to make a tape recording of the metronome cadence; by turning up the sound on the player, the cadence can be heard easily. The beat of a drum can be used for this purpose.

Pulse counts can be made in various ways. The most reliable pulse is taken with a stethoscope placed on the chest below the left nipple at a point halfway between the sternum and the left nipple. Lacking a stethoscope, either the carotid or radial pulse may be utilized. For the carotid pulse, place three fingers on the carotid artery at the side of the neck below the jaw. For the radial pulse, place three fingers on the radial artery on the thumb side of the wrist.

Blood Pressure Measurement

The systolic blood pressure is needed for the Crampton Blood-Ptosis Test, the Barach Energy Index, and the Schneider Test; the diastolic blood pressure is necessary for the Barach Energy Index. Blood pressure measurements are made with a mercury sphygmomanometer; a stethoscope is also needed. The cuff is wrapped snugly around the upper part of the left arm just above the elbow joint. The stethoscope earphone is placed in the tester's ears; the stethoscope bell is placed firmly over the brachial artery just above the elbow slightly toward the inside of the arm. The cuff is pumped up with the instrument bulb until no pulse beat can be heard. The tester, then, slowly releases the pressure, watching the mercury column as he does so. When the first pulse sound is heard, the mercury column is read. This is the *systolic pressure*, recorded in millimeters of mercury (mm. Hg.). The tester continues slowly to release the pressure in the cuff. When a dull, forceless beat is noted, the pressure on the mercury column is again read. This is the *diastolic pressure.* Blood pressure is recorded with the systolic reading first. Thus, a recording of 122/72 means a systolic pressure of 122 and a diastolic pressure of 72 mm. Hg. Considerable practice is necessary in order to take blood pressure measurements accurately.

FUNCTIONAL ENDURANCE MEASURES

In defining circulatory-respiratory endurance, the stamina of the body to maintain a run involving a definite aerobic expenditure was aptly used as an illustration of this component of physical fitness. Therefore, it is not surprising that physical educators and others concerned with developing this component have turned to various runs for its evaluation. Initially, short distances, which were more of a sprint than a distance run were used. For example, the 300-yard shuttle run was utilized by the United States Army and Air Forces during World War II. The aerobic requirements for short runs have been questioned, although some endurance is certainly involved. Currently, two runs have come into wide use, the 600-yard run-walk and the 12-minute run.

600-Yard Run-Walk

The 600-yard run-walk is one of the test items comprising the AAHPER Youth Fitness Test,[60] as presented in Chapter 9. Both boys and girls from age 10 years through college are included in the test. Percentile norms for each age 10 through 17 years and college are available and appear in Appendix Table B.10.

Directions for taking this test are: the subject used a standing start, with the forward foot toeing the starting line; at the signals, "Ready?" and "Go," he or she starts running the 600-yard distance; running may be interspersed with walking. It is suggested that a dozen subjects can run at one time by having them pair off before the start of the event. Then, each pupil listens for and notes his partner's time as the latter crosses the finish line; the timer merely calls out the time as each subject crosses the finish. The scoring is in minutes and seconds (fractions of a second are not recorded).

Reliability coefficients for the 600-yard run-walk have been variously reported; a coefficient of 0.90 seems possible, although lower ones have been obtained. Some evidence suggests that greater test-retest reliability occurs with younger than with older subjects, differences in motivation seemingly being a factor.

Several investigators have related time in the 600-yard run-walk to relative maxVO₂; the correlations cluster mostly between -0.62 and -0.71. Davis[61] obtained correlations ranging from -0.67 and -0.79 between the run-walk and the 12-minute run for boys in each grade, fifth through eighth. For girls, the correlations between the two runs had marked differences: respectively, for grades six and seven, -0.83 and -0.85; for five and eight, -0.52 and -0.45. Manahan and Gutin[62] reported a correlation of -0.82 for ninth grade girls between the run-walk and a two-count step test in which the girls performed as many steps on an 18-inch bench as possible in one minute.

[60]*AAHPER Youth Fitness Test Manual,* Rev. Ed. (Washington, D.C.: American Alliance for Health, Physical Education, and Recreation, 1975).

[61]Paul Davis, "Relationships Between the 12-minute Field Test and the 600-Yard Run-Walk for Elementary School Children," Master's Thesis, American University, 1972.

[62]Joan E. Manahan and Bernard Gutin, "The One-Minute Step Test as a Measure of 600-Yard Run Performance," *Research Quarterly,* **42,** No. 2 (May 1971), p. 173.

12-Minute Run

The distance an individual can run in 12 minutes was proposed and popularized by Cooper[63] as a test of circulatory-respiratory endurance; the basic research was conducted with United States Air Force personnel. Subsequently, he and his wife[64] utilized the same test for women. The distance run is recorded in miles. Based on a points system, the adequacy of the individual's circulatory-respiratory training regimen is determined; activities in the training system include running, swimming, cycling, stationary running, and various sports activities. Distance means and standard deviations for younger boys and girls have been reported in miles by Davis,[65] as follows.

	Boys		*Girls*	
Grade	*Mean*	*S.D.*	*Mean*	*S.D.*
Fifth	1.51	0.19	1.34	0.14
Sixth	1.42	0.20	1.42	0.16
Seventh	1.54	0.19	1.25	0.14
Eighth	1.71	0.20	1.30	0.15

Reliability coefficients between 0.90 and 0.94 have consistently been obtained for the 12-minute run for men and women, boys and girls. Conflicting correlations between the distance run and relative maxVO2 have been reported. The highest correlations were around 0.90 in studies by Cooper for men and women, studies by Doolittle and Bigbee[66] for high school boys, and studies by Doolittle, Dominic, and Doolittle[67] for high school girls. However, studies by Maksud and Coutts[68] for boys 11 through 14 years of age, Gregory[69] with college men, and Burris[70] with college women reported lower correlations. Burris obtained correlations of 0.73 and 0.77 between this distance run and relative maxVO2 on a treadmill run and maximum performance on the treadmill, and with optimum work capacity determined from several physiological criteria. A low correlation of 0.42 was obtained by Dunn[71] between the distance run and performance on the Ohio State University Step Test. Burris found a significant improvement between trials one and two on the 12-minute run, so concluded that practice trials should be given before the test score is recorded.

Alternative Runs

Some investigators have questioned the straight-out run, such as the 300-yard run, as an adequate indicator of circulatory-respiratory endurance, largely because these runs do not consider differences in the basic speed of the subjects. As a consequence, alternative procedures for runs have been proposed.

[63]Kenneth H. Cooper, *The New Aerobics* (New York: M. Evans and Company, Inc., 1970).

[64]Mildred Cooper and Kenneth H. Cooper, *Aerobics for Women* (New York: M. Evans and Company, Inc., 1972).

[65]Davis, "The 12-Minute Field Test and the 600-Yard Run-Walk."

[66]T. D. Doolittle and Rollin Bigbee, "The Twelve-Minute Run-Walk: a Test of Cardiorespiratory Fitness of Adolescent Boys," *Research Quarterly,* **39,** No. 3 (October 1968), 491.

[67]T. L. Doolittle, Jo Ann C. Dominic, and Jan Doolittle, "The Reliability of Selected Cardiorespiratory Field Tests with Adolescent Female Populations," *American Corrective Therapy Journal,* **23,** No. 5 (September–October 1969), 135.

[68]Michael G. Maksud and Kenneth D. Coutts, "Application of the Cooper Run-Walk Test to Young Males," *Research Quarterly,* **42,** No. 1 (March 1971), 54.

[69]John D. Gregory, "The Relationship of the Twelve-Minute Run to Maximum Oxygen Intake," Master's Thesis, Mankato State College, 1970.

[70]Barbara J. Burris, "Measurement of Aerobic Capacity of Women," Doctoral Dissertation, University of Wisconsin, 1970.

[71]John M. Dunn, "An Investigation of the Ohio State University Step Test as an Instrument for Assessing the Cardiovascular Efficiency of 13–18 Year Old Boys," Master's Thesis, Northern Illinois University, 1969.

Endurance Ratio.   The endurance ratio is the proportion between times in short and long runs. This technique is intended to account for the individual's basic speed in the short event; the ratio indicates how well this speed is carried over the longer distance. McCloy[72] computed a factor analysis on 12 athletic events, administered to 400 men. Four factors were found and identified as follows: circulo-respiratory endurance, velocity, muscular endurance, and mesomorphic body build (tentatively identified). An endurance ratio, obtained as the ratio between the 300-yard and six-seconds runs, had a factor weighting of 0.88 with circulo-respiratory endurance.

Drop-off Index.   In the drop-off index the slowing up in seconds for various parts of a long run is recorded. Cureton[73] utilized this technique in the 100-yard swim by recording the slowing up cumulatively from lap to lap throughout the distance. Another form of the drop-off index is the difference between the time required for a relatively long run and the time that would have been made had the runner maintained the speed he established in the sprint.

Residual Index.   Henry and Kleeberger[74] objected to such indices as the above because the index scores of their subjects

[72]C. H. McCloy, "A Factor Analysis of Tests of Endurance," *Research Quarterly,* **27,** No. 2 (May 1956), 213.

[73]Thomas K. Cureton, "A Test for Endurance in Speed Swimming," *Supplement to the Research Quarterly,* **6,** No. 2 (May 1935), 106.

[74]Franklin M. Henry and F. L. Kleeberger, "The Validity of the Pulse-Ratio Test of Cardiac Efficiency," *Research Quarterly,* **9,** No. 1 (March 1938), 32.

showed a considerable correlation with times on the short distance, indicating that the indices did not achieve their purpose. As a result of their experimentation, a residual index was proposed consisting of the ratio between time on the 70-yard dash, less the time for the first 10 yards (to eliminate variability in starting time) and time in the 220-yard sprint. These investigators also proposed a variation of the residual index in which the effect of speed was partialed out by statistical procedure.

SELECTED REFERENCES

CLARKE, H. HARRISON, *Physical Fitness Research Digest,* President's Council on Physical Fitness and Sports: "Circulatory-Respiratory Endurance," **3,** No. 3 (July 1973); "Circulatory-Respiratory Endurance Improvement," **4,** No. 3 (July 1974).

CLARKE, H. HARRISON, and DAVID H. CLARKE, *Developmental and Adapted Physical Education.* Englewood Cliffs, N.J.: Prentice-Hall, Inc., 1963, Ch. 4.

CURETON, THOMAS K., and L. F. STERLING, "Factor Analysis of Cardiovascular Tests," *Journal of Sports Medicine and Physical Fitness,* **4,** No. 1 (March 1964), 1.

HENRY, FRANKLIN M., and DANIEL S. FARMER, "Condition Ratings and Endurance Measures," *Research Quarterly,* **20,** No. 2 (May 1949), 126.

LARSON, LEONARD A., "Cardiovascular-Respiratory Function," *Supplement to the Research Quarterly,* **12,** No. 2 (May 1941), 456.

McCLOY, C. H., "A Factor Analysis of Tests of Endurance," *Research Quarterly,* **27,** No. 2 (May 1956), 213.

CHAPTER 9

Motor
Fitness Tests

The term motor fitness came into being during World War II. Actually, motor fitness is a limited phase of general motor ability, with emphasis placed on the underlying elements of vigorous physical activity, but does not include the primary elements of coordination and skills. It is also a more general fitness designation than physical fitness. The relationships between the three concepts may best be explained in terms of their basic elements, as shown in Figure 9.1. Thus, organic soundness and proper nutrition undergird the entire physical structure. The basic physical fitness elements are muscular strength, muscular endurance, and circulatory endurance. Muscular power, agility, speed, and flexibility are added to compose motor fitness; then, kinesthetic arm-eye foot-eye coordinations are needed for general motor ability.

Definitions of the various elements designated in the motor fitness concept presented above are as follows.

Muscular Strength. Muscular strength refers to the maximum contraction power of the muscles. How strong muscles are is usually measured with dynamometers or tensiometers, which record the amount of force particular muscle groups can apply in a single effort.

Muscular Endurance. Muscular endurance is the ability of muscles to perform work. Two manifestations of muscular endurance are recognized: *isometric,* whereby a maximum static muscular contraction is held; and *isotonic,* whereby the muscles continue to raise and lower a submaximal load, as in weight training or performing push-ups. In the isometric form, the muscles maintain a fixed length; in the isotonic form, they alternately shorten and lengthen. Muscular endurance must assume some muscular strength. However, there are differences between the two; muscle groups of the same strength may possess different degrees of endurance.

Circulatory-Respiratory Endurance. Circulatory-respiratory endurance is characterized by moderate contractions of large muscle groups for relatively long periods of time, during which maximal adjustments of the circulatory-respiratory system to the activity are necessary, as in distance running and swimming. Obviously, strong and enduring muscles are needed. However, by themselves, they are not enough; they do not guarantee well-developed circulatory and respiratory functions.

Muscular Power. Muscular power is the ability to release maximum muscular force in an explosive manner, that is, in the shortest possible time. Example: standing broad jump.

Agility. Speed in changing body positions or in changing direction. Examples: squat thrusts; dodging run.

Speed. Rapidity with which a movement or successive movements of the same kind may be performed. Examples: flexing the forearm; 50-yard dash.

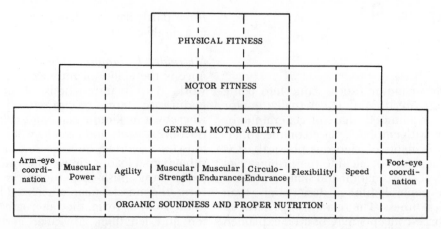

FIGURE 9.1. *Chart of Physical Elements*

Flexibility. Range of movement in a joint or a sequence of joints. Examples: knee extension movement; touching fingers to floor without bending the knees.

In the above discussion, only the most fundamental elements in physical and motor fitness and general motor ability are indicated. Many other elements could be mentioned and are considered by other authors. McCloy[1] gives a much more complete coverage of these elements, presenting 9 physical qualities and 18 "motor educability" factors. For the purpose of this text, however, the smaller, basic number is considered adequate.

OREGON MOTOR FITNESS TEST

On two different occasions, Oregon motor fitness tests[2] have been constructed. Research on the most recent of these tests was conducted separately for boys and girls each at the elementary, junior high, and senior high school levels by graduate students at the University of Oregon and Oregon State University. The motor fitness elements and suggested test items for each element were proposed by a statewide committee. The elements selected for this test were: arm and shoulder girdle strength and endurance, abdominal strength and endurance, muscular power, running speed and endurance, agility, and trunk flexibility.

The construction of the tests followed essentially the same pattern for both sexes at the three school levels. Potentially useful test items were assembled for each of the several motor fitness elements. These test items were administered twice, each time by a different tester, to a random sample of subjects who were representative of the sex and age group for which the test was intended. Objectivity coefficients were computed based on the repeated tests. At this point, those test items were discarded which had low objectivity coefficients and which did not discriminate between levels of performance. A composite of the remaining test items served as the criterion of motor fitness; the test items to compose each motor fitness battery were selected by multiple correlation procedures. The multiple correlations for three-item batteries ranged from 0.91 to 0.95.

[1]C. H. McCloy and Norma D. Young, *Tests and Measurements in Health and Physical Education,* 3rd ed. (New York: Appleton-Century-Crofts, Inc., 1954), pp. 4–11.

[2]*Motor Fitness Tests for Oregon Schools* (Salem, Oregon: State Department of Education, 1962).

Boys' Batteries

Upper Elementary School. The test items for boys in grades four, five, and six are: standing broad jump, floor push-ups, and sit-ups. These tests are illustrated in Figure 9.2.

1. Standing broad jump: A take-off line is drawn on the floor, ground, or mat. At a distance all can jump, but at an even number of feet for convenience, a second line is drawn; additional parallel lines two inches apart are drawn to a point exceeding the farthest jump anticipated. The boy takes a position with toes just touching the take-off line, feet slightly apart. Taking off from both feet simultaneously, he jumps as far as possible, landing on both feet; in jumping, he crouches slightly and swings the arms to aid the jump. Scoring is the distance to the nearest inch from take-off line to the closest heel position; if the pupil falls back, he should retake the test. The best of three trials is recorded.

2. Floor push-ups: The boy takes a front-leaning rest position with body supported on hands and balls of feet; the arms are straight and at right angles to the body. He then dips or lowers the body so that the chest touches or nearly touches the floor, then pushes back to the starting position by straightening the arms, and repeats the procedure as many times as possible. In performing floor push-ups, only the chest should touch the floor; the arms must be completely extended with each push-up; the body must be held straight throughout. Scoring consists of the number of correct push-ups.

3. Knee-touch sit-ups: The boy lies on his back, knees straight, feet about 12 inches apart, and hands clasped behind his head. A scorer kneels on the floor and holds the feet, pressing firmly. The pupil performs the following movement as many times as possible: (a) raise the trunk rotating it somewhat to the right, and bend forward far enough to touch the right elbow to the left knee; (b) lower the trunk to the floor; (c) sit up again, but rotate the trunk to the left and touch the left elbow to the right knee; (d) again, lower the trunk to the floor. The knees may be slightly bent as the boy sits up. However, he must not pause during the test, and bouncing from the floor is not permissible. In scoring, one point is given for each complete movement of touching elbow to knee.

Junior and Senior High Schools. The test items for boys in both junior high school and senior high school are the same: jump and reach, pull-ups, and 160-yard potato race.

1. Pull-ups: See page 132.

2. Jump and reach: Same as vertical jump, page 241.

3. 160-yard potato race: Three circles, each one foot in diameter, are drawn on the floor in line with each other. Circle 1 is behind and tangent to a starting line. The center of circle 2 is 50 feet from the starting line, and circle 3 is 70 feet from the starting line. (See Figure 9.3.) One two by four inch block, or eraser, is placed in circle 2, and a second one is placed in circle 3. From a standing start, the subject (a) runs to circle 2, picks up the block, returns to circle 1 and places it in the circle; (b) he then runs to circle 3, picks up the block and carries it to circle 1; (c) he immediately picks up the first block, carries it back to circle 2; (d) he then returns to circle 1, picks up the second block and carries it to circle 3; (e) finally, he races back across the starting line. The blocks must be placed, not dropped or thrown, in the proper circle each time.

Three or four stations are possible in giving this test so that a number of students may compete at once. In this instance, a comparable number of spotters are necessary. As the first runner approaches the finish line, the starter counts the seconds in a loud voice. Each spotter observes his contestant and records the time as he crosses the finish line. The score is the elapsed time in seconds.

T-scale scoring charts for the boys' Oregon Motor Fitness Tests appear in Appendix Table B.8A. T-score scales are also available in the Oregon state manual and on state score cards.

Girls' Batteries

The Oregon Motor Fitness Test items for girls are: hanging in arm-flexed position, standing broad jump, and crossed-arm curl-ups. These tests are given as follows.

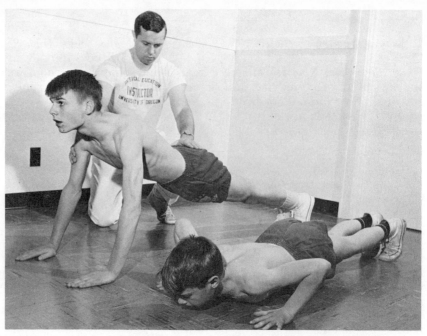

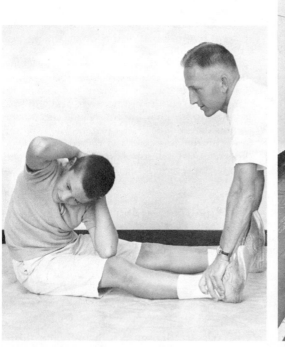

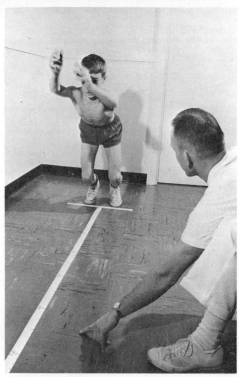

FIGURE 9.2. *Oregon Motor Fitness Tests for Elementary School Boys.* Top: *Push-ups.* Right: *Standing broad jumps.* Left: *Knee-touch sit-ups.*

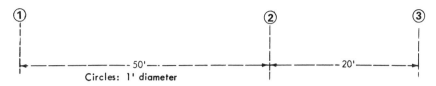

FIGURE 9.3. *Oregon Boys' 160-Yard Potato Race*

1. Hanging in arm-flexed position (Figure 9.4A). The girl stands on a stool or other support, placing her hands shoulder width apart, palms outward, on a one-inch standard horizontal bar or ladder with elbows flexed to permit the chin to be level with the bar. The support is removed. The girl holds her chin at the level of the bar as long as she can do so. (The legs should remain extended throughout.) The score is the number of seconds the student is able to maintain some flexion in the elbow, preventing the elbow from straightening. The chin should not rest on the bar.

2. Standing broad jump. Same as for boys' test.

3. Crossed-arm curl-ups. (Figure 9.4B). The subject assumes a lying position on her back with knees bent at approximately a right angle, soles of the feet flat on the floor, hip width apart; the arms are folded and held against the chest. The girl's feet should be held down firmly by a partner. The test consists of raising the trunk to an erect sitting position and returning to a back-lying position as many times as possible. The feet must remain on the floor throughout the test; the elbows must be kept down and the arms not used to help the body sit up; bouncing from the floor is not permissible; resting during any phase of the performance is not allowed. The score is the number of times the girl raises herself correctly to a sitting position.

T-scale scoring charts for the girls' Oregon Motor Fitness Tests are provided in Appendix Table B.8B.

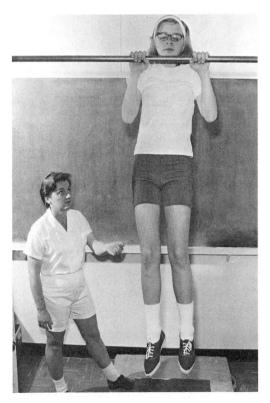

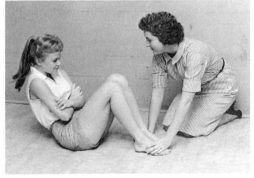

FIGURE 9.4. *Oregon Girls' Motor Fitness Tests.* Left: *Hanging in arm-flexed position.* Above: *Crossed-arm curl-ups.*

CALIFORNIA PHYSICAL PERFORMANCE TESTS

A new revision of the California Physical Performance Test[3] for boys and girls from 10 through 18 years of age was announced in 1971. The test items were designated by physical educators and research specialists in the state. A single battery of six physical performance test events was adopted, consisting of standing long jump, knee bent sit-ups for one minute, chair push-ups, side steps, pull-ups, and jog-walk. In a subsequent memorandum, the flexed arm hang was allowed as an alternate test for girls who cannot perform one pull-up.[4] Directions for these tests follow.

1. Standing long jump. Same as for standing broad jump. Oregon Motor Fitness Test (page 175, Figure 9.2).

2. Knee bent sit-ups for time. The pupil assumes a supine lying position, knees bent to an angle less than 90 degrees, and hands clasped behind neck. The feet are held down by a partner. To perform the sit-ups, the pupil brings his head and elbows forward in a curl-up motion, touching elbows to knees. In returning to the supine position, the elbows should touch the floor each time. *Scoring:* number of correctly executed sit-ups performed in one minute.

3. Side step. A set of three parallel lines, each five feet long, are needed; the distance from the middle of the center line to the outer borders of each outside line is four feet. The test: the pupil takes a standing position astride the center line; on signal to start, he sidesteps to the left until his left foot completely crosses the left line; he then sidesteps to the right across the center line and touches the floor outside the right line with the right foot; this maneuver continues as rapidly as possible. *Scoring:* one point each time a line is crossed, left, center, or right, in 10 seconds.

[3]Genevie Dexter, *The Physical Performance Test for California,* rev. ed. (Sacramento, Calif.: Bureau of Physical Education, Health Education, Athletics, and Recreation, California State Department of Education, 1971).

[4]John J. Klumb and Genevie Dexter, "Designation of the Physical Performance Test for California by the California State Board of Education for the 1974–1975 School Year," Communication, Department of Education, State of California, April 1974.

4. Chair push-ups. The pupil grips the front corners of a chair, assumes a front leaning rest position with arms and body forming a right angle, legs together, and with both feet against a wall, toes supporting the legs; the chair is held securely by a partner. In performing push-ups, the body should be lowered until the chest touches the nearest edge of the chair seat, which is the starting position for the test; the body should be kept straight throughout. *Scoring:* number of push-ups correctly performed; the pupil is stopped after the 50th push-up.

5. Pull-ups. Same as in Rogers' Strength Index test (page 132, Figure 7.5). An alternative test, the flexed-arm hang, is provided for girls who cannot perform one pull-up. This test is performed in the same manner as for "hanging in arm-flexed position," Oregon Motor Fitness Test (page 177, Figure 9.4). However, the time is terminated when the girl's chin touches the bar, or her head tilts backward to keep chin above bar, or her chin falls below the level of the bar. *Scoring:* time in seconds chin is held above bar.

6. Jog-walk. The jog-walk area, whether it be an oval, a circle, or a rectangle, should be a multiple of 110 yards, in order to mark out equal segments of this length; thus, a 440-yard track would have four 110-yard distances. The subject covers as much distance as possible in six minutes; walking is permitted if necessary. *Scoring:* number of 110-yard segments completed, plus the one the pupil is in when time is terminated. A spotter for each participant should be assigned to count the number of segments completed.

A separate percentile table for boys and for girls at each age 10 through 18 years is available for each test, as shown in Appendix Table B.9 for all tests but the flexed-arm hang. The norms for the latter test are the same as contained in the AAHPER Youth Fitness Test (Appendix Table B.10).

AAHPER YOUTH FITNESS TEST

Under the chairmanship of Paul A. Hunsicker, University of Michigan, a committee of the American Alliance for Health, Physical Education, and Recreation, as now known, selected test items to compose the AAHPER Youth Fitness Test. Percentile Norms, based both on age and on the Neilson-Cozens (California) Classification Index, were initially presented in 1957; some revisions of test items and new norms were developed in 1965. Some 9200 children from 10 to 17 years of age inclusive participated in the revision of the norms. A representative United States sample was drawn by the Survey Research Center of the University of Michigan. Subsequently, norms were constructed for college men and women respectively by Hunsicker and by Dorothy R. Mohr, then at the University of Maryland.

In 1975, a second revision of the AAHPER test was announced, proposed jointly by the AAHPER and the President's Council on Physical Fitness and Sports.[5] The following changes were made over the preceding revision: softball distance throw eliminated; bent-knee sit-ups for one minute replaced the unlimited straight-knee sit-ups; the 600-yard run-walk retained, but two optional runs added, 1 mile or 9-minute run for ages 10-12 and 1½ miles or 12-minute run for ages 13 and over. Percentile norms for boys and girls at each age 10 through 18 and for college men and women appear in Appendix Table B.10. In using the norms, age is recorded to the last birthday. Percentile norms based on the Neilson-Cozens Classification Index are not given here, inasmuch as Espenschade[6] found that height and weight did not appreciably influence the scores on the tests beyond the influence of age alone. Instructions for giving the tests follow.

1a. Pull-ups (boys). Same as in Strength Index, without use of rings (page 132, Figure 7.5).

1b. Flexed-arm hang (girls). This test is comparable to "hanging in arm-flexed position," as

contained in the girls' Oregon Motor Fitness Test, although administered differently. The height of the bar is adjusted to equal each girl's standing height. An overhand grasp is used, as in the Oregon test. With the assistance of two spotters, one in front and one behind, the pupil raises her body to a position where the chin is above the bar; the elbows are flexed and the chest is close to the bar. The girl holds this position as long as possible. Time is started as soon as the hanging position is taken. The watch is stopped when (a) pupil's chin touches the bar, (b) pupil's head tilts backward to keep chin above the bar, (c) pupil's chin falls below the level of the bar. Time is recorded to the nearest second the hanging position is held.

2. Bent-knee sit-ups (one minute). Same as in California Physical Performance Test (page 178).

3. Shuttle run (boys and girls). Two blocks of wood two by two by four inches are used; the pupils wear sneakers or run barefooted. Two parallel lines are marked on the floor 30 feet apart. The blocks are placed behind one of the lines; the subjects start from behind the other, or starting, line. The test consists of running to the blocks and bringing them to the starting line one at a time and *placing* them behind the starting line. Two trials are allowed with some rest between. Record the time of the best of the two trials to the nearest tenth of a second.

4. Standing broad jump. Same as in the Oregon Motor Fitness Test (page 175, Figure 9.2). Indoors, a tape measure may be taped to the floor; the pupil may then jump along this tape, as shown in the illustration.

5. 50-yard dash. The pupil takes a position behind the starting line. The starter uses the commands "Are you ready?" and "Go!" The word "Go" is accompanied by a downward sweep of the starter's arm as a signal to the timer. More than one pupil may run at a time if sufficient stop watches are available. The score is recorded in seconds to the nearest tenth of a second.

6. 600-yard run-walk. The pupil uses a standing start. At the signals "Ready?" and "Go!" the subject starts running the 600-yard distance; the running may be interspersed with walking. Time is recorded in minutes and seconds.

Alternate Runs. As indicated above, alternate runs may be used in place of the 600-yard run-walk: 9 minutes or 1 mile for ages 10 through 12 years and 12 minutes or 1½ miles for older ages.

[5]*AAHPER Youth Fitness Test Manual*, rev. 1975 ed. American Alliance for Health, Physical Education, and Recreation, 1201 Sixteenth Street, N.W., Washington D.C. 20036.

[6]Anna S. Espenschade, "Restudy of Relationships Between Physical Performance of School Children and Age, Height, and Weight," *Research Quarterly,* **34,** No. 2 (May 1963), 144.

Hunsicker and Reiff[7] compared the average achieved by boys and girls in the 1958 and 1965 surveys for each youth fitness test item at each age 10 through 17. The averages for the girls were higher in 1965 in all instances, except for the softball distance throw at ages 16 and 17 years; 39 comparisons were significant at the 0.05 level and 9 were not. The boys' averages at each age were high in 1965 for all comparisons; in all but two instances, the differences between averages were significant. This improvement in youth fitness over a seven-year period is attributed to increased efforts by school physical educators throughout the nation to enhance the physical fitness of boys and girls in their classes. This effort was rigorously stimulated and abetted by the President's Council on Physical Fitness and Sports.

The AAHPER Youth Fitness Test has been subjected to research by several investigators. Corroll[8] related relative maxVO2 to the test items plus height and weight with 11-year-old boys as subjects. His highest multiple correlation was 0.78 with 600-yard run-walk and weight as the test items. For boys ages 16 and 17, Olree and associates[9] obtained a multiple correlation of 0.615 for relative maxVO2 versus 600-yard run-walk, shuttle run, and 50-yard dash. These investigators also formed a criterion consisting of the mean percentile on the 1965 seven-item AAHPER tests. Multiple correlations reported were 0.93 with pull-ups, sit-ups, and 50-yard dash as the test items and 0.90 with 600-yard run-walk and standing broad jump as the

items. Mohr[10] obtained insignificant to low correlations between test items for college women.

The AAHPER Youth Fitness Test has been officially adopted by the President's Council on Physical Fitness and Sports as part of its motivational and evaluation processes. And, the test items form the basis for the President's Physical Fitness Award, which has been won by over a million boys and girls since its inception in March, 1966. To earn an award, a girl or boy must achieve the 85th percentile or better on all tests.

PCPFS SCREENING TESTS

The President's Council on Physical Fitness and Sports has recommended that all pupils receive a screening test[11] at the beginning of the school year and be retested each six weeks on tests failed until they are passed. Four such tests, which measure levels of cardiovascular endurance, muscular endurance, and agility, are presented. The "Recovery Index Test," a step test, is included—this test was described in Chapter 8. The other tests consist of the following:

Pull-ups for boys and flexed-arm hang for girls: arm and shoulder muscular endurance.

Sit-ups for boys and girls: abdominal muscular endurance.

Squat thrusts for 10 seconds: agility.

Instructions for administering boys' pull-ups, girls' flexed-arm hang, and sit-ups are the same as in the AAHPER Youth Fitness Test. The squat-thrust test is given in the following manner:

---

[7]Paul A. Hunsicker and Guy G. Reiff, "A Survey and Comparison of Youth Fitness 1958 to 1965," *Journal of Health, Physical Education, and Recreation,* **37,** No. 1 (January 1966), 23.

[8]Victor A. Corroll, "AAHPER Youth Fitness Test Items and Maximum Oxygen Intake," Doctoral Dissertation, University of Illinois, 1967.

[9]Harry Olree and others, "Evaluation of the AAHPER Youth Fitness Test," *Journal of Sports Medicine and Physical Fitness,* **5,** No. 2 (June 1965), 67.

[10]Dorothy R. Mohr, "Interrelationships Between Physical Fitness Scores," *Research Quarterly,* **38,** No. 4 (December 1967), 725.

[11]*Youth Physical Fitness: Suggestions for School Programs,* rev. ed. (Washington, D.C.: U.S. Government Printing Office, 1973).

Starting Position. Pupil stands erect.

Action, by Four-Count Movement. (1) Bend knees and place hands on floor in front of feet; arms may be outside, inside, or in front of knees. (2) Thrust legs back until the back is straight from shoulder to feet (push-up position). (3) Return to squat position. (4) Return to standing position.

Rule. Pupil should be instructed how to do a correct squat thrust and encouraged to do as many as possible in a 10-second time limit. The pupil must come to erect standing position at the completion of each squat thrust.

To pass the screening test items, the following standards are provided:

Girls' Screening Standards

Test	Age	Standard
Flexed-Arm Hang	10–17	3 sec.
Sit-ups	10–14	20
	15	19
	16–17	18
Squat Thrusts	10–17	3

Boys' Screening Standards

Test	Age	Standard	Age	Standard
Pull-ups	10–13	1	16	4
	14	2	17	5
	15	3		
Sit-ups	10	25	14	45
	11	26	15	49
	12	30	16	50
	13	38	17	45
Squat-Thrusts	10–17	4		

NSWA PHYSICAL PERFORMANCE TEST

The National Section on Women's Athletics (NSWA)[12] proposed a motor fitness test[13] for high school girls consisting of eight items designed to evaluate muscular control and coordination, speed, agility, and "strength to move the body and implements used in work and play." The following five-item battery is suggested when circumstances do not permit use of all eight tests: standing broad jump, basketball distance throw, potato race *or* 10-second squat thrusts, unlimited sit-ups, and push-ups *or* pull-ups. For the eight-item battery, the 30-second squat thrust test is added and both the potato race and 10-second squat thrusts and both push-ups and pull-ups are included. Descriptions of the test techniques follow.

Standing Broad Jump. Same as in Oregon Motor Fitness Test (page 175, Figure 9.2).

Basketball Distance Throw. The girl throws from behind a throwing line. Only one step is allowed, but both feet must remain behind the throwing line until the ball has left the hand. The score is the distance in feet, to the nearest foot, that the ball travels in the air; the best of two trials is recorded. Scoring may be facilitated by marking parallel lines on the floor or field, at intervals of five feet, starting at the shortest and ending at the longest throws anticipated.

Potato Race. Two lines are drawn on the floor 30 feet apart, the width of a volley ball court. Two blocks or erasers are placed beyond the second line. The subject stands behind the first line; on signal, she runs to the second line, picks up one block, runs back to the first line, and places (not throws) the block behind the line; she then returns to the second line, picks up the second block, and runs back over the first line with the block in her hand. The best of two trials is recorded in seconds and fifths of seconds.

[12]The National Section on Women's Athletics has had name changes. For some time, it was known as the Division of Girls' and Women's Sports of the American Association for Health, Physical Education, and Recreation; currently, the designation is the National Association for Girls' and Women's Sports of the American Alliance for Health, Physical Education, and Recreation.

[13]Eleanor Metheny, "Physical Performance Levels for High School Girls," *Journal of Health and Physical Education*, **16**, No. 6 (June 1945), 32.

Modified Pull-ups. Modified pull-ups are performed from a 3½ foot high horizontal bar. For the starting position, the girl grasps the bar with both hands, palms upward, bends her arms and moves her body under the bar until it is parallel with the floor when the knees are bent at a right angle and the feet flat on the floor. From this position, she pulls up until her chest touches the bar, the body must move from the knees, without bending the hips or rounding or hollowing the back. Then, the body is lowered to the starting position. This movement is repeated as many times as possible. The score is the number of completed pull-ups.

Knee Push-ups. The girl kneels on a mat and places her hands on the floor in position for push-ups. In this position, body support is borne by the knees and hands; the body is straight with hands below shoulders and shoulder width apart; the feet are raised. The body is lowered until the chest touches the floor, then pushing up until the arms are straight; the body should remain straight throughout. The score is the number of times correct push-ups are performed.

Knee Touch Sit-ups. Same as in the Oregon Motor Fitness Test (page 175, Figure 9.2).

10-Second and 30-Second Squat Thrusts. Squat thrusts are performed by the same procedure described in the PCPFS Screening Test, page 180. The score is the number of complete squat thrusts plus extra quarter movements.

A six-sigma scoring chart, three standard deviations both sides of the mean, for each item on this test appears in Appendix Table B.11.

NEW YORK STATE PHYSICAL FITNESS SCREENING TEST

The New York state test is designed to provide schools with a convenient instrument for periodic evaluation of status and progress in motor fitness of boys and girls in grades four through twelve; the intent, too, was to use the test to identify physically underdeveloped children, so that appropriate steps could be taken to provide for their improvement. Two batteries of tests are proposed, the total test[14] and a screening test. The total test has seven items, one for each of the following components: posture, accuracy, strength (muscular endurance), agility, speed, balance, and endurance. Only four of these components are represented in the screening test; these tests and their descriptions follow.

Agility Test, Sidesteps. Same as in California Physical Performance Test (page 178).

Strength Test, Sit-ups. Sit-ups start from a back-lying position, knees straight, feet about one foot apart, hands behind the neck. On each sit-up, the elbow is alternately touched to the opposite knee. *Scoring:* Number of sit-ups in one minute.

Speed Test, Shuttle Run. Turning markers, such as Indian clubs or rubber cones should be placed 15 yards apart. The pupil traverses this distance, going around the markers each time. The distances run vary for different grades as follows:

No. of Laps	No. of Yards	Grade Group
1½	45	All pupils, grades 4–6
2	60	Girls in grades 7–12
3	90	Boys in grades 7–9
4	120	Boys in grades 10–12

Score: The pupil's score is the time to the nearest half second that it takes to run the indicated number of laps for his or her grade group.

Endurance Test, Squat Thrusts. Same as in PCPFS Screening Test (page 180). *Scoring:*

[14]*New York State Physical Fitness Screening Test,* rev. ed. (Albany: Division of Health, Physical Education, and Recreation, New York State Education Department, 1968).

For all pupils in grades four through six and all girls in grades seven through twelve, number of squat thrusts completed in 30 seconds; for boys in grades seven through twelve, number of squat thrusts in one minute.

Two types of normative information, achievement levels and percentile ranks, are supplied, as shown in Appendix Table B.12. Separate tables are provided for boys and girls at each grade, four through twelve. Achievement levels represent 11 equal units along a scale of physical fitness; the average level is 5 and the high and low extremes are 0 and 10, respectively. Percentile equivalents corresponding to each achievement level are given in the table. A Total Physical Fitness Score is the sum of the achievement levels for the four components of the screening test; this score can be converted to an achievement level by referring to the appropriate column in the table. The New York State Division of Health, Physical Education, and Recreation provides a test manual, a pupil score card, a cumulative record form, and a class record sheet.

The selection of the motor fitness components and the tests to represent each were chosen after consulting research data available in the literature. Test items for the screening test were evaluated on the basis of their validity, reliability, and ease of administration. The reliability coefficients for the total test for boys and girls in the various grades clustered between 0.90 and 0.94. The correlations between each test item and the total fitness score range from 0.65 to 0.76. The norms were obtained by testing 11,145 pupils in 30 school districts throughout New York State, excluding New York City.

GLOVER BATTERY FOR
PRIMARY GRADE CHILDREN

Most motor fitness tests have not included the primary grades within their purview, which is unfortunate as physical educators should not wait until the fourth grade be-

fore effectively dealing with the fitness of their pupils. Glover[15] constructed a test battery which helps fill this gap.

After examining performance items that could be utilized in a motor fitness battery, 18 tests were chosen. These tests were evaluated on two occasions by individuals familiar with physical fitness and with primary school children. On the first occasion, the judges indicated either selection, need for revision, or rejection of each test; as a result, 12 items were retained for further consideration. On the second occasion, the judges made evaluations while the tests were being administered to children. As a consequence, seven tests composed the final selection. Percentile norms were developed for all seven items for all grades combined. However, the following four tests were found to be most valid, reliable, and discriminatory. Barrow[16] developed percentile norms for the four items, boys and girls combined at each age, six, seven, eight, and nine, as shown in Appendix Table B.13.

Standing Broad Jump. Same as in Oregon Motor Fitness Test (page 175, Figure 9.2).

Sit-ups. Sit-ups are performed with knees bent and hands clasped behind the head. The score is the number performed in 30 seconds.

Shuttle Race. Two parallel lines 40 feet apart are marked with masking tape (indoors) or lime (outdoors); two objects, such as waste paper baskets, are placed, one inside and touching the starting line and the other inside and touching the other line (these should be weighted so they will not tip over). The subject is timed in seconds and tenths of a second for two round trips.

[15]Elizabeth G. Glover, "Physical Fitness Test Items in the First, Second, and Third Grades," Master's Thesis, Women's College, University of North Carolina, 1962.
[16]Harold M. Barrow and Rosemary McGee, *A Practical Approach to Measurement in Physical Education,* 2nd. ed. (Philadelphia: Lea & Febiger, 1971), p. 215.

Seal Crawl.   Two parallel lines are drawn 20 feet apart; a ribbon is held by two helpers over the finish line. The subject in a prone position raises and supports his chest and shoulders by placing his hands behind the starting line, fingers facing backward and with elbows straight; the ankles are extended and the body is moved by pulling it along with the arms; if the subject falls, he lifts his body again and continues to crawl. The subject is timed in seconds and tenths of a second, until the hands cross the finish line.

MOTOR FITNESS TESTS OF
THE ARMED FORCES

Starting with World War II, motor fitness tests have been used extensively by the various branches of the armed forces. While these military tests may not be applicable for the elementary and secondary schools, they do have implications for college physical education.

Marine Corps Physical Fitness Tests

The U.S. Marine Corps has designed tests[17] for women between ages 18 and 35 years and for men between ages 17 and 44 years. Older men and women may voluntarily take the tests. Testing is done on a quarterly basis for all Marines.

Female Marines.   Five tests compose the battery for women Marines. For each test, passing scores are indicated. Women failing one or more of the tests are placed in a supervised physical fitness program and retested monthly until the passing standards are met.

1. Shuttle run. Two parallel lines are marked on the ground 30 feet apart; four blocks of wood, two by four by four inches, are placed two feet behind one line; testee stands behind the other line. The test: run to the blocks, pick one up,

[17]Marine Corps Order, 6100. 3 F, 17 December 1971.

run back to the starting line and place the block behind the line; continue for all four blocks; in each instance, both feet must be across the line when placing the block. *Passing:* 27 seconds.

2. Knee push-ups.   Same as in the NSWA Physical Performance Test, page 181. *Passing:* 30, ages 18–25; 25, ages 26–35.

3. Bent knee sit-ups. This test is given with knees bent to an angle of approximately 65 degrees, feet flat on the floor about 12 inches apart and held at ankles by a partner, elbows bent, hands on shoulders. In performing the sit-up, the elbows should alternately touch the opposite knee. *Passing:* 28, ages 18–25; 23, ages 26–35.

4. Jump and reach. Same as described for the vertical jump, page 241, Figure 12.2. *Passing:* 11 inches.

5. 600-yard run-walk. Same as in AAHPER Youth Fitness Test (page 179). *Passing:* 2 minutes, 42 seconds, ages 18–25; 3 minutes, ages 26–35.

Male Marines.   The motor fitness test for male Marines consists of three events: pull-ups, bent knee sit-ups, and three-mile run. These events were selected to test the strength and stamina of the upper body, abdomen, and lower body.

1. Pull-ups. Same as in Strength Index battery (page 132, Figure 7.5).

2. Bent knee sit-ups. The knees are bent at a 90-degree angle, legs spread shoulder width apart, and hands interlocked behind head; the feet are held to the ground by another person. In performing sit-ups, the trunk is raised until the head is directly over the knees; lower the body until the hands touch the ground.

3. Three-mile run. Complete a three-mile measured course on a flat surface as rapidly as possible.

To successfully pass this test, male marines must complete the minimum repetitions or time listed for each of the three events, plus earn the required additional points listed by age group on a performance chart. Additional points may be earned in any of the three events of the test. The required minimum acceptable performance standards appear in Table 9.1. The point system is set out in Appendix Table B.14.

TABLE 9.1. *Male U.S. Marine Corps Test*

A. Required Minimum Performance Standards

Age	Pull-ups	Sit-ups	3-Mile Run (Minutes)	Sub-total Points	Required Added Points	Passing Score
17–26	3	40	28	95	40	135
27–39	3	35	29	84	26	110
40–45	3	35	30	78	7	85

B. Required Minimum Scores

Age	Unsatis-factory	Third Class	Second Class	First Class
17–26	0–134	135	175	225
27–39	0–109	110	150	200
40–45	0–84	85	125	175

To illustrate use of the scoring system, assume a subject 20 years of age performs 7 pull-ups and 40 sit-ups and runs three miles in 23.5 minutes. Looking at Table 9.1A, this 20-year-old man achieved or exceeded minimum performances on all tests. Turning to Appendix Table B.14, the points for these performances are: 6 pull-ups, 30; 40 sit ups, 40; 23.5 minutes, 65. Total points = 135. The passing score for his age group in Table 9.1A is 135, so he just reaches this amount. From Table 9.1B, his total points of 135 places him in third class.

Other U.S. Armed Forces Tests

Department of the Navy. [18] The Navy has adopted the Aerobics Program developed by Kenneth H. Cooper. The latest presentation appears in his book, *The New Aerobics,* published by M. Evans and Company, Inc., New York. During World War II, the Navy had a comprehensive motor fitness testing program. Five items composed the battery: squat thrusts for one minute, knee-touch sit-ups, floor push-ups, pull-ups, and squat jumps. [19]

United States Naval Academy. [20] The physical fitness status of midshipmen is graded on the mile run and three muscular endurance tests, chins, bent-knee sit-ups, and parallel bar dips.

Coast Guard Academy. [21] A physical fitness test battery is administered in the fall and spring each year. Four items comprising the test are pull-ups, bent-knee sit-ups for two minutes, standing long jump, and 300-yard shuttle run (60-yard distance). Also, biannually, a 12-minute run is administered. Scoring tables for all tests are provided. Based on points achieved, cadet physical fitness status is classified as remedial, weak, average, honor, and "Max Club." The points required for these classifications increase each of the four years of Academy tenure. As an absolute minimum, a cadet must score 175 points out of a total of 500, or he will be dismissed from the Academy. Under 250 points, he is added to a remedial physical fitness course and is required to spend free hours working on his personal fitness. [22]

Department of the Air Forces. [23] Physical fitness categories in the Air Forces are based upon time for a 1.5-mile run; adjustments are made for altitude. The airmen are classified in five fitness categories:

[18]Letter from L. E. Belter, Lieutenant Commander, MSC, USN, Assistant to Head of Physical Standards Branch, Bureau of Medicine and Surgery, Department of the Navy, September 30, 1974.

[19]*Physical Fitness Manual for the U.S. Navy,* Bureau of Naval Personnel, Training Division, Physical Section, 1943, Ch. 4.

[20]Department of Physical Education, United States Naval Academy, Annapolis, Md.

[21]"Instructions for Administering Cadet Physical Fitness Evaluation," Department of Physical Education, United States Coast Guard Academy, 1972.

[22]Letter from C. W. Selin, Director, Department of Physical Education, United States Coast Guard Academy, New London, Conn., September 13, 1974.

[23]*USAF Aerobics Physical Fitness Program (Male),* Air Force Pamphlet 50–56, 31 July 1974.

poor, fair, average, good, and excellent. When lack of suitable facilities or adverse weather conditions prohibit using the run, a stationary running test may be substituted to determine the fitness category. The stationary running test is a sustained in-place run at the rate of 80–90 steps per minute, counting only when the left foot strikes the floor. The knees must be brought up in front, raising the feet at least eight inches. The use of a metronome is encouraged to assist in maintaining the proper pace. The score is the length of time in minutes and seconds the pace is maintained.

Army Physical Fitness Tests

During World War II, the Army developed a seven-item Physical Efficiency Test[24] which required two days to administer. Subsequently, this test was reduced to the following five items: pull-ups, squat-jumps, floor push-ups, sit-ups, and 300-yard shuttle runs. Substitution of one-minute squat thrusts was provided for the shuttle run when adequate space for the run was unavailable. Since then, the Army has made changes in motor fitness testing procedures. In 1965, three tests were authorized for use in measuring the physical fitness of male personnel within the Army.

Physical Combat Proficiency Test. This test is standard for evaluating the physical qualities of running, crawling, throwing, climbing, dodging, and jumping. Basically, these skills require agility, coordination, strength, and endurance. There are five events: 40-yard low crawl, horizontal ladder travel by hands, dodge run and jump, grenade throw, and one-mile run. A more recent form of this battery substituted 15-yard man carry for the grenade throw.[25]

Army Minimum Physical Fitness Test. This test is used to determine the physical ability of those active Army personnel who are assigned to duties which preclude participation in a physical fitness program that will prepare them for the Physical Combat Proficiency Test or who cannot be tested on the combat test due to lack of facilities. The test battery consists of selecting one test from each of six categories, as follows: (a) flexibility: squat bender or squat stretch; (b) shoulder girdle: push-ups or 8-count push-ups; (c) abdomen: sit-ups or body twist; (d) back: leg over or leg spreader; (e) legs: squat thrust or mountain climber; (f) endurance: stationary run or half-mile run.

Airborne Trainee Physical Fitness Test.[26] The Airborne Trainee Physical Fitness Test is used as a means of determining the physical ability of the applicant for acceptance to and retention in the Army airborne course. The test items consist of pull-ups, knee bender, floor push-ups, knee-bent sit-ups, and one-mile run.

United States Military Academy.[27] A Physical Aptitude Examination of the motor-fitness type is used for admission to and retention at the United States Military Academy. Four test items are utilized: pull-ups, standing broad jump, modified basketball throw (from the knees), and 300-yard shuttle run (25-yard distance).

Evaluation of Service Tests

In constructing the World War II Air Force motor fitness test, 15 items were selected as measuring the elements to be included in the test. The three items finally selected correlated 0.86 with the 15

[24]Department of the Army Technical Manual 21–200, Change No. 3, *Physical Conditioning* (Washington, D.C.: Government Printing Office, July 11, 1963).

[25]R. M. Mance, "The United States Army Physical Fitness Program," *Physical Educator*, **25**, No. 3 (October 1968), 103.

[26]Department of the Army Technical Manual 21–200, Change No. 4, *Physical Conditioning* (Washington, D.C.: Government Printing Office, May 26, 1965).

[27]"Physical Aptitude Examination," United States Military Academy, West Point, N.Y., 1974 (Robert W. Stauffer, Director of Research and Evaluation, Office of Physical Education, USMA).

items.[28] Validity for an Army physical fitness test utilized during World War II was studied by Esslinger and McCloy[29] with 220 troops who had completed intensive basic training at Fort Knox, Kentucky, and 324 men of the 125th Infantry Regiment. Test items selected for the test battery showed high critical ratios between the upper and lower 25 percent of these troops.

Mathews, Shay, and Clarke,[30,31] as part of pack-carrying studies conducted for the Climatic Research Laboratory, Army Quartermaster Corps, determined the relationships between muscular fatigue caused by carrying military packs under field conditions and various motor-physical fitness tests. The college men serving as subjects were conditioned from six marches carrying the combat load of the rifleman. On the final march, the subjects carried 61 pounds with a rucksack for 7.5 miles at a rate of 2.5 miles in 50 minutes. The highest multiple correlation obtained was. -0.92 between the strength loss of major muscle groups involved and the Strength Index; the correlations between World War II Navy, Air Force, and Army motor fitness tests were -0.57, -0.51, and -0.49 respectively. In terms of predictive index, the Strength Index had 3.4 times greater predictive value than did the Navy test, while the Navy test exceeded the Army test by 38 percent.

In this study, too, the Army motor fitness test correlated well with the other two tests for conditioned subjects, as follows: 0.88 with the Navy test and 0.86 with

the Air Force battery. The correlation between the Navy and Air Force tests was much lower (0.48). The correlations of the Strength Index with the three service tests ranged from 0.32 to 0.50. The correlations of the Physical Fitness Index with the service tests were 0.80 with the Army test, 0.63 with the Air Force test, and 0.49 with the Navy test.

OTHER MOTOR FITNESS TESTS

A large number of other motor fitness tests have been proposed. While many of them are worthy instruments, space does not permit their complete presentation in this text. However, several are briefly described below. The references may be consulted for more detail.

University of Illinois Motor Fitness Tests[32]

In developing motor fitness criteria, Cureton recognized six components, as follows: endurance, power, strength, agility, flexibility, and balance. Fourteen-item and 18-item test batteries were developed, validated against a 30-item criteria. A validity coefficient of 0.87 is reported for the 18-item test. Subsequently, a seven-item motor fitness test was proposed for use when greater administrative simplicity is desired. The items in this battery are: dive and roll, medicine ball put, bar vault, chinning, leg lifts and sit-ups (agility run may be substituted), breath-holding, and man-lift. Scoring is simplified by using the pass or fail plan. This procedure screens out the subjects poor in ability, and does not require a severe effort on the part of the majority of subjects.

Motor fitness tests were also constructed for high-school girls.[33] A single-period test

[28]Leonard A. Larson, "Some Findings Resulting from the Army Air Forces Physical Training Program," *Research Quarterly*, **17**, No. 2 (May 1946), 144.

[29]Arthur A. Esslinger, University of Oregon, unpublished data.

[30]Donald K. Mathews, Clayton T. Shay, and H. Harrison Clarke, "Relationship Between Strength Loss in Pack Carrying and Certain Motor-Physical Fitness Criteria," *Research Quarterly*, **26**, No. 4 (December 1955), 426.

[31]H. Harrison Clarke, Donald K. Mathews, and Clayton T. Shay, "Strength Decrements from Carrying Various Army Packs on Military Marches," *Research Quarterly*, **26**, No. 3 (October 1955), 253.

[32]Thomas K. Cureton, *Physical Fitness Appraisal and Guidance* (St. Louis: The C. V. Mosby Co., 1947), Ch. 13.

[33]Mary E. O'Connor and Thomas K. Cureton, "Motor Fitness Tests for High School Girls," *Research Quarterly*, **16**, No. 4 (December 1945), 302.

of six items and a double-period test of 12 items are available.

The JCR Test

The JCR Test[34] is a three-item battery consisting of the vertical jump (J), chinning (C), and 100-yard shuttle run (R). In the shuttle run, the subject covers a ten-yard course ten times, with the aid of bankboards to assist him in making the turn. The test is intended to measure the ability of the individual to perform fundamental motor skills, such as jumping, chinning, running, and dodging, which involve the basic elements of power, speed, agility, and endurance. Reliability coefficients ranging from 0.91 to 0.97, and validity coefficients from 0.59 to 0.90, are reported for the test. Six-sigma scale scoring tables for college-age men are available. In a subsequent study, a low but definitely positive relationship was found between the JCR Test and success in primary and advanced levels of pilot training.[35]

Elder Motor Fitness Test[36]

Elder developed a motor fitness test designed to evaluate the following eight basic components: strength, endurance, power, agility, flexibility, speed, balance, and body size and age. The composite score on 14 motor fitness items served as the criterion for the selection of tests to compose the final battery. The tests thus selected were: floor push-ups, standing broad jump, trunk flexion forward, Cozens'

dodge run, and 20-second squat thrusts. This battery was found to differentiate well between eight groups considered to be different in terms of their "physical fitness," ranging from "top athletes" to boys who were absent because of illness 15 or more days during a 20-week period. Six-sigma scale norms are available for six divisions of the California Classification System, which is based on the boy's age, height, and weight.

Indiana Motor Fitness Test

Motor fitness tests have been constructed at Indiana University for the following groups: college men,[37] high school boys[38] and girls,[39] and elementary school children.[40] The test items for elementary and high school boys and girls are straddle chins, floor push-ups, vertical jump, and squat thrusts for 20 seconds. For college men, the items are pull-ups or straddle chins, floor push-ups, and vertical jump or standing broad jump. For college men, norms are based on the six-sigma scale for each of the tests. Norms for the other age groups are based on McCloy's Classification Index.

Washington Motor Fitness Test

An elementary school motor fitness test was developed by Glenn Kirchner for the Washington Association for Health, Physi-

---

[34]B. E. Phillips, "The JCR Test," *Research Quarterly,* **18,** No. 1 (March 1947), 12.

[35]B. E. Phillips, "Relationships Between Certain Aspects of Physical Fitness and Success in Pilot Training," *Journal of Aviation Medicine,* **19** (June 1948), 186.

[36]Haskell P. Elder, "Appraising the Physical (Motor) Fitness of Junior High School Boys," Doctoral Dissertation, Springfield College, 1958. Materials obtained from author, 12002 Weatherby Rd., Los Alametose, Calif.

[37]Karl W. Bookwalter and Carolyn W. Bookwalter, *A Measure of Motor Fitness for College,* Bulletin of the School of Education, Indiana University, **19,** No. 2 (September 1943).

[38]State of Indiana, *Physical Fitness Manual for High School Boys,* Bulletin No. 136 (Indianapolis: Department of Public Instruction, 1944).

[39]State of Indiana, *Physical Fitness Manual for High School Girls,* Bulletin No. 137 (Indianapolis: Department of Public Instruction, 1944).

[40]C. C. Franklin and N. G. Lehsten, "Indiana Physical Fitness Tests for the Elementary Level (Grades 4 to 8)," *Physical Educator,* **5,** No. 3 (May 1948), 38.

cal Education, and Recreation;[41] this test was adopted by the Washington State Department of Physical Education and Recreation. It is one of the few tests which include the primary school grades. The test items are: standing broad jump, bench push-ups, curl-ups, squat jumps, and 30-yard dash. T-score norms are available for each sex at each age 7 through 12 years.

Purdue University Motor Fitness Test

At Purdue University, Arnett[42] developed short motor fitness test batteries for high school girls. The battery found best was composed of three items: modified pull-ups, 600-yard run, and standing broad jump. This battery had a validity coefficient of 0.755 and an estimated reliability coefficient of 0.848. In addition, at Purdue University, Ismail and associates[43] have studied motor fitness tests for college men based upon factor analysis of a comprehensive coverage of components and test items.

North Carolina Fitness Test[44]

A motor fitness test was developed for the elementary and secondary schools of North Carolina. The test item consists of 30-second bent-knee sit-ups, 30-second side stepping, standing broad jump, and 30-second squat thrusts for both boys and girls. In addition, boys perform full pull-ups and girls perform a modified form of

pull-ups performed in 30 seconds (from a bar 30 inches from floor). Percentile norms separately for boys and girls at age nine through 17 years are available in the test manual. This test is in process of revision.

Fleishmen Test[45]

Based upon a factor analysis of motor fitness test items with Navy recruits at the Great Lakes and San Diego naval training centers as subjects, test items were selected to construct tests for boys and girls from 12 to 18 years of age. Percentile tables are available in the reference. The test items included in this battery are: extent flexibility, dynamic flexibility, shuttle run, softball throw, hand grip, pull-ups, leg lifts, cable-jump test, and 600-yard run-walk. Percentile tables are available in the reference.

EVALUATION OF MOTOR FITNESS TESTS

The wide use of a motor-fitness type of test has evolved since World War II. These tests are designed to secure ease of operation; little training is required to master the testing techniques involved; with good administration, large numbers can be given the tests in a short time by a few testers; and self-scoring is, in some instances, encouraged. In other words, a major consideration has been to test as easily, as economically, and as simply as possible. Such practices are desirable, provided, of course, that the validity and accuracy of the test are not sacrificed. Although much remains to be studied in relation to the effectiveness of these tests as fitness appraisal instruments, several researches have been reported which throw some light on this problem.

---

[41]*Physical Fitness Test Manual for Elementary Schools* (Olympia, Washington: State Office of Public Instruction, 1966).

[42]Chappelle Arnett, "The Purdue Motor Fitness Test Batteries for Senior High School Girls," *Research Quarterly,* **33,** No. 3 (October 1962), 323.

[43]I. H. Ismail, Pudue University, Lafayette, Indiana.

[44]State of North Carolina, *North Carolina Fitness Test* (Raleigh: State Department of Public Instruction, 1961).

[45]Edwin A. Fleishman, *The Structure and Measurement of Physical Fitness* (Englewood Cliffs, N.J.: Prentice-Hall, Inc., 1964).

Number of Test Items

Two general approaches have been made to the construction of motor fitness tests. One approach is to decide upon the components that comprise motor fitness and to select by research or judgment a test item to represent each. The AAHPER Youth Fitness Test is an example: for the current (1975) issue of the test, six components were chosen; consequently, the battery consists of six items. The second approach also starts with a determination of the components of motor fitness. But, a minimum number of tests is designated to represent all the components, irrespective of whether each component has a corresponding specific test. To accomplish this end, several test items are selected, hopefully an even number for each component to weight them evenly; these are combined into a composite score. By multiple correlation with this composite as a criterion, the fewest and most significant tests to reflect the criterion are selected. The Oregon Motor Fitness Test is an example: seven components were designated; three tests were chosen to comprise the battery, so obviously, all components are not represented by a test. The first approach permits a more diagnostic follow-up of testing, since pupils' weaknesses and strengths in the various components can be identified.

Test Item Evaluations

Sit-ups. The widely used sit-up test is proposed as a measure of the endurance of the abdominal muscles. This test, however, has been the subject of some controversy. For example, does a person who can perform 100 sit-ups have proportionately greater abdominal endurance than one who can do only 50? And how account in fitness terms for the phenomenal records of 500, 1000, 2000 and more sit-ups?

Both DeWitt[46] and Wedemeyer[47] studied two-minute and unlimited sit-ups, and concluded that no markedly significant relationships existed between sit-ups and abdominal strength and endurance. DeWitt's criterion of abdominal strength was a direct pull upward on a dynamometer when lying supine on a table with shoulders over the edge to permit anchoring the instrument to the floor; his criterion of abdominal endurance was the length of time the body could be held clear of the floor while in a sitting position, hands clasped back of head, and feet on floor under bottom rung of stall bars. As a criterion of abdominal strength, Wedemeyer tested his subjects with the Martin "breaking" method while each was in a sitting position, trunk at an angle of 45 degrees with the floor; as a criterion of endurance, the subjects went through a training period and the initial and final results were compared. In this latter study, after strength reached a certain level, further improvement in the number of sit-ups was not accompanied by significant increases in strength. Also, the endurance factor appeared to improve more than did strength.

With college men, Berger[48] compared results obtained from three methods of scoring sit-ups: two-minute, unlimited, and 1-RM (amount of weight a barbell held behind the neck can be raised in a single sit-up.) Sit-ups were performed

[46]R. T. DeWitt, "A Study of the Sit-up Type of Test as a Means of Measuring Strength and Endurance of the Abdominal Muscles," *Research Quarterly,* **15,** No. 1 (March 1944), 60.

[47]Ross Wedemeyer, "A Differential Analysis of Sit-ups for Strength and Muscular Endurance," *Research Quarterly,* **17,** No. 1 (March 1946), 40.

[48]Richard A. Berger, "Evaluation of the 2-Minute Sit-Up Test as a Measure of Muscular Endurance and Strength," *Journal of Association for Physical and Mental Rehabilitation,* **20,** No. 4 (July–August 1966), 140.

with knees bent to a right angle; the sit-up movement was to a vertical position. The correlations between two-minute and unlimited sit-ups was 0.71; these two forms correlated 0.51 and 0.52 with 1-RM sit-up.

While the validity of the sit-up test as an indicator of the condition of the abdominal muscles is doubtful, Mathews[49] questions the use of the straight-leg sit-up from a kinesiological point of view. He points out that the test performed in this position is performed primarily with the iliopsoas muscles, particularly if the back is arched. Thus, as this muscle is attached to the bodies of the lumbar vertebrae, it may, in persons with weak abdominal muscles, cause serious strain at the lumbosacral joint. As a consequence of these observations, Mathews urges that the sit-up test with knees flexed be used.

Squat Jumps. Squat jumps as a motor fitness test item has been used sparingly, which is probably just as well, as some apprehension has been expressed relative to the effect on the knee joint from projecting the body upward from a full squat position. Klein[50] conducted extensive studies of this type of exercise utilizing anatomical analysis, knee dissection studies, knee joint instability found in knee injuries resulting from athletics, and the instability of the knees of weight lifters and paratroopers (who use squat jumps extensively in training). He demonstrated that extensive use of this exercise resulted in frequent knee joint instability; the ligaments especially involved were the lateral and anterior cruciates. As a consequent, Klein recommended that such exercises be avoided. This recommendation has received the support of the National Federation of State High School Athletic Associations and the Committee on the Medical Aspects of Sports of the American Medical Association.

Klein has proposed that squat jumps be performed with the rear foot far enough back so that the knee comes in contact with the floor. In this way, the knee joint is not compressed; the forward leg, which is not less than a right angle of flexion at the knee, takes the stress of the exercise. The effect of this modification on scoring squat-jump performances is uncertain; probably adjustment of norms may be necessary. Additional instructions for administering the test provide for: (a) a warm-up calisthenic drill preceding the testing; (b) instruction in and demonstration of the exact techniques for performing each test item correctly; (c) sufficient number of practice trials in preceding class periods to insure proper understanding of test procedures; and (d) five-minute rest period between the events of the test.

Pull-ups. DeWitt[51] compared the average number of chins college men could do grasping the bar with palms in, with palms out, and with kipping and kicking. He found that his subjects averaged two more chins with the palms-in than with the palms-out grip. The kick-kip method produced slightly more chins than the palms-in method. This study points to the need for indicating the specific grip to be used in pull-ups when including this test in a test battery.

[49]Donald K. Mathews, *Measurement in Physical Education,* 4th ed. (Philadelphia: W. B. Saunders Company, 1973), p. 110.

[50]Karl K. Klein, "The Deep Squat Exercise as Utilized in Weight Training for Athletics and Its Effect on the Ligaments of the Knee," *Journal of Association for Physical and Mental Rehabilitation,* **15,** No. 1 (January-February 1961), 6.

[51]R. T. DeWitt, "A Comparative Study of Three Types of Chinning Tests," *Research Quarterly,* **15,** No. 3 (October 1944), 249.

Reliabilities. McCraw and McClenney[52] administered three motor fitness tests— floor push-ups, pull-ups, and two-minute sit-ups—on four separate occasions to elementary, junior high, and senior high school boys to determine the reliabilities of using a single trial, better of two trials, and average of two trials. A trend analysis of the data revealed significant score increases during the four trials; scores increased significantly from trial to trial on push-ups. Neither the better of two trials nor the average of two trials was found to be any more reliable than a single trial. The range of reliability coefficients for sit ups (0.69 to 0.75) was generally lower than for the other tests (0.83 to 0.97).

With college women as subjects, Dobson[53] obtained the following objectivity coefficients for motor fitness test items: 0.81, squat thrusts for 30 seconds; 0.93, knee push-ups; 0.97, unlimited sit-ups; 0.91, vertical jump; and 0.99, flexed arm hang. With a composite of motor fitness items, she obtained a multiple correlation of 0.90 with flexed arm hang, 30-second squat thrusts, and knee push-ups; when sit-ups and vertical jump were added, the multiple correlation increased to 0.95.

Inter-Relationships

Brown[54] studied the relative effectiveness of 12 physical-motor test batteries, with college men at Southern Methodist University as subjects. A criterion score consisting of performances on the 12 batteries was established. The highest correlations obtained with this criterion were:

0.84 with McCloy's Motor Ability Test, 0.84 with Rogers' Strength Index, 0.81 with Larson's (Outdoor) Motor Ability Test, and 0.80 with the Indiana Motor Fitness Test. Several of these tests are classified in this text as general motor ability tests, as presented in Chapter 12. However, the relationships reported by Brown show the close relationship existing between motor fitness and motor ability. This relationship was pointed out at the beginning of this chapter.

Mathews, Shay, and Clarke[55] obtained various correlations between the World War II service motor fitness tests and the test items composing these tests with conditioned college students. The most significant of these relationships were as follows:

1. Time in 300-yard shuttle run: −0.81 with Army test, −0.74 with Air Force test, −0.72 with Strength Index, −0.66 with Physical Fitness Index, and −0.61 with Navy test.

2. Number of squat thrusts in one minute: 0.79 with Navy test and 0.62 with the Army test.

3. The following multiple correlations were obtained:

   a. Physical Fitness Index, 0.99: leg lift, squat thrusts, and sit-ups.

   b. Strength Index, 0.98: leg lift and squat thrusts.

   c. Army Physical Efficiency Test, 0.95: 300-yard shuttle run, sit-ups, and squat jumps (0.92 without squat jumps).

   d. Navy Standard Physical Fitness Test, 0.93: squat thrusts, squat-jumps, and 300-yard shuttle run.

   e. Air Force Physical Fitness Test, 0.82: 300-yard shuttle run and sit-ups.

Self-Scoring

Self-scoring, as suggested for some of the tests, may be seriously questioned. There is a large chance for error in catching one's time or a partner's time at the

[52]Lynn W. McCraw and Byron N. McClenney, "Reliability of Fitness Strength Tests," *Research Quarterly,* **36,** No. 3 (October 1965), 289.

[53]Margaret J. Dobson, "An Evaluation of the Portland State College Women's Physical Education Classification Test," Doctoral Dissertation, University of Oregon, 1965.

[54]Howard S. Brown, "A Comparative Study of Motor Fitness Tests," *Research Quarterly,* **25,** No. 1 (March 1954), 8.

[55]Mathews, Shay, and Clarke, "Strength Loss and Motor-Physical Fitness Criteria," p. 426.

finish of the runs as the seconds are called off by the timer. The practice of appointing a judge for each individual is much better. Also, unless carefully checked, such tests as chinning or dipping will result in many partial movements being scored as complete. Securing straight elbows in the pull-up test and sufficient elbow bend in dipping is difficult even with competent testers present. And, too, if the individual knows that important decisions affecting his status depend upon his scores, the tendency is to become lax in carrying out the exact requirements of the tests.

SELECTED REFERENCES

AAHPER Youth Fitness Test Manual, rev. ed. Washington, D.C.: American Alliance for Health, Physical Education, and Recreation, 1975.

BROWN, HOWARD S., "A Comparative Study of Motor Fitness Tests," *Research Quarterly,* **25,** No. 1 (March 1954), 8.

CURETON, THOMAS K., *Physical Fitness and Dynamic Health,* rev. ed. New York: The Dial Press, 1973, Part 1, Sec. 2.

HUNSICKER, PAUL A., and GUY G. REIFF, "A Survey and Comparison of Youth Fitness, 1958 to 1965," *Journal of Health, Physical Education, and Recreation,* **37,** No. 1 (January 1966), 23.

MCCLOY, CHARLES H., and NORMA D. YOUNG, *Tests and Measurements in Health and Physical Education,* 3rd ed. New York: Appleton-Century-Crofts, 1954.

MATHEWS, DONALD K., CLAYTON T. SHAY, and H. HARRISON CLARKE, "Relationship Between Strength Loss in Pack Carrying and Certain Motor-Physical Fitness Criteria," *Research Quarterly,* **26,** No. 4 (December 1955), 426.

PART THREE

SOCIAL EFFICIENCY

Social efficiency was defined in Chapter 1 as the development of desirable standards of conduct and of the ability to get along with others. Too frequently in physical education this development is considered merely as a concomitant of the activity program, functioning automatically and requiring neither special planning nor definite programs designed to achieve these results. Character development does continuously take place in all life's activities. This constitutes an obligation and a challenge to physical educators to *see to it* that social development takes the right direction; carefully planned programs should be instituted to realize this objective of physical education.

The physical educator may utilize a number of procedures to achieve the greatest benefits from his efforts to improve the social efficiency of his pupils. In Chapter 3, evidence was presented pertaining to the relationships between physical-motor traits and personal-social traits, and so will not be repeated here. An extensive review of this evidence has been published by the author.[1] In this chapter

[1]H. Harrison Clarke, "The Totality of Man Continued," *Physical Fitness Research Digest*, **2,** No. 1 (January 1972).

Physical Education and Social Efficiency

several such expedients are listed, and the uses of measurement in their development process are pointed out.

ATHLETICS

In the physical educator's attempt to improve social efficiency, special emphasis should be given to sports activities. All kinds of competitive athletics provide many situations requiring individual and social responses. However, team sports should be included in the physical education program for their unique social value, if for no other reason, and no pupil who is physically able to participate should be exempt from the valuable experience of team sports.

While one must consider relative merits, close-knit team sports, such as basketball, soccer, lacrosse, football, water polo, and field and ice hockey offer a unique opportunity through their maximum reliance on team play, for the development of such desirable social traits as co-operation, voluntary suppression of self for the good of the group, leadership, and followership. Most athletics foster such traits as loyalty, quick thinking, initiative, courage, self-control, and a host of other equally desirable characteristics. The realization of such social outcomes is achieved by setting up standards of conduct and applying proper motivation to carry them through. Mores of conduct can be developed by the application of good educational procedures. Such positive slogans as "Play the game," "Play fair," "Hit the line hard," "Follow through," "Play together," "One for all and all for one," are examples of a realistic language for human conduct, indicating the direction and dynamic appeal of such training when properly conducted.

Furthermore, as expressed by Goodwin Watson: "There is no more fundamental human longing than the desire to be an accepted member of a social group."[2] The individual who feels himself isolated, or an outcast, may develop all sorts of undesirable behavior traits. Team sports provide opportunities for all individuals to be members of a group, to participate in group activities, to strive with others toward the accomplishment of desirable goals of achievement. For most pupils, the opportunity itself will be a sufficient incentive. For the reticent pupil, however, wise guidance is essential if he is to experience emotionally the merging of himself with the group.

As an example of the significance of athletic participation, a study by Werner[3] will be cited. On the basis of secondary school histories of athletic participation, he formed two groups of men entering the United States Military Academy; the groups were designated as athletes and nonparticipants. The Cattell Sixteen Personality Factor test was administered to all subjects. The entering cadet athletes were significantly more sociable, dominant, enthusiastic, adventurous, tough, group dependent, and conservative than the cadets with little or no prior competition in sports. Further, the proportion of athletes who graduated from the Academy was significantly greater than for the nonparticipants who graduated.

That many boys and girls do not compete in sports on organized teams may be inferred from an adult physical fitness survey of the American public by the Opinion Research Corporation, Princeton, N.J., for the President's Council on Physical Fitness and Sports.[4] According to

the survey, 38 percent of the men and 60 percent of the women did not compete in athletics either on between schools or within schools teams. Opportunities for such competition should be increased. For men, especially, a great imbalance was found between the two forms of competition; if men competed in school, they invariably had to be good enough to make a school team. Much smaller numbers of women had played sports while in school, even though a balance existed between the inter-school and intramural types, so such programs should be enhanced for them.

Girls and women have been reluctant to develop fully their athletic potentials and to compete in vigorous athletic activities. For many years, women physical education teachers frowned on their competition on inter-school teams. According to Harris,[5] a review of the literature produced no evidence to support the notion that active participation in competitive sports may harm the healthy female, but an unwritten decree seems to exist that only certain sports have a desirable effect on the feminine image. Stereotypes, prejudices, and misconceptions have served to curtail the participation of girls and women in vigorous, competitive activities for too many years. Without question, this situation is changing: more girls are competing and are doing so more frequently. Harris indicated that a revolution in attitudes concerning athletic competition for girls has begun in spite of all the problems involved. The Division of Girls and Womens Sports of the American Association for Health, Physical Education, and Recreation, however, has gone on record as opposed to the exploitation of girls in athletics, as has frequently been the case for boys. This group has indicated that, "The enrichment of the life of the partici-

[2]Goodwin Watson, "Personality Growth Through Athletics," *Journal of Health and Physical Education,* **9,** No. 7 (September 1938), 408.

[3]Alfred C. Werner, "Physical Education and the Development of Leadership Characteristics of Cadets at the United States Military Academy," Doctoral Dissertation, Springfield College, 1960.

[4]H. Harrison Clarke, "National Adult Physical Fitness Survey," *Physical Fitness Research Digest,* **4,** No. 2 (April 1974).

[5]Dorothy V. Harris, "The Sportswoman in Our Society." *DGWS Research Reports: Women in Sports* (Washington, D.C.: American Association for Health, Physical Education, and Recreation, 1971), p. 1.

pant should be the focus and the reason for athletic programs."[6]

SOCIAL ACCEPTABILITY

Social acceptance is an important requisite for satisfactory personal and social adjustment. Lack of social status frequently results in discontent and unhappiness; attainment of status once lacking may produce marked changes in an individual's personality and feeling of well-being. Obtaining and maintaining social acceptability is particularly important during adolescence, as an emerging interest in social, especially heterosexual, relationships is characteristic of this age.

The learning of motor skills is an important element in social adjustment. It often constitutes the difference between the development of social, well-integrated individuals and unsocial, retiring types. The physical education program, therefore, has "a strategic position for contributing to the development of individual students in their personal-social relations."[7]

In connection with the Berkeley Growth Studies, Harold E. Jones[8] reported that boys high in physical strength tend to have good physiques, to be physically fit, and to enjoy a favored social status in adolescence. Boys who are low in strength show a tendency toward asthenic physiques, poor health, social difficulties and lack of status, feelings of inferiority, and personal maladjustment in other areas. In interpreting this social phenomenon, the "pile-up" effect of associated biological

factors should be considered. Individuals low in strength are frequently found to have an accumulative assortment of handicaps and those high in strength frequently show an imposing variety of physical advantages. Thus, those at the strength extremes were deficient or superior not in one but in many aspects of size, build, health, and fitness, each of which makes its additive contribution. It is not surprising that these multiple defects or advantages should be reflected, not merely in physical activity, but also in social participation and in the individual's own attitudes and self-appraisal.

ABILITY GROUPINGS

In this text, equating the powers of opposed individuals and groups has been classified primarily as a phase of the social development program. Other values, however, have not been lost sight of, as there are at least three purposes to be served by ability grouping in physical education: (a) pedagogical advantages; (b) desirable attitudes toward physical education; and (c) social development.

Pedagogical Advantages

Ability grouping is an important pedagogical procedure; class instruction is more efficient when the abilities of groups are similar. Heterogeneous grouping presents a serious problem in class instruction, as class work may well be geared to the ability of the less able pupils. Instruction adapted to the ability of the average student becomes too difficult for the poor performers and too easy for the good ones. Equating, however, brings together pupils of near equal ability, all of whom are ready for instruction on approximately the same level. Skills may thus be taught effectively and efficiently.

Homogeneous grouping, too, may be far more important in physical education

[6]"Policies on Women Athletes Change," *AAHPER Update,* May 1973.

[7]Lois H. Meek, Chairman, *The Personal-Social Development of Boys and Girls with Implications for Secondary Education.* (New York: Committee on Workshops, Progressive Education Association, 1940), p. 204.

[8]Harold E. Jones, "Physical Ability as a Factor in Social Adjustment in Adolescence," *Journal of Educational Research,* **40** (December 1946), 287.

than in scholastic phases of the educational program, as the manner of an individual's participation in many physical activities—what he does, how he reacts—depends to a large extent upon the *actions* of those participating with him. For example, the greatest football player cannot catch a forward pass if the ball is badly thrown, or make long runs against comparable opposition if his own line and blocking backs do not function efficiently in removing potential tacklers from his path; the basketball player cutting for the basket cannot shoot effectively unless the ball is thrown to him in a way in which he can handle it, and unless he can avoid defensive guards attempting to block the shot. Correlative and oppositive efforts of this sort are not required in English, mathematics, and other academic classes.

Ability grouping has been fairly well done in classroom work. Within certain limits, of course, academic grade classification is a reasonably satisfactory arrangement for mental activities. The fact that pupils have been promoted to a certain grade, although differing in such factors as social maturity, intelligence, interest, and industry, is at least partial evidence that they have attained a certain academic level. To use grades in school as the only means of classifying pupils for physical education, however, as is frequently done, is grossly unsatisfactory, as such important elements as physique type, body size, physiological maturity, physical fitness, strength, speed, and ability to learn new skills bear little relationship to academic abilities. Also, especially in high school and college, previous experience and training in physical education activities differ far more widely than they do in academic subjects. It may be assumed, for example, that an entering freshman in college has had certain definite educational training in such subject-matter fields as English, science, social studies, and so forth. In physical education, nothing can be taken for granted, as many college freshmen have had little—or even no—training in physical skills. Such differences, therefore, unless equated in some way, markedly handicap the physical education program.

Desirable Attitudes

Physical educators desire to insure real and lasting interest in physical education activities, not only that their program may be more attractive, but that their pupils may carry on desirable physical activities during their leisure time and engage in them after graduation. But the development of desirable attitudes depends upon the amount of individual skill acquired by the participant and upon satisfying experiences in the activities themselves. By grouping students according to their abilities, opportunity for individual success is increased. Under such conditions pupils compete with approximate equals and thus have the satisfaction of extending themselves and their opponents and of winning a *fair share* of contests. The interest of all participants is therefore largely assured, neither contestant (or team) winning easily or losing badly.

That matching the competing powers of teams is an essential factor in conducting a successful intramural program has been demonstrated repeatedly. One need only observe the practices of professional sports promoters to have a convincing argument: the achievement of initial equality and great doubt of the outcome is their prime aim in boxing, baseball, hockey, and the like. In horse racing, even weight handicaps are added to insure exciting—that is, fair, equal—chances.

During the writer's several years of experience in conducting high school and university intramural programs, the equating of competing teams was carefully planned, with deliberate scheduling of opposing teams of similar ability. In intramural sports, a close game should be regarded as a successful one from the standpoint of the director, for, above all, the interest of all competitors is maintained and return matches are the rule. A lopsided score represents failure, especially failure to maintain the interest of the players on the losing team.

With intramural teams, many of the most exciting and interesting games (for the contestants) have been played by "dub" teams previously classified by competitive abilities. One has only to observe the interest in these leagues to be completely convinced of the value of ability grouping. All players realize that the contests remembered the longest, exciting the greatest interest, and discussed in later years with the greatest enthusiasm were the ones played against opponents of equal ability, where the game was hard fought and the score close. To be sure, winning the game is important; but, when the game is played against decidedly inferior opponents, it is a victory devoid of lasting satisfaction. For the intramural director, loss of interest due to uneven contests should be a matter of serious concern.

Social Development

The third value of ability grouping is in providing a setting for desirable social experiences. When competing individuals or teams are evenly matched, players are more active, cooperation is essential, and initiative and courage are necessary requisites to playing the game successfully. In fact, all of the physical, mental, emotional, and social qualities of the individual are at a premium when playing hard-fought, closely contested matches. In unequal contests, the winning players are not required to exert themselves, teamwork is nor particularly important, "grandstand" players may perform without jeopardizing the success of their teams, individuals are not stimulated to display initiative, and head work, loyalty, and fortitude are not essential elements of the game. The losing team

may either fight through under great odds, a desirable outcome, or, as is sometimes the case, lose interest and coast through in any way to complete the contest. When each new effort is met with overwhelming superior power and ends in disappointment, or when the slightest effort produces success, there is little encouragement for continuing.

It may be argued that certain advantages result from heterogeneous situations. The excellent performer may benefit socially from helping those who are less skilled, thus developing a tolerant and understanding attitude toward beginners. The poor performer, on the other hand, is given a better concept of possible excellence in physical activities and is perhaps extended beyond his ordinary performance by participating with more highly skilled contestants. Physical educators, therefore, may wish to provide opportunities for participation of this sort. As a regular practice, however, the advantages of homogeneous grouping in physical education outweigh the disadvantages.

PLAYER CONTROL OF CONTESTS

Pupil responsibility and initiative are essential to the development of pupil leadership. Physical education is especially rich in opportunities for the exercise of these qualities. Every game provides a setting for developing pupil leadership by permitting the players themselves to plan, direct, and control their own contests. The extensiveness of this opportunity is especially apparent when one considers the large number of contests conducted in physical education classes and in intramural leagues.

The guidance of the physical educator, however, should be a very definite part of this plan. He should capitalize on opportunities to drive home in this natural setting important lessons in citizenship. A democratic state, one that is particularly rich in social experiences, may thereby be approached.

SUCCESS EXPERIENCES

An important factor in developing confidence and poise in students, which will in turn pave the way for wider personality adjustments, is for them to realize success experiences. Physical education activities should be so selected and arranged that the individual has a chance to succeed, and will do so a fair share of the time. To be met constantly with defeat or to be subjected repeatedly to activities beyond one's ability to perform can only result in feelings of impotence and inferiority, culminating in defeatism and withdrawal from people and from life situations. On the other hand, to present the pupil with an activity he can learn, despite its possible elementary nature, to face him with a situation he can master, or to place him with and against others of his own ability will result in his increased interest, self-assurance, and willingness to attempt progressively more difficult assignments. The application of the success principle may well be the starting point in the unfolding of full personalities of many hitherto retiring introverts.

SOCIAL EDUCATION

The development of the individual for social living is an essential task of education; in this task, physical education naturally shares. Students must be prepared to live in a complex, highly interdependent society, to participate responsibly in a democracy which is no longer only nationally oriented but envisages an international society based on the brotherhood of man, and to be committed irrevocably to a moral and spiritual way of life. Accomplishment of these very vital objectives is the greatest need apparent in life today.

All of our science, all of our technology, all of the truly great achievements of the mind, and all the physical fitness and athletic skills will be ineffectual in the face of a society with unrestricted competition and with a world based upon unrestricted power politics.

Social stability and progress in a democracy is dependent upon the conviction that self-interest is interwoven with the social good and the social welfare. Cooperation is developed as common interests and common activities are carried out by the team or group.[9] Voluntary cooperation, contrary to the idea of the survival of the fittest, is essential to all forms of life. Fundamentals of such social development are an appreciation of individual personality, an assumption of responsibility for the consequences of one's own conduct, an acceptance of the concept of moral equality, and a desire to achieve excellence.

The mere participation in activities, no matter how potentially useful, will not automatically result in desirable social outcomes. Any sport can be presented in a manner to develop either desirable or undesirable modes of conduct. Good sportsmanship may be obvious in some athletic contests, while unsportsmanlike acts may be rife in others; well-coordinated team play may be evident in the way some teams compete, while a collection of individual stars, each playing for his own glory, may characterize other teams. The teacher or coach is the key to social education. Social growth can be no better than the understanding and ability of the teacher to develop those qualities needed in men today for the sake of the years to come. As expressed by the Educational Policies Commission: ". . . the teacher of sports is usually one of the most influential members of the school community in the shaping of moral and spiritual values."[10]

[9]Charles C. Cowell, *Scientific Foundations of Physical Education* (New York: Harper & Row, 1953), p. 119.

[10]Educational Policies Commission, *Moral and Spiritual Values in the Public Schools* (Washington: National Education Association, 1951), p. 68.

Many of the activities of physical education may be used to provide a realistic laboratory experience in democratic living. Sports participation knows no racial barriers, national restrictions, or differences in creed. Sports achievement is widely recognized and acclaimed regardless of the origins of the competitor; the code of a sportsman is realistic and universal and knows no special privileges; "fair play" is an experience in the application of law and justice; each competitor recognizes and accepts his appropriate role in the team effort. In order to realize these goals, the welfare of the participant, not the athletic record of the school, must always be the first consideration.

Nixon and Jewett[11] have indicated that awareness of responsibility toward others and toward society as a whole is increasingly necessary in a free society. These authors stress that every society establishes some limitations upon individual behavior in the interests of the public welfare; and, that a basic social responsibility is a "willingness to accept properly constituted authority and to respect reasonable limitations set up for the common good." The rules established for games and sports can be viewed similarly. "Physical education settings can be useful in guiding students toward a recognition of the role of authority in a democracy, provided the learning climate is genuinely democratic, attention is focused on the need for rules and the proper role of officials, and there is satisfying participation for all."

Students need to know what respect for authority means; they should be given a vision of a more desirable state toward which to strive and of which they themselves may not be cognizant; and they must learn to make wise choices and to develop *for themselves* worthy standards of conduct. The physical educator deals many times with emotionalized attitudes developed under the stress of actual pressure; character may thus be emphasized as underlying and integrating all behavior of the individual. Wise guidance is essential if best results are to be attained.

MENTAL HEALTH

Over a million mental patients are treated annually in hospitals in the United States. In addition, an estimated half million persons receive services in outpatient psychiatric clinics, and a substantial number are treated by private psychiatrists.[12] And this is far from the whole picture. Estimates suggest that as many as 17,000,000 people in this country are suffering from some sort of mental illness. Not all of these need to be hospitalized, but the figures do represent a staggering national problem.

Experienced health educators and physical educators, as well as other teachers, are acquainted with the so-called "troublemakers" and other maladjusted boys and girls in school. They are concerned with those children who show abnormal behavior, who are "problem cases" in education, who may respond to guidance, to whom physical activities may become an outlet for aggressive or antisocial behavior, or whose withdrawal indications may be counteracted by group participation. Health and physical educators need to be alert to observe early symptoms of deviant behavior and to take what steps they can to arrest them and to improve the mental health of these children.

Emma McCloy Layman[13] has written a comprehensive book on mental health through physical education. She presents ten ways by which physical education and athletics can contribute to the attainment

[11]John E. Nixon and Ann E. Jewett, *An Introduction to Physical Education*, 7th ed. (Philadelphia: W. B. Saunders Company, 1969), p. 219.

[12]*Facts on Mental Health and Mental Illness*, Public Health Service Publication No. 543 (Washington, D.C.: U.S. Government Printing Office, 1962).

[13]Emma McCloy Layman, *Mental Health through Physical Education and Recreation* (Minneapolis: Burgess Publishing Co., 1955), pp. 190–204.

of mental health goals, as follows: (a) acceptable channels for satisfaction of fundamental needs and desires are provided; (b) emotions can find an outlet; (c) release from strain is provided; (d) motor skills and physique are related to spontaneity of expression; (e) the individual can find a means to success in and mastery of something which he considers important and real; (f) a sufficiently wide range of activities are available so that individual differences in abilities and interests may be met; (g) the intrinsic nature and presentation of physical education and athletic activities are conducive to the overt expression of personality traits; (h) the student-teacher relationship is sufficiently informal that the teacher can readily establish rapport with the boy or girl; (i) classes in this field provide situations which more nearly approximate that of natural social groups than any other in the school; (j) physical education and athletics form the basis for the development of recreational interests which are particularly significant for mental health in adult life.

Meeting individual needs

Individuals vary in social characteristics and needs as widely as they do in the physical characteristics and needs discussed in earlier chapters of the text. Too frequently, however, school pupils are treated en masse, with occasional reprimands and punishments meted out to the few incorrigibles and the overly mischievous, no matter how different their temperaments, how varied their interests, how peculiar their social characteristics, or how pressing their social problems may be. No attempt is made to understand the individual; he is lost in the shuffle.

If the individual is to develop socially in such a way as to indicate high probability of a social rather than a self-centered or predatory career, individual needs must be determined; treatment must be based upon measurement of the individual pupil, recorded regularly during the successive phases of his maturation. For those with social problems, individual diagnosis to discover the cause of the condition should be made and appropriate steps for its correction instituted. Retests from time to time should be given in order to determine the progress being made. If no progress is recorded as a result of the retests, the case should again be reviewed, gone into even more thoroughly, and possibly referred to psychologists or psychiatrists.

Need for objective tests

Measurement in relation to the social development of boys and girls may take a number of directions. Most significant among these are the following:

1. Measurement of social efficiency. Health and physical education teachers should utilize the better tests of social efficiency and conduct appropriate follow-up procedures for those in need. They should develop ability to recognize behavior problems and to know their meaning. They should take steps to discover the origin of the child's behavior disturbances, looking for dominant behavior tendencies. Their chief concern, however, should be with the appearance of these unsocial attitudes and psychic anomalies which at first seem insignificant but which later may lead to neurotic or serious social maladjustment. Tests to aid health and physical education teachers in measuring personality and character traits are presented in the next chapter.

2. Ability grouping. Ability grouping as a means of improving interpersonal relations is a concern of the physical educator, as discussed earlier in this chapter. He may accomplish this roughly by judgment or by "choosing sides."

However, it is also possible to use tests for this purpose; tests are presented in Chapter 12.

3. Physical fitness. The causes of many cases of social maladjustment have been traced to physical sources. Obviously, one is not a very social being when he has a splitting headache or when he is fatigued. Eyestrain may be the cause of irritation, lack of attention, and disciplinary problems in the classroom. Organic defects, resulting in lowered physical vitality and general bodily weakness, may result in poor grades and inability to take part in the activities of the school, thus promoting failure and retardation, with their attendant undesirable effects upon the social development of the pupil. A foundation of abundant health and vitality is a major asset in the development of a socially adjusted individual. Physical fitness measurement was considered in Part II of this text.

4. Individual competence. Competence in physical skills, resulting in the development of confidence and poise, involves acquiring a satisfactory degree of proficiency in various physical education activities. Tests of such activities appear in Chapter 14.

SELECTED REFERENCES

CLARKE, H. HARRISON, "Totality of Man Continued," *Physical Fitness Research Digest,* **2,** No. 1 (January 1972).

COOK, LLOYD and ELAINE, *School Problems in Human Relations.* New York: McGraw-Hill Book Company, 1957.

COWELL, CHARLES C., and HELDA M. SCHWEHN, *Modern Principles and Methods in High School Physical Education.* Boston: Allyn and Bacon, Inc., 1958.

EDUCATIONAL POLICIES COMMISSION, *Moral and Spiritual Values in the Public Schools.* Washington: National Education Association, 1951.

LAYMAN, EMMA McCLOY, *Mental Health through Physical Education and Recreation.* Minneapolis: Burgess Publishing Co., 1955.

NIXON, JOHN E., and ANN E. JEWETT, *An Introduction to Physical Education,* 7th ed. Philadelphia: W. B. Saunders Company, 1969.

CHAPTER 11

In the preceding chapter it was pointed out that the field of physical education is particularly rich in opportunities for social experiences, since pupils participate actively and wholeheartedly in activities requiring many and varied social responses. These experiences develop social traits. Further, definite programs can be devised to develop desirable traits and to suppress undesirable ones.

A major obstacle to rapid progress in the development of social efficiency, however, is the difficulty of measuring social character. Without adequate tests, a really strong program of social development is impossible, regardless of the number and nature of the general procedures employed to realize this objective. In fact, without measurement, the physical director cannot tell whether he is actually developing desirable social traits in any or all of his pupils. An understanding of pupil social characteristics is thus the base upon which this aspect of the physical education program must be built. Moreover, determining the effects of such programs upon the individual can be done only by re-tests of these individuals from time to time. Thus, like the physical fitness program, the social efficiency program of the physical educator must be essentially an individual program, the physical educator adapting procedures to meet individual needs *after such needs have been determined through measurement.*

Moreover, in the development of social efficiency, physical educators should be interested in two fundamental aspects of this problem. First, does physical education develop desirable behavior in relation to physical activities in which the pupils participate? Second, are these same qualities carried over into school and life activities? The real success of any physical educator's attempt to improve pupils' social efficiency may very well be identified with the degree of transfer achieved. But particularly he should be familiar with the actual social problems of his pupils as a means of directing his teaching toward specific individual problems.

In measurement, therefore, consideration should be given to social traits functioning in physical education, in school, and in out-of-school situations. As physical education tests of social efficiency are confined primarily to behavior responses in physical education activities without reference to individual traits in other school and life activities, tests in the fields of education and psychology measuring similar qualities will be included in this chapter. The physical educator, consequently, who uses the latter type of test will be in a position to meet the broad needs of his pupils and to plan definitely for the carry-over of specific traits in individual case.

Measurement of Social Efficiency

BEHAVIOR RATING SCALES

A number of behavior rating scales have been proposed for use by physical educators. These tests are typically based upon ratings of behavior frequencies. Thus, such a test contains statements classified under subheads of a general trait; the ratings are based upon whether the behavior occurs "never," "seldom," "fairly often," "frequently," and "extremely often."

McCloy's Behavior Rating Scale

McCloy[1] proposed one of the first behavior rating scales in physical education. In this scale, nine traits are listed: leadership, active qualities, attitudes, self-control, co-operation, sportsmanship, ethics, efficiency, and sociability. A total of 37 typical trait actions are listed under the nine traits, each of which is rated by the judges on a scale of 5 to 1, with 5 representing "good" behavior. The assurance of the rater is also indicated opposite each trait action, as follows: 0, a mere guess; 1, slight inclination; 2, fair assurance; and 3, positive assurance.

In utilizing McCloy's scale with boys 8 to 12 years of age in the University of Illinois Sports Fitness Summer Day School, Orban[2] found a lack of consistency between raters. Further, he observed a strong tendency for the raters to rate the boys high on the traits. By contrast, the use of Sheldon's Temperament Scale showed satisfactory rater consistency as a behavior rating scale.

Blanchard's Scale

Blanchard[3] utilized 85 trait actions classified under the nine traits suggested by McCloy. These trait actions were evaluated by 16 physical education teachers; the 45 receiving the highest ratings were selected as the basis for his study. Three major criteria were used in the selection of the final trait actions, as follows: (a) median of the average deviations of the total scores of four teacher and eight student raters (indicating consistency of ratings); (b) the reliability of teacher and student scores per trait action; and (c) the intercorrelations of each trait with the remainder of its category.

Twenty-four trait actions were finally selected for the behavior frequency rating scale. The reliability of this battery is 0.71 and the intercorrelation of one trait action with the rest of the items in its category is 0.93. The complete scale appears in Figure 11.1.

Cowell Social Behavior Trend Index

In identifying a socially well-adjusted student, Cowell[4] presented the following description: "One who has a feeling of social security as the result of his social skills, his social 'know how,' and because he is accepted and 'fits into the group.' One who feels 'at home in the group' and does not feel that he differs markedly from the ways the group feels are important. He has group status and is accepted by the group. One interested in the games, hobbies, and activities favored by the majority of his classmates."

After studying factors which differentiate junior high school boys who tend to participate wholeheartedly in physical education and those who are reticent to so participate, Cowell developed 12 pairs of behavior "trends" representing good and poor adjustments. As a result of a factor analysis, 10 of the pairs of positive and negative behavior trends were retained as common denominators underlying good and poor adjustment. These positive and negative scales (forms A and B respectively) appear in Figure 11.2.

Cowell recommends that three teachers

[1]C. H. McCloy, "Character Building in Physical Education," *Research Quarterly,* **1,** No. 3 (October 1930), 42.

[2]William A. R. Orban, "An Item Analysis of Temperament and Behavior Ratings of Young Boys," Master's Thesis, University of Illinois, 1953.

[3]B. E. Blanchard, "A Behavior Frequency Rating Scale for the Measurement of Character and Personality in Physical Education Classroom Situations," *Research Quarterly,* **7,** No. 2 (May 1936), 56.

[4]Charles C. Cowell, "Validating an Index of Social Adjustment for High School Use," *Research Quarterly,* **29,** No. 1 (March 1958), 7.

Name:................................Grade:......................Age:..................Date:................

School:..Name of Rater:...

BEHAVIOR RATING SCALE

Personal Information	No Opportunity to Observe	Never	Seldom	Fairly Often	Frequently	Extremely Often	Score
Leadership							
1. Popular with classmates.................		1	2	3	4	5	
2. Seeks responsibility in the classroom.......		1	2	3	4	5	
3. Shows intellectual leadership in the classroom		1	2	3	4	5	
Positive Active Qualities							
4. Quits on tasks requiring perseverance......		5	4	3	2	1	
5. Exhibits aggressiveness in his relationship with others..........................		1	2	3	4	5	
6. Shows initiative in assuming responsibility in unfamiliar situations.................		1	2	3	4	5	
7. Is alert to new opportunities..............		1	2	3	4	5	
Positive Mental Qualities							
8. Shows keenness of mind.................		1	2	3	4	5	
9. Volunteers ideas........................		1	2	3	4	5	
Self-Control							
10. Grumbles over decisions of classmates......		5	4	3	2	1	
11. Takes a justified criticism by teacher or classmate without showing anger or pouting..		1	2	3	4	5	
Co-operation							
12. Is loyal to his group.....................		1	2	3	4	5	
13. Discharges his group responsibilities well...		1	2	3	4	5	
14. Is co-operative in his attitude toward his teacher		1	2	3	4	5	
Social Action Standards							
15. Makes loud-mouthed criticism and comments		5	4	3	2	1	
16. Respects the rights of others..............		1	2	3	4	5	
Ethical Social Qualities							
17. Cheats		5	4	3	2	1	
18. Is truthful		1	2	3	4	5	
Qualities of Efficiency							
19. Seems satisfied to "get by" with tasks assigned		5	4	3	2	1	
20. Is dependable and trustworthy............		1	2	3	4	5	
21. Has good study habits...................		1	2	3	4	5	
Sociability							
22. Is liked by others........................		1	2	3	4	5	
23. Makes a friendly approach to others in the group		1	2	3	4	5	
24. Is friendly		1	2	3	4	5	

FIGURE 11.1. *Blanchard's Behavior Rating Scale*

rate each pupil on both forms at different times; a pupil's social adjustment score is the total of the ratings of the three teachers combining the two forms. Thus, a socially well-adjusted pupil would get a high positive score, a socially maladjusted pupil would receive a high negative score. These raw scores can be transposed to percentile values as prepared by Cowell from testing 222 junior high school boys. This scale appears in Appendix Table B.15.

Cowell has reported correlations of 0.50 and 0.62 between teachers' judgments of social status and scores on Cowell's Personal Distance Scale and Who's Who Ballot respectively. He also obtained a biserial correlation of 0.82 between teachers' ratings of the best and worst socially adjusted boys.

For 13-year-old boys in the Medford Boys' Growth Study, Broekhoff[5] obtained a correlation of −0.793 between the positive and negative scales of the Trend Index; he also found low but significant correlations with strength and motor tests. For boys of the same age, Howe[6] reported correlations of −0.536 and −0.527 between the negative index and the Physical Fitness Index and standing broad jump, respectively.

Rating Precautions

Considerable care should be exercised in making ratings, as they are merely the opinions of one person in respect to the quality being considered. Masoner[7] has recommended that schools should use behavior ratings only when pupils can be observed carefully and when established principles of rating can be followed. Such factors as the experience of the raters, their understanding of the traits being rated, and their acquaintance with the subject affect the results of the ratings. Traits of character cannot be seen, but action can. However, the motive behind action may not be understood. Raters should be carefully trained in habits of observation, the qualities to be rated being clearly pointed out so that the possibility of misunderstanding is reduced to a minimum. Also, the reliability of ratings can be increased by combining the ratings of several judges of the same pupil.

The degree of assurance of the rater should be recorded. O'Neel[8] found that ratings were usually reliable when the rater had fair or positive assurance, and that the reverse was true when he was guessing. Blanchard on the other hand, concluded that raters' assurance columns may be eliminated, as the assurance of raters is only an index of the range of personal contact and acquaintance of the judge with the student. The best procedure for the rater is not to judge a trait action unless he has a fair acquaintance with the subject. If not reasonably sure, he should observe the subject for a time before making the ratings.

Caution must be exercised also against the "halo effect" in rating pupils, as raters tend to rate individuals whom they like, or who have fine reputations, too highly in everything, whereas the reverse is true for those whom they dislike, or who have unsavory reputations, even if such reputations are due to single-trait deficiencies. The idea of "love is blind" is indicative of this situation. Langlie[9] found this situation, and also discovered that sex differences in ratings exist, as both men and

[5]Jan Broekhoff, "Relationships Between Physical, Socio-Psychological, and Mental Characteristics of Thirteen Year Old Boys," Doctoral Dissertation, University of Oregon, 1966.

[6]Bruce L. Howe, "Longitudinal Analyses of the Relationships Within Measures of Personality and Social Status and Between These Measures and Physical Variables for Boys Ages Between Twelve and Seventeen Years," Doctoral Dissertation, University of Oregon, 1973.

[7]Paul Masoner, "A Critique of Personality Rating Scales," Doctoral Dissertation, University of Pittsburgh, 1949.

[8]F. W. O'Neel, "A Behavior Frequency Rating Scale for the Measurement of Character and Personality in High School Physical Education for Boys," *Research Quarterly,* **7,** No. 2 (May 1936), 67.

[9]T. A. Langlie, "Personality Ratings. I: Reliability of Teachers' Ratings," *Journal of Genetic Psychology,* **50** (June 1937), 339.

Cowell Social Behavior Trend Index (Form A)

Date: _____ Grade: ___

School: _____ Age: _____

Describer: _____

Last Name   First Name

INSTRUCTIONS:--Think carefully of the student's behavior in group situations and check each behavior trend according to its degree of descriptiveness.

	Descriptive of the Student			
Behavior Trends	Markedly (+3)	Somewhat (+2)	Only Slightly (+1)	Not at All (0)
1. Enters heartily and with enjoyment into the spirit of social intercourse ____				
2. Frank; talkative and sociable, does not stand on ceremony ____				
3. Self-confident and self-reliant, tends to take success for granted, strong initiative, prefers to lead ___				
4. Quick and decisive in movement, pronounced or excessive energy output ____				
5. Prefers group activities, work or play; not easily satisfied with individual projects ____				
6. Adaptable to new situations, makes adjustment readily, welcomes change ____				
7. Is self-composed, seldom shows signs of embarrassment ____				
8. Tends to elation of spirits, seldom gloomy or moody ____				
9. Seeks a broad range of friendships, not selective or exclusive in games and the like ____				
10. Hearty and cordial, even to strangers, forms acquaintanceships very easily ____				

FIGURE 11.2. *Cowell Social Behavior Trend Index*

women teachers tend to rate girls as superior to boys, even though test records do not verify this trend. Also, according to Grant,[10] the "halo effect" results from the failure of a rater to discriminate between the traits of the person he is rating. This effect is recognized by the existence of high positive intercorrelations between the items in a rating scale.

McCloy[11] suggests that the "halo effect" may be partially avoided by rating each item for all individuals separately, rather than rating one individual completely before proceeding to the next. Again, care

[10]Donald L. Grant, "An Exploratory Study of the Halo Effect in Rating." Doctoral Dissertation, Ohio State University, 1952.

[11]McCloy, "Character Building," p. 42.

Cowell Social Behavior Trend Index (Form B)

Date: _____ Grade: ____

School: _____ Age: _____

Describer: _____

Last Name   First Name

INSTRUCTION:--Think carefully of the student's behavior in group situations and check each behavior trend according to its degree of descriptiveness.

	Descriptive of the Student			
Behavior Trends	Markedly (-3)	Somewhat (-2)	Only Slightly (-1)	Not at All (-0)
1. Somewhat prudish, awkward, easily embarrassed in his social contacts _____				
2. Secretive, seclusive, not inclined to talk unless spoken to ___				
3. Lacking in self-confidence and initiative, a follower _____				
4. Slow in movement, deliberative or perhaps indecisive. Energy output moderate or deficient ___				
5. Prefers to work and play alone, tends to avoid group activities___				
6. Shrinks from making new adjustments, prefers the habitual to the stress of reorganization required by the new _____				
7. Is self-conscious, easily embarrassed, timid or "bashful"___				
8. Tends to depression, frequently gloomy or moody___				
9. Shows preference for a narrow range of intimate friends and tends to exclude others from his association _____				
10. Reserved and distant except to intimate friends, does not form acquaintanceships readily ___				

---

and concentration on traits and their meanings will do much to counteract this effect. It will also be advantageous to confine these ratings to behavior in physical activities, without attempting to complicate the situation by introducing academic or out-of-school behavior. Behavior evaluation in the latter activities should be the result of separate ratings, or other measurement procedures designed for this specific purpose.

SOCIAL ACCEPTANCE EVALUATION

Cowell[12] has pointed out that teachers' judgments of social behavior are apt to be based on mature adult standards and to be largely indicative of the child's adjustment in dealing with adults in classroom situations. Such judgments, then, may or not reflect the standards which students apply

[12]Cowell, "Index of Social Adjustment," p. 7.

to each other. Teachers' standards may not always be realistic; they may even be oppositive to those of the students. In some instances, the teachers' set of values may be the more desirable, as they may be based upon the broader goals of society, rather than upon possible ill-conceived goals of occasional unworthy student leaders. Nevertheless, the acceptance of students by their peers may frequently be an important form of personality evaluation. So, it may logically be contended that both forms of evaluation are desirable.

Two types of social acceptance evaluation have come into use in education. These may be designated as the social distance scale and the sociometric questionnaire. Both of these will be presented in this section.

Social Distance Scale

Social distance scales have been used in research pertaining to social psychology since 1925 when Bogardus published his *Social Distance Scale*. The Bogardus-type instrument has been used to study race attitudes and indicate social distance toward professions, religious groups, conscientious objectors, and so on. Although modified for specific purposes, the general format has been maintained.

The concept of social distance has been used in education to evaluate the closeness of personal relationships. A test of this type, proposed for physical education, is the *Cowell Personal Distance Ballot.*[13] In Cowell's report, this ballot was used to represent boys' attitudes toward accepting boys. As he points out, it is possible also to determine girls' attitudes toward girls, boys' attitudes toward girls and vice-versa by various methods of balloting. A student's index on this scale depends largely on his degree of social participation in his own group and, therefore, on his own "individual stimulus value."

[13]Ibid.

The Cowell Personal Distance Ballot appears in Figure 11.3. The ballot is prepared by listing the names of all classmates, or other acquaintances to be evaluated. Each boy answers the ballot by checking on the seven-point scale how near to his family he would like to have each classmate or acquaintance listed. A Personal Distance Score is derived by adding the total *weighted* scores given the subject by the class or group and dividing by the total number of respondents. Division is carried to two places and the decimal point dropped. The low score is the desirable score. Cowell's percentile scale scores for boys appears in Appendix Table B.16.

In a study of the social integration of a college football squad, Trapp[14] reported reliability coefficients of 0.91, 0.88, and 0.93 between Cowell's balloting on the same participants at three different times during the football season. In the validation of the Cowell Personal Distance Ballot as a social adjustment instrument, Kurth and Cowell obtained a correlation of 0.84 with student "who's who in my group" ratings and 0.90 with Dean's Guidance Office Ratings.

For ten-year-old boys, Clarke and Greene[15] reported correlations of -0.739 and -0.517 between the Cowell Personal Distance Ballot and the Friends and Homework categories, respectively, of the sociometric questionnaire described in the next section. Other significant correlations with the ballot were reported as follows: 0.288 for 60-yard shuttle run, -0.257 for standing broad jump, 0.267 for ectomorphy, and -0.236 for mesomorphy.[16]

[14]Ibid.

[15]H. Harrison Clarke and Walter H. Greene, "Relationships Between Personal-Social Measures Applied to 10-Year-old Boys," *Research Quarterly*, **34**, No. 3 (October 1963), 288.

[16]Inasmuch as low scores are considered desirable on the Cowell ballot, negative correlations have positive connotations and vice versa. Such connotations are not true for the shuttle run, as low scores on both tests are desirable.

What To Do:	I would be willing to accept him:						
	Into my family as a brother	As a very close "pal" or "chum"	As a member of my "gang" or club	On my street as a "nextdoor neighbor"	Into my class at school	Into my school	Into my city
If you had full power to treat each student on this list as you feel, just how would you consider him? How near would you like to have him to your family? Check each student in one column as to your feeling toward him. Circle your own name.	1	2	3	4	5	6	7
1.							
2.							
3.							
4. etc.							

NOTE: The Personal Distance Score is determined by adding the total *weighted* scores given the subject by members of the class or group and dividing by the total number of respondents. Division is carried to two places and the decimal point dropped. The low score is the desirable score. The percentile scale scores in the appendix represent boys' attitudes toward accepting boys. It is possible also to determine girls' attitudes toward girls, boys' attitudes toward girls and vice-versa by various methods of balloting.

FIGURE 11.3. *Cowell Personal Distance Ballot*

In a 1970 study by Dietrick,[17] contrary findings were obtained for ninth- and eleventh-grade girls. She found that stronger girls were regarded with less status on the Cowell ballot by girls of their own age than were girls who were not as strong.

Sociometric Questionnaire

Sociometry is a promising evaluative technique for determining social status and group integration. This form of systematic determination of group structure and the individual's place in it had its chief origin in the work of Moreno,[18] published in 1934. The sociometric test consists of asking a boy (or girl) to choose his associates for any group of which he is or might become a member. For example, the individuals within a group might be asked to choose those members whom they would wish to have with them in the formation of some new group, whether it be one of recreation, work, or study.

Medford   Questionnaire. A sociometric questionnaire was utilized in the Medford Boys' Growth Study, on which each boy lists as many other boys in his homeroom as he wishes in each of the following five categories:

Friends: List your good boy friends and boys you would like for friends.

Movies: List the boys you would like to go to the movies with.

Sports: List the boys you would like to play sports with.

Homework: List the boys you would like to study homework with.

Party: List the boys you would like to invite to a birthday party.

The scoring of this questionnaire consists simply of tabulating the number of times a boy is chosen by his classmates. Where different numbers of boys are involved, the percentage of choices may be utilized. For eleven-year-old boys, Devine[19] found that this questionnaire might well be reduced to two categories, Friends and Homework. Friends correlated above 0.90 with Movies, Birthday, and Sports; the correlation with Homework was 0.76.

Such a questionnaire may be used by restricting to three the number of choices that may be made, and, also, listing the names of any individuals with whom association is not wanted. Breck[20] investigated four methods of scoring her questionnaire as applied to college women; she found the following two methods to be of practical value: (a) tabulating only expressions of choice, assigning one point to each expression; (b) tabulating expressions of choice and deducting expressions of rejection, assigning one point for each acceptance and subtracting one point for each rejection.

Sociograms may be developed in order to show the basic social structure of a group. In plotting it, a common practice is to place the popular pupils in the center of the diagram and the unpopular ones toward the outer edges. Lines can be drawn with arrows pointing to a person chosen from the person making the choice; when two individuals choose each other, the line would have an arrow designation at each end. Thus, reciprocal and unreciprocal choices would be revealed. Of course, those with many arrows pointing toward them have greatest acceptance by their peers; and vice versa for those with few or

---

[17]Judith A. Dietrick, "The Relationship Between Strength and Social Status in Ninth- and Eleventh-Grade Girls," Master's Thesis, Western Illinois University, 1970.

[18]J. L. Moreno, *Who Shall Survive?* (New York: Beacon Press, 1934).

[19]Barry M. Devine, "Analysis of Responses on a Sociometric Questionnaire and the Re-Examination of Structural and Strength Relationships for Nine- and Eleven-Year-Old Boys," Master's Thesis, University of Oregon, 1960.

[20]Sabina J. Breck, "A Sociometric Measurement of Status in Physical Education Classes, *Research Quarterly,* **21,** No. 2 (May 1950), 75.

no arrows. Concentrations of reciprocal arrows may indicate some form of cohesive group. If boys and girls are both involved in the choices, boys could be represented by squares and girls by circles. If rejections are included, acceptances could be designated by solid lines and rejections by broken lines. The number of the choice, whether first, second, or third, may be indicated by numerals on the line at the end near the person chosen. Examples:

Joe chooses Ann as a first choice, but is not reciprocated:

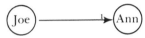

Joe chooses Bill as a second choice and Bill reciprocates as a first choice

Mary rejects Sue; as a third rejection:

Peer status measures, by use of the Medford sociometric questionnaire, have low but significant relationships with physical tests. For boys nine to eleven years of age, Clarke and Clarke[21] found that those in high sociometric groups had higher McCloy and Rogers arm strength scores than did boys in low groups. For eleven-year-old boys, Devine[22] obtained similar results with the Rogers arm strength score. With ten-year-old boys, Clarke and Greene[23] reported that the Friends category of the questionnaire correlated negatively with ectomorphy and positively with

mesomorphy. Greene[24] obtained the following significant correlations: 0.472 between Sports and standing broad jump; 0.404 and 0.420 between Movies and Party respectively and the average of 11 cable-tension strength tests; −0.387 and 0.393 between Sports and 60-yard shuttle run and Physical Fitness Index respectively.

Dunn's Questionnaire.[25] Dunn applied a "peer popularity" questionnaire to 369 boys in grades five through twelve. The questionnaire consisted of each boy listing the following:

1. His three best friends.

2. The three boys he most admired.

3. The three boys he would most want to be like.

The peer status of the boys, as thus revealed, was related to muscular strength, muscular endurance, and muscular power tests: static arm strength by pressing upward on a bar from a bench-press position; leg lift, utilizing a dynamometer with belt; pull-ups; and vertical jump. Static strength was found to have a higher overall relationship with peer status than did either muscular endurance or muscular power.

The use of a sociometric questionnaire permits physical educators to gain understanding of the interpersonal relationship within a class of pupils and to discover which boys and girls are accepted and not accepted by their peers. Those in the latter category usually need special help in making wholesome social adjust-

[21]H. Harrison Clarke and David H. Clarke, "Social Status and Mental Health of Boys as Related to Their Maturity, Structural, and Strength Characteristics," *Research Quarterly,* **32,** No. 3 (October 1961), 326.

[22]Devine, "Responses on a Sociometric Questionnaire."

[23]Clarke and Greene, "Personal-Social Measures," p. 288.

[24]Walter H. Greene, "Peer Status and Level of Aspiration of Boys as Related to Their Maturity, Physique, Structural, Strength, and Motor Ability Characteristics," Doctoral Dissertation, University of Oregon, 1964.

[25]John P. Dunn, "The Relationship Between Strength and Selected Social and Personality Factors," Doctoral Dissertation, Texas A & M University, 1970.

ments. Such improvements can be brought about, as was demonstrated by Todd[26] with high school girls. By use of a sociometric instrument, she showed greatly increased acquaintanceship and a significant decrease in the number of unpopular and unwanted girls in a single semester.

LEVEL OF ASPIRATION

As defined by Frank,[27] level of aspiration is "the level of future performance in a familiar task which an individual, knowing his level of past performance in that task, explicitly undertakes to reach." Studies involving level of aspiration have utilized mental and personality traits more than physical and motor tasks for test situations, although an increasing number in the latter field is becoming evident. Aspiration investigations in psychology have dealt with such broad topics as effects of success or failure on personality traits, effects of success or failure on the initial setting of the level of aspiration, generalities in the discrepancy scores of different tasks, the transfer of level of aspiration, and sex and age differences. In physical education, the aspiration studies have been directed toward knowledge of previous scores in task performances, the effects of athletic success and failure on aspiration, aspiration as related to motor skill learning, and the relationships between aspiration measures and physical and motor traits.

A level of aspiration test, utilized in the Medford Boys' Growth Study, is based on maximum grip strength efforts of the right hand, as follows.

1. After instructing the subject in grip testing techniques, his grip strength is taken. This score is recorded as his first grip strength (P-1). The subject is informed of his score.

2. The pupil is then asked to estimate what score he believes he can attain on a second grip strength effort. This score is recorded as his first aspiration score (A-1).

3. A second grip strength test is administered and recorded (P-2). The subject is informed of this score.

4. Steps 2 and 3 are repeated to obtain a second aspiration score (A-2) and a third grip strength performance (P-3).

The attitude of the tester throughout this process is one of encouragement, urging the subject to do his best. At no time is the pupil criticized for making a poor showing or for failing to reach his stated aspiration.

Several level of aspiration scores have been utilized in various Medford analyses; the more meaningful scores are given here, as Aspiration Discrepancies (AD), M-score, and D-score. They are as follows:

AD.1　　= A.1 - P.1

AD.2　　= A.2 - P.2

AD.3　　= A.2 - P.1

D-score　= average of all AD scores.

M-score　= average of all AD scores, but direction of differences disregarded.

Second Aspiration Discrepancy (AD-2). The difference between P-2 and A-2. With nine-year-old boys, Clarke and Stratton[28] found that this score correlated well, relatively, with performance discrepancy, other aspiration discrepancies, and grip strength scores. Greene[29] obtained a correlation of 0.48 between AD-2 and skeletal age at nine years of age; however, for the same boys one year later, this rela-

[26]Frances Todd, "Sociometry in Physical Education," *Journal of American Association for Health, Physical Education, and Recreation,* **24,** No. 5 (May 1953), 23.

[27]Jerome D. Frank, "Individual Differences in Certain Aspects of Level of Aspiration," *American Journal of Psychology,* **47** (January 1935), 119.

[28]H. Harrison Clarke and Stephen T. Stratton, "A Level of Aspiration Test Based on the Grip Strength Efforts of Nine-Year-Old Boys," *Child Development,* **33,** No. 4 (December 1962), 897.

[29]Greene, "Peer Status and Level of Aspiration."

tionship was insignificant. He also found that boys in a high AD-2 group had significantly superior means than did boys in a low AD-2 group at one or more ages on the following tests: body weight, cable-tension strength average, Wetzel physique channel, mesomorphy, standing height, and standing broad jump.

First Aspiration Discrepancy (AD-1). The difference between P-1 and A-1. Clarke and Clarke[30] found that nine-year-old boys in a high AD-1 group had a signifi-cantly greater Physical Fitness Index mean than did boys in zero and low AD-1 groups. Where high and zero (P-1 and A-1 being the same) groups were compared, the high group was significantly superior in the following five additional tests: stand-ing height, body weight, McCloy's Classifi-cation Index, McCloy's arm strength score, and Strength Index.

D- and M-Scores. For the same boys at 13, 15, and 17 years of age, Venables[31] re-ported that the most meaningful aspira-tion measures were D-score, M-score, and AD.3, in that order. His criterion of mean-ingfulness was the degree of interrela-tionships among the aspiration measures. Generally, however, the aspiration mea-sures correlated low and mostly insignifi-cantly with physical and motor tests. More correlations with the M-score were signifi-cant than for the other aspiration mea-sures, as follows: at 13 years, the three somatotype components, weight, and height times chest girth; at 15 years, height, weight, height times chest girth, cable-tension strength average, and stand-ing broad jump times weight; at 17 years,

shuttle run and standing broad jump times weight (negative).

Apparently, young boys who strive to at-tain higher goals (express higher levels of aspiration) are physically superior in size and strength to other boys their ages who are not willing to risk the chance of failure and who, thereby, choose the aspiration level that seems to ensure some measure of continued success. It would seem that this technique does provide a means of studying behavior, for the selection of a level of aspiration appears to reflect a boy's previous success or failure which he associates with the risk.

SELF-CONCEPT

Investigators have hypothesized that a person's self-concept, which includes body image, affects both the type of activity he chooses and his success in the activity. Not only does the individual's view of physique play an important role in the development of self-concept, but so does the view of the psyche. Several investigations have contributed to the validation of this as-sumption. Consequently, an understand-ing of the self-concept of students may well assist physical educators in providing adequate learning experiences for them. Thus, some self-concept instruments will be presented here.

Davidson-Lang Adjective Check List

The Davidson-Lang Adjective Check List[32] was utilized in the Medford Boys' Growth Study to provide an understand-ing of each boy's self-concept. From an original pool of 200 trait names, 50 were retained by Davidson and Lang. The bases

[30]Clarke and Clarke, "Social Status and Mental Health," p. 326.

[31]C. E. Hugh Venables, "Longitudinal Analyses of Level of Aspiration Measures and Their Relationship to Growth and Development Variables of Boys Ages Thirteen, Fifteen, and Seventeen Years," Doctoral Dissertation, University of Oregon, 1973.

[32]Helen H. Davidson and Gertrude Lang, "Chil-dren's Perceptions of Their Teacher's Feelings To-ward Them Related to Self-Perception, School Achievement, and Behavior," *Journal of Experimental Education,* **29,** No. 2 (December 1960), 107.

for retention were: words commonly used to describe people's feelings toward self and others; words easy enough to read and comprehend from ages 10 to 16 years; and about an even division of words connoting positive and negative concepts. The 50 adjectives in this check list appear in Figure 11.4.

This check list is not a test in the usual sense, in that the individual does not achieve a score and self-concept status is not identified by application to norms.

Name: _____ School: _____

Age: _____ Grade _____ Date: _____

Directions: These are words that are often used to describe children. Check the ones that apply to you.

_____ Afraid	_____ Loving
_____ Bad	_____ Mean
_____ Bossy	_____ Neat
_____ A brat	_____ Nervous
_____ A bully	_____ Noisy
_____ Careless	_____ Not alert
_____ Cheerful	_____ Outstanding
_____ Clean	_____ A pest
_____ Clever	_____ Polite
_____ Clumsy	_____ Quiet
_____ A copy cat	_____ Selfish
_____ A cry-baby	_____ A show off
_____ Dependable	_____ Silly
_____ Fair	_____ A sissy
_____ Forgetful	_____ A sloppy worker
_____ Friendly	_____ A smart aleck
_____ Generous	_____ A sore loser
_____ A good pupil	_____ Smart
_____ A good sport	_____ Stupid
_____ A hard worker	_____ A time waster
_____ Helpful	_____ A trouble maker
_____ Honest	_____ Unhappy
_____ Kind	_____ Not eager to
_____ Lazy	study
_____ A leader	_____ Willing
_____ Not eager to learn	

FIGURE 11.4. *Davidson-Lang Adjective Check List (Original Form)*

Rather, each student checks those adjectives that apply to their respective concept of self. In Medford analyses, the mean differences in physical and motor traits for boys who checked and who did not check each adjective were tested for significance. Two major studies with the check list were completed by Reynolds[33] and by Flynn[34] with 13 and 16 year old boys, respectively. Among their findings were the following:

1. Significant differences between means on physical and motor tests were obtained for 34 and 20 adjectives by 13- and 16-year-old boys, respectively. Nineteen of the adjectives were significantly related to the tests at both ages, although the patterns of relationship with physical and motor tests were not the same. The largest numbers of significant differences were eight for Cry-baby and seven for Stupid by 13-year-olds, and ten for Clumsy, nine for Leader, eight for Good sport, and seven for Sissy by the 16-year-olds.

2. The physical and motor tests with greatest frequency of significant differences at both ages were skeletal age, endomorphy, shuttle run, and standing broad jump. Other tests with relatively more significant differences were ectomorphy and Physical Fitness Index at 13 years and cable-tension strength and Strength Index at 16 years.

3. Examples of the results obtained by Reynolds and Flynn are limited here to muscular strength tests. The 13-year-old boys with low relative strength (Physical Fitness Indices) checked the negative adjectives of Clumsy, Nervous, Sissy, and Unhappy significantly more times than did boys with high PFI's; the reverse was true for Leader. At 16 years of age more low PFI boys checked Sissy and more high PFI boys checked Leader and Good sport.

[33]Robert M. Reynolds, "Responses on the Davidson Adjective Check List as Related to Maturity, Physical, and Mental Characteristics of Thirteen Year Old Boys," Doctoral Dissertation, University of Oregon, 1965.

[34]Kenneth W. Flynn, "Responses on the Davidson Adjective Check List as Related to Maturity, Physical, and Motor Ability Characteristics of Sixteen Year Old Boys," Doctoral Dissertation, University of Oregon, 1967.

For gross strength (cable-tension average), more low strength boys at 13 years checked Cry baby and Careless than did high strength boys; the reverse occurred for Stupid. At 16 years, more low strength boys marked Not eager to learn, Quiet, Silly, and Sissy, while the high strength boys checked Dependable and Friendly. Thus, at these ages, boys with low relative and low gross strength revealed negative self-concepts, while boys high on these tests indicated positive self-concepts. It may be suggested that enhancement of self-concept may be related to the improvement of such developmental physical fitness traits as muscular strength.

The adjective check list may be used to identify boys and girls with personal problems by noting the adjectives each one checks and/or by identifying such problems common to an entire class. Appropriate approaches on an individual or class basis could then be applied to improve their self-concepts. Negative adjectives checked point to obvious deficiencies in self-concept. However, unchecked positive adjectives may also provide leads for follow-up attention.

Gough's Adjective Check List

The Gough Adjective Check List[35] was developed jointly by Gough and Heilbrun for college students; the instrument contains 300 adjectives commonly used to describe attributes of a person. It may be administered to an individual to elicit self-evaluation (or his characterization of anyone he knows) or it may be used by raters, judges, or observers as a convenient way of evaluating personality traits of men and women. Twenty-four scales and indices are available for use with this instrument. Among the scales are the following: Self-Confidence, Self-Control, Liability, Personal Adjustment, Dominance, Affiliation, Exhibition, Autonomy, Aggression, Succorance, Abasement, and Deference.

How I See Myself Scale

Two forms, elementary and secondary, of the *How I See Myself Scale*[36] were developed by Gordon for use with boys and girls, grades three through twelve; the forms contain 40 and 42 items respectively. Instead of treating each item as a dichotomy, it applies or does not apply, the statements are placed on a five-point scale. For example:

I am a poor athlete

$$1 \quad 2 \quad 3 \quad 4 \quad 5$$
I am a good athlete

The scale was developed through a factor analysis process. The factor structure identified several sub scales, including Teacher-School, Physical Appearance, Interpersonal Adequacy, Autonomy, Academic Adequacy, Emotions, Physical Adequacy, and Body Build.

SOCIAL OUTCOMES OF SPORTS

Cowell[37] has stressed that goals of personal and social development in sports participation must be made clear to the student. These goals should receive individual and group acceptance; they should be visible in printed form. Cowell has proposed an evaluation check-sheet on the outcomes of sports for this purpose, as shown in Figure 11.5. This instrument suggests 20 ways in which, through learning experiences in athletics, students may

---

[35]Harrison G. Gough and Alfred B. Heilbrun, *The Adjective Check List Manual* (Palo Alto, Calif.: Consulting Psychologists Press, Inc., 1965).

[36]Ira J. Gordon, *A Test Manual for the How I See Myself Scale* (Gainsville, Fl.: Florida Educational Research and Development Council, 1968).

[37]Charles C. Cowell, "Our Function Is Still Education!" *The Physical Educator,* **14,** No. 1 (March 1957), 6.

OUTCOMES OF SPORTS: AN EVALUATION CHECK-SHEET

To What Extent Did I Learn:	(5) A Very Great Deal	(4) A Great Deal	(3) Somewhat	(2) Very Little	(1) Not at All
1. To sacrifice my own personal "whims" or desires for the good of the group or team?					
2. To test myself—to see if I could "take it," endure hardship and "keep trying" to do my best even under adversity?					
3. To overcome awkwardness and self-consciousness?					
4. To recognize that the *group* can achieve where the *individual* alone cannot?					
5. That each team member has a unique or special contribution to make in the position he plays?					
6. To share difficult undertakings with my "buddies" (teammates) because of struggling together for a goal?					
7. To respect the skill and ability of my opponents and be tolerant of their success?					
8. To make friendships with boys from other schools and to maintain good guest-host relationships in inter-school games?					
9. To feel that the school team helped break up "cliques" and factions in the school by developing common loyalty and community of interests?					
10. To consider and practice correct health and training routine such as proper eating, sleeping, avoidance of tobacco, etc.?					
11. To "take turns" and to "share"?					
12. To develop physical strength, endurance and a better looking body?					
13. To be loyal and not "let my buddy, the coach, team, or school down"?					
14. To give more than I get—not for myself but for an ideal or for one's school, town, or country?					
15. To develop a sense of humor and even to be able to laugh at myself occasionally?					
16. To think and act "on the spot" in the heat of a game?					
17. To understand the strategy—the "why" of the best methods of attack and defense in games?					
18. To understand and appreciate the possibilities and limitations of the human body with respect to skill, speed, endurance, and quickness of reactions?					
19. That in sports there is no discrimination against talent? It is performance and conduct and not the color of one's skin or social standing that matters.					
20. That nothing worthwhile is accomplished without hard work, application, and the "will to succeed"?					

FIGURE 11.5. *Cowell Outcomes of Sports: An Evaluation Check List*

be motivated to change. These represent "some of the organic-physical, mental-emotional, and self-social components of the total personality." Cowell states that a perfect score on the check-sheet is 100.

PERSONALITY INVENTORIES

The various tests discussed in the section on "Social Acceptance Evaluation" are especially useful in judging how well boys and girls fit into the group: how well they are accepted by their peers and how well they impress teachers and others in authority who judge them. However, these evaluative instruments largely neglect another equally valuable criterion of social worth—the complex of traits such as individuality, initiative, personal integrity in the face of social disapproval, and individual creativity. While tests do not exist to measure all facets of this phase of personal and social adjustment, consideration of these traits should not be neglected. In some instances, the tests presented below are helpful in this form of evaluation.

A large number of attempts have been made to construct character, personality, or social adjustment tests in the fields of education and psychology. As early as 1937, Strang[38] demonstrated that if this bibliography were extended to include not only studies in which measuring devices themselves were evaluated, but all studies concerned with the analysis and measurement of social qualities, the whole list would contain approximately 4000 titles. Although many of these tests have been hastily constructed, empirically established, and poorly standardized, a sufficient number are now available to make a reasonably scientific approach to this type of measurement.

In selecting tests for this section of the chapter, the following criteria have been kept in mind:

1. The correlative value. General efficiency tests to be utilized by the physical educator in determining transfer values and transfer needs of social programs should measure traits developed in physical education. Thus, tests that measure social adjustment, emotional adjustment, confidence, leadership, responsibility, initiative, and so forth, have been selected.

2. The scientific value. Only tests that have a reasonably satisfactory degree of validity and accuracy have been considered.

3. Comprehensiveness. Tests representing a narrow field or involving only one or two character traits have been avoided. The comprehensiveness of the test, or the range of social behavior covered by the test, was therefore a factor in its selection.

4. Normality. Primary consideration has been given to normal application of the tests; tests utilized to evaluate abnormal behavior or neurotic cases were avoided, as were those designed especially for psychiatrists in dealing with advanced behavior problems. Tests selected are primarily useful in detecting incipient social problems found among so-called "normal" pupils.

5. Recognition in the field. In surveying the immense amount of material in the field of character and personality tests, a preliminary screening of the better tests was made by consulting test-evaluation studies in this area. The various Mental Measurements Yearbooks[39] were especially useful in making this evaluation. After the preliminary selection was made, these tests were studied to determine their applicability to health and physical education.

6. Availability. At the time of the revision of this book, all tests listed were available through commercial sources. As a consequence, two tests prominently considered in previous editions do not appear. These tests are the *Washburne Social Adjustment Inventory* and the *Mental Health Analysis.*

Bell Adjustment Inventory

The initial Student Form of the Bell Adjustment Inventory[40] was constructed in 1934; a revision of this form was published in 1962. The 1962 revision provides six measures of personal and social adjustment, as follows: Home Adjustment, Health Adjustment, Submissiveness, Emotionality, Hostility, and Masculinity-Fem-

[38]Ruth Strang, *Behavior and Background of Students in Colleges and Secondary Schools* (New York: Harper & Row, Publishers, 1937).

[39]Oscar K. Buros, ed., *The Seventh Mental Measurements Yearbook* (Highland Park, N.J.: Gryphon Press, 1972).

[40]Hugh M. Bell, *Bell Adjustment Inventory,* Revised 1962 Student Form (Palo Alto, Calif.: Consulting Psychologists Press, Inc., 1962).

ininity. High scores on the parts of the test indicate an unsatisfactory adjustment; low scores, a satisfactory adjustment.

The revised Student Form contains 200 statements to be marked as "yes," "no," or "?." A new, reusable booklet is available, along with an IBM answer sheet and scoring stencils for either hand or machine scoring. The revision also produced a Manual, summarizing the results of 30 years of research with the Inventory and containing a guide to interpretation and use of the instrument. The reliability of this test is satisfactory: all reliability coefficients are above 0.80. About 35 minutes are required to take the test. An Adult Form of the Bell Inventory is also available, which includes an additional scale for Occupational Adjustment but does not contain the Hostility and Masculinity-Femininity scales.

Bernreuter Personality Inventory

The Bernreuter Personality Inventory[41] is a group test for high school and college students and adults. It consists of 125 questions adapted largely from Laird's C2 Test of Introversion-Extroversion, Allport's A-S Reaction Study, Thurstone's Neurotic Inventory, and Bernreuter's Self-Sufficiency Test. The questions are answered by circling "yes," "no," or "?." About 30 minutes are required to take the test. Six separate scoring keys are applied to the questionnaire, one for each trait tested. The six traits are as follows: Neurotic Tendency, Self-Sufficiency, Introversion-Extroversion, Dominance-Submission, Confidence in Oneself, and Sociability. The intercorrelations among the Neurotic Tendency, Introversion-Extroversion, and Confidence in Oneself scales are very high, between 0.90 and 0.95. As a consequence, little would be

gained by applying more than one of these scales, so the use of four scales only on this test is adequate. Percentile norms are provided separately for adult men and women, college men and women, and high school boys and girls.

The correlation between the first four traits listed and the corresponding four criterion tests varied from 0.84 to approximately 1.00. For validity coefficients, these correlations are spuriously high, since the Bernreuter inventory consists largely of items taken from the criterion tests, and the items are weighted on the basis of these tests. The validity of the inventory, therefore, is dependent upon the validity of the four criterion tests, and may be used in place of the four separate tests previously constructed by Thurstone, Bernreuter, Laird, and Allport.

Sixteen Personality Factor Questionnaire

The Sixteen Personality Factor Questionnaire (16 PF)[42] was developed over a quarter century by Cattell. The latest manual, the fourth edition, was authored jointly with Eber and Tatsuoka. The test was designed to give broad coverage of the personality of individuals aged 16 years and over. Four forms of the test are available for those whose education is roughly equivalent to the high school level; other forms are designed for persons with marked educational and reading deficits. For other ages, the following comparable instruments are available through the same source, the Institute for Personality and Ability Testing: *Early School Personality Questionnaire*, 6 to 8 years; *Jr.-Sr. High School Personality Questionnaire*, 11 or 12 years through 17 or 18 years. Brief descriptions of the 16 personality factors in the 16 PF follow.

[41]Robert G. Bernreuter, *Manual for the Personality Inventory* (Palo Alto, Calif.: Consulting Psychologists Press, Inc., 1959).

[42]Raymond B. Cattell, Herbert W. Eber, and Maurice M. Tatsuoka, *Handbook for the 16 PF*, 4th ed. (Champaign, Ill.: Institute for Personality and Ability Testing, 1972).

A, *Cyclothymia:* good natured, easy-going, ready to cooperate, attentive to people, soft-hearted, kindly, trustful.

B, *General Intelligence:* intellectual, cultured.

C, *Ego Strength:* calm, emotionally mature and stable, realistic about life, absence of neurotic fatigue, placid.

E, *Ascendance:* assertive, hard, stern, self-assured, independent-minded, solemn, unconventional, attention-getting.

F, *Surgency:* talkative, cheerful, serene, happy-go-lucky, frank, expressive, quick and alert.

G, *Character:* perservering, determined, responsible, conscientious.

H, *Parmia:* adventurous, responsive, friendly, impulsive and frivolous, carefree.

I, *Premia:* demanding, impatient, attention-seeking, anxious.

L, *Protension:* jealous, suspicious, brooding, tyrannical, irritable.

M, *Autia:* unconventional, self-absorbed, imaginative, creative.

N, *Shrewdness:* socially alert, calculating mind, aloof, emotionally disciplined, ambitious, expedient.

O, *Guilt Proneness:* worrying, anxious, sensitive, depressed, strong sense of duty, moody.

Q_1, *Radicalism:* well-informed, more inclined to experiment than to moralize, leading and persuading people, breaking custom and tradition.

Q_2, *Self-Sufficiency:* resourceful, extroverted, dissatisfied with group integration.

Q_3, *Self-Sentiment Formation:* controlled, exacting will-power.

Q_4, *Ergic Tension:* tense, excitable, irritable, in turmoil.

For the most part, Cattell's *Sixteen Personality Factor Questionnaire* resulted from factor analyses of behavior ratings, although the last four factors (Q_{1-4}) were based on inventory studies. His factor analysis method was based on the theory that all personality traits are unique, but in a population with common cultural backgrounds, a majority are so nearly common that they can be treated as common traits, and can be measured on a common axis.

A number of studies have been conducted to determine relationships between Cattell's factors and various physical measures, with encouraging results. For example, Betz[43] obtained significant correlations between Ego Strength, Premia, and Autia and the Schneider test, 100-yard drop-off swim test, and five-minute step test. In addition, Ego Strength, Ascendance, and Shrewdness, normally associated with mature, aggressive, sophisticated individuals, correlated significantly, but negatively, with length of a treadmill run. Apparently, according to the author, college men with these traits resist being persuaded to run to exhaustion.

Also, with college men Gottesman[44] obtained significant multiple correlations between Cattell's factors as dependent variables and physique, structure, strength, and motor tests as independent variables. The highest multiple coefficient was 0.587; General Intelligence was the dependent variable and ectomorphy, mesomorphy (negative), and standing height were the independent variables. Other dependent variables with significant multiple correlations were Shrewdness, Autia, Premia, Surgency, Radicalism, and Character. The 60-yard shuttle run was an independent variable in six of these relationships.

Attempting to relate the significance of personality measures to physique and physical performance, Cattell[45] offers the

[43]Robert Betz, "A Comparison Between Personality Traits and Physical Fitness of College Males," Master's Thesis, University of Illinois, 1956.

[44]Donald T. Gottesman, "Relationships Between Cattell's Sixteen Personality Factor Questionnaire and Physique, Structure, Strength, and Motor Traits of College Men," Doctoral Dissertation, University of Oregon, 1964.

[45]Raymond B. Cattell, "Some Psychological Correlates of Physical Fitness and Physique," *Exercise and Fitness* (Chicago: The Athletic Institute, 1959), p. 145.

following hypotheses: (a) that a high level of physical fitness reduces anxiety and neuroticism and favors aggressive and extrovert adjustment; (b) that the mind affects the body, so that an absence of neuroticism and anxiety leads to improved physical performance; and (c) that among persons of a high level of physical fitness, only those who possess personality traits of stability and low anxiety do well in intense training and competitive situations.

California Psychological Inventory

The California Psychological Inventory,[46] based largely on the Minnesota Multiphasic Personality Inventory, is a 480-item true-false questionnaire applicable to normal individuals (that is, without pathological manifestations) 13 years of age and older. The Inventory contains 18 scales, identified as follows: Dominance, Capacity for Status, Sociability, Social Presence, Self-Acceptance, Sense of Well-Being, Responsibility, Socialization, Self-Control, Tolerance, Good Impression, Communality, Conformance, Achievement via Independence, Intellectual Efficiency, Psychological-Mindedness, Flexibility, and Femininity. The Inventory scales have been repeatedly cross-validated; most scales are based on the test responses of persons considered to exhibit various kinds of effective behavior. Norms are based on over 13,000 cases distributed through 30 states.

Edwards Personality Inventory

The Edwards Personality Inventory[47] is designed to measure a large number of personality characteristics of normal people in grades 11 to 16 and adults. Edwards developed a pool of 2824 descriptive statements of personality by asking acquaintances to describe individuals they knew. These phrases were grouped by intuitive procedures and by factor analysis to provide scales composing the test. The complete inventory consists of five booklets which together provide measurement of 53 personality variables; each booklet contains 300 true-false items. Such traits as the following are included: persistent, self-confident, enjoys being center of attention, carefree, conforms, is a leader, kind to others, likes to be alone, interested in behavior of others, desires recognition, cooperative, feels superior, assumes responsibility, self-centered, and makes friends easily.

Mooney Problem Check List

The Mooney Problem Check List[48] is not a test in the usual sense, but is a listing of brief statements describing personal problems boys and girls have. Forms are available for junior high school, high school, college, and adult populations. In the Junior High School Form, 30 items are presented in each of seven problem areas: Health and Physical Development; School; Home and Family; Money, Work, and the Future; Boy and Girl Relations; Relations to People in General; and Self-Centered Concerns. The Senior High School and College Forms contain 30 items for each of 11 problem areas: Health and Physical Development; Finances, Living Conditions, Employment; Social and Recreational Activities; Social-Psychological Relations; Personal-Psychological Relations; Courtship, Sex, Marriage; Home and Family; Morals and Religion; Adjustment to School Work; The Future, Vocational

[46]Harrison G. Gough, *California Psychological Inventory* (Palo Alto, Calif.: Consulting Psychologists Press, Inc., 1956).

[47]Allen L. Edwards, *Edwards Personality Inventory* (Chicago: Science Research Associates).

[48]Ross L. Mooney and Leonard V. Gordon, *The Mooney Problem Check Lists* (New York: Psychological Corporation, 1950).

and Educational; Curriculum and Teaching Procedures. In using this instrument, the individual underlines all problems that trouble him; he then circles the numbers in front of those items which are of most concern to him.

This check list can be utilized effectively in health and physical education to locate the various problems boys and girls feel they possess. It has been used successfully in identifying personal and social maladjustments of boys and girls with unsatisfactory levels of physical fitness, in those cases where both situations are associated.

Precautions in the Use of Personality Tests

Although there have been many studies of personality tests, they have not yet reached the stage where their validity can be completely accepted. The criteria utilized have been mostly ratings by judges, which are not highly reliable, even when the characteristic to be rated is well understood. When the trait is intangible and difficult to grasp, still less confidence can be placed in the ratings. Also, many of these tests are only sufficiently reliable for group use (0.70 to 0.85). As a consequence of these factors, the results of personality tests should not be considered infallible, but rather as aids in locating boys and girls who need help and guidance in making personal and social adjustments.

As most personality tests depend upon answers given by the subjects, the ability to obtain frank responses becomes a major problem. The desire for social acceptance results in a temptation for the subject to give answers which present him in a favorable light. Also, in contemplating his own adjustment, the individual is likely to be biased or prejudiced. It is therefore necessary in administering personality tests to make every effort to establish rapport with each pupil, so that he will be willing to reveal extremely personal informa-

tion about himself. Assurance must be given that the replies will be kept confidential. The pupil must be made to feel that honest answers are necessary in order that the health and physical education programs may serve him best.

Personality is an extremely complex phenomenon with many traits acting and re-acting in numerous ways and in many combinations. Yet testing procedures must necessarily sort out and identify single traits, attempting to withdraw each from the setting in which it naturally resides. The need to reserve judgment on the status of individual traits and to attempt the association of such traits with the total personality should be kept in mind.

Not only should the individual's achieved score on each trait in a personality test be considered, but the way in which he answered each of the questions should be examined. This procedure is particularly important in studying the problems of individual students, as it provides many leads to be followed. For example: if a student gives a negative reply to the question "Do you make friends easily?" an excellent lead is provided for additional informal questions resulting ultimately in a better understanding of the individual and a sounder basis for providing a proper educational program for him.

As with the physical self, specialized knowledge is required to evaluate, understand, and treat the social and psychological self. Medicine has been developed to care for extreme deviates from normal physical states; psychology and psychiatry have been likewise developed in the personality field. In neither of these is the physical educator qualified to practice. As a result, when pronounced deviations in social and personal adjustment are suspected from testing or other procedures, the physical educator should refer them to appropriate specialists, just as readily as he now refers students with physical abnormalities to the physician.

CONCLUSION

In physical education, rating scales, social distance tests, and sociometric questionnaires have been more effective in identifying boys and girls with personality difficulties and social problems than have the inventory-type tests. The results of several reported in Chapter 3, for example, show significant relationships of physical and motor fitness measures to peer status, leadership qualities, and personal and social traits.

As a further example, Popp[49] found no significant differences on the Washburne Social Adjustment Inventory between boys grouped by highest and lowest 20 percent on Rogers' Physical Fitness Index; also, the boys lowest on the Rogers test expressed fewer problems on the Mooney Problem Check List than did boys high on the Rogers test. Yet, when five representative administrators and teachers, who knew the boys, each independently selected the ten boys "most nearly like sons they would like to have" and the ten boys "least like sons they would like to have," the results were dramatically different. Of the boys selected in the desirable category ("most nearly like sons"), 69 percent had high PFI's; of the boys in the undesirable category ("least like sons"), 75 percent had low PFI's.

[49]James Popp, "Case Studies of Sophomore High School Boys with High and Low Physical Fitness indices," Master of Science Thesis, University of Oregon, 1959.

SELECTED REFERENCES

BRECK, SABINA J., "A Sociometric Measurement of Status in Physical Education Classes," *Research Quarterly,* **21,** No. 2 (May 1950), 75.

BUROS, OSCAR K., ed. *The Seventh Mental Measurements Yearbook.* Highland Park, N.J.: The Gryphon Press, 1972.

CATTELL, RAYMOND B., "Some Psychological Correlates of Physical Fitness and Physique," *Exercise and Fitness.* Chicago: Athletic Institute, 1959, p. 145.

COWELL, CHARLES C., "Our Function Is Still Education!" *Physical Educator,* **14,** No. 1 (March 1957), 6.

McCLOY, C. H., "Character Building in Physical Education," *Research Quarterly,* **1,** No. 3 (October 1930), 42.

McCLOY, C. H., and TERENCE HEPP, "General Factors of Components of Character as Related to Physical Education," *Research Quarterly,* **28,** No. 3 (October 1957), 269.

TODD, FRANCES, "Sociometry in Physical Education," *Journal of American Association for Health, Physical Education, and Recreation,* **24,** No. 5 (May 1953), 23.

CHAPTER 12

The social objective in physical education was discussed in Chapter 10, together with suggested procedures for its realization. With respect to these procedures, it was pointed out that equating the powers or abilities of individuals and groups provides a desirable setting for the optimum development of personal and social traits. Attitudes toward participation in physical education activities may also be enhanced. Further, ability grouping is an important pedagogical procedure, as it brings together pupils of like ability, all of whom are ready for instruction on approximately the same level. Skills may then be taught effectively and efficiently. The present chapter deals with tests that may be used to group students according to their general abilities.

CONCEPT OF GENERAL MOTOR ABILITY

Traditionally, general motor ability has been considered as one's level of ability in a wide range of activities. It has been thought of as an integrated composite of such individual traits as strength, endurance, power, speed, agility, balance, reaction time, and coordination, traits underlying performance in many motor complexes. In successful motor performances, these traits function in a coordinated manner and in effective sequence to achieve an accurate and efficient movement, whether it be a single effort, as in the golf drive, or in a series of complex and rapidly changing movements, as in basketball.

Studies by Henry[1] and his associates have demonstrated that motor skills and large muscle psychometric abilities are far more specific than had previously been realized. Henry contends that it is largely a matter of chance whether an individual who is highly coordinated in one type of performance will be well or poorly coordinated in another. Thus, the "natural athlete" is endowed with a large number of specifics rather than with a great amount of general motor ability. Further, successful patterns of specific traits will not be the same for all athletes. In constructing profile charts of outstanding upper elementary and junior high school athletes, Clarke and associates[2] demonstrated that, while such athletes have some common characteristics, the pattern of these characteristics varies from athlete to athlete; where a successful athlete is low on a significant trait, he compensates for strength in another.

The concept of specificity as contrasted with generality in motor performance must be recognized. The measurement of all specifics entering into complex motor activities of many types is the most desirable approach to their evaluation. However, this process becomes intricate and time-consuming, if not impossible. An acceptable alternative is to sample the many specifics entering into such

General Motor Abilities

---

[1]Franklin M. Henry, "Coordination and Motor Learning," *59th Annual Proceedings*, College Physical Education Association, 1956, p. 68.

[2]H. Harrison Clarke, *Physical and Motor Traits in the Medford Boys' Growth Study* (Englewood Cliffs, N.J.: Prentice-Hall, Inc., 1971), p. 255.

performances; actually, this has been the traditional approach. High multiple correlations result between a small number of specifics and the composite of many specifics serving as a motor ability criterion. Henry[3] has indicated that the resulting sample represents general motor ability when the concept is restricted to this sense.

BASES FOR ABILITY GROUPINGS

Homogeneous grouping of individuals for participation in a physical activity program, whether it be accomplished by judgment or by objective measurement, may follow two major procedures: (a) equating by specific activities, or (b) equating by general abilities. Each of these methods has its place in physical education; the one selected, however, will depend upon the type of program being conducted in the school.

Equating by Specific Activities

In ability grouping by specific activities, the abilities of the pupils are evaluated and the classification of the participants changed for each activity included in the program. A simple example of this procedure is the process of "choosing sides" for a game of basketball, or any other sport, during the physical education class, or informally during free-play periods. Tests might also be used to determine such groupings.

This basis for ability grouping is useful when a single physical education activity is being taught to the same group for a considerable period of time, as is often done in college programs where students elect the same activity for a quarter of the year or longer. In this situation, skill-testing of the specific activity being taught could well be a part of the instruction program, the results of which could be used for equating or classifying purposes. Sufficient time is available to make this procedure worth while and even essential for good teaching practice. Tests of this sort are discussed in Chapter 14.

Equating by General Abilities

In grouping by general abilities, a measure of all-round athletic or motor ability is given, and groups are arranged on this basis. A test of all-round ability does not measure skill in any particular sport. An individual with a high score on such a test, however, should perform well, or have capacity for good performance after a period of instruction, in a number of athletic events. These measures do not consider previous experience in specific activities, nor do they measure such character qualities as interest, persistence, courage, and initiative. Consequently, in applying them, the best results will be obtained if some judgment is also used in placing pupils in the various groups, the physical educator being guided by his knowledge of the abilities of the different individuals, or by his subsequent observation of their performances, to make necessary adjustments and to insure proper equation.

General motor ability is complex. Physical, mental, emotional, and social factors enter into efficient motor performance. It is a *Gestalt,* with the whole personality dynamically organized, that results in top-flight performance. To identify physical and motor traits involved in general motor ability, a number of factor analysis studies have been conducted.

McCloy[4] lists the following ten factors as prerequisite to effective learning of motor skills: muscular strength, dynamic energy, ability to change direction, flexibility, ability, peripheral vision, good vision, concentration, understanding of the mechanics of the techniques of the activities,

[3]Franklin M. Henry, "Specificity vs. Generality in Learning Motor Skills," *61st Annual Proceedings,* College Physical Education Association, 1958, p. 127.

[4]C. H. McCloy, "A Preliminary Study of Factors in Motor Educability," *Research Quarterly,* **11,** No. 2 (May 1940), 28.

and absence of disturbing or inhibiting emotional complications. Other factors in motor educability he summarizes as: insight into the nature of the skill; ability to visualize spatial relations; ability to make quick and adaptive decisions; sensory-motor coordination relations of eye to head, hand, or foot; sensory-motor coordination related to weight and force; judgment of the relationship of the subject to external objects in relation to time, height, distance, and direction; accuracy of direction and small angle of error; general kinesthetic sensitivity and control; ability to coordinate a complex unitary movement; ability to coordinate a complex series or combination of movements that follow one another in rapid succession; arm control; factors involved in the function of balance; timing; motor rhythm; sensory rhythm; and esthetic feeling.

McCloy's findings demonstrate clearly the conclusion reached earlier that it is obviously too difficult and too complicated for the physical educator "on the job" to attempt to measure all the elements contributing to general motor ability. He must select general or cross-section tests that have been shown to possess a high relationship with motor ability and that measure the elements of greatest significance.

Ability grouping by general abilities is a very useful method of classification in physical education, as individuals or groups may be equated for a wide range of activities without changing the grouping. It is particularly valuable in that type of physical education program where the activities may vary either within a single class period or from day to day, or where the same activity does not continue on consecutive days for more than a week or two at the most. Classification by individual activities would be cumbersome in these situations, as it would necessitate changing the groupings repeatedly. The great amount of time spent in testing or evaluating pupils for a number of frequently changing activities does not seem justifiable when a measure of general ability may be applied satisfactorily.

EARLY MEASURES OF GENERAL MOTOR ABILITIES

From the early days of physical education in the United States, physical educators have attempted to classify individuals roughly into equivalent groups, both for physical education class activity and for athletic competition. The change from the early emphasis on gymnastics and calisthenics to the later stress on games and sports created a need for general ability testing, which has continued to the present time.

A typical example of an early test of the general motor ability type, and one which has been revised in recent years, is the Sigma Delta Psi Test. In 1912, a national athletic fraternity, known as Sigma Delta Psi, was started. In order to obtain membership in the fraternity, the following achievements were required:[5]

1. 100-yd. dash: $11^{3}/_{5}$ sec.

2. 120-yd. low hurdles: 16 sec.

3. Running high jump: 5 ft.

4. Running broad jump: 17 ft.

5. 16-lb. shot put: according to a man's weight; 30 ft. for a man weighing 160 lbs. or over.

6. Rope climb: 20 ft. in 12 sec.

7. Baseball distance throw: 250 ft.

8. Football distance punt: 120 ft.

9. 100-yd. swim: 1 min. 45 sec.

10. One-mile run: 6 min.

11. Tumbling: (a) Front handspring (b) fence vault with bar at chin height (c) handstand, 10 sec.

12. Posture: erect carriage

13. Scholarship: C grade average or better

Note: If the candidate has won a letter in a varsity sport, he may substitute this for any of the above requirements except swimming.

[5]National Fraternity, Care of the School of Health and Physical Education, Indiana University, Bloomington, Indiana.

The rules of the National Collegiate Athletic Association are followed for the various track and field events. In the 120-yard low hurdle race, five standard low hurdles, 20 yards apart, are used. For the test to count, all hurdles must remain upright after the test.

In the rope climb, the contestant starts from a sitting position on the floor; the rope is climbed without the use of the legs. The legs, however, may be used in the descent.

In the timed handstand, the contestant is not allowed to advance or retreat more than three feet during the test.

Other early tests of this general type include: Detroit Decathlon utilized to select the best all-round athletes in the city of Detroit; Athletic Badge Tests devised for boys and girls in 1913 by the National Playground and Recreation Association of America; Richard's Efficiency Tests for grade schools proposed in 1914; Philadelphia Public School Age Aim Charts; Reilly's Scheme of Rational Athletics for boys and girls; California Decathlon; and Los Angeles Achievement Expectancy Tables. Later the California Pentathlon was proposed.

In the initial stages of motor or physical ability testing, the aim was to use the tests primarily to arouse the interest of boys and girls in all-round physical proficiency. Standards of achievement were set up and scoring tables were devised, on a point basis in many instances, with divisions into junior and senior groups or into various combinations of age, height, and weight.

STRENGTH INDEX

In discussing Rogers' Physical Fitness Index test in Chapter 7, the Strength Index[6] was described, and its use to determine general athletic ability was mentioned. Rogers' hypothesis was that an individual with a high SI would perform well, or have potentialities for good performance after a training period in a number of activities, and that an individual with a low SI would have athletic capabilities on a lower level. There is considerable evidence to support this hypothesis.

Rogers[7] utilized two different methods to determine the validity of the SI as a measure of general athletic ability. In the first method, a correlation of 0.76 was obtained between the SI and the weighted score on the 100-yard dash, the running high jump, the running broad jump, and the bar vault. This correlation was found to be nearly twice as significant for predictive purposes as that obtained by the best combination of age, height, and weight. A second correlation between the SI and ability in a 2-lap run, standing broad jump, running high jump, 8-pound shot-put, basketball foul throw, and throwing baseballs and footballs at a specially marked target raised the coefficient to 0.81.[8]

Assuming that success in "making the school team" is a criterion of athletic ability, Rogers, as a second method of obtaining validity for the SI, compared the Strength Indices of major sports athletes with those scored by all other boys in the school from which the data were obtained. The resultant relationships are significant: (a) not more than five boys in 100, including the football men themselves, reached the median SI for football letter men; (b) ten football players achieved SI's higher than 371 of the 390 boys in the school, including themselves, and (c) no single score was recorded above the median score

---

[6]Directions for administering these tests appear in Chapter 7; the Oregon Simplification of this test is also applicable.

[7]Frederick Rand Rogers, *Physical Capacity Tests in the Administration of Physical Education* (New York: Bureau of Publications, Teachers College, Columbia University, 1925).

[8]All studies concerned with strength tests reported in this chapter, except for the Medford Series, used the old method of measuring leg lift (without the belt).

TABLE 12.1 *Contrasting Strength Index Means of Nonparticipants and Outstanding Athletes by Sports*

Groups	School levels and ages		
	Ele-mentary: 12 yrs.	Junior High: 15 yrs.	Senior High: 17 yrs.
Nonparticipants	1089	2043	2723
Football	1430	2903	3338
Basketball	1264	2761	3123
Track	1389	2768	3190
Baseball	1159		3123

achieved by the "five best athletes" or school team captains by any boy not a member of some major sports team.

In the Medford Boys' Growth Study, Clarke and associates[9] reported that strength was a consistent differentiator of the athletic success of upper elementary, junior high, and senior high school boys as revealed in interschool competition. For the single ages of 12, 15, and 17 years, the SI means of nonparticipants and outstanding athletes in various interscholastic sports are shown in Table 12.1. The means were generally much higher than the means of the nonparticipants in all sports at the three school levels. The football athletes had the highest means throughout. Their means were higher than the means of the nonparticipants by 32 percent for elementary school, 42 percent for junior high school, and 23 percent for senior high school boys.[10] Mel Thompson, head football coach, Central Washington State College, reported the following SI distribution for his 1965 team: high, 4686; third quartile, 3979; median, 3655; first quartile, 3264; low, 2593.

[9]Clarke, *Medford Boys' Growth Study*, p. 240.

[10]H. Harrison Clarke, "Characteristics of Athletes," *Physical Fitness Research Digest*, President's Council on Physical Fitness and Sports, **3**, No. 2 (April 1973), 7.

As subsidiary evidence of the relationship between strength and general athletic ability, significant relationships have been found with the learning of motor skills. For example, Shay[11] found the following correlations between ability or speed in learning the kip or upstart on the horizontal bar:

0.83, Physical Fitness Index

0.76, Strength Index

0.52, Brace Test of Motor Ability

Although objective experimental evidence is essential in determining the value of the Strength Index as a measure of general athletic ability, it is also important to "try it out" in actual practice by equating groups and recording the results of formal contests between them. This has been done in a number of situations with satisfying results. Illustrations of such applications follow.

Oesterich[12] equated basketball teams by means of the Strength Index and compared the results with the choose-up method. The largest difference in team scores was 16, as compared with 30 for the choose-up method; the median difference was 3.4 as compared with 6. Eleven of the 26 games played by the test-equation method, or 44 percent, ended either in a tie score or with a 1-point difference. The results of this study are surprising, inasmuch as the SI is not intended as a measure of basketball ability or as a measure of any other *specific* skill.

Clarke and Bonesteel[13] utilized the Strength Index to equate two teams in

[11]Clayton T. Shay, "The Progressive Part Versus the Whole Method of Learning Motor Skills," *Research Quarterly*, **5**, No. 4 (December 1934), 66.

[12]Harry G. Oesterich, "Strength Testing Program Applied to Y.M.C.A. Organization and Administration," *Research Quarterly*, **6**, No. 1 (March 1935), 197.

[13]H. Harrison Clarke and Harold A. Bonesteel, "Equalizing the Abilities of Intramural Teams in a Small High School," *Supplement to the Research Quarterly*, **6**, No. 1 (March 1935), 193.

each of three physical education classes. Games in touch football, speedball, field hockey, and indoor soccer were scheduled between the teams in each class. Previous experience in game skills was negligible. The number of games won and lost by the equated teams was very evenly divided. Of 64 games played by all teams in the four sports, 29, or 45 percent, ended with tie scores. The greatest scoring difference between any two teams in all four sports was eight points, or 2.4 percent of the total number of points scored by both teams. The least difference was three points, or 0.9 percent of the combined score of the two teams.

The use of the Strength Index for equating motor abilities of girls has not been so extensive as for boys. In conducting one such study, however, Hinton and Rarick[14] obtained a correlation of 0.81 between the SI and scores on the Cubberly and Cozens Girls' Basketball Achievement Test, utilizing college women as subjects. These investigators recommended lung capacity, back lift, and Rogers' arm strength score as a test for girls that relates well to basketball ability. The multiple correlation of these test items with the basketball test was sufficiently high to predict basketball achievement with a 10 percent limit above or below the basketball score.

Anderson[15] studied the athletic performance of high-school girls, utilizing the following strength tests: items in McCloy's Strength Index, push, pull, vertical jump, forward bends, squats, and thigh flexors. A correlation of 0.65 was obtained between the McCloy SI with vertical jump and a criterion composed of ratings of the athletic ability of 300 girls made by the investigator.

[14]Evelyn A. Hinton and Lawrence Rarick, "The Correlation of Rogers' Test of Physical Capacity and the Cubberly and Cozens Measurement of Achievement in Basketball," *Research Quarterly,* **11,** No. 3 (October 1940), 58.

[15]Theresa Anderson, "Studies in Strength Testing for High School Girls," *Research Quarterly,* **8,** No. 3 (October 1937), 69.

STRENGTH COMPOSITE

In Chapter 7, Oregon Cable-Tension Strength Test batteries were presented for boys and girls at each school level, upper elementary, junior high, senior high, and college. Each battery consisted of three strength tests; the sum of the tests was called the Strength Composite (SC). The SC could well be used for the same purpose as the Strength Index. A major difference between the two batteries is that the SC is composed entirely of muscular strength tests, while the SI contains both muscular strength and muscular endurance items.

McCLOY'S GENERAL MOTOR ABILITY AND CAPACITY TESTS

General Motor Ability

McCloy[16] constructed a test of general motor ability composed of a simple test of strength and a number of track and field events. The elements are as follows.

For Boys. The strength test included is the pull-up or chinning test computed for arm strength, using McCloy's formula (see Chapter 7). The track and field events may vary according to the age and experience of the group, the selection being made by the physical educator, provided scoring tables are available for the event. However, the events selected should include one sprint (varying from 50 to 100 yards), one broad jump (either running or standing), the running high jump, and a weight-throwing event (shot-put, basketball throw, or baseball throw). These four events are scored on McCloy's scoring tables, the sum of which is combined by special formula with chinning strength as follows:

[16]C. H. McCloy and Norma D. Young, *Tests and Measurements in Health and Physical Education,* 3rd ed. (New York: Appleton-Century-Crofts, 1954), Ch. 17.

General Motor Ability Score =
0.1022 (track and field point) +
0.3928 (chinning strength).

For Girls. The actual number of push-ups, rather than pull-up strength, is used in the girls' General Motor Ability Test. Three track and field events are included: a sprint, a broad jump, and a throw, scored on McCloy's scoring tables for boys. The formula for combining these elements is:

General Motor Ability Score =
0.42 (track and field point) +
9.6 (number of chins)

In the development of the General Motor Ability Tests, results on individual test elements were correlated with the total score on a large battery of achievement tests. The elements finally selected to form the test gave as high a prediction of general motor ability as was given by any other combination of events. Other items added to this battery gave no significant additional predictive value.

McCloy correlated total track and field points with technical skill in soccer and basketball of physical education professional students, as determined by student ratings, each student in the group rating each other individually. The resulting correlations were: with soccer, 0.84; with basketball, 0.92.

General Motor Capacity

McCloy also worked out an ingenious relationship between general motor ability and general motor capacity that may prove useful to the physical educator who wishes to analyze the individual motor problems of his students. The General Motor Capacity Test, the basis for this analysis, is designed to measure innate or inherent motor potentialities—the limits to which an individual may be developed. In this respect, the General Motor Capacity Test may be compared to an intelligence test. It is not designed to test present developed ability in any one activity, but to predict potential levels that the individual may be expected to attain. The following test items, together with the elements they purport to measure, compose this test.

1. Classification Index: general size and maturity.

2. Sargent Jump: "explosive" power of the large muscles.

3. Iowa Brace Test: motor educability.

4. Burpee (squat-thrust) Test: large-muscle speed test.

The items on the McCloy Motor Capacity Test are weighted differently for each school level. For girls it was found that the Classification Index was of little value, and it was eliminated from the battery. The correlation of the final weighted batteries with the ratings made by competent teachers was 0.51 for boys and 0.73 for girls, and with a criterion score 0.97 for boys and 0.91 for girls. The test battery may be used in a number of different ways, as follows.

1. General Motor Capacity Score. The GMCS is the total score on the test and is proposed as the measure of innate or inherent motor potentialities of the individual. By analogy, it may be compared with the raw score on an intelligence test.

2. Motor Quotient. The GMCS may be divided by a norm based on the Classification Index for boys and on age for girls, giving the Motor Quotient. This quotient may be compared to the Intelligence Quotient in the mental field.

3. General Motor Achievement Quotient. The GMAQ is a quantitative statement comparing the individual's developed motor ability and his innate motor capacity. Instead of the average GMAQ being placed at 100, the formulae for its computation were weighted so that 100 is located two "standard deviations" of estimate above the average GMCS, or at a "practical maximum." Thus, a percent relationship of actual ability to the predicted or standard ability has been worked out. An AMAQ of 85, there-

fore, indicates that the individual's performance is only 85 percent of what it would be if he
were developed to his capacity.

4. Individual analysis. It is possible to analyze an
individual's test results by transmitting the various elements to T-scores and studying the
comparative scores of the individual on each
item of the test.

Following the pattern established by
McCloy, Carpenter[17] developed formulae
for predicting general motor ability and
general motor capacity for boys and girls
in the first three grades. The items included in the GMAS are standing broad
jump, 4-pound shot-put, and body weight.
For the GMCS, the items are Sargent
(vertical) jump, Burpee (squat-thrust) test,
six Brace-type tests, and McCloy's Classification Index III. In this latter battery, five
of the Johnson-type tests may be used in
place of the Brace stunts. These tests are
used in the same manner as described
above for the McCloy batteries. Tables for
ready computation of all formulae are
available in the reference.

LARSON TESTS

In a study of strength tests utilizing the
Rogers battery, the MacCurdy Test, and
a new test composed of chinning, dipping, and the vertical jump, Larson[18] obtained significant correlations, as shown
in Table 12.2, with a criterion of motor
ability composed of the following 15 motor skills: bar-snap, feet-to-bar, half-lever,
bar-vault, rope-climb, frog-stand, standing
broad jump, running broad jump, standing
hop-step-jump, football punt for distance,

[17]Aileen Carpenter, "The Measurement of Gen-
eral Motor Capacity and General Motor Ability in the
First Three Grades," *Research Quarterly,* **13,** No. 4
(December 1942), 444.

[18]Leonard A. Larson, "A Factor and Validity
Analysis of Strength Variables and Tests with a Test
Combination with Chinning, Dipping, and Vertical
Jump," *Research Quarterly,* **11,** No. 4 (December
1940), 82.

TABLE 12.2 *Correlation of Strength Tests with
a Criterion of 15 Motor Ability Items*

| | High School | |
Strength Tests	Data	College Data
Rogers Si	0.84	0.59
MacCurdy test	—	0.52
Larson test	0.83	0.68

football pass for distance, baseball throw
for distance, shot-put, dodging-run, and
440-yard run. For high-school boys, the
correlations obtained between the criterion and the SI were slightly higher than
those obtained between the criterion and
the Larson tests. With the college data, the
Larson test had an advantage.

The measurement procedures for the
Larson test are the same as those described elsewhere in the text: chinning
and dipping, as in the SI test, and the
vertical jump, as in the McCloy General
Motor Capacity Test appearing in this
chapter. In scoring, the raw scores must be
changed into "weighted scores"; the sum
of these equals the "Index Score." Scoring
tables appear in Larson's study, together
with a five point classification chart for the
college age group.

Subsequently, Larson[19] constructed the
following two general motor ability tests,
one as an indoor test and the other as an
outdoor test, after experimenting with 25
motor ability items:

Indoor test	*Outdoor test*
1. Dodging run	1. Baseball throw for distance
2. Bar-snap	2. Chinning
3. Chinning	3. Bar-snap
4. Dipping	4. Vertical jump
5. Vertical jump	

[19]Leonard A. Larson, "A Factor Analysis of Motor
Ability Variables and Tests with Tests for College
Men," *Research Quarterly,* **12,** No. 3 (October 1941),
499.

The multiple correlations with the criterion measure were: for the Indoor Test, $R = 0.97$; for the Outdoor Test, $R = 0.98$. According to Larson, the tests do not predict or indicate specific qualities, such as endurance, coordination, sports skills, and so forth. They are valuable in that they do indicate ability in the basic elements underlying sports skills.

CARPENTER-STANSBURY TEST FOR CHILDREN IN FIRST THREE GRADES

In an attempt to find a simple substitute for the Rogers Strength Index as a measure of motor ability for boys, Stansbury[20] established a criterion, known as "total points," composed of: vertical jump, 16-pound shot-put, obstacle race, baseball throw, 8-pound shot-put, 20-foot rope climb, and standing broad jump. The final selected test items consist of the following, as presented in his regression equation of weighted scores:

$$1.4 \text{ (8-pound shot-put in feet)} + \text{(standing broad jump in inches)} + \text{(body weight in pounds)}.$$

Norms are available in the reference based upon McCloy's Classification Index for high school boys.

Carpenter[21] experimented with the Stansbury test items as applied to children in the first three grades. As a result, the following formulae were developed:

Boys: (standing broad jump in inches) + 2.3 (4-pound shot-put in feet) + (body weight in pounds).

[20]Edgar Stansbury, "A Simplified Method of Classifying Junior and Senior High School Boys into Homogeneous Groups for Physical Education Activities," *Research Quarterly*, **12**, No. 4 (December 1941), 765.

[21]Aileen Carpenter, "Strength Testing in the First Three Grades," *Research Quarterly*, **13**, No. 3 (October 1942), 328.

Girls: .5 (standing broad jump in inches) + 3 (4-pound shot-put in feet) + (body weight in pounds).

Norms for this test are based upon McCloy's Classification Index III, with the following weightings:

Girls' norm $0.2549 CI - 27.91$
Boys' norm $0.3009 CI - 64.60$

In computing the "Physical Efficiency Index," the achieved score on the test, multiplied by 100, is divided by the individual's norm. A "PEI" of 100 indicates that the child has just the amount of motor ability that would be expected of him for his age, height, and weight. The norms for this test appear in Appendix Table B.17.

NEWTON MOTOR ABILITY TEST FOR HIGH SCHOOL GIRLS

Experimenting with ten test items, Powell and Howe developed the "Newton" test of motor ability for high school girls,[22] composed of the standing broad jump, a "baby" hurdle race, and a "scramble" test. The multiple correlation of these with a composite criterion of 18 items, selected on the basis of strength, power, speed, and coordination, is 0.91. Other criteria were also used, in which these same items occupied a favored position.

Directions for giving the Powell and Howe items are given below. Six-sigma standard score achievement scales for each of the three tests in the battery and for "total points" appear in Appendix Table B.18. In obtaining total points, the unweighted scale scores on the three tests are added directly. The decile locations for the various parts of the tests and the total achievement are given in the table, as an additional aid in judging performance.

[22]Elizabeth Powell and E. C. Howe, "Motor Ability Tests for High School Girls," *Research Quarterly*, **10**, No. 4 (December 1939), 81.

Standing Broad Jump. The subject toes a starting line, two feet from the end of a gymnasium mat held firmly in place against the wall, and jumps as far as possible. The best of three trials is recorded to the nearest inch.

Baby Hurdles. Ten gymnasium benches and five split bamboo sticks are used for setting up the hurdles. The first hurdle is five yards from the starting line; the others are at three-yard intervals; an Indian club, or substitute, is placed three yards beyond the last hurdle. The subject runs over the hurdles, around the Indian club, and back over the hurdles to the starting line. Penalties are not imposed for displacing hurdles. Time is recorded to the nearest fifth of a second.

Scramble. A jumping standard is arranged with a small shelf (four feet above the floor) upon which a tap bell is fastened securely; it is placed ten feet from a wall. The subject starts from a back-lying position on the floor with both feet against the wall and the arms stretched sideways at shoulder level, palms down. At the starting signal, she gets up, runs and taps the bell twice, returns to the starting position and claps the hands on the floor twice; this performance is repeated until she has made the fourth double tap of the bell. The time is recorded to the nearest fifth of a second.

MOTOR ABILITY TESTS FOR COLLEGE MEN

Cozens Athletic Ability Test

One of the early tests of general athletic ability for college men was constructed by Cozens.[23] in order to obtain a composite idea of the elements that comprise general athletic ability. Cozens secured judgments from 52 representative physical educators, and selected the seven deemed most important by the judges. Over 40 possible tests were collected and classified under the seven elements previously chosen, one test for each element being retained after experimentation. These elements and tests appear in Table 12.3.

In scoring this test, the raw scores are transposed into sigma scores,[24] and these are multiplied by the weights given in Table 12.3, to obtain the relative value that each test contributes to the general quality of athletic ability. The validity and reliability of the test are high.

Barrow Motor Ability Test

In constructing a motor ability test for college men, Barrow[25] used expert opinion in order to select eight factors of motor ability and 29 items as potential measures of these factors. On the basis of multiple correlations against a criterion consisting of the sum of performances on the 29 tests, two test batteries were chosen. For the first battery, the correlation was 0.95; for the second test battery, 0.92. The two test batteries were as follows:

First Battery	*Second Battery*
Standing broad jump	Standing broad jump
Softball distance throw	Medicine ball put (6 lb.)
Zigzag run	Zigzag run
Wall pass	
Medicine ball put (6 lb.)	
60-yard dash	

[23]Frederick W. Cozens, *The Measurement of General Athletic Ability in College Men* (Eugene, Oregon: University of Oregon Press, 1929).

[24]Sigma scoring tables based on Cozens' Classification Index are available in the following reference: F. W. Cozens, *Achievement Scales in Physical Education for College Men* (Philadelphia: Lea & Febiger, 1936).

[25]Harold M. Barrow, "Test of Motor Ability for College Men," *Research Quarterly,* **25,** No. 3 (October 1954), 253.

TABLE 12.3 *Elements and Test Items Comprising the Cozens Test of General Athletic Ability for College Men*

Test Elements	Test Items	Score Multi-plication
1. Arm and shoulder-girdle strength	Dips	0.8
2. Arm and shoulder-girdle coordination	Baseball throw for distance	1.5
3. Hand-eye foot-eye, arm-eye coordination	Football punt for distance	1.0
4. Jumping strength, leg strength, and leg flexibility	Standing broad jump	0.9
5. Endurance	Quarter-mile run	1.3
6. Body coordination, agility, and control	Bar-snap for distance	0.5
7. Speed of legs	Dodging run	1.0

Directions for administering the items in this motor ability test and norms appear in the reference.

MOTOR EDUCABILITY

As intelligence testing occupies an important place in education, a number of experimenters in physical education have attempted to construct tests of "motor intelligence." McCloy's General Motor Capacity Test, described above, is an important attempt of this sort. Other investigators have proposed tests of "motor educability," a term popularized by McCloy and referring to the "ease with which an individual learns new motor skills."

Iowa-Brace Test

In 1927, Brace[26] published the first test designed to measure inherent motor skill. The test was composed of 20 stunts, each of which was scored in terms of success or failure. Later, McCloy[27] revised the Brace Test, experimenting with 40 different stunts and retaining 21 of them, 10 of which were in the old Brace battery. From

these 21 stunts, six batteries of ten stunts each were drawn up for the upper three grades of the elementary school, for the junior high school, and for the senior high school, one set on each level being for boys and one for girls. Two trials of each test are allowed, with absolutely no practice being permitted in advance. The stunts are scored on a pass-or-fail basis. If the pupil succeeds on the first trial, he receives two points; if he fails on both trials, no points. The highest possible score for the 10 stunts in any battery, therefore, is 20. T-score tables for the test have been prepared by McCloy.

In preparing the Iowa Revision of the Brace Test, three criteria were applied to the selection of stunts, as follows.

1. The percentage of individuals passing it increased with age.

2. It had a relatively low correlation with strength, with the Classification Index, and with the Sargent Jump. In other words, it was not a measure of strength, size, maturity, or power.

3. It correlated relatively highly with track and field athletic ability when the Classification Index (or age alone for girls), the Sargent Jump, and strength were held constant to the athletic events but not to the stunt; consideration was thus given to greater skill (or a greater degree of motor educability).

[26]David K. Brace, *Measuring Motor Ability* (New York: A. S. Barnes & Co., Inc., 1927).

[27]McCloy and Young, *Tests and Measurement,* p. 85.

In the validation of both the Brace and the Iowa-Brace tests, the criterion was achievement, not ability to learn. In a later study with high school girls,[28] a different approach to this problem was made. Various measures of motor educability were correlated with the rate of learning basketball, volleyball, and baseball skills. The highest relationship was found with the Brace Test, the next with the Iowa-Brace Test, and the last with the Johnson Test. Brace[29] reported similar results in studies which he conducted in speed of learning field hockey, tennis, and aquatic skills with girls.

In later studies, Brace[30] investigated motor ability in relation to learning skills, as indicated by the following six tests: "tangle" (stunt-type) test, rhythm test, wall volley with a volleyball, ball bounce with a basketball, kick test, and target toss. The learning situation involved 90 performances of each test. He concluded that the Brace motor ability test does not measure motor learning to an extent that would justify its being classified as a test of motor educability, although it was slightly superior to the Iowa Revision in this respect. For college men, Darby[31] obtained a correlation of 0.51 between the Brace test and the Arkansas State College Motor Fitness Test, a ten item battery.

Metheny-Johnson Test

In 1932, Johnson[32] proposed a test designed to measure "native neuro-muscular skill capacity." The test consists of performing ten stunts down the length of a five by ten foot gymnasium mat, specially marked for this purpose. Johnson reported a validity coefficient of 0.69, but did not indicate the criterion. Koob[33] obtained a correlation of 0.95 between this test and the number of trials required for junior high school boys to learn a series of ten tumbling stunts. A reliability coefficient of 0.97 was indicated by Johnson with college men as subjects. Other experiments, however, have not found the same accuracy for the test when administered to girls. Gire and Espenschade[34] report a reliability of 0.61 with high school girls. Hatlestad[35] concludes, after administering the test to college women, that greater objectivity is needed.

Metheny[36] studied the Johnson Test and found that, with boys, four of the tests alone correlated 0.98 with the total Johnson score, and 0.93 with a criterion of learning tumbling stunts. For girls, a combination of three of the Johnson items gave a correlation of 0.86 with the total Johnson score.

With the elimination of six of the original Johnson items, Metheny was able to simplify the mat used in the performance of the test, as shown in Figure 12.1. A lane 2 feet wide is marked down the center of a 15-foot mat. This lane is divided into two equal narrow lanes by a center line, and into ten equal sections lengthwise by lines placed every 18 inches. These lines are alternately 3 inches wide and ¾ inch wide, the 18-inch sections being measured to the middle of the line in each case.

[28]Eugenia Gire and Anna Espenschade, "The Relationship Between Measures of Motor Educability and the Learning of Specific Skills," *Research Quarterly,* **13,** No. 1 (March 1942), 43.

[29]David K. Brace, "Studies in the Rate of Learning Gross Bodily Motor Skills," *Research Quarterly,* **12,** No. 2 (May 1941), 181.

[30]David K. Brace, "Studies in Motor Learning of Gross Bodily Motor Skills," *Research Quarterly,* **7,** No. 4 (December 1946), 242.

[31]Jake Darby, "A Comparison of Results Obtained on the Arkansas State College Motor Fitness Test with Results from Selected Tests of Physical Abilities," Master's Thesis, Arkansas State College, 1965.

[32]Granville B. Johnson, "Physical Skill Tests for Sectioning Classes into Homogeneous Units," *Research Quarterly,* **3,** No. 1 (March 1932), 128.

[33]Clarence G. Koob, "A Study of Johnson Skills Test as a Measure of Motor Educability," Master's Thesis, University of Iowa, 1937.

[34]Gire and Espenschade, "Motor Educability and Specific Skills," p. 43.

[35]L. Lucile Hatlestad, "Motor Educability Tests for Women College Students," *Research Quarterly,* **13,** No. 1 (March 1942), 10.

[36]Eleanor Metheny, "Studies of the Johnson Test as a Test of Motor Educability," *Research Quarterly,* **9,** No. 4 (December 1938), 105.

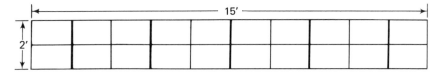

FIGURE 12.1. *Canvas Markings for Metheny-Johnson Test of Motor Skill*

On this mat, the selected Johnson Test items are performed. The first three tests are used for both boys and girls; the fourth test, "jumping full turns," is included for boys only. The tests are described as follows:

Front Roll. Perform rolls in the 2-foot lane. Start with feet outside of chart. Perform two front rolls, the first within the limits of the first half of the lane (not going beyond the middle 3-inch line); the second within the limits of the second half, never touching or overreaching the lanes. *Scoring:* Count five points for each roll. Deduct two for overreaching side-line right or left for each roll; one for overreaching end limit on each roll; and five for failure to perform a true roll.

Back Roll. Perform two back rolls in entire 2-foot lane, one in each half of the lane. Start with feet outside of chart. *Scoring:* Score as for front roll.

Jumping Half-Turns, Right and Left Alternately. Start with feet on first 3-inch line. Jumping with both feet to second 3-inch line, executing a half-turn either right or left; jump to third 3-inch line, executing half-turn in opposite direction; continue the length of the mat, alternating directions of rotation. *Scoring:* Deduct two points for each jump in which the subject does not land with both feet on the 3-inch line, or turns the wrong way, or both.

Jumping Full Turns. Start with the feet outside the chart at about the center of the lane. Jump with feet together to second rectangular space, executing a full turn with the body right or left; continue across the mat, executing full turns, rotating in

the same direction, landing on both feet in every second rectangular space. *Scoring:* Score as for preceding test, deducting two points if the subject fails to land on both feet, oversteps the square, turns too far or not far enough, or loses balance before starting the next jump.

Gross, Greisel, and Stull[37] obtained low correlations between both the Metheny Revision of the Johnson Test (0.33) and the Iowa-Brace Test (0.46) and the ability of college men to learn wrestling. They also found that the correlation between the Metheny-Johnson and Iowa-Brace tests to be low (0.40), thus concluding that the two tests were "not measures of the same ability." Cooper[38] also obtained a low correlation between these two tests with high school girls as subjects.

In arranging sections for physical education on the basis of this test, Johnson suggests dividing the scores either into units based on the normal curve or into equal parts, depending upon the number of sections desired.

Adams Sport-Type Test

From a study of the literature, Adams[39] concluded that there are two types of motor educability tests, stunt-type and sport-type, and that these are not highly

[37]Elmer A. Gross, Donald C. Greisel, and Alan Stull, "Relationships Between Two Motor Educability Tests, a Strength Test, and Wrestling Ability after Eight Weeks' Instruction," *Research Quarterly,* **27,** No. 4 (December 1956), 395.

[38]Bernice Cooper, "The Establishment of General Motor Capacity for High School Girls," Doctoral Dissertation, State University of Iowa, 1945.

[39]Arthur R. Adams, "A Test Construction Study of Sport-Type Motor Educability Test for College Men," Doctoral Dissertation, Louisiana State University, 1954.

related. From a study of 49 "sport-type" learning test items, he selected four, which had a multiple correlation of 0.79 with the total of all tests for college men. These tests were as follows:

Wall Volley Test.   Subject stands three feet from a wall and volleys a volleyball above a line on the wall 10½ feet above the floor. The score on each trial is the number of consecutive volleys above the line, up to 10; the total score is the sum of the scores on seven trials.

Lying Tennis Ball Catch.   Subject lies flat on his back, holding a tennis ball. He throws the ball six feet or higher in the air and catches it in either hand, while remaining in the lying position. The score is the number of successful catches in 10 trials.

Ball Bounce Test.   Subject stands in middle of a six-foot circle and attempts to volley a volleyball on the top end of a bat without leaving the circle. The score on each trial is the number of consecutive volleys up to 10; the total score is the sum of scores on 10 trials.

Basketball Shooting Test.   Subject shoots 20 free throws from the foul line. The score is the number of baskets made.

The following regression equation is a rounded-off version of the one presented by Adams:

Sport Educability Score =
7.2 (wall volley) + 17.3 (tennis ball catch) + 2.7 (ball bounce) + 19.2 (foul shooting).

T-scale norms are presented in Appendix Table B.19.

Muscular power

Muscular power was defined in Chapter 9 as the ability to release muscular force in the shortest time. As a mathematical model, it may be considered the product of force and distance divided by time, or

$$\frac{F \times D}{T}$$

Pure power tests are not utilized in physical education testing, nor are pure power movements encountered in athletics. A pure power movement of the leg muscles, for example, would restrict the take-off for a jump to a stationary position, such as a crouch, and would prohibit use of the arms to assist the jump. Such positions have been used by investigators as power criteria; functionally, however, the movement is unnaturally restricted.

The most common muscular power tests in use are the vertical jump and the standing broad jump. At least one of these tests is found in most motor ability and motor fitness batteries. Actually, distance jumped should be considered a relative power test, as the amount of body weight projected is not included in the score. For example, a distance of 60 inches in a standing broad jump by 100-pound and 150-pound boys is scored the same for both boys; yet, one boy projected 50 percent more weight than did the other.

Vertical Jump

The Sargent Jump, named after its originator, Dr. Dudley A. Sargent,[40] consists of a vertical leap into the air, and is primarily a test of the ability of the body to develop power in relation to the weight of the individual himself. In this jump, the individual swings his arms downward and backward, taking a crouch position with knees bent approximately to a right angle. The subject pauses in this position, to eliminate the possibility of a double jump, and leaps upward as high as possible, swinging the arms forcefully forward and upward.

[40]Dudley A. Sargent, "Physical Test of a Man," *American Physical Education Review*, **26,** No. 4 (April 1921), 188.

Just before the highest point of the jump is reached, the arms should be swung forward and downward, motion being timed to coincide with the height of the jump. The specified arm movements in executing the jump are extremely important, the test developing serious inaccuracies without them.[41] The best of three trials should be recorded.

The distance on the vertical jump may be measured in several ways. Three useful methods are described.

1. A jump board about two feet wide and five feet long, marked with horizontal lines one centimeter (or one inch) apart is fastened to the wall so that the lower edge is just below the standing height of the shortest subject to be tested; the distance between standing height and the top of the head at the height of the jump is recorded. Recording the distance jumped can be facilitated, and a shorter board can be used, by arranging a jump board that can be adjusted for height; the zero line can then be located at the standing height of each subject.

2. An adjustable jump board can be mounted on the wall near the floor; an elastic band with a button attached is placed on the subject's ankle and adjusted to the zero line on the board; the record of the jump is the point reached by the button when the subject jumps (knees must be kept straight).[42]

3. A simple method, known as the "chalk jump," consists in having the subject make two chalk marks (chalked or wet fingers may be substituted for an actual piece of chalk) on a dark, clean wall: one made standing with the arm fully extended and the other at the height of the jump; the distance between the two marks is recorded. The technique for the vertical jump is shown in Figure 12.2.

It is generally agreed by experimenters that best results are obtained with this test after the technique of the jump has been

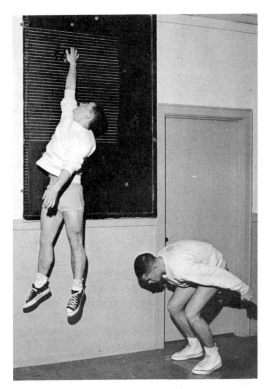

FIGURE 12.2. *Vertical Jump Technique*

taught and the subjects have practiced its execution. Under these conditions, objectivity coefficients in the 0.90s have been reported for both boys and girls by several investigators. Martin and Stull[43] studied the technique of vertical jumping by having college men perform the jump with all combinations (48) of knee angles of 65, 90, and 115 degrees and lateral and posterior foot spacings of 0, 5, 10, and 15 inches. The most effective stance was with a knee angle of 115 degrees, the feet spread from 5 to 10 inches, and the back foot about 5 inches behind the front foot. Interestingly, the knee angle of 115 de-

[41]Deobold Van Dalen, "New Studies in the Sargent Jump," *Research Quarterly,* **11,** No. 2 (May 1940), 112.

[42]Thomas K. Cureton, "Fitness of Feet and Legs," *Supplement to the Research Quarterly,* **12,** No. 2 (May 1941), 368.

[43]Thomas P. Martin and G. Alan Stull, "Effects of Various Knee Angle and Foot Spacing Combinations on Performance of the Vertical Jump," *Research Quarterly,* **40,** No. 2 (May 1969), 324.

grees was found to be the strongest position in the range of motion for knee extension in cable-tension strength testing, as noted in Chapter 7.

Gray, Start, and Glencross[44] analyzed the vertical jump from the standpoint of foot-pounds of work done. This measure was established on the physical sciences definition of power; leg power was evaluated in units of horsepower. Subsequently, these investigators[45] simplified their power evaluation based on the vertical jump, utilizing the following formula:

$$\text{work} = \frac{\text{body weight (lbs)} \times \text{distance jumped (in.)}}{12}$$

The Jump, itself, is performed from a full squat; extraneous movements of the hands are eliminated by securing one hand behind the back, while the preferred arm is raised vertically and held steadily against the side of the head.

Standing Broad Jump

The standing broad jump has also been used as a leg power test. This jump is performed in a manner similar to the vertical jump, except the jump is in a horizontal direction. Techniques for administering the standing broad jump appear on page 175.

Four methods of scoring the standing broad jump were investigated by Flynn[46] in the Medford boys' growth study. The

TABLE 12.4 *Contrasting Standing Broad Jump Means in Inches of Nonparticipants and Outstanding Athletes by Sports*

| Groups | School Levels and Ages | | |
	Elementary: 12 yrs.	Junior High: 15 yrs.	Senior High: 17 yrs.
Nonparticipants	62.4	77.5	85.7
Football	68.5	88.5	91.6
Basketball	68.4	88.1	94.0
Track	70.4	89.4	94.7
Baseball	67.1		87.2

following multiple correlations were obtained with 12-year-old boys:

1. Distance × weight: 0.902 with weight, Strength Index, and skinfold.

2. Weight/distance: 0.908 with abdominal girth, Physical Fitness Index, and skinfold.

3. Leg length/distance: 0.717 with Physical Fitness Index, leg length, 10-foot run, and skinfold.

4. Distance jumped: 0.690 with Physical Fitness Index, 10-foot run, sitting height, skinfold, and cable-tension strength.

In the Medford series, too, standing broad jump distance was found to be a consistent differentiator of the athletic ability of upper elementary, junior, and senior high school boys as demonstrated in interscholastic competition. The broad jump means of nonparticipants and athletes in various sports appear in Table 12.4. The means of the athletes in all sports were considerably higher than nonparticipants at the three school levels.[47]

Clarke[48] reported relationships between the standing broad jump and various strength and anthropometric measures

[44]R. K. Gray, K. B. Start, and D. J. Glencross, "A Test of Leg Power," *Research Quarterly,* **33,** No. 1 (March 1962), 44.

[45]R. K. Gray, K. B. Start, and D. J. Glencross, "A Useful Modification of the Vertical Power Test," Unpublished report, University of Western Australia, Perth.

[46]Kenneth W. Flynn, "Relationship Between Various Standing Broad Jump Measures and Strength, Speed, Body Size, and Physique Measures of Twelve-Year-Old Boys," Master's Research Paper, University of Oregon, 1966.

[47]Clarke, *Medford Boys' Growth Study,* p. 219.

[48]H. Harrison Clarke, "Relationships of Strength and Anthropometric Measures to Physical Performances Involving the Trunk and Legs," *Research Quarterly,* **28,** No. 3 (October 1957), 223.

with college men as subjects. The highest correlations obtained were −0.59 and −0.52 with adipose tissue over the abdomen and ilium respectively. A multiple correlation of 0.66 resulted between the jump and adipose tissue over the abdomen and hip extension strength. With 12-year-old boys, Clarke and Degutis[49] reported a multiple correlation of 0.69 with standing broad jump; the variables were elbow flexion, hip extension, and ankle plantar flexion strengths and weight. With adolescent boys as subjects, Espenschade[50] obtained a correlation of 0.64 between this jump and the 50-yard dash; when correlated for attenuation, this correlation rose to 0.80. Hester[51] reported correlations of 0.76 and 0.69 between the jump and the 60-yard dash and a distance ball throw for junior high school boys; the correlation between the standing broad jump and the Sargent jump was 0.65.

Power Tests of Arms and Shoulders

Power tests of the arm and shoulder muscles have seldom been used in motor ability and motor fitness test batteries and research centered on such tests has been meager. A notable exception was the softball throw for distance contained in earlier versions of the AAHPER Youth Fitness Test, described in Chapter 9. Other power tests for this body region are medicine ball put, shot put, and basketball throw. The puts and throws are frequently from a

standing or sitting position in order to concentrate the effort on the muscles involved and to reduce the influence of other muscles and body momentum when steps or a run are permitted.

PULL-UPS

Pull-ups, or chinning the bar for boys and modified pull-ups or the bent-arm hang for girls are commonly included as arm-shoulder muscular endurance tests in motor fitness and motor ability batteries. The usual method of scoring pull-ups is simply the number of chins the person can do. This procedure provides a relative muscular endurance measure, since only the number of repetitions is counted. The weight of the subject and the distance his or her weight is pulled are not considered in the score; heavy-tall and light-short persons receive the same credit. As a consequence, gross arm-shoulder endurance series, which provide for these factors, have been proposed. An example of such gross measures is the Rogers arm strength score, included in his Strength Index battery as described in Chapter 7.

A question frequently posed regarding administration of the pull-up test concerns the grip to be used: supinated (palms rear) or pronated (palms forward). On the average, one or two more chins are performed with hands in the supinated position; a contributing reason for the difference may be a greater tendency to leave a bend in the elbows each time the body is lowered. However, differences do exist in muscle involvements, as shown through electromyographic studies. Randall[52] found no differences in action potentials of the brachialis and brachioradialis muscles, but the pronator teres and biceps brachii muscles were more active when the

[49] H. Harrison Clarke and Ernest W. Degutis, "Relationships Between Standing Broad Jump and Various Maturational, Anthropometric, and Strength Tests of 12-Year-Old Boys," *Research Quarterly*, **35**, No. 3 (October 1964), 3.

[50] Anna S. Espenschade, "Motor Performance in Adolescence," *Monograph of Society for Research in Child Development*, **5**, 1940.

[51] Robert A. Hester, "The Relationship Between Performance of Junior High School Boys in the Standing Broad Jump and Achievement in Selected Tests of Motor Ability," Master's Thesis, University of Wisconsin, 1955.

[52] Nellie G. Randall, "An Electromyographic Study of Selected Muscles Involved in Two Methods of Chinning," Doctoral Dissertation, State University of Iowa, 1963.

hands were in the supinated position. This investigator concluded that the most favorable position in which to perform pull-ups was with a supinated grasp. In studying the two hand positions for girls, Gala[53] recommended the supinated grip for Roger' modified pull-up test and the pronated grip for bent-arm hang.

In the Medford boys' growth study, the correlations between arm and shoulder endurance tests with endomorphy and body size measures were negative and mostly insignificant; low positive correlations, mostly insignificant, were obtained with maturity and gross strength measures. These results could be expected inasmuch as pull-ups and bar push-ups are relative endurance measures while the tests correlated with them are gross in nature. Junior high school athletes rated by their coaches as outstanding when 15 years of age had significantly higher mean Rogers' arm strength scores than did nonparticipants not only at age 15 years but at all ages traced back to 12 years; the same was true in football, basketball, and track and field.[54]

AGILITY RUNS

Various agility runs have been utilized in motor ability and motor fitness tests batteries. The 60-yard shuttle run (10-yard distance) was included in the Medford boys' growth study as a measure of speed and agility in a running situation. The justification for choosing this agility run was based on research by Gates and Sheffield,[55] who experimented with 18 tests, 15 of which involved change of direction while running and three of which were other motor ability items. A criterion measure was established consisting of the total T score of the subjects on all tests. For boys in the seventh, eighth, and ninth grades, the 60-yard shuttle run correlated 0.81 with this criterion at each grade. The reliability coefficient was 0.93: Lawson[56] obtained similar results with a 40-yard shuttle run for girls aged seven through 12 years; her criterion consisted of Hull-scale totals on 12 obstacle and shuttle runs.

Problems can be encountered in administering shuttle runs in order to obtain consistency and comparability of results. Two such problems are stabilizing of the running surface and provision for a sharp turn by the runner at the end of each traverse. For the Medford study,[57] these problems were solved and the conditions for the shuttle run remained constant over the 12-year period of the study by providing a common running surface of a prescribed width. Two strips of rubberized matting, each 38 feet by 3 feet were laid side by side on the gymnasium floor; thus, the running surface was 38 feet long and 6 feet wide. The strips were secured to the floor and held together with adhesive tape. Four feet from each end and at the junction of the two mats, thus 30 feet apart, an erect wand was located (this wand was held upright by use of a "plumber's helper"). The subjects were required to stay on the mat while performing the shuttle run; and they ran in their bare feet. Zieger[58] studied surface and footwear in performing the Illinois Agility Run. He found that significantly faster times were made when running on

[53]Rosemary Gala, "The Effect of Two Gripping Positions on Performance of College Women on the Modified Pull-up and the Bent-Arm Hang as Indicated by Electromyography," Master's Thesis, University of Washington, 1965.

[54]Clarke, *Medford Boys' Growth Study,* p. 206.

[55]Donald D. Gates and R. P. Sheffield, "Tests of Change of Direction as Measurement of Different Kinds of Motor Ability in Boys of the Seventh, Eighth, and Ninth Grades," *Research Quarterly,* **11,** No. 3 (October 1940), 136.

[56]Patricia A. Lawson, "An Analysis of a Group of Motor Fitness Tests which Purport to Measure Agility as They Apply to Elementary School Girls," Master's Thesis, University of Oregon, 1959.

[57]Clarke, *Medford Boys' Growth Study,* p. 225.

[58]Patricia A. Zieger, "Influence of Warm-up, Running Surface, and Different Types of Obstacles on Performance of the Illinois Agility Run," Master's Thesis, University of Washington, 1964.

asphalt as contrasted with the gymnasium floor, when running in bare feet as contrasted with wearing tennis shoes, and when wearing tennis shoes without treads as contrasted with tennis shoes with treads.

Kistler[59] obtained a multiple correlation of 0.93 between a dodging run and squat thrusts for 12 seconds, shot put, and McCloy's Classification Index. For 14-year-old boys, the highest correlations obtained by Radcliff[60] with the Medford 60-yard shuttle run were −0.57 for standing broad jump and −0.53 for Physical Fitness Index. He also reported a multiple correlation of 0.65 for the shuttle run with standing broad jump. Physical Fitness Index, and total body reaction time as the independent variables. The shuttle run had a good application to the performance of athletes in the Medford series. In football, basketball, and track, the superior athletes had faster times than nonparticipants for most ages and at all school levels, upper elementary, junior high, and senior high.

AGE-HEIGHT-WEIGHT INDICES

Age-height-weight indices have been proposed for the classification of boys and girls for participation in the general physical education program. These indices are not as satisfactory for this purpose as are the general motor ability tests presented in this chapter. This is true for several reasons, chief of which is that chronological age does not relate well with physiological maturation. Boys and girls of the same chronological age, tested within two

months of their birthdays, differ by as much as six and seven years in skeletal age. The standard deviation by single chronological ages is around one year.[61] Body weight, within limits at least, does relate reasonably well to strength and motor performances. However, age-height-weight indices are simple to obtain; they do not require special testing equipment, other than weight scales, and they can be administered in a minimum of time.

McCloy's Classification Indices

McCloy[62] proposed classification indices based on the best combinations of age, height, and weight for boys at elementary school, high school, and college levels. These indices are as follows:

High School Boys

Classification Index I =
$(20 \times \text{age}) + (6 \times \text{height}) + \text{weight}$

College Men

Classification Index II = $(6 \times \text{height}) + \text{weight}$

Elementary School Boys

Classification Index III $(10 \times \text{age}) + \text{weight}$

Classification Index III is particularly significant on the elementary-school level, as height was found to be a negligible factor with this group and is omitted from the formula. Classification Index I is more significant for the high-school level, where height seems of greater importance. Classification Index II is used with college men, as it was found that after the age of 17, age ceased to make a further contribution.

[59]Joy W. Kistler, "The Establishment of Bases for Classification of Junior and Senior High School Boys into Homogeneous Groups," *Research Quarterly,* **8,** No. 4 (December 1937), 11.

[60]Robert A. Radcliff, "Relationships Between the Sixty-yard Shuttle Run and Various Maturity, Physique, Structural, Strength, and Motor Characteristics of Fourteen Year Old Boys," Master's Thesis, University of Illinois, 1965.

[61]Clarke, *Medford Boys' Growth Study,* p. 19.

[62]Charles W. McCloy and Norma D. Young, *Tests and Measurements in Health and Physical Education,* 3rd. ed. (New York: Appleton-Century-Crofts, 1954), p. 58.

Neilson-Cozens Classification Indices

Neilson and Cozens[63] also studied the problem of classifying pupils on the basis of age, height, and weight. Their results differ somewhat from those of McCloy, but interpreted in the same terms for high school boys, their formula is:

Classification Index =
(20 × age) + (5.55 × height) + weight.

The McCloy and Neilson-Cozens indices correlate 0.98, indicating that either one may be used for high school boys with equal satisfaction. In Appendix Table B.20, a chart is presented for easy computation of this index and the classifications by means of it.

SELECTED REFERENCES

CLARKE, H. HARRISON, "Characteristics of Young Athletes," *Physical Fitness Research Di-*

gest, President's Council on Physical Fitness and Sports, **3,** No. 2 (April 1973).

CLARKE, H. HARRISON, *Physical and Motor Tests in the Medford Boys' Growth Study.* Englewood Cliffs, N.J.: Prentice-Hall, Inc., 1971.

ESPENSCHADE, ANNA S., "Motor Performance in Adolescence," *Monograph of Society for Research in Child Development,* **5,** 1940.

GIRE, EUGENIA, and ANNA ESPENSCHADE, "The Relationship Between Measures of Motor Educability and the Learning of Specific Skills," *Research Quarterly,* **13,** No. 1 (March 1942), 43.

HENRY, FRANKLIN M., "Specificity vs. Generality in Learning Motor Skills," *61st Annual Proceedings,* College Physical Education Association, 1958, 127.

McCLOY, C. H., and NORMA D. YOUNG, *Tests and Measurement in Health and Physical Education,* 3rd ed. New York: Appleton-Century-Crofts, 1954, Part III.

ROGERS, FREDERICK RAND, "It Has Been Done," *Journal of Health and Physical Education,* **9,** No. 2 (February 1938), 77.

WILLGOOSE, CARL E., "Use of Strength Tests in Team Equalization," *The Physical Educator,* **6,** No. 1 (March 1949), 4.

[63]N. P. Neilson and Frederick W. Cozens, *Achievement Scales in Physical Education Activities for Boys and Girls in Elementary and Junior High School* (New York: A. S. Barnes & Co., Inc., 1934), p. 161.

PART FOUR

PHYSICAL EDUCATION
SKILLS AND APPRECIATIONS

As has been stressed consistently throughout this text, the major concern of the physical educator should always be the realization of educational objectives. The methods he adopts, the activities he selects, and the tests he uses should be based upon the specific objectives he is determined to meet. In previous chapters, procedures for meeting the physical fitness and the social objectives were presented. Part IV is devoted to measurement for the development of skills and appreciations, and to procedures for conducting effective programs in these areas.

PHYSICAL EDUCATION SKILLS

Physical education has a history that extends back many centuries, beginning with early Greek civilization. While they were not continuous over this entire period, physical education activities nevertheless have a rich heritage in the evolution of present-day civilization. The basis for this form of education is the learning and practice of skills in order to achieve worthwhile objectives. For example, gymnastics, the pentathlon, boxing, pankration, swimming, riding, fighting in armor,

Importance of Skills and Appreciations

military maneuvers, archery, hunting, and athletic games were used by the Athenians during the fourth and fifth centuries B.C. to develop the body, an essential phase of the education of Greek youth.[1] Stunts on the horizontal bar and parallel bars and other forms of gymnastics and athletics were the basis of Jahn's system of physical exercise designed to develop a physically strong nation for Germany's wars.[2] A great variety of physical activities are included in present-day physical education programs in order to develop a physically and socially fit nation. The true basis of all physical education is to learn skills essential for physical fitness, for building character, and for use during leisure time.

Physical activities differ not only in their educational content, but also in the contributions they make to specific objectives. Moreover, the contributions that any one physical activity can make are not confined to a single objective, but apply in some degree to them all. In selecting activities for his program, therefore, the physical educator should understand the various values of these activities and should keep in mind the purposes to be served by their use. For example, all physical activities have some recreational value. When this quality is to be *specifically* developed, however, activities like tennis, swimming, bowling or golf, which are high in recreational content, should be taught.

Physical Fitness

Many types of physical activities develop strength, endurance, and body flexibility, essential components of physical fitness. It is true that these qualities may be developed through activities requiring little skill, such as calisthenics and running. However, these activities are not

[1]Kenneth S. Freeman, *Schools of Hellas*, 3rd ed. (London: Macmillan & Co., Ltd., 1922), p. 299.

[2]Friedrich Ludwig Jahn and Ernst Eiselen, *Die Deutsche Turnkunst* (Berlin: Auf Kosten der Herausgeber, 1816), p. 315.

sufficiently interesting to some people for continuance as a regular habit in their daily lives. Activities requiring skill, on the other hand, when once acquired, may be practiced much more consistently and zealously. Thus, some activities require skill and result in more general use, such as gymnastics, tumbling, wrestling, and various forms of dancing for strength, flexibility, agility, and balance. Soccer, basketball, tennis, and swimming are good for endurance and stamina. The danger in the use of sports activities for the development of physical fitness lies in their competitive nature. Competition provides a temptation to maximal exertion, to go the limit. Such exertion is desirable for many, but may be undesirable for those not in condition and for those men and women well beyond school and college age who have become sedentary.

NEUROMUSCULAR COORDINATION

The neuromuscular coordination of the individual, which includes his ability to learn new skills and finally to achieve competency in physical activities, is essential to all phases of physical education. Activities for developing such coordination, therefore, should be considered. The following factors are involved.

1. Nerve-eye-muscle coordination. Skills requiring the coordination of hand and eye, as in throwing at targets, goals, and so forth, and on foot and eye, as in kicking a ball.

2. Agility. Skills requiring rapid movement of the entire body, in different directions and in response to unexpected circumstances, as dodging in football, pivoting in basketball, and agile stunts in tumbling.

3. Rhythm. Skills requiring smooth, rhythmic, and relaxed motion, as in the club swing in golf, in the rhythmic movement of the dance, and in performing an "effortless" crawl stroke in swimming.

4. Precision of movement. Skills requiring precise performance, in which every detail must be executed with exactness, as in apparatus exercises and in diving.

5. Speed. Skills requiring coordination while moving at considerable speed, as in soccer, basketball, and hockey.

6. Poise. Skills resulting in the well-poised individual, the final culmination of the entire physical being, strong, enduring, well-coordinated, and highly skilled.

Social Acceptability

Studies have shown that competitive athletic skills are among the chief sources of social esteem for boys in the period preceding maturity. The development of skills in sports and games is influential as an entree into acceptance by their peers. Physical prowess is pre-eminent in establishing prestige, and, as such, becomes an important factor in a boy's feeling of confidence in himself. Outstanding athletic skill can maintain the prestige of a boy even though he may have few other assets. To illustrate relevant evidence, two reports from the Medford boys' growth study will be mentioned.

Anderson[3] reported that, when a sociometric technique was used, successful elementary school athletes had a higher degree of peer status and social adjustment than had boys with less success or no competition in inter-school athletics. When boys answered the Mental Health Analysis, the better athletes indicated greater social participation in both elementary and junior high schools and closer personal relationships in elementary school. From the Dreese-Mooney Interest Inventory, the elementary school athletes showed a greater interest in people.

Broeckhoff[4] examined individual profiles of ten 13-year-old boys having unusual scores on physical tests. Some of

[3]Robert B. Anderson, "A Study of Personal Adjustment and Social Status Measures of Nonparticipants and Athletic Groups of Boys Ten to Fifteen Years of Age," Doctoral Dissertation, University of Oregon, 1965.

[4]Jan Broekhoff, "Relationships Between Physical, Socio-Psychological, and Mental Characteristics of Thirteen-Year-Old Boys," Doctoral Dissertation, University of Oregon, 1966.

his observations were: (a) the extreme endomorph and the predominant ectomorph are at a distinct disadvantage in the dynamic physical world of the early adolescent, because of the weakness inherent in their body types; and (b) in the expansive, vital environment of this age group, the boy with high relative strength and motor ability has a social as well as a physical advantage over boys with low scores. Boys with high scores were more popular among peers and teachers than boys with low scores.

Jones[5] attributed this phenomenon not merely to the high premium which adolescents place upon the athletic efficiency of boys, but also to the fact that strength and other aspects of physical ability are closely joined to such favorable traits as activity, aggressiveness, and leadership. The situation for girls has been quite different, since athletic ability has not been a primary source of gaining social status for them. However, a changing attitude toward girls and their participation in sports is sweeping the country. Therefore, such studies if repeated now and in the future would logically produce different results for girls.

Various factors have influenced the full acceptance of sports by women in their societal value system. One factor has been fear of injury, especially to the reproductive organs and the breasts. Evidence does not support this fear; rather, the normal healthy female may participate in any athletic endeavor for which training and experience adequately prepare her. Quite obviously, either boys or girls may be injured in athletic activity, but, basically, a person's organs are quite well protected. When the body receives a severe blow, the force transmitted to the internal organs is much less than on the surface of the body.[6] A second factor has been the belief

that sports participation tends to masculinize the appearance and behavior of girls. This myth has been exploded, as evidenced by the shapeliness and grace of women in gymnastics, swimming and diving, figure skating, skiing, and the like at the very highest levels of Olympic and international competitions. Judi Ford, a physical education major at the University of Illinois with a trampoline routine as her talent act, was Miss America 1969. A third factor has been that women physical educators of an earlier day frowned upon inter-school sports for girls and women and society did not rank women athletes high on the social scale. Both of these situations are changing, accelerated by the so-called "women's liberation movement." A period of transition is in progress.

The present trend is toward more encouragement and greater opportunities for girls to participate in intramural, extramural, and inter-school sports. The National Association for Girls and Women's Sports of the American Alliance for Health, Physical Education, and Recreation[7] has given strong leadership to procedures and programs related to participation in sports at all levels by girls and women. In 1971, the first national conference on girls' sports programs for secondary schools[8] was held; the first Delegate Assembly of the Association for Intercollegiate Athletics for College Women,[9] an autonomous organization established to provide a governing body and leadership for initiating and maintaining standards in women's intercollegiate programs, was held in 1973.

[5]Harold E. Jones, "Physical Ability as a Factor in Social Adjustment in Adolescence," *Journal of Educational Research*, **40** (December 1946), 287.

[6]Clayton L. Thomas, "The Female Sports Participant: Some Physiological Questions," *DGWS Research Reports: Women in Sports* (Washington, D.C.:

American Association for Health, Physical Education, and Recreation, 1971), p. 37.

[7]Until 1974, the name was Division of Girls and Women's Sports of the American Association for Health, Physical Education, and Recreation.

[8]Alice A. Barron, "Report of the First DGWS National Conference on Girls Programs for the Secondary Schools," *Journal of Health, Physical Education, Recreation*, **42**, No. 9 (November–December 1971), 14.

[9]Joan Hult, "First AIAW Delegate Assembly," *Journal of Health, Physical Education, Recreation*, **45**, No. 3 (March 1974), 79.

There is little doubt that the changing roles of women in today's society provide a significant element of social discontinuity that must affect sport. According to Jan Felshin, for a time, girls and women will seek access to existing teams in light of their established legal rights to do so. "By the twenty-first century, women will have liberated sport both as a male domain and from its contemporary models."[10]

Recreational Efficiency

Much of the skill instruction in physical education is "education through the physical," in which participation in physical activities has for its purpose the development of such qualities as strength, stamina, speed, individual and group character traits, and neuro-muscular coordination. In preparing for the wise use of leisure, however, the physical educator teaches skills as ends in themselves—to be used as a part of the individual's avocation. The outcome desired is recreational efficiency, or the acquisition of skills and their use as after-school and after-graduation activities.

The recreation movement came into being at the turn of the century in order to counteract the boredom effects of man's long tedious day at the factory, mill, or shop. Today, however, as expressed by Levy,[11] "recreation is at the crossroads," due to drastically changing needs introduced by a technological and affluent society. In the past century, reduction of the average workweek by about 13 hours has netted the American worker 675 hours of free time annually; added to increased vacation time and more paid holidays, this amounts to a total gain in time free of work of nearly 800 hours annually, or roughly one month a year, according to

J. H. Hodgson, U.S. Secretary of Labor.[12] During the past decade alone, he said further, the average American worker has gained about 50 hours a year in free time—15 hours in additional holiday time and the balance in reduced working hours. Another way of expressing leisure situation is provided by Nanus and Adelman[13] of the Center for Futures Research, University of Southern California: Leisure absorbed 26.5 percent of the average person's day in 1900 and 34 percent in 1950; at this rate of progress, it could account for 44 percent by the year 2000. A panel of 60 experts in the manpower field was formed by the Center in conjunction with the Manpower Administration of the U.S. Department of Labor. This panel foresaw a considerable increase in leisure time available, a much more highly educated populace having this leisure, and a greatly expanded government interest in all aspects of manpower planning.

In "Charter for Leisure" by the Recreation Division, American Association for Health, Physical Education, and Recreation,[14] leisure and recreation are joined to create a basis for compensating for many of the demands placed upon man by today's way of life. More important, it presents the enrichment of life through participation in physical relaxation and sports and through the enjoyment of art, science, and nature. As an entity, of course, recreation is extremely broad, including many types of activities, and a host of leisure-time pursuits. However, sports and games constitute a large segment of America's recreational pursuits. In 1963, The Athletic Institute[15] reported on a sports par-

[10]Jan Felshin, "The Triple Option for Women in Sport," *Quest*, Monograph XXL, Winter Issue (January 1974), 36.

[11]Joseph Levy, "Recreation at the Crossroads," *Journal of Health, Physical Education, Recreation*, **42**, No. 7 (September 1971), 51.

[12]J. D. Hodgson, "Leisure and the American Worker," *Journal of Health, Physical Education, Recreation*, **43**, No. 3 (March 1972), 38.

[13]Burt Nanus and Harvey Adelman, "Forecast for Leisure," *Journal of Health, Physical Education, Recreation*, **44**, No. 1 (January 1973), 61.

[14]"Charter for Leisure," *Journal of Health, Physical Education, Recreation*, **43**, No. 3 (March 1972), 48.

[15]*The Athletic Institute Sportscope*, December 30, 1963.

ticipation survey for the years 1956, 1961, and 1963. Here are just a few figures showing the tremendous growth in such participation: volleyball, from 20 million in 1956 to 60 million in 1963; tennis, from 6.5 million in 1956 to 7.5 million in 1961 to 8 million in 1963; archery, from 4.6 million in 1956 to 5.5 million in 1961 to 7 million in 1963. Other participation figures for 1963 are: boating 37.5 million; bowling, 32 million; cycling, 55 million; table tennis, 20 million; and horseshoes, 9 million.

In a later report by The Athletic Institute,[16] 11,149,000 elementary-through-college-age individuals took part in some form of scheduled or recorded sports activities in 1967. The highest participant numbers were 3,134,700 in swimming, 2,688,100 in baseball, 1,221,200 in football, 1,129,000 in basketball, and 724,100 in track and field.

In a recent issue, *Sportscope*[17] stressed: "Women are no longer content to sit on the sidelines and watch men exhibit their prowess." The passive role to which women were relegated in sports or were content to accept has become one of involvement, at the high school and college levels and beyond. To support this surge in girls' and women's sports participation, *Sportscope* reported that 746,000 girls participated in 24 prep sports during 1972–73, nearly triple the number for the previous year.

In the selection of specific physical skills for recreation, the following factors should be kept in mind:

1. Enjoyment. The activity should give the participant pleasure, so that he will seek opportunities to continue with it from time to time. Frequently, one's enjoyment of an activity is largely dependent upon his acquired skill in it, as he usually prefers to do that which he can do well, and avoids those activities in which he performs poorly.

[16]*The Athletic Institute Sportscope*, December 10, 1968.

[17]*The Athletic Institute Sportscope*, November-December, 1973.

2. Companionship. The activity should be one in which friends like to participate, or one that is universally popular. Included among these activities should be some that can be played with the opposite sex.

3. Number of participants. The activity should preferably be one that requires only a few participants to play. The best recreational sports are those that can be played alone or with from one to three companions, such as golf, tennis, swimming, and so forth. When more players are required, as in softball and volleyball, participation suffers owing to the difficulty of getting a large group together.

4. Vigor. The age, sex, and physical condition of the participant should be considered in selecting recreational activities. High-school boys and college men frequently choose vigorous sports, such as basketball, touch football, and baseball. Older men, however, require milder activities, especially those that may be adaptable in dosage; for example, nine holes of golf today, perhaps eighteen next week. On the other hand, activities requiring little physical exertion or skill frequently are not challenging enough for the majority as a regular participant activity.

5. Skill. The activity should require skill to perform it satisfactorily. Individuals are more interested when they are learning and obtain greater satisfactions when they can note their own improvement and measure their own attainments.

6. Competition. Generally speaking, the activity should be competitive in nature. Many people, however, prefer hikes in the woods, ski trips, nature study, horseback riding, and the like, where competition is absent. Nevertheless, for most, the oppositive element in sports is one of its most intriguing aspects.

7. Facilities. Facilities for the activity should be generally available. Obviously, one cannot swim without water or take ski hikes without snow. The more generally accepted recreational sports are those for which facilities may be found in most communities.

CULTURAL POTENTIALITIES OF PHYSICAL EDUCATION

Culture has been defined as "training or discipline by which man's moral and intellectual nature is elevated." As indicated in

Chapter 1, the concept of culture in society has been traditionally related to classical areas of human thought: literature, philosophy, art, music, and the humanities. In this text a broader definition has been given to the culture concept: the extension of "one's stock of appreciations" to include all aspects of living that will improve one's understanding and enjoyment of people and events in his civilization.

Cozens and Stumpf[18] have produced a scholarly and penetrating tome on sports in American culture. The following passage colorfully presents this cultural orientation: "Sports and physical recreation activities belong with the *arts* of humanity. Such activities have formed a basic part of all cultures, including all racial groups and all historical ages, because they are as fundamental a form of human expression as music, poetry, and painting. Every age has had its artists and its amateurs, its adherents and its enemies. While wars, systems of government, plagues, and famines have come and gone in the long record of mankind, these fundamental things have always been present in greater or lesser degree."[19] In discussing the origins of the Olympic games, Ryan[20] asks this interesting question: "What is the nature of these contests, which draw the attention and participation of men and women from all over the world every four years and which can override serious and fundamental political differences to the extent that East and West Germany can unite to send a single team?" In the ancient Olympiad, the Greek city-states shared control of the games, even when at war with each other, and would declare a "truce of the Gods" so that the contests could be held.

Perhaps the most surprising and dramatic use of a sport was in international relations, when, in 1971, the People's Republic of China invited a United States ping pong team to play exhibition matches with their world championship team. Characterized as "ping-pong diplomacy," it signalled a thaw in the cold war between the two countries. A year later, a table tennis team from Communist China toured the United States for two weeks playing matches with teams in Detroit, Washington, New York City, Memphis, and Los Angeles. The Chinese players, who started their international matches in Canada and went to Mexico from the United States, viewed their mission more as an exhibition of good will than as a show of sports superiority.

Huizinga[21] has shown that play is older than culture, for culture always presupposes human society, and animals have not waited for man to teach them their playing. Further, contests in skill, strength, and perseverence have always occupied an important place in every culture, either in connection with ritual or simply for fun and festivity. Cowell and France[22] include games with language, customs, laws, and music among the many manifestations of our social inheritance, which gives the picture of our culture. Nowhere in early American culture is the pioneer spirit more evident than in the rugged nature of the period's games and sports.

Aesthetic Potentialities

Down through the ages, the human body has been the subject of art masterpieces. Athletic youth has frequently been

---

[18]Frederick W. Cozens and Florence S. Stumpf, *Sports in American Life* (Chicago: University of Chicago Press, 1953).

[19]Ibid., p. 1.

[20]Allen J. Ryan, "The Olympic Games and the Olympic Ideals," *Journal of American Medical Association*, **162**, No. 12 (November 17, 1956), 1105.

[21]J. Huizinga, *Homo Ludens: A Study of the Play-Element in Culture* (London: Routledge & Kegan Paul, Ltd., 1944), p. 1.

[22]Charles C. Cowell and Wellman L. France, *Philosophy and Principles of Physical Education* (Englewood Cliffs, N.J.: Prentice-Hall, Inc. 1963), pp. 78–79.

portrayed, particularly in sculpture. In all the world's history, none have equaled the Greeks in making statues of exquisitely formed athletes. In recent times, R. Tait McKenzie, physician and director of physical education at the University of Pennsylvania before his death, approached nearest to Greek achievements. Beginning with a figure of a sprinter, whose proportions were determined from nearly a hundred sprinters, he made statue after statue of young men in various athletic activities, beautiful in form and expressing the full "joy of effort." McKenzie had a greater scope of subject than did the Greeks centuries ago. Many athletic events today in which great grace and beauty of the human body in action are shown, such as diving, skating, pole vaulting, hurdling, and numerous other games and sports, were unknown to the Greeks. A runner in a relay race, a boxer, a shotputter, a diver, a flight of hurdlers, and an early team of football players massed in an onslaught are some of McKenzie's subjects. Whether looked upon as studies in anatomy or as charming sculptured figures embodying the vigor and beauty of youth, they are satisfying.[23]

Today, Joseph Brown, resident sculptor at Princeton University, and former track athlete, football halfback, and boxer, has turned his artistic talents and athletic experiences toward "art through sports."[24] His athletic masterpieces include the line buck in football, the basketball dribbler, boxers, runners, swimmers, and many others. Brown maintains that art through sport is logical in contemporary society, since vital art grows out of the way people live, how they treat each other, and the insights gained from life's experiences. Play is nature's greatest school.

Miller and Russell[25] have shown the artist's use of sports paintings by Picasso to convey a feeling of movement through distortion through a runner in his *By the Sea* and to give a "visceral shock" in his painting of welterweight Sugar Ray Robinson mashing the jaw of Kid Gavilan in 1948. Similar impressions of force, speed, and energy of movement, as well as the excitement of the event, are to be found in the paintings of artists commissioned by *Sports Illustrated*, including portfolios by Bob Stanley of the Indianapolis 500 car race, by Bernie Fuchs of the Masters and U.S. Open Golf tournaments, by Cliff Condak of the tall men who play basketball, by Bob Peak of the thunder of the conflict in professional football, by Harvey Schmidt of the cadence and power of oarsmen, by Jim Jonson of the mechanical perfection of the track and field athlete through vaulting and hurdling, by Jerome Martin of the din, color, and mood of track, and by André Francois of the bold lines and flashing colors of hockey.

Anne Ingram[26] has indicated four major sources for information and materials on sport and art, which are currently available: the National Art Museum of Sport, the AAHPER film strip *Art and Sport*, slide collections of college and university art departments, and originals in museums throughout the country. The National Art Museum originated in 1959 as a publicly supported, nonprofit educational corporation located in Madison Square Garden, New York City. Its primary goal is to help strengthen the sound art tradition in America by taking advantage of the public's knowledge of and en-

---

[23]Christopher R. Hussey, *R. Tait McKenzie: A Sculptor of Youth* (Philadelphia: J. B. Lippincott Co., 1930). The February 1944 issue of the *Journal of Health and Physical Education* was devoted to McKenzie's life and works.

[24]Joseph Brown, "Art Through Sports," *Journal of Health, Physical Education, and Recreation,"* **34,** No. 2 (February 1963), 27.

[25]Donna Mae Miller and Kathryn R. E. Russell, *Sport: A Contemporary View* (Philadelphia: Lea & Febiger, 1971), p. 91.

[26]Anne Ingram, "Art and Sport," *Journal of Health, Physical Education, Recreation,* **44,** No. 2 (February 1973), 24.

thusiasm for sport. It is the best source of information on sport art in the United States. The museum has a permanent collection of paintings, drawings, and sculpture and has staged numerous exhibitions with works from their own and other collections.

Millions of people today witness innumerable athletic events, yet their eyes and minds are trained to see the action, the competitive aspect of the sport, and their thoughts and emotions are concerned with whether "their" team wins. An appreciation of the beauty of polished, graceful, effortless performance, for its own sake, is lost on many. Physical educators can well consider a renewal of aesthetic appreciation in presenting the various aspects of their programs to boys and girls. Four factors involved in an aesthetically perfect performance are noted below.

1. Bodily proportion. The body should be well proportioned physically, should be carried in pleasing posture, and should be well-developed and vigorous.

2. Rhythm. Body movement in physical action should be graceful, poised, rhythmic; the action should be effortless in appearance and synchronized with the movement of others if involved in the same movement.

3. Precision. The action should be well executed; it must be technically correct in its performance.

4. Color. The surroundings in which the action takes place should be appropriate to the activity and, also, pleasing to the eye; unsightly objects and unhygienic conditions detract from an otherwise aesthetic performance.

Activities rating high in aesthetic contribution are those that require the greatest precision of movement, that show the human body to best advantage, and that necessitate a rhythmic, polished performance. Such activities as the following, therefore, are rated high in aesthetic values: various forms of the dance, gymnastics and tumbling, diving, track and field, fencing, skiing, archery, free exercise, and skating. Yet many, if not all sports, as depicted by McKenzie and Brown, have their moments of great beauty, showing the body in highly coordinated, graceful action.

Contemporary Interest

Sports and games have become an integral part of the great American scene. From the largest metropolitan centers to the smallest rural communities, men and women participate in athletics of all sorts. From the professional baseball, football, and boxing events to the purely amateur football and basketball games of the small hamlets of the nation, men and women witness these contests. The scene is a colorful one with intense local loyalties, bands, parades, and "million-dollar gates." Great businesses have been developed to provide the facilities, equipment, and supplies needed; radio and television devote regular programs to sports news and conduct play-by-play broadcasts and telecasts of many of the great athletic contests over the country and around the world; and the sports section in newspapers is a regular feature and special sports reporters are engaged to insure adequate and up-to-the-minute coverage.

Although physical educators are primarily concerned with activity and with encouraging people to participate, they also should develop good spectators. To appreciate an excellent performance, to understand the rules, to be tolerant toward the difficulties of the official's position in these contests, to converse intelligently on athletic subjects, therefore, becomes a function of the physical education program and constitutes a phase of the cultural heritage of our present-day civilization.

Activities high in "contemporary interest" are those given the greatest coverage in the newspapers, those broadcast on radio and televised with greatest frequency, and those which stimulate interesting conversations. Baseball, football, basketball, boxing, golf, ice hockey, and track and field have high ratings.

History and Literature

As indicated above, athletes were portrayed in early Greek sculpture. Athletic contests were also described in the Greek literature of that time. For example, in Homer's *Iliad,* several athletic events were contested at the funeral of Patroclus, over which Achilles presided, including chariot races, boxing, wrestling, foot races, spear fights, weight-throwing, archery, and spear-throwing for distance. Even in Homer's story, one contestant in the chariot race fouled another, causing considerable discussion about his disqualification. Some time later, in Homer's *Odyssey,* an interesting contest took place. Odysseus, after being provoked by Leodamus: ". . .sprang and seized a discus larger than the rest and thick, heavier by not a little than those which the Phaeacians were using for themselves. This with a twist he sent from his stout hand. The stone hummed as it went; down to the ground crouched the Phaeacian oarsmen, notable men at sea, at the stone's cast. Past all the marks it flew, swift speeding from his hand."

Both ancient and medieval literary masterpieces have included descriptions of athletic events; for example, archery contests in *Robin Hood,* jousting in *Ivanhoe,* and fencing in *The Three Musketeers.* Modern literature is no exception. Many books have been written and many moving pictures have been filmed either with athletics as their background or with athletic contests occupying important places in the plot.

Dancing is also a part of the physical education program and occupies an important place in the cultural contributions of this field. Dancing has its roots in the very origins of civilization, portraying the customs and emotions of primitive man and civilized man alike. It has been recognized as an art form through the ages. Folk dances, taught by physical educators, also include a presentation of the origins and purposes of the dance in its native land, with a discussion of the customs of the people and a display of the costumes worn.

Under "History and Literature," activities with high ratings have their origin in antiquity, are mentioned prominently in ancient, medieval, and modern literature, and are among the early activities included in the physical education programs of the United States and other countries. Thus, the following are particularly important: archery, track and field, dance, boxing, wrestling, fencing, and stunts and tumbling.

MEASUREMENT

As in all measurement, tests of skill are made for the purpose of determining status and measuring improvement; certain of these skill tests may be related to the recreational competency of boys and girls. A large number of skill tests are available; many of them are presented in the next chapter. Tests designed to measure knowledge of rules, techniques, and strategy of various physical education activities have been constructed; these appear in Chapter 15. Unfortunately, however, tests of cultural appreciation in physical education are comparatively undeveloped.

SELECTED REFERENCES

AMERICAN ASSOCIATION FOR HEALTH, PHYSICAL EDUCATION, AND RECREATION, "Leisure Today," *Journal of Health, Physical Education, Recreation,* **43,** No. 3 (March 1972), 33–56; **44,** No. 1 (January 1973), 35–64; and **44,** No. 9 (November-December 1973), 33–59.

COZENS, FREDERICK W., and FLORENCE S. STUMPF, *Sports in American Life.* Chicago: University of Chicago Press, 1953.

HARRIS, DOROTHY V., ed., *DGWS Research Reports: Women in Sports.* Washington, D.C.: American Association for Health, Physical Education, and Recreation, 1971.

HUIZINGA, J., *Homo Ludens: A Study of the Play Element in Culture.* London: Routledge & Kegan Paul, Ltd., 1944. (Tr. from German in 1949 by R. F. C. Hull.)

JONES, HAROLD E., "Physical Ability as a Factor in Social Adjustment in Adolescence," *Journal of Educational Research,* **40** (December 1946), 287.

MCKENZIE, R. TAIT, *Journal of Health and Physical Education,* **15,** No. 2 (February 1944).

CHAPTER 14

In discussing the importance of skills in the preceding chapter, it was pointed out that the learning of desirable skills is the very foundation of physical education. It is through the development of skills and subsequent practice in them that physical educators realize their objectives. Accomplished performance in skills provides incentive for their continuance. Without sufficient skill for satisfactory participation in physical activities, the physical benefits from vigorous strength and endurance activities, the social values from group activities and team sports, the personal-social competence from skill in any socially accepted activity, the recreational competence from activities of value for leisure time, and the appreciation of skilled performance wherever observed, are not realized. In fact, skill in physical activities is essential for the well-integrated personality. To evaluate status and progress in the acquisition of skills, therefore, is an important phase of measurement in physical education.

Actually, skill testing accomplishes three major purposes in physical education, as follows:

Skill Tests

1. The achievement and progress made by pupils in the various activities included in the program may be determined, thus evaluating the progress of each pupil and increasing his interest in the program.

2. Pupils may be classified according to levels of ability in each activity. Groups in specific sports may also be equated for class and intramural competition.

3. Progress toward educational objectives may be measured. In the area of skill tests, this is especially true of the recreational objective, where the learning of specific activities becomes an end in itself. And, too, in physical education programs calling for "minimum standards" in activities high in recreational content, achievement levels may be established in terms of skill-test scores.

AAHPER SKILL TEST MANUALS

In addition to the skill tests constructed by independent investigators, many of which are presented in this chapter, test manuals in several sports were developed by the Sports Skills Project Committee of the Research Council of the American Alliance for Health, Physical Education, and Recreation under the chairmanship of Frank D. Sills, Pennsylvania State College, East Stroudsburg, Pennsylvania. The manuals presently available are:[1]

Archery for Boys and Girls, 1967
Basketball for Boys, 1966
Basketball for Girls, 1966
Football, 1965
Softball for Boys, 1966
Softball for Girls, 1966
Volleyball for Boys and Girls, 1969

David K. Brace was the Test Consultant and author for all manuals but the one on volleyball; Clayton T. Shay performed

[1]The manuals may be obtained from the American Alliance for Health, Physical Education, and Recreation, 1201 Sixteenth Street, N.W., Washington, D.C. 20036.

these functions for the latter manual. The manuals contain illustrated instructions for administering and percentile norms for scoring each test item; in addition suggested score and record cards are provided.

The initial test items for the various sports were selected by the Project Committee; the selected items were given a preliminary trial to approximately 100 college and university men and women. These data were analyzed, especially for the reliability of test items and the improvement of test directions, by the Project Chairman; the final tests were selected based on these analyses. The final test items were then administered by city directors of physical education throughout the United States to appropriate subjects in their schools. Percentile norms for all test items were constructed based on 600 to 900 scores for each sex at each age 10 through 18 years.

ARCHERY

Hyde Archery Test

Hyde[2] established norms for archery achievement of college women in shooting the Columbia Round, a standard event in archery competition. The Columbia Round consists of shooting 24 arrows at a 48-inch target at three distances, 30, 40, and 50 yards. The shooting is conducted in the following manner.

1. Standard 48-inch target faces are used, so placed that the center of the gold is four feet from the ground.

2. Arrows are shot in ends of six arrows each, one practice end only being allowed at each distance.

3. The entire round need not be completed on the same day; however, at least one distance should be completed at each session.

4. The target values are: Gold, 9; Red, 7; Blue, 5; Black, 3; White, 1; outside of white or missing target, 0.

5. An arrow cutting two colors counts as having hit the inner one; an arrow rebounding from, or passing through the scoring face of the target shall count as one hit and 5 in value.

The archery achievement scale,[3] based on the six-sigma scale, appears in Appendix Table B.21. This scale consists of three parts, as follows:

1. Scale for first Columbia Round shot by a student. Before administering this round, the beginning student should be permitted a minimum of practice, 120 arrows at each distance being suggested as sufficient.

2. Scale for total score made in the Columbia Round after an unlimited amount of practice in the event. This scale would normally be used toward the end of the archery season to determine the student's achievement in the activity.

3. Three separate scales for each of the distances included in the round, to be used during any practice period when 24 arrows are shot at one of the three distances. As this part of the scale was constructed from the final or highest Columbia Round scores, the achievement level for beginners will naturally fall relatively low on the scale.

Bohn's Archery Test

Bohn[4] proposed an archery test for college men, which consists of shooting 30 arrows from a 30-foot distance. Based upon data obtained during the last week of an eight-week instruction period, he obtained a reliability coefficient of 0.79 for the test. For validity, the test correlated 0.93 when corrected for attenuation against a criterion of scores made in a collegiate archery tournament.

AAHPER Archery Test Manual

In the AAHPER skills test manual, the distances for the archery shoot are 10 and

[2]Edith I. Hyde, "National Research Study in Archery," *Research Quarterly,* **7,** No. 4 (December 1936), 64, and "The Measurement of Achievement in Archery," *Journal of Educational Research,* **17,** No. 9 (May 1934), 673.

[3]Edith I. Hyde, "An Achievement Scale in Archery," *Research Quarterly,* **8,** No. 2 (May 1937), 109.

[4]Robert W. Bohn, "An Achievement Test in Archery," Master's Thesis, University of Wisconsin, 1962.

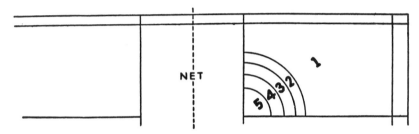

FIGURE 14.1. *Target for French's Badminton Serve Test*

20 yards for both boys and girls and an additional distance of 30 yards for boys. The same distances were originally proposed for both sexes. However, when scores obtained from the preliminary trials were analyzed, shooting at 30 yards was found to be too difficult for many girls, so that distance was dropped for them. Sixty-five percent of girls at ages 17 and 18 were unable to score at that distance. The target is the standard 48-inch size with the center of the gold four feet from the ground. Each subject shoots two ends of six arrows each at each distance. Four practice shots are allowed at each distance. Percentile tables are provided for each distance and for all distances combined at the following ages: 12–13, 14, 15, 16, and 17–18 years. These skill tests are regarded as "practice tests," as they are intended for use in improving ability in the fundamental skills of archery. Girls and boys are urged to practice the skill tests and chart their own progress from the percentile scales.

BADMINTON

French-Stalter Badminton Test

French[5] constructed a satisfactory badminton test for women, and restudied it with Stalter.[6] It contains two elements, a

[5]M. Gladys Scott, "Achievement Examinations in Badminton," *Research Quarterly,* **12,** No. 2 (May 1941), 242.

[6]Esther French and Evelyn Stalter, "Study of Skill Tests in Badminton for College Women," *Research Quarterly,* **20,** No. 3 (October 1949), 257.

serve test and a clear test. Reliability coefficients ranging from 0.77 to 0.98 were obtained. For validity, a correlation of 0.85 was obtained in a preliminary study between the test and a combination of subjective estimates and standings in tournament play.

The Serve Test. The subject serves 20 birds at the target diagrammed in Figure 14.1 and described as follows: (a) a clothesline rope is stretched 20 inches directly above the net and parallel to it; (b) a series of four arcs is drawn within the right service court at distances of 22 inches, 30 inches, 38 inches, and 46 inches from the intersection point of the short service line and the center line (the use of different-colored lines helps in scoring). *Scoring:* Zero is recorded for each trial that fails to go between the rope and the net or that fails to land in the service court for the doubles game. Score each of the other birds as shown in the figure. Any bird landing on a line dividing two scoring areas shall receive the higher score. The score of the entire test is the total of 20 trials. Illegal serves shall be repeated.

The Clear Test. The subject returns a serve, attempting to score on the target shown in Figure 14.2 and described as follows: (a) a clothesline rope is stretched across the court 14 feet from the net and parallel to it, 8 feet from the floor; (b) the following floor markings are made: 2 lines across the court and 4 feet nearer the net than the rear service line in the doubles game, and a line across the court 2 feet farther from the net than the rear service

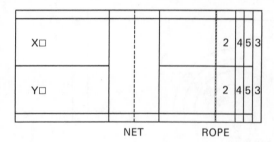

NET   ROPE

FIGURE 14.2. *Target for French's Badminton Clear Test*

line in the singles game. The subject stands between the two square marks, *X* and *Y,* which are 2 inches square and located 11 feet from the net and 3 feet from the center line. The service shall be made from the intersection of the short line and the center line on the target side of the net; the bird must cross the net with enough force to carry it to the line between the two squares before it touches the floor. As soon as the bird is hit, the subject may move about as she wishes. *Scoring:* A zero is recorded for each trial that fails to go over the rope or that fails to land on the target. Score each of the other birds as shown in the diagram. Any bird landing on a line dividing two scoring areas shall receive the higher score. The score on the entire test is the total of 20 trials. If the stroke is "carried" or "slung," it is considered a foul, and the trial is repeated.

The following grading plan for the badminton skill test was proposed:

Beginners		Advanced	
A	115–145	A	170–180
B	85–114	B	110–169
C	40–84	C	55–109
D	15–39	D	25–54
F	0–14	F	0–24

A T-score scale is also available and appears in Scott's report. This scale is useful in checking improvement and in motivating performance.

Lockhart-McPherson Badminton Test

Lockhart and McPherson[7] proposed a badminton test for college women, which consists of volleying a shuttlecock against a wall. While intended for college women, Mathews[8] has reported that it is equally satisfactory for college men. In the validation of the test, the originators obtained the following correlations: 0.71 between the test results and the evaluation of badminton playing ability by three experienced judges, and 0.60 between the test results and percentage of total games won in a round-robin badminton tournament. The test-retest reliability correlation for the volleying test was 0.90.

The following wall and court markings, as shown in Figure 14.3, are needed for this test. *Wall markings:* An unobstructed wall space at least 10 feet high and 10 feet wide is needed; across this space a one-inch net line is marked 5 feet above and parallel to the floor. *Floor markings:* Two floor lines parallel to the wall are necessary; a starting line is drawn 6½ feet from the wall and a restraining line is drawn 3 feet from the wall. Other items of equipment needed are a badminton racket, shuttlecock, stop watch, and score sheets.

To start the test, the subject stands behind the starting line with a badminton racquet in one hand and a shuttlecock in the other; on the signal to start, she serves the shuttlecock against the wall above the net line. The shuttlecock is volleyed against the wall as many times as possible in 30 seconds; three trials are given interspersed with short rests of about a half minute. The subject's score is the total number of legal hits made for the three

[7]Aileene Lockhart and Frances A. McPherson, "The Development of a Test of Badminton Playing Ability," *Research Quarterly,* **20,** No. 4 (December 1949), 402.

[8]Donald K. Mathews, *Measurement in Physical Education* 4th ed. (Philadelphia: W. B. Saunders Company, 1973), p. 202.

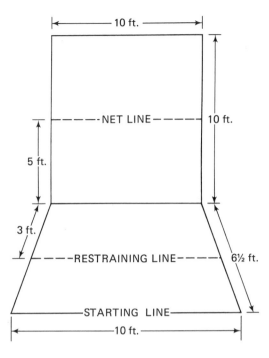

FIGURE 14.3. *Lockhart-McPherson Badminton Target*

trials. A legal hit is one made on or above the net line without crossing the restraining line in making the play. If the shuttlecock is missed, the player must retrieve it and put it back in play with a serve from behind the starting line.

The score is the total number of legal hits made on or above the net line in the time allowed. T-scales for college women appear in the reference. However, any physical educator using the test may easily construct scales of his or her own in accordance with instructions in Appendix A.

Miller Wall Volley Test

From a count of the strokes utilized in a United States Amateur Badminton championship, Miller[9] found that both the

men's and women's finalists employed clears more than any other stroke in all of their games. After analyzing movies of the various types of clears, she devised a badminton test based on this stroke.

On a wall at least 15 feet high and 10 feet wide, a one-inch line is drawn at a height of 7 feet 6 inches from and parallel to the floor. A line is drawn on the floor 10 feet from the wall and parallel to it. After one minute of practice, the subject puts a sponge-end shuttlecock into play with a legal serve from behind the 10-foot floor line. The bird is volleyed against the wall with clear strokes as many times as possible in 30 seconds. Three 30-second trials are given with at least 30 seconds of rest between them. The score consists of the sum of the three trials. Rebounds count only when the bird is hit legally from behind the 10-foot floor line and hits the wall above the 7½-foot line. The play may be stopped at any time and restarted with a legal service.

With 100 college women as subjects, a reliability coefficient of 0.94 was obtained with the test-retests given one week apart. A validity coefficient of 0.83 was reported. The criterion was the standing of the subjects after round-robin badminton play.

BASEBALL

Kelson Baseball Classification Plan

Kelson[10] proposed a baseball classification plan for boys. His subjects were 64 boys, ages 8 to 12 years, who participated in the 1951 Little League Baseball Program at Las Vegas, New Mexico. His criterion of baseball ability consisted of a composite of the following baseball qualities: seasonal batting averages and the evaluation by 12 judges of distance accu-

[9]Frances A. Miller, "A Badminton Wall Volley Test," *Research Quarterly,* **22,** No. 2 (May 1951), 208.

[10]Robert E. Kelson, "Baseball Classification Plan for Boys," *Research Quarterly,* **24,** No. 3 (October 1953), 304.

racy in throwing, catching of fly balls, and fielding ground balls. A correlation of 0.85 was obtained between this composite criterion and the distance the boys could throw a baseball. Multiple correlations involving other tests did not appreciably increase the amount of this correlation.

Directions for administering the baseball distance throw are as follows. Lines, five feet apart, are marked off from 50 feet to 200 feet beyond a starting line. Scorers are stationed on the lines 25 feet apart. The subjects are permitted a run before throwing, but are not allowed to cross the starting line. Using Little League baseballs, the score is the best throw in feet of three trials. The following scoring plan is presented by Kelson:

Classification	Distance of Throw
Superior ability	177 feet and over
Above average ability	145–176 feet
Average ability	113–144 feet
Below average ability	80–112 feet
Inferior ability	79 feet and under

BASKETBALL TESTS FOR BOYS

Johnson Basketball Test

Johnson[11] experimented with 19 basketball test items, checking each for validity and reliability. Two batteries of tests were finally proposed, to measure the following: (a) *basketball ability,* composed of three test items: field-goal speed test, basketball throw for accuracy, and dribble; (b) *potential basketball ability,* composed of four test items, none of which requires ball handling: footwork, jump and reach, dodging run, and Iowa Revision of the Brace Test. The battery reliability and validity for the ability test were 0.89 and 0.88, respectively; for the potential ability test,

[11]L. William Johnson, "Objective Test in Basketball for High School Boys," Master's Thesis, State University of Iowa, 1934.

0.93 and 0.84, respectively. Individual items on the ability test, however, had reliability coefficients ranging from 0.73 to 0.80. In securing validity, a biserial correlation of 0.88 was obtained between test scores and "good" and "poor" groups of basketball players; the good group was composed of boys who made a high school basketball squad and the poor group was composed of those who did not make the squad.

A brief description of the items on the Johnson Basketball Ability Test follows.

1. Field-goal speed test. Starting close under the basket in any position he desires, the subject throws as many baskets as he can in 30 seconds. One point is given for each basket made.

2. Basketball throw for accuracy. The target, as shown in Figure 14.4, is a series of rectangles of various sizes, arranged one inside of the other, the dimensions as follows: 60 inches by 40 inches, 40 inches by 25 inches, and 20 inches by 10 inches. The target is either marked or hung on the wall with the length of the rec-

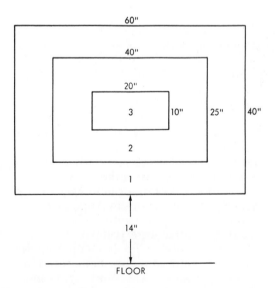

FIGURE 14.4. *Johnson Basketball Accuracy Target*

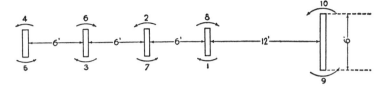

FIGURE 14.5. *Diagram of Zones for Johnson's Dribble Test*

tangle in a horizontal position, the bottom 14 inches from the floor. The subject has ten trials, from a distance of 40 feet, using either the baseball or the hook pass. *Scoring:* 3 points, inner rectangle and line; 2 points, middle rectangle and line; and 1 point, outer rectangle and line.

3. Dribble. Four hurdles are placed in a line 6 feet apart, with a distance of 12 feet from the starting line to the first hurdle. The subject starts from one end of the starting line (which is six feet long), dribbles around through the hurdles and back to the other end of the starting line. *Scoring:* the number of zones passed in 30 seconds, as shown in Figure 14.5.

The three tests are scored as a battery by adding the three obtained scores. The total score range was 16 to 68, with the median at 42.

Knox Basketball Test

Knox[12] developed a basketball battery composed of speed dribble, wall bounce, dribble-shoot, and "penny-cup" tests. Reliability coefficients for various test items ranged from 0.58 to 0.90; for the total battery the coefficient was 0.88. The criterion for validating the test was success in making a ten-man high-school varsity basketball squad competing in an Oregon district tournament. Three divisions of basketball ability, nonplayers, substitutes, and first-team members, were compared at eight "B" league high schools composing the district organization. The tests were given to all boys in these schools during the sec-

ond week after regular basketball practice had started.

The results of the study are as follows.

1. There was 89 percent agreement between the results of the basketball test and squad membership for tournament play, and 81 percent agreement with membership on the first team.

2. The six members of the "all-star" team achieved total scores on the test that were not reached by 95 percent of the 254 boys included in the study.

3. Of the 24 members of the Eugene high school basketball squad, the total scores obtained on the test agreed with the eventual selection of players taken to the Oregon State Tournament in five out of seven cases as to squad membership and five out of five cases as to membership on the first team. Loose[13] related the Knox test to the members of "A" and "B" basketball teams of six high schools in northern California. Significance was obtained between the two performances, but not to the same degree as reported by Knox.

Scoring of the test is accomplished by adding together directly the scores made on the four tests. The score in each instance is the number of seconds required to complete the test. The probable range of initial scores before extensive coaching and practice is from 34 to 58; low scores are the better scores. Directions for administering the test items follow.

1. Speed dribble test. Four chairs are placed in a straight line so that the first one is 20 feet from

[12]Robert D. Knox, "Basketball Ability Tests," *Scholastic Coach,* **17,** No. 3 (March 1947), 45.

[13]W. A. Robert Loose, "A Study to Determine the Validity of the Knox Basketball Test," Master's Thesis, Washington State University, 1961.

the starting line and the others 15 feet apart. The subject dribbles around the chairs as in the Johnson dribble test.

2. *Wall bounce test.* The subject stands with his toes behind a line five feet from a wall. The object of the test is to ascertain how long it will take him to chest-pass (no batting) the ball against the wall and catch it 15 times.

3. *Dribble-shoot test.* As diagramed in Figure 14.6, three chairs are arranged in a straight line diagonally from the basket to the right side-line of the court. The starting line is 65 feet from the basket; the first chair is 20 feet from starting line and the others are 15 feet apart. The subject dribbles around the chairs;

shoots until he makes a basket; and dribbles back around the chairs to the starting line.

4. *Penny cup test.* A course is set up, as follows (Figure 14.7): 8 feet from and parallel to a starting line (A), a signal line is drawn (B); 12 feet farther is a finish line 10 feet long; three tin cups, painted red, white, and blue, are placed on this line, one in the center and one at each end. The subject stands behind the starting line with his back to the cups and with a penny in his hand; at the signal "Go," he pivots and races toward the cups; as he crosses the "signal line," the tester calls out one of the cup colors; the subject must drop his penny into the cup so designated. The test is repeated four times, the total elapsed time representing the score.

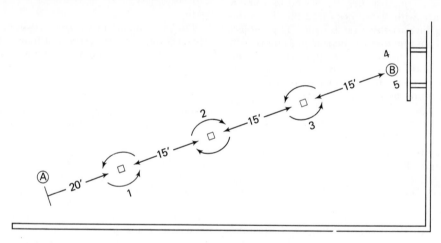

FIGURE 14.6. *Knox Dribble-Shoot Basketball Test*

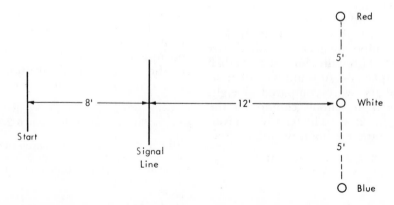

FIGURE 14.7. *Knox Penny-Cup Basketball Test*

Glines and Petersen[14] used the Knox test to equate students for basketball teams within university men's physical education service classes. The competition between equated teams was very close. They also obtained a correlation of 0.89 between scores on the basketball test and the total points the participants scored in competition throughout the course. Glines[15] also administered the Knox test early in the season to all boys in the high school at Hamilton City, California. Seventeen of the twenty highest boys on the test made either the varsity or junior varsity basketball teams; the five boys with the highest scores on the tests eventually formed the starting lineup on the varsity team.

Boyd, McCachren, and Waglow[16] administered the Knox test to 42 candidates for the University of Florida junior varsity basketball squad. A bi-serial correlation of 0.96 was obtained between scores on the test and those who made and those who were eventually cut from the squad. The correlations, however, between test scores and the coach's ratings of each squad member's basketball ability were low.

Stroup Basketball Test

Stroup[17] used the scores made by competing teams as a criterion for validating his basketball skill test. The subjects were 121 students enrolled in college physical education service courses. Each time their class met, they were randomly placed on basketball teams; 82 such teams were formed throughout the study. These teams played a total of 41 ten-minute basketball games. At the end of this competition, they were given tests of goal shooting, wall passing, and dribbling. Approximately 84 percent of the games were won by the team with the high skill score average.

Descriptions of the techniques used in administering the three items of the Stroup test are as follows:

1. Goal shooting. Starting at any position on the floor, the subject shoots as many baskets as possible in one minute, retrieving the ball each time himself.

2. Wall passing. The subject stands behind a line six feet from a wall and passes the ball against the wall as many times as possible in one minute. A pass is not counted if the ball is batted instead of caught and passed and if the subject moves over the restraining line when making a pass.

3. Dribbling. The subject dribbles alternately to the left and right of bottles placed in a line 15 feet apart for a 90-foot distance, circles the end bottle each time, and continues for one minute. A miss is counted if a bottle is knocked over or if the bottle is not passed on the proper side. The score is the number of bottles properly passed in the time limit.

Scale scores with letter grade equivalents for performances on each item were proposed, based on population divisions of the normal curve. Each subject's raw scores on the three items are converted to scale scores, which are then averaged to obtain his basketball *skill* score. A table used for this conversion is shown in Appendix Table B.22. The letter equivalents of the average of the scale scores appear below, along with the population percentage falling in each letter category.

[14]Don Glines and Kay Petersen, University of Oregon, informal report, 1956.

[15]Correspondence from Don Glines.

[16]Clifford A. Boyd, James R. McCachren, and I. F. Waglow, "Predictive Ability of a Selected Basketball Test," *Research Quarterly,* **26,** No. 3 (October 1955), 364.

[17]Francis Stroup, "Game Results as a Criterion for Validating Basketball Skill Test," *Research Quarterly,* **26,** No. 3 (October 1955), 353.

Skill Score	Letter Grade	Population Percentage
91–100	A	7
81–90	B	24
71–80	C	38
61–70	D	24
60–below	F	7

Harrison Basketball Test

Harrison[18] developed a four-item basketball test for boys in grades seven through ten. The four items are field goal shooting, speed pass, dribble, and rebounding. The subjects were 100 boys in each of the grades. Test-retest correlations for the separate tests ranged from 0.72 to 0.96; for the total battery, the coefficients clustered between 0.91 and 0.96. The validity of the test was established as correlations between scores on the test and three criterion measures, as follows: 0.82 with the Johnson Basketball Test; 0.86 with peer ratings of basketball playing ability; and 0.77 with expert jury ratings. A correlation of 0.89 was reported between the test and the average of the three basketball criterion measures.

Each of the test items is performed for 30 seconds; two trials are given with the score recorded as the best of the two. Descriptions of the four tests follow.

Goal Shooting.   Shoot the ball at a basketball goal in any fashion from any distance starting close under the goal. The score is the number of goals made in 30 seconds.

Speed Pass.   Establish a restraining line on the floor parallel to and eight feet from a wall. Pass the ball, any pass allowed, against the wall as many times as possible in 30 seconds. Passes to count must be thrown and received from behind the restraining line.

Dribble.   Establish a dribble course as shown in Figure 14.8. The obstacles shown in the diagram are chairs, placed ten feet apart, the first one being on a level with the starting line. The score is the number of midpoints passed in 30 seconds of dribbling; the numerals shown alongside of the obstacles help in making this count. Thus, each round trip counts 10 points.

[18]Edward R. Harrison, "A Test to Measure Basketball Ability for Boys," Master's Thesis, University of Florida, 1969.

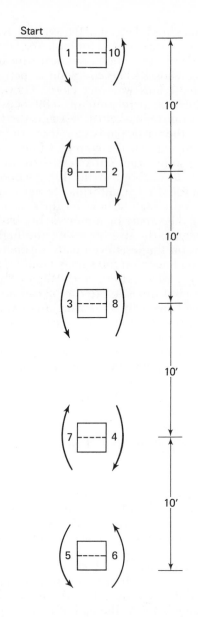

FIGURE 14.8. *Dribble Course for Harrison Basketball Test*

Rebounding.   The subject stands near a basketball backboard with a basketball in his hands. The test consists of tossing the ball against the backboard and returning it as rapidly as possible in 30 seconds; catching and returning the ball to the backboard while the feet are off the floor are encouraged. The score is the number of times the ball hits the backboard in 30 seconds.

T-scale norms were constructed for each of the four test items for each of the four school grades, seven through ten, as presented in Appendix Table B.23. The subjects tested for the norms had received a unit of basketball instruction prior to the administration of the battery.

AAHPER Basketball Test Manual for Boys

Instructions for the administration of and percentile norms for nine basketball skills are presented in the AAHPER basketball test manual for boys. These skill tests are: front shot, side shot, foul shot, underbasket shot, speed pass, jump and reach, overarm pass for accuracy, push pass for accuracy, and dribble.

BASKETBALL TESTS FOR GIRLS

In the women's field, Young and Moser[19] have constructed a satisfactory test of basketball ability. Their battery is composed of wall-bouncing speed test, accuracy throw at a moving target, free jump, Edgren ball handling test, and bounce and shoot. The test has a validity coefficient of 0.86, with ratings by expert judges of each player's ability in a game situation as the criterion measure. Schwartz[20] has worked out a battery of basketball tests for high school girls, validating them through critical analysis by experts, and has constructed scoring tables for each element of

the test. Validity and reliability coefficients are not given in the report. Colvin, Glassow, and Schwartz[21] have also constructed a test which includes five items with satisfactory reliability coefficients. A validity coefficient of 0.66 is given for three of the tests, the best combination that the authors found.

Leilich Basketball Test

In a factor analysis study of the primary components of selected basketball tests for college women, Leilich[22] found four factors to be basic for these tests: basketball motor ability, speed, ball handling involving passing accuracy and speed, and ball handling involving accuracy in goal shooting. On the basis of this analysis, the following three tests were proposed: bounce and shoot, half-minute shooting, and push-pass. Achievement scales on these tests have been constructed by the Professional Studies and Research Committee of the Midwest Association of College Teachers of Physical Education for Women,[23] as presented in Appendix Table B.24.

Directions for administering the three women's basketball tests are as follows:

1. Bounce and shoot. Two dotted lines are drawn on the floor in a "V," with the apex at the middle of the endline under the basket and extending at 45-degree angles for 18 feet on both sides of the court. A 24-inch solid line is centered at the end of each dotted line and at right angles to them. One foot behind and 30 inches to the outside of the 18-foot lines, 18-inch lines are drawn; at each of these, forward legs touching the line, a chair is located and a basketball is

[19]Genevieve Young and Helen Moser, "A Short Battery of Tests to Measure Playing Ability in Women's Basketball," *Research Quarterly*, **5**, No. 2 (May 1934), 3.

[20]Helen Schwartz, "Knowledge and Achievement Tests in Girls' Basketball on the Senior High School Level," *Research Quarterly*, **8**, No. 1 (March 1937), 143.

[21]Ruth B. Glassow and Marion R. Broer, *Measuring Achievement in Physical Education* (Philadelphia: W. B. Saunders Co., 1938), p. 103.

[22]Avis Leilich, "The Primary Components of Selected Basketball Tests for College Women," Doctoral Dissertation, Indiana University, 1952.

[23]Wilma K. Miller, Chairman, "Achievement Levels in Basketball Skills for Women Physical Education Majors," *Research Quarterly*, **25**, No. 4 (December 1954), 450.

placed on it. These markings are diagramed in Figure 14.9.

In taking the test, the subject starts behind the 24-inch line at the right of the basket. At the signal, she picks up the ball from the chair, bounces it once, shoots for the basket, recovers the rebound, and passes the ball to a catcher behind the chair from which she got the ball (the catcher replaces the ball on the chair). She then runs to the chair on the left side and repeats as before. This performance is continued, alternating five times on each side. Each bounce must start from behind a 24-inch line. Fouls consist of running with the ball, double bouncing, and failure to start each time at the 24-inch line. The test terminates when the subject has retrieved the ball after the tenth shot at the basket. In scoring, the subject receives two scores, as follows:

a. Time score: Time is taken to the nearest tenth of a second from the starting signal until the girl has caught or retrieved the ball following the tenth attempted shot at the basket; one second is added to this time for each foul committed.

b. Accuracy score: Two points are awarded for each basket made, one point for hitting the rim but not making the basket, and no point for missing both the basket and the rim.

2. Half-minute shooting. Starting at any position she chooses on the court, the subject shoots as many baskets as possible in 30 seconds. If the ball has left her hands at the end of 30 seconds, the basket counts if made. The score is the largest number of baskets made in two trials.

3. Push-pass. As shown in Figure 14.10, a three-ring concentric target is drawn on the wall, with the lower edge of the outer ring 24 inches from the floor; one-half-inch lines are used and are included within the diameter of each circle. The radii for the rings are: inner ring, 10 inches; middle ring, 20 inches; outer ring, 30 inches. The contestant stands behind a restraining line 10 feet from the wall. The test consists in passing a basketball with a two-hand chest pass to the target, recovering the pass, and continuing to pass for 30 seconds. All passes must be made from behind the restraining line. The subject is scored 5, 3, and 1 for hitting within the inner, middle, and outer circles respectively. Line hits are counted for the inner circle area.

AAHPER Basketball Test Manual for Girls

The AAHPER basketball test manual for girls contains instructions for administering and percentile norms for nine skill tests. The skill tests are the same as in the boys' manual: front shot, side shot, foul shot, underbasket shot, speed pass, jump and reach, overarm pass for accuracy, push shot for accuracy, and dribble.

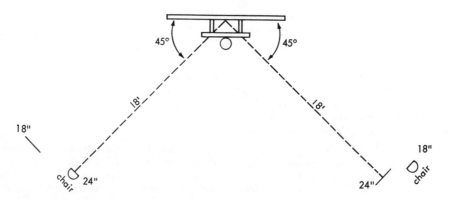

FIGURE 14.9. *Leilich Bounce-Shoot Basketball Test*

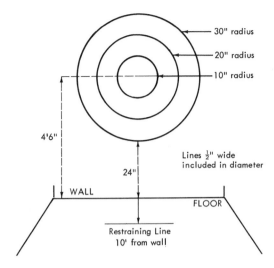

30" radius
20" radius
10" radius

4'6"

Lines ½" wide
included in diameter

24"

WALL

FLOOR

Restraining Line
10' from wall

FIGURE 14.10. *Leilich Push-Pass Basketball Target*

BOWLING NORMS

Six-sigma bowling scales were developed for college women by Phillips and Summers,[24] based on scores obtained from 3634 students in 22 colleges. These norms are available in the reference for eight ability groups.

Martin and Keogh[25] established bowling norms separately for inexperienced and experienced men and women in elective physical education classes at the University of California, Los Angeles. Students were classified as nonexperienced if they had bowled 10 lines or less and had received no previous formal instruction; all other students were classified as experienced. Norms are presented for both initial and

final performances. Initial scores were obtained after four to six class periods for the inexperienced bowlers and after four class periods of regular games for the experienced bowlers; for all groups, final scores were taken at the end of one semester of bowling instruction. Each set of norms consist of five categories, each based upon 1.2 standard deviations of the distribution. The categories are designated as superior, good, average, poor, and inferior. These norms appear in Appendix Table B.25.

FIELD HOCKEY

In 1940, Schmithals and French[26] constructed a field hockey test which consisted of three performances, as follows: the dribble, dodge, circular tackle, and drive; goal shooting; and fielding and drive. Twenty years later, Strait[27] also proposed a field hockey test. For both of these tests, special equipment is needed and the maneuvers performed are elaborate. Illner[28] presented a single-item test based on the drive, which she considered the most important skill in field hockey.

Friedel[29] proposed a single-item field hockey test for high school girls, which she called "pass receiving, fielding, and drive while moving." A test area is necessary, as shown in Figure 14.11. There are ten trials from each side, right and left; each

[24]Marjorie Phillips and Dean Summers, "Bowling Norms and Learning Curves for College Women," *Research Quarterly*, **21**, No. 4 (December 1950), 377.

[25]Joan Martin and Jack Keogh, "Bowling Norms for College Students in Elective Physical Education Classes," *Research Quarterly*, **35**, No. 3, Part 1 (October 1964), 325.

[26]Margaret Schmithals and Esther French, "Achievement Tests in Field Hockey for College Women," *Research Quarterly*, **11**, No. 3 (October 1940), 84.

[27]Clara J. Strait, "The Construction and Evaluation of a Field Hockey Skill Test," Master's Thesis, Smith College, 1960.

[28]Jules A. Illner, "The Construction and Validation of a Skill Test for the Drive in Field Hockey," Master's Thesis, Southern Illinois University, 1968.

[29]Jean E. Friedel, "The Development of a Field Hockey Skill Test for High School Girls," Master's Thesis, Illinois State Normal University, 1956.

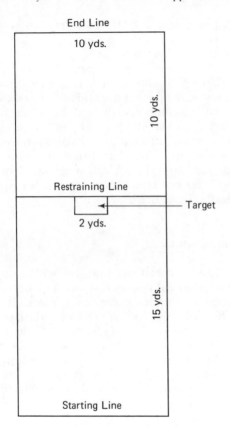

FIGURE 14.11. *Friedel Field Hockey Test*

use of the Spearman-Brown formula, reliability coefficients are 0.90 for the left side and 0.77 for the right side. For validation, the test correlated 0.87 with the Schmithals-French ball control test.

FOOTBALL

An AAHPER test manual was devoted to ten basic fundamentals of football; the usual percentile norms are presented for each skill. The skills are: forward pass for distance, 50-yard dash with football, blocking, forward pass for accuracy, football punt for distance, ball changing zigzag run, catching the forward pass, pull-outs, kick-off, and dodging run.

GOLF

Although the game of golf may be considered its own best test, a number of attempts have been made to measure the various elements involved, especially for indoor use. These tests usually have the added advantage of being good practice media.

Clevett Golf Test

Clevett[30] proposed empirical indoor tests for accuracy with the brassie, mid-iron, mashie, and putter. Although not scientifically constructed and lacking in norms, these tests have sufficient interest and practical value to warrant brief descriptions.

1–2. Brassie and midiron tests. These tests are given in a cage. The target is ten feet square, marked off into 25 areas, each of which is 20 inches square, and placed 21 feet from the tee. The point values of the various squares are given in Figure 14.12A. Balls striking to the left

trial is timed with a stop watch. To field a pass from the right side, the subject moves forward from behind the starting line on the signals "Ready" and "Go;" at the same time, the ball is rolled from the right corner toward the target. The subject receives the pass on her right in the target area, carries the ball by dribbling to the end line, reverses direction, and drives the ball back to the starting line. If the ball is not driven hard enough to reach the starting line, the subject must follow up the drive. Time is terminated when the ball crosses the starting line. When the test is from the left side, the ball is rolled from the left corner and the subject receives it on her left side.

By the split-half method corrected by

[30]Melvin A. Clevett, "An Experiment in Teaching Methods of Golf," *Research Quarterly,* **2,** No. 4 (December 1931), 104.

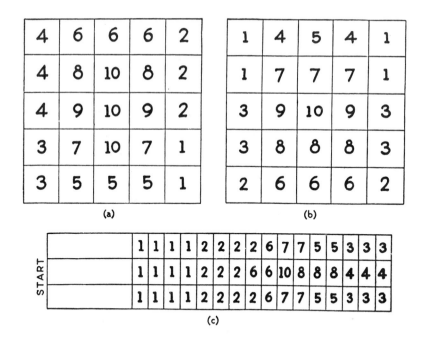

FIGURE 14.12. *Targets for Clevett's Golf Test: Brassie-Midiron, Mashie, and Putter*

of the target are scored higher than those striking to the right (for right-handed players), as Clevett maintains that a ball which strikes the right side of the target would slice, an outstanding error in golf. Each individual plays ten shots with the brassie and ten with the midiron. No preliminary practice or instruction is permitted.

3. Mashie test. The mashie test is designed to ascertain the individual's ability to make a short approach shot to the green. The approach is from 15 feet from the nearest edge of a target, composed of gymnasium mats, marked off into 25 areas each of which is four feet square. The point values of the various squares are given in Figure 14.12B. Ten shots are permitted, each being scored according to the spot where the ball lands rather than where it rolls or bounces.

4. Putting test. The putting test is made on smooth carpets 27 inches wide and 20 feet long, securely fastened to the floor. The putting line is 15 feet from the "hole." Forty-eight scoring areas, each nine inches square, are marked off on the carpet as shown in Figure

14.12C. Balls that stop slightly short of the hole are considered to be lower in point value than balls that travel slightly beyond the hole, as on an irregular green such a ball often rolls into the hole. The score is counted as the point where the ball stops. Ten trials are permitted.

Benson Golf Test

Benson[31] developed an outdoor golf test utilizing a single club, the number five iron, based on the belief that skill with this club reflects total golf-playing ability. Both the flight distance and the deviation from the intended flight of the golf ball are scored; in order to obtain these scores, the test area is marked out according to Figure 14.13. Distance signs are placed 25

[31]David W. Benson, "Measuring Golf Ability Through Use of a Number Five Iron Test," Unpublished paper, Research Section, California Assn. for Health, Physical Education, and Recreation Convention, April 7, 1963.

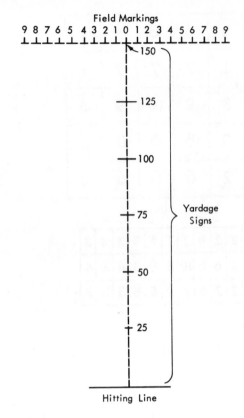

Field Markings
9 8 7 6 5 4 3 2 1 0 1 2 3 4 5 6 7 8 9

150

125

100

75 — Yardage Signs

50

25

Hitting Line

FIGURE 14.13. *Benson 5-Iron Golf Test Layout*

shot toward the 150-yard sign. The average of the 20 trials provides a distance score and a deviation score.

The reliability coefficients by odd-even correlations corrected by application of the Spearman-Brown prophecy formula are approximately 0.90 for the distance score and 0.70 for the deviation score. With uncorrected validity coefficients, the multiple correlation between actual golf scores and the distance and deviation scores was 0.75. When corrected estimates were used, the multiple correlation was 0.94.

Green Golf Test

With college men as subjects, Green[32] developed tests for six golf shots under field conditions, that is, the shots are made on a golf course. While this test is too lengthy for routine use, it does have merit for testing purposes in a golf course; the various tests provide satisfactory practice sessions. The shots were as follows.

Short Putt. Distance, 4 feet; shots taken from 12 positions around a circle with radius of 4 feet; measure by distance from cup on first putt and by the number of putts required to enter cup.

Long Putt. Distance, 25 feet; shots taken from 20 positions around a circle with radius of 25 feet; measurements, same as for short putt.

Chip Shot. Distance, 35 feet; use any iron; 20 shots; measure by distance from cup that shot comes to rest.

Pitch Shot. Distance, 40 yards; use either 7, 8, or 9 iron; 20 trials; measure same as for chip shot.

yards apart from the hitting line. At right angles to the distance signs at a distance of 150 yards, nine deviation signs five yards apart and numbered from 1 to 9 are placed at each side. Additional flags or signs may be placed on the field to assist the scorers in estimating distance.

In administering the test, the subject is provided with 25 golf balls. With a number five iron, he is allowed 5 practice shots; he then takes 20 shots that are scored. The scorer stands approximately three yards behind the hitting line, in line with the 150-yard sign. For each of the 20 trials, the scorer records two numerical values, an estimate of the distance the ball travels in flight, and the deviation from a straight

[32]Kenneth N. Green, "The Development of a Battery of Golf Skill Tests for College Men," Doctoral Dissertation, University of Arkansas, 1974.

Middle-Distance Shots. Distance, 140 yards; use any iron; 20 shots; measure by distance from cup and by lateral deviation from a straight line to the cup from the point the shot was taken.

Drive Shot. Distance, 300 yards; use any wood; 20 trials; measure, same as for middle-distance shot.

A criterion measure was established as the golf score for 36 holes of play. The highest correlations with this criterion were 0.66 for the middle-distance shot and −0.65 for the drive. A multiple correlation of 0.724 was obtained with two of the shots, the middle distance and the pitch. Diagrams for efficient administration of the various tests are given in the thesis.

Vanderhoof Golf Test

Vanderhoof[33] developed a number of indoor golf tests utilizing plastic practice golf balls. The tests involved the drive, the five-iron approach, the seven-iron approach, and a combination of these tests. Special targets are needed and timing the golf ball in flight is necessary in some instances. The drive and approach tests correlated around 0.70 with form ratings.

GYMNASTICS

As form plays such a large part, the construction of objective tests for the evaluation of gymnastic ability is difficult. Zwarg,[34] however, has given excellent suggestions for judging competitive gymnastic exercises. Hunsicker and Loken[35] analyzed the judging of the 1951 National Collegiate Athletic Association Gymnastic Meet and found that the objectivity coefficients were reasonably high. Judging on the horizontal bar was most and tumbling was least consistent. Only one correlation between judges was below 0.80; nine correlations were between 0.80 and 0.84; and the remaining 50 correlations were 0.85 and above. However, Faulkner and Loken[36] reported lower interjudge correlations at the 1961 NCAA Gymnastic Meet. Of the 120 such correlations, 26 were below 0.76; the coefficients decreased in the judging of the parallel bars and tumbling. Since these studies NCAA introduced compulsory routines into its championship meets. For the 1970 meet, Johnson[37] reported that 11 of 72 correlations between judges were below 0.80; 13 were between 0.80 and 0.84; and 48 were above 0.85. Of the 11 correlations below 0.80, eight were from judging compulsory routines; six of the eight were from judging the long horse vault. All but one of the 24 correlations between judges for the parallel bar and horizontal bar were above 0.90.

Wettstone[38] studied the factors underlying potential ability in gymnastics and tumbling. A list of the qualities of a good gymnast was developed and tests for 15 of those qualities with highest ranking by gymnastic coaches were devised. With 22

[33]Ellen R. Vanderhoof, "Beginning Golf Achievement Tests," Master's Thesis, State University of Iowa, 1956.

[34]Leopold F. Zwarg, "Judging and Evaluation of Competitive Apparatus for Gymnastic Exercises," *Journal of Health and Physical Education,* **6,** No. 1 (January 1935), 23.

[35]Paul Hunsicker and Newt Loken, "The Objectivity of Judging at the National Collegiate Athletic Association Gymnastic Meet," *Research Quarterly,* **22,** No. 4 (December 1951), 423.

[36]John Faulkner and Newt Loken, "Objectivity of Judging at the National Collegiate Athletic Association Gymnastic Meet: A Ten-Year Followup Study," *Research Quarterly,* **33,** No. 3 (October 1962), 485.

[37]Marvin Johnson, "Objectivity Judging at the National Collegiate Athletic Association Gymnastic Meet," *Research Quarterly,* **42,** No. 4 (December 1971), 454.

[38]Eugene Wettstone, "Tests for Predicting Potential Ability in Gymnastics and Tumbling," *Research Quarterly,* **9,** No. 4 (December 1938), 115.

active gymnasts at the University of Iowa as subjects, a correlation of 0.79 was obtained between ratings of their abilities by gymnastic coaches and the following three elements: (1) thigh circumference divided by height; (2) strength test, consisting of chinning, dipping, and thigh flexion; and (3) the Burpee (squat-thrust) test for ten seconds. In the strength test, the three test items are added together. Thigh-flexion strength is measured by having the subject hang from stall bars and flex the leg and thigh to a horizontal position as many times as possible. The following regression equation is used to predict the subject's potential gymnastic ability, PGA (the X-numerals refer to the numbered variables above):

$$PGA = 0.355X_1 + 0.260X_2 + 0.035X_3 + 13.990$$

HANDBALL

Since 1935, proposals have been made for testing handball playing ability. Some of these tests have been empirical in nature, while others have shown low validity. In recent years, the typical criterion of handball ability for use in validating tests has been the round-robin tournament. Two handball batteries with best relationships to this criterion are presented below.

Oregon Handball Test

Four graduate students at the University of Oregon[39] administered 17 strength, motor ability, and handball skill tests to 37 college men. The highest correlations of single variables with round-robin play were 0.71 for a service test, 0.68 for 30-second volley, and 0.66 for total wall volley

[39]Gary G. Pennington, James A. P. Day, John N. Drowatzky, and John F. Hanson, "A Measure of Handball Ability," *Research Quarterly,* **38,** No. 2 (May 1967), 247.

score. A multiple correlation of 0.80 was obtained with these tests. A multiple regression equation was computed for three tests, as follows:

Criterion =
1.75 service placement + 2.27 total wall volley + 1.59 back-wall placement + 0.29.

Descriptions of these tests follow.

Service Placement. The handball court is divided into areas that are assigned numerical values, as shown in Figure 14.14A. Serving in a regulation manner, the student attempts to place the service into the area having the highest numerical value. Each subject is given 10 trials.

Total Wall Volley. The subject's score on this test is the sum of items 1 and 2 below.

1. Thirty-second Wall Volley: The subject stands in the center of the court behind the short service line, drops the ball to the floor, and strokes it against the front wall repeatedly for 30 seconds. He is permitted to step ahead of the line for one return, but the next must be played behind the line. If he violates this rule or loses control, he must recover the ball and begin a new series in the same way as at the start. The score is the number of times the ball is legally stroked against the front wall.

2. Thirty-second Wall Volley, Nondominant Hand: This test is given in the same manner as the previous test, but the subject may not strike the ball with the dominant hand.

Back-Wall Placement. The front wall is divided into different areas with assigned numerical values, as shown in Figure 14.14B. The subject throws the ball high and hard against the front wall and, after it hits the floor and rebounds off the back wall, attempts to stroke it into the high scoring areas of the front wall. The number of trials is five each with the right and left hands.

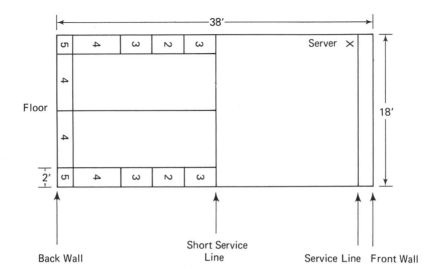

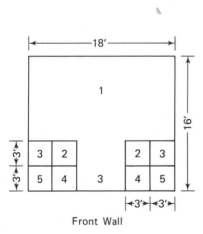

FIGURE 14.14. *Oregon Handball Test Targets.* Above: *Service placement test.* Left: *Wall placement test.*

play, the handball ability of each player was determined as the average of his scores minus the average his opponents scored against him. The highest correlations with this handball criterion were 0.87 for 30-second volley and 0.84 for front wall kill with dominant hand; a multiple correlation of 0.90 was obtained with these tests as the independent variables. Descriptions of these tests follow.

Thirty-second Volley. The subject stands at any point behind the short service line; at the signal to start, he puts the ball in play with an easy toss to the front wall. He, then, volleys the ball against the front wall as many times as possible in 30 seconds. To count in the score, the ball must be stroked from behind the service line; the ball may be hit from over the service line, but such hits do not count. If the player loses control of the ball, the ball is replaced immediately by the tester.

Tyson Handball Test

Tyson[40] set up round robin handball competition in four physical education classes consisting of a total of 64 college men. At the end of a semester of such

[40]Kenneth W. Tyson, "A Handball Skill Test for College Men," Master's Thesis, University of Texas at Austin, 1970.

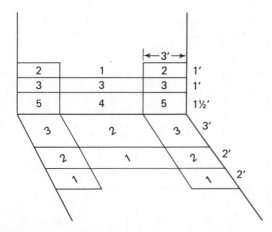

FIGURE 14.15. *Tyson Target for Handball Front-Wall Kill*

Front Wall Kill, Dominant Hand. In this test, attempts are made to place the ball in a target on the front wall, as shown in Figure 14.15 with the numerical values for the various target areas. The subject stands in the doubles service box against the left side wall if he is right-handed or against the right side wall if he is left-handed. The tester stands in the service lane midway between the side walls and tosses the ball so that it rebounds to his right if the subject is right-handed or to his left if the subject is left-handed. As soon as the ball leaves the tester's hand, the player may leave his starting position and, crossing behind the tester, move into a position to attempt the hit. The subject's score is the total number of points scored in five attempts.

RHYTHM

Several efforts have been made to measure motor rhythms and dance. For the most part, however, these have not as yet advanced to the practical stage. Annett[41]

obtained a low correlation of 0.47 between the Seashore Rhythm Test and a criterion consisting of expert judgment of skill in motor rhythm. Lemon and Sherbon,[42] after studying the Seashore Rhythm Test and others of their own device, concluded that tests of this quality more useful to physical education were possible and deserved further study. Briggs[43] used the Rhythmic Imagery Section of the Gordon Aptitude Musical Profile as a criterion of rhythmic response. This criterion correlated 0.657 with her test of Motor Rhythmic Performance, which contained two sections involving walking and skipping respectively.

Over a period of five and one-half years, Ashton[44] developed a gross motor rhythm test using simple movement initiated by the student. This test consists of three sections: directed walk, run, and skip; musical excerpts for improvisation; derived or combined dance steps, in which the step is identified but the subject initiates the movement for polka, waltz, and schottische. Rating scales for the sections of the test appear in the reference. Ashton concluded that the administration of this test had proven feasible and economical of time when varied forms of dance have to be judged without excessive staff training and with the use of only one period of class time.

In preparing a social dancing test, Waglow[45] had a record transcribed for the following rhythms: waltz, tango, slow fox trot, jitterbug, rhumba, and samba. The

[41]Thomas Annett, "A Study of Rhythmic Capacity and Performance in Motor Rhythm in Physical Education Majors," *Research Quarterly*, **3,** No. 2 (May 1932), 183.

[42]Eloise Lemon and Elizabeth Sherbon, "A Study of Relationships of Certain Measures of Rhythmic Ability and Motor Ability in Girls and Women," *Supplement to Research Quarterly*, **5,** No. 1 (March 1934), 82.

[43]Ruth A. Briggs, "The Development of an Instrument for Assessment of Motoric Rhythmic Performance," Master's Thesis, University of Missouri, 1968.

[44]Dudley Ashton, "A Gross Motor Rhythm Test," *Research Quarterly*, **24,** No. 3 (October 1953), 253.

[45]I. F. Waglow, "An Experiment in Social Dance Testing," *Research Quarterly*, **24,** No. 1 (March 1953), 97.

test consists of an evaluation of the subject's ability to perform each of the dance steps to the recorded music. The reported objectivity coefficient for the test is 0.79.

Benton[46] studied not only elements of rhythm, but factors basic to dance movement techniques, including Johnson-type tests, McCloy Physical Fitness Index, Seashore Series A Rhythm Test, Brace-type tests, Motor Rhythm Test, and Static Balance Test. A criterion of the judgment of three dance experts, who observed the subjects on selected dance movements, was established. Multiple correlations between 0.77 and 0.93, when corrected for attenuation, were reported for five regression equations using various combinations of variables found significant in the research.

Soccer

McDonald Volleying Soccer Test

McDonald[47] studied the use of volleying a soccer ball against a backboard as a test of general soccer ability. With college men as subjects, he obtained the following correlations between scores on the test and the ratings of playing ability by their coaches: 0.94 for varsity players, 0.63 for junior varsity players, 0.76 for freshmen varsity players, and 0.85 for the combined groups.

The backboard for the test is 30 feet wide and 11½ feet high. A restraining line is drawn 9 feet from the backboard and parallel to it. Three soccer balls are used; one is placed on the restraining line, the other two are located 9 feet behind this line in the center of the area. The test consists of kicking the soccer ball against the backboard as many times as possible in 30 seconds. Any type kicks may be used; both ground balls and fly balls which hit the backboard count. To count, however, all balls must be kicked from the ground with the supporting leg behind the restraining line. Rebounds may be retrieved in any manner, including use of the hands. If a ball is out of control, the subject may play one of the spare balls, but must bring the ball by use of hands or feet to a position at the restraining line before kicking against the backboard (no penalty other than the lost time in getting the ball in position to kick). The score is the number of legal kicks in the time period; the best of four trials is recorded.

Mitchell[48] modified the McDonald Volleying Soccer Test for upper elementary school boys. The modifications were as follows: (a) the backboard target is 8 feet wide by 4 feet high; (b) the restraining line is placed 6 feet from the backboard; (c) the test consists of three trials of 20 seconds each; (d) the hands may not be used in retrieving a ball or in securing a new one; and (e) a retriever service is instituted for balls kicked out of play. A rank-difference correlation of 0.84 was obtained between scores on this test and teacher-coach's ratings. The test-retest coefficient is reported as 0.89.

Johnson Soccer Test

Johnson[49] also developed a wall-volleying soccer test for college men. The test area is diagramed in Figure 14.16; as will be noted, the target dimensions are the same as for the regulation soccer goal. The essential rules for this test are as follows:

1. In starting the test, the subject holds a soccer ball behind the restraining line and puts it

[46]Rachel Jane Benton, "The Measurement of Capacities for Learning Dance Movement Techniques," *Research Quarterly*, **15**, No. 2 (May 1944), 137.

[47]Lloyd G. McDonald, "The Construction of a Kicking Skill Test as an Index of General Soccer Ability," Master's Thesis, Springfield College, 1951.

[48]J. Reid Mitchell, "The Modification of the McDonald Soccer Test for Upper Elementary School Boys," Master's Thesis, University of Oregon, 1963.

[49]Joseph R. Johnson, "The Development of a Single-Item Test as a Measure of Soccer Skill," Master's Thesis, University of British Columbia, 1963.

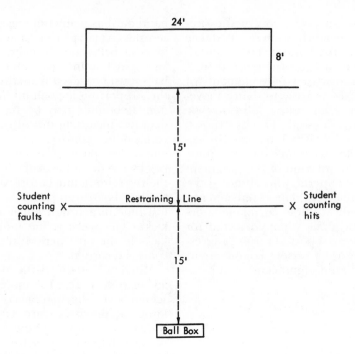

FIGURE 14.16. *Johnson Soccer Wall-Volley Test*

in play by kicking it against the backboard. The ball can be kicked on "the fly" or dropped to the ground and kicked. A test bout is 30 seconds; three such bouts are performed.

2. A hit is counted when a ball played legally from behind the restraining line strikes the target area and rebounds across the restraining line.

3. Faults are counted for any infringement over the restraining line by the subject or illegal playing of the ball according to soccer rules. No penalty is counted for the use of spare balls. A tester-assistant is employed to retrieve any ball abandoned by the subject.

4. The subject's score is the aggregate number of hits on the three trials less the number of faults. The following scale was developed:

	Number of Hits
Superior	42–over
Good	37–41
Average	31–36
Below average	25–30
Poor	24–below

The reliability coefficient for the Johnson test was 0.92 for consecutive trials. Validity was determined by rank-difference correlations between scores on the test and investigator rankings of soccer ability at various performance levels. These correlations were 0.98 for men in required physical education soccer classes, 0.94 for physical education major students, and 0.81, 0.84, and 0.58, respectively, for third, second, and first team varsity soccer players.

Crew Soccer Test

Crew[50] related several soccer skills to the soccer ability of college men. The criterion of soccer ability consisted of the opinions of competent judges formed during competitive play. Correlations of test

[50]Vernon N. Crew, "A Skill Test Battery for Use in Service Program Soccer Classes at the University Level," Master's Thesis, University of Oregon, 1968.

items with this criterion were 0.96 for ball control, 0.95 for aerial accuracy, 0.92 for dribbling, and 0.88 for wall volley. A multiple correlation of 0.97 was reported with the ball control and dribbling tests. T-scores for these tests appear in Appendix Table B.26. Descriptions of their administration follow.

Ball Control.   The subject tosses the ball in the air and then proceeds to keep the ball clear of the ground by use of his head, feet, thighs, or any other legal body part. Each trial score is the number of times the subject legally connects with the ball before it touches the ground. Three trials are allowed; the score is the total of the two best trials.

Dribble.   Five wire baskets are placed upside down in a straight row nine feet apart with the first basket nine feet from the starting line. The subject dribbles in a weaving fashion around these baskets, as in the basketball dribble test (Figure 14.5). Time for completing the circuit once is recorded to the nearest tenth of a second; the individual's score is the total of the two trials.

SOFTBALL

As has been true for other team sports, such as basketball and soccer, efforts have been made to measure fundamental skills involved in playing softball. For the most part, however, the skill tests have not correlated highly with softball playing ability as judged by competent observers. Several of the skill tests are presented below.

Cale Softball Test Items

While Cale[51] did not construct a softball test, she did determine the reliability of softball test items as performed by college

[51]Audrey A. Cale, "The Investigation and Analysis of Softball Skill Tests for College Women," Master's Thesis, University of Maryland, 1962.

women. She experimented with ten such items, selected as being associated with the most important skills of softball. Three items had reliability coefficients above 0.80; the items with their respective coefficients are repeated throws (0.81), distance throw (0.91), and batting off a tee (0.96). Directions for giving these tests follow.

Repeated Throws.   A line 15 feet long is drawn on an unobstructed wall 13 feet above and parallel to the floor. A second 15-foot line is drawn on the floor 10 feet from and parallel to the wall; this is a restraining line. To start the test, the subject stands behind the restraining line with the ball; she throws it against the wall above the 13-foot line and catches the rebound as many times as possible in 30 seconds. One point is scored each time the ball hits above the 13-foot line, provided it is thrown from behind the restraining line. If the ball has been released when time is up, the throw is counted if made. Balls out of control must be recovered by the subject. The score is the total number of hits in four trials of 30 seconds each.

Distance Throw.   A throwing zone is marked out with a restraining line and a second line six feet back of and parallel to it; down field, lines five yards apart are provided and marked with distance from the restraining line. The subject throws a softball overhand from the throwing zone. The point where the ball lands is marked with a small stake. Two more trials are taken and the stake adjusted to any longer distances. After the third throw, the longest distance is measured from the nearest five-yard line toward the restraining line.

Batting Tee Test.   For this test, 15 parallel lines five yards apart are drawn on an area at least 35 by 75 yards. An adjustable batting tee is placed on the center of the first parallel line. Before batting, the subject may adjust the height of the tee to her satisfaction. After five practice trials, 20 batting trials are taken. The point at which the ball comes to rest after it is hit is estimated to the nearest yard. If the batter swings and misses or swings and hits only the tee, the trial is scored as a zero. The score for the test is the total yardage the ball is batted in the 20 trials.

Shick's Defensive Softball Skills

Also for college women, Shick[52] proposed three tests of defensive softball skills. These tests with their test-retest reliability coefficients are repeated throws, 0.86, fielding, 0.89, and target 0.88. A multiple correlation of 0.74 was reported between judgments of softball playing ability by competent observers and the repeated throw and target tests; for all three tests, the coefficient was 0.75. Description of the test follows.

Repeated Throws.   This test is conducted in the same manner as in the Cale battery, except for the following: (a) the wall line is 10 feet above the floor; (b) the restraining line is 23 feet from the wall; and (c) the ball must be thrown using either an overhand or sidearm motion.

Fielding Test.   A line is drawn on the wall four feet from the floor and parallel to it; another line is drawn on the floor 15 feet from the wall and parallel to it. The test consists of four 30-second trials. This test is conducted in the same manner as for repeated throws with two exceptions: (a) the type of throw is not specified, and (b) the subject attempts to hit the wall below the line drawn on it. The scoring is also the same as for repeated throws, except that no ball which hits above the line on the wall is counted.

Target Test.   Wall and floor targets for this test are shown in Figure 14.17. The wall target is 66 inches square and its center is 36 inches from the floor. To aid in recording scores, the following colors are suggested: 5, red; 4, medium blue; 3, bright yellow; 2, pale aqua; and 1, black. A restraining line is drawn on the floor 40 feet from the wall and parallel to it. The test consists of two trials of 10 throws each. Each throw is given two scores, a score for the hit on the wall and a score for the hit on the floor, first bounce only.

AAHPER Softball Test Manuals

Softball AAHPER Test Manuals are available separately for boys and girls. The same eight skill tests appear in both manuals, as follows: throw for distance, overhand throw for accuracy, underhand pitching, speed throw, fungo hitting, base running, fielding ground balls, and catching fly balls.

SWIMMING

Hewitt's Swimming Scales

Hewitt has done some very practical work in the construction of swimming achievement scales for men in the armed forces, for college men, and for high school boys and girls. The test items for the various groups are as follows:

High School Boys and Girls.[53]   Time for the 25-yard flutter kick while holding a regulation water polo ball; time for the 50-yard crawl; and number of strokes to cover 25 yards each with the elementary back, side, and breast strokes (glide and relaxation tests).

[52]Jacqueline Shick, "Battery of Defensive Softball Skill Tests for College Women," *Research Quarterly,* **41,** No. 1 (March 1970), 82.

[53]Jack E. Hewitt, "Achievement Scales for High School Swimming," *Research Quarterly,* **20,** No. 2 (May 1949), 170.

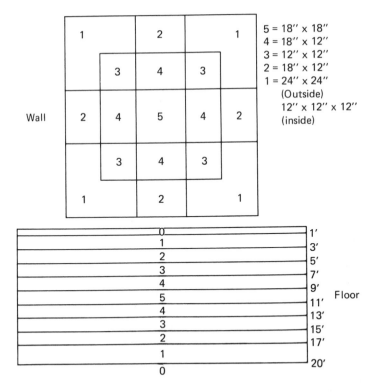

FIGURE 14.17. *Target Areas for Shick Softball Test*

College Men.[54] Time for 20- and 25-yard underwater swims; distance covered during 15-minute swim for endurance; time for 25- and 50-yard swims each with the crawl, breast, and back-crawl strokes; and number of strokes to cover 50 yards each with the elementary back, side, and breast strokes (glide and relaxation tests).

Men in the Armed Forces.[55] Time for the 20- and 25-yard underwater swims; distance covered during 15-minute swim for endurance; and number of strokes to cover 50 yards each with elementary back, side, and breast strokes (glide and relaxation tests).

The reliability of the tests at the college and high school levels was checked with satisfactory results. The coefficients for the various tests ranged from 0.89 to 0.95. At these levels, too, criteria of over-all swimming ability were established, consisting in each situation of the total accomplishment in all events. Short batteries of swimming tests to be used for classification purposes were then determined. For college men, the 25- or 50-yard crawl plus the three gliding strokes correlated 0.87 with the criterion; for high school boys and girls, the side-stroke gliding test correlated 0.94 with the total score.

[54]Jack E. Hewitt, "Swimming Achievement Scales for College Men," *Research Quarterly,* **19,** No. 4 (December 1948), 282.

[55]Jack E. Hewitt, "Achievement Scales for Wartime Swimming," *Research Quarterly,* **14,** No. 4 (December 1943), 391.

Fox Swimming Power Test

An objective test of swimming power for the front crawl and side strokes was developed by Fox.[56] The reliability coefficients for the two tests are 0.95 and 0.97 respectively. T-scores were prepared, based on the performance of college women ranging in ability from beginning to advanced swimmers. These norms appear in Appendix Table B.27. Directions for administering the test follow.

A rope approximately 20 feet longer than the width of the pool is tied at one end to some firm object two feet from one end of the pool; the other end remains free directly across the pool. A weight is suspended from the rope at a point half way across the pool, so that the rope will drop when the free end is released. Starting at the position of the rope, the deck of the pool is marked off in five-foot intervals with adhesive or masking tape; distances from the start may be marked on these walls with waterproof material.

In taking the test, the rope is pulled taut enough so that it is about a foot under water at the point the subject is to start. The swimmer assumes the appropriate floating position for the stroke (i.e., side float for side stroke, face float for crawl stroke), and rests the feet on the rope with the malleoli at rope level. At the start, the rope is dropped; the swimmer takes five complete strokes with glides. The distance covered for the side stroke is measured from the rope to the position of the ankles at the beginning of the recovery of the legs for the sixth stroke. For the crawl stroke, the distance traversed by the swimmer is measured by noting where the ankles are at the moment the fingers enter the water to begin the sixth arm cycle. The distance measurement is made to the nearest foot from the five-foot distance markers on the deck.

Rosentswieg[57] revised the Fox swimming test for college women by making the following changes: (a) the test is started by having a helper stand by the side of the swimmer, who uses her forearms as a cradle to hold the legs of the swimmer at the surface of the water; (b) the subject sculls or floats in the appropriate position for a given stroke with her shoulders parallel to the starting line; thus, measurements for the revision are made from the shoulders rather than the ankles; (c) when the subject is ready, she swims away from the helper using the designated arm stroke; if a kick is made prior to the stroke, the trial is immediately stopped; (d) twelve strokes, or six cycles, are used for the power test; and (e) power tests for five strokes are proposed: front crawl, side, elementary back, back crawl, and breast. Reliability coefficients for the revised power strokes ranged between 0.89 and 0.97. The revised strokes correlated between 0.63 and 0.83 with ratings of swimming form by at least two judges for each subject.

Connor Swimming Testing Methods

Connor[58] has proposed the following two swimming tests for elementary school children, ages 5 to 12 years inclusive:

50-Yard Prone Swim.   Push-off in the water; swim 50 yards in prone position without stopping.

50-Yard Combined Swim.   Push-off in water; swim 25 yards in prone position; without stopping, turn over and swim 25 yards on back.

The tests designated for boys and girls at different ages are as follows:

[56]Margaret G. Fox, "Swimming Power Test," *Research Quarterly,* **28,** No. 3 (October 1957), 233.

[57]Joel Rosentswieg, "A Revision of the Power Swimming Test," *Research Quarterly,* **39,** No. 3 (October 1968), 818.

[58]Donald J. Connor, "A Comparison of Objective and Subjective Testing Methods in Selected Swim-

Sex	Age	Test	Scoring
Girls	5–9 years	50-yd. prone swim	Time
		50-yd. combined swim	Count strokes
	10–12 years	50-yd. prone swim	Time or count strokes
Boys	5–9 years	50-yd. prone swim	Time
	10–12 years	50-yd. combined swim	Count strokes

Rating of Synchronized Swimming

A method for rating synchronized swimming stunts was developed by Durrant.[59] Six judges rated 24 subjects on seven selected swimming stunts, using an analytical method developed by the investigator. High correlations were obtained on all stunts; the correlations were higher and showed less variation among the raters for those stunts that had the higher total point values. The rating scale appears in the reference.

TABLE TENNIS

A table-tennis test, patterned after the Dyer tennis test procedure, described later in this chapter, was developed by Mott and Lockhart.[60] For the test, a table-tennis table is needed, hinged in the middle and arranged so that one-half of it is propped against a post or wall above and perpendicular to the playing surface, so serve as a backboard. A chalk line is marked on the perpendicular half of the table, six inches above the playing surface of the table; a kitchen match box is thumbtacked to the edge of the table and even to its end (place on the right side for right-handed players, on the left side for left-handed players). A stop watch, table-tennis racket, and three table-tennis balls are also necessary.

The testing procedure is as follows: At the signal "Go," the player drops a ball to the table and rallies it against the perpendicular table surface as many times as possible in 30 seconds. Any number of bounces on the playing surface is permitted. If the player loses control of the ball, another may be taken from the match box, dropped to the playing surface, and played. Hits on the perpendicular surface do not count if the ball is volleyed (that is, the ball must bounce at least once), the player puts the free hand on the table during or immediately preceding a hit, or the ball strikes the perpendicular surface below the chalk line. The test score is the best score of three trials.

A reliability coefficient of 0.90 for the table-tennis backboard test with college women as subjects was obtained. A validity coefficient of 0.84 is also reported, but the criterion is not given. T-scales for college women were constructed and appear in Appendix Table B.28.

TENNIS

Dyer Tennis Backboard Test

A backboard volleying test of general tennis ability was constructed by Dyer.[61] The test does not analyze the various strokes and elements of the game. It has been used extensively as a classification device for tennis and as a means of determining the progress being made in the

---

ming Skills for Elementary School Children," Master's Thesis, Washington State University, 1962.

[59]Sue M. Durrant, "An Analytical Method of Rating Synchronized Swimming Stunts," *Research Quarterly,* **35,** No. 2 (May 1964), 126.

[60]Jane A. Mott and Aileen Lockhart, "Table Tennis Backboard Test," *Journal of Health and Physical Education,* **17,** No. 9 (November 1946), 550.

[61]Joanna T. Dyer, "The Backboard Test of Tennis Ability," *Supplement to the Research Quarterly,* **6,** No. 1 (March 1935), 63, and "Revision of Backboard Test of Tennis Ability," *Research Quarterly,* **9,** No. 1 (March 1938), 25.

game as a whole. The test consists merely of volleying a tennis ball as rapidly as possible against a backboard. Directions for administering the test are as follows:

1. A backboard or wall, approximately 10 feet in height and allowing about 15 feet in width for each person taking the test at one time, is used. A line 3 inches in width, to represent the net, is drawn across the backboard so that the top of the line is 3 feet from the floor.

2. A restraining line, 5 feet from the base of the wall, is drawn on the floor.

3. Two balls and a racquet are provided for each subject taking the test at one time. A box containing extra balls, about 12 inches long, 9 inches wide, and 3 inches deep, is provided and placed on the floor at the junction of the restraining line and the left side-line for right-handed players, and at the right for left-handed players.

4. In starting the test, the subject drops the ball and lets it hit the floor once, then plays it against the wall as rapidly as possible for 30 seconds. There is no limit to the number of times the ball may bounce before it is hit. Also, with the exception of the start and when a new ball is put into play, the ball need not touch the floor before being played. Any stroke or combination of strokes may be used, but all balls must be played from behind the restraining line. The line may be crossed to retrieve balls, but any hits made while in such a position do not count. Any number of balls may be used. If the subject loses control of the ball, the second that was supplied may be used after which, if necessary, other balls may be taken from the box.

5. Each ball striking the wall on or above the net line before the end of the 30 seconds counts as a hit and scores one point. Three trials are given, the final score being the sum of the scores on the three trials.

6. For efficient administration of the test, divide the group into units of four players each, numbered from one to four. Their duties are as follows:

Number 1 takes the test.

Number 2 counts the number of balls that strike the wall on or above the net line.

Number 3 checks the number of violations at the restraining line.

Number 4 collects and returns all balls to the box.

7. After each person in the entire group has had one trial, the test is repeated in the same order, until everyone has had three trials in all.

Scoring tables for the Dyer test have been computed and appear in Appendix Table B.29. T-score and percentile rank norms for this test as applied to women physical education students have been prepared by Miller, and will be found in her reference.[62]

Dyer reported a correlation of 0.92 between scores on her test and the positions of the subjects following round-robin play, in which each match consisted of 20 points (the probable equivalent of three or four games). Fox[63] obtained a correlation of 0.53 between scores of college women beginning players on the Dyer test and subjective ratings of their ability to execute the forehand drive, the backhand drive, and the serve. Using a restraining line of 28 feet (instead of 5 feet), Koski[64] obtained correlation coefficients ranging from 0.51 to 0.68 between wall rally results and tournament play, with college men as subjects. He also constructed norms for beginning and intermediate levels of tennis ability.

An account of the use of the Dyer Tennis Test in a field situation was kept by Leon Doleva, when coaching and instructing tennis at Williston Academy.[65] Sixty boys were tested and arranged into three groups: the first squad was considered the

[62]Wilma K. Miller, "Achievement Levels in Tennis Knowledge and Skill for Women Physical Education Major Students," *Research Quarterly,* **24,** No. 1 (March 1953), 81.

[63]Katharine Fox, "A Study of the Validity of the Dyer Backboard Test and the Miller Forehand-Background Test for Beginning Tennis Players," *Research Quarterly,* **24,** No. 1 (March 1953), 1.

[64]Arthur Koski, "A Tennis Wall Rally Test for College Men," mimeographed report.

[65]Clayton T. Shay, "An Application of the Dyer Tennis Test," *Journal of Health and Physical Education,* **20,** No. 4 (April 1949), 273.

varsity and had 12 boys; the other two groups had 24 boys each. Ladder tournaments within each group were organized, and an opportunity was provided for boys to change from one group to the other on the basis of competitive merit. Certain of the results were reported as follows: the six boys with the highest test scores became the first six players on the school team and were never displaced; the number one man on the test became the number one man on the team; and only two members from the intermediate group were able to advance to the first squad.

A number of revisions of the Dyer backboard tennis test have been proposed. Studies by Fox[66] and Hewitt[67] indicate that this test does not discriminate sufficiently at the beginner's level and that it discriminates tennis ability best after the subjects are sufficiently advanced to volley. The changes in the test have been largely confined to the distance of the restraining line from the backboard and the length of time for volleying.

As a consequence of his research, Hewitt revised the Dyer test for college men by increasing the distance of the restraining line from the wall to 20 feet and by starting each volley with a serve. Reliability coefficients were 0.82 for beginning players and 0.93 for advanced players. The rank-order correlations between scores on the test and the rank of players as determined from round-robin play ranged from 0.67 to 0.72 for four beginning tennis classes and 0.83 and 0.88 for two advanced tennis classes.

In studying the Dyer tennis test also for college men, Ronning[68] experimented with restraining lines 5, 15, 25, and 35 feet

from the wall, and with volleying times of 30 and 60 seconds. The combination of the 35-foot restraining line and three 60-second trials was best, although the 30-second time was nearly as satisfactory for tennis service-course men. The correlations between the 30-second and 60-second tests and round-robin play in the service classes were 0.87 and 0.90, respectively. For varsity players, however, the 60-second trials were definitely superior. The correlations with round-robin play were 0.60 for the 30-second test and 0.97 for the 60-second test.

Broer-Miller Tennis Test

Broer and Miller[69] designed a test to measure the ability of college women to place forehand and backhand drives into the backcourt area. One regulation net is used, with a rope stretched four feet above the top of the net. Special tennis court markings are needed, as illustrated in Figure 14.18.

In taking this test, the subject stands behind the baseline, bounces the ball to herself, and attempts to hit it into the back nine feet of the opposite court. Fourteen trials are taken each with forehand and with backhand strokes. Each ball is scored depending upon the area in which it lands, as shown in Figure 14.18. Balls that go over the rope score half the value of that area in which they land. If the player misses the ball in attempting to strike it, it is considered a trial. "Let" balls are taken over.

Broer and Miller obtained a reliability coefficient for this test of 0.80 for both beginning and intermediate tennis players. The validity of the test was determined by correlating the ratings given the subject by various judges with the subject's performance on the test. For the intermediate

---

[66]Fox, "Validity of the Dyer and Miller Tests," p. 1.

[67]Jack E. Hewitt, "Revision of the Dyer Backboard Tennis Test," *Research Quarterly*, **36**, No. 2 (May 1965), 153.

[68]Hilding E. Ronning, "Wall Tests for Evaluating Tennis Ability," Master's Thesis, Washington State University, 1959.

[69]Marion R. Broer and Donna Mae Miller, "Achievement Tests for Beginning and Intermediate Tennis," *Research Quarterly*, **21**, No. 3 (October 1950), 303.

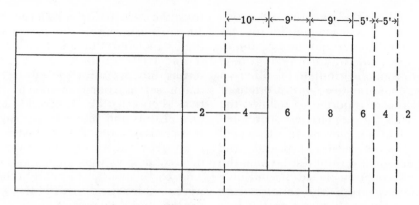

FIGURE 14.18. *Court Markings for Broer-Miller Forehand-Backhand Drive Test*

group, this correlation was 0.85; for the beginning group, it was 0.61. Fox[70] reported a correlation of 0.69 between the Dyer and Broer-Miller tests, with college women as subjects.

Hewitt's Tennis Test Items

Hewitt[71] constructed tests of four tennis skills for university men and women. The skills are forehand drive placement, backhand drive placement, service placement, and speed of service (as indicated by distance ball bounces). Special markings on a tennis court are necessary for these tests. The Dyer wall volley test was also given, but with the restraining line at 20 feet as proposed above by Hewitt. Test-retest reliability coefficients for the four skill tests were service placement, 0.94; speed of service, 0.84; backhand drive placement, 0.78; forehand drive placement, 0.75.

For validation of the tests, round-robin tennis competition was conducted separately at three levels of tennis ability: var-

sity and junior varsity men, advanced service course men and women, and beginning men and women. The correlations between the round-robin play and the various tests of tennis skill appear in Table 14.1. As can be seen, the highest correlation at each of the tennis skill levels were: 0.93 with serrvice placement for varsity/junior varsity, 0.84 with Dyer wall volley for advanced, and 0.89 with speed of service for beginning players. Achievement scale norms, based on grades F to A, are given in the reference for Hewitt's four tests at each of the three levels of tennis ability.

TABLE 14.1 *Rank Order Play Ability in Tennis Versus Hewitt's Tennis Achievement Test Scores*

	Varsity/ Jr. Varsity	Advanced	Beginners
Forehand drive placement	0.57	0.62	0.67
Backhand drive placement	0.52	0.61	0.62
Service placement	0.93	0.63	0.72
Speed of service	0.86	0.72	0.89
Dyer Wall Test (with 20-foot restraining line)	0.87	0.84	0.73

[70]Fox "Validity of the Dyer and Miller Tests," p. 1.

[71]Jack E. Hewitt, "Hewitt's Tennis Achievement Test," *Research Quarterly,* **37,** No. 2 (May 1966), 231.

Kemp-Vincent Tennis Rally Test

The Kemp-Vincent rally test of tennis ability[72] was constructed to overcome such criticisms of existing tennis skills as: current tests do not measure skills under game conditions; require the use of special equipment or line markings; and the time required for their administration is prohibitive. In this rally test, two players of similar ability take positions on opposite sides of the net on a singles tennis court, and rally the ball as in a game situation as many times as possible within a three-minute time period. Directions for and scoring of the rallies appear in the reference. Correlations of the test with round-robin play were 0.84 for beginning and 0.93 for intermediate players. With the Dyer test, the correlation was 0.80.

TOUCH FOOTBALL

Borleske[73] has proposed a test designed to measure ability to play touch football composed of five items, as follows: forward pass for distance, catching forward passes, punting for distance, 50-yard dash carrying the ball, and zone pass defense. In constructing the test, Borleske experimented with 18 individual objective tests, obtaining a validity coefficient of 0.85 with the opinion of experts using a check sheet for subjectively rating performance. The battery of five tests finally selected has a correlation of 0.93 with the larger objective battery of which the five tests were a part. A short battery of three tests (forward pass for distance, punting for distance, and 50-yard dash with the ball) correlated 0.88 with the criterion. A T-score table for the three tests appear in Appendix Table B.30.

A description of the short battery of touch football tests is given below. The omission of the pass-catching and pass-defense items simplifies the test considerably and reduces the amount of time required for its administration.

Forward Pass for Distance. The field is marked with lines every five yards and with markers every ten yards, so that the subjects can throw in pairs from both ends of the field. From one to six pairs of passers, depending on the width of the field, can throw together. Each passer checks the spot where the ball hits the ground when his partner throws, and estimates the distance to the nearest yard. Each participant is allowed three throws after warming up for one minute. The best throw of the three trials is counted. Each throw must be preceded by the catch of a pass from center.

Punt for Distance. The punt for distance is executed in much the same way as the pass for distance described above, the punters working in pairs, each punter being allowed three trials, the punt being preceded by a pass from center. The ball must be kicked within two seconds after receiving the center pass.

Running-Straightaway, Speed, or Sprint. The subject starts on snap of ball by center and from a backfield three-point stance, catches the ball, and carries it by any form used in football for a distance of 50 yards, running as fast as possible. One minute is allowed for warm-up.

[72]Joann Kemp and Marilyn F. Vincent, "Kemp-Vincent Rally Test of Tennis Ability," *Research Quarterly,* **39,** No. 4 (December 1968), 1000.

[73]Frederick W. Cozens, "Ninth Annual Report of Committee on Curriculum Research of the College Physical Education Association: Part III," *Research Quarterly,* **8,** No. 2 (May 1937), 73.

VOLLEYBALL

The items usually found in volleyball tests include the following: serving, return over net, volleying, passing, spiking or killing, set-up, and playing out of the net. French and Cooper[74] experimented with four test elements: repeated volleys, serving, set-up and pass, and recovery from net. They found that the best combination of measures for girls in grades nine to twelve was the serving test and repeated volleys. The validity coefficient of this combination, with ratings of volleyball ability as the criterion, was found to be 0.81. Bassett, Glassow, and Locke[75] studied the reliability and validity of two volleyball test items, serving and volleying, with college women. Reliability of the serving test was 0.84, and of the volleying test, 0.89. Validity coefficients, using the composite ratings of three judges as criterion, were 0.79 for the serving test and 0.51 for the volleying test.

Russell-Lange Volleyball Test

Russell and Lange[76] studied the two test items recommended by French and Cooper, serving and repeated volleys, as applied to girls in grades seven, eight, and nine. They concluded that these tests, with slight modifications, were adequate for use with girls in the junior high school. Validity and reliability ratings were about the same as those reported by French and Cooper. Brief descriptions of the serving and volleying tests as given by Russell and Lange are as follows.

[74]Esther L. French and Bernice I. Cooper, "Achievement Tests in Volleyball for High School Girls," *Research Quarterly,* **8**, No. 2 (May 1937), 150.

[75]Gladys Bassett, Ruth Glassow, and Mabel Locke, "Studies in Testing Volleyball Skills," *Research Quarterly,* **8**, No. 4 (December 1937), 60.

[76]Naomi Russell and Elizabeth Lange, "Achievement Tests in Volleyball for High School Girls," *Research Quarterly,* **11**, No. 4 (December 1940), 33.

Serving Test. The subject serves ten times in a legal manner into a target on the court across the net. "Let" serves are repeated. Special court markings, as shown in Figure 14.19: (1) Chalk line across court five feet inside and parallel to end line. (2) Chalk line across court parallel to and 12½ feet from the line under the net. (3) Chalk lines five feet inside and parallel to each sideline, extending from line under the net to line (1). Each service is scored according to the value of the target area in which the ball lands, as shown in the diagram. A ball landing on a line separating two areas is given the highest value. A ball landing on a side or the endline scores the value of the area adjacent. Trials in which foot faults occur score zero. (This test is identical with the one proposed by French and Cooper.)

Volleying Test. In this test, the subject volleys as rapidly as possible against a wall. Special court markings are as follows: (1) A line 10 feet long marked on the wall at net height, 7½ feet from the floor. (2) A line on the floor 10 feet long and 3 feet from the wall. The subject starts the volley from behind the 3-foot line, with an underhand movement tosses the ball to the wall, and then volleys the ball repeatedly against the wall above the net line for 30 seconds. The ball may be set up as many times as desired or necessary; it may be caught and re-started with a toss as at the beginning. If the ball gets out of control, it must be retrieved by the subject and put

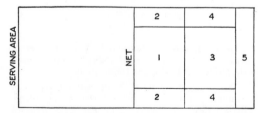

FIGURE 14.19. *Diagram of Zones for Russell-Lange Volleyball Serving Test*

into play at the 3-foot line as at the beginning. The score consists of the number of times the ball is clearly batted (not tossed) from behind the 3-foot line to the wall above or on the net line. The best score of three trials is recorded. Rest periods between trials should be allowed. (In the French-Cooper volleying test, each trial is for 15 seconds and a total of ten trials is completed by each subject, the score for the test being the sum of the five best trials.) Russell and Lange have provided scoring tables for these two tests applied to junior high school girls, as shown in Appendix Table B.31.

Brady Volleyball Test

A volleying test has been proposed by Brady[77] as a measure of general volleyball playing ability for college men. In this test, a simple target is marked on a smooth side wall, consisting of a horizontal chalk line 5 feet long and 11½ feet from the floor; vertical lines are extended upward toward the ceiling at the ends of the horizontal line. In the test, the subject stands where he wishes and throws the ball against the wall, he then volleys it as many times as possible in one minute. Only legal volleys are counted, that is, they must be volleys, not thrown balls, and they must hit the wall within the boundaries of the target. If the ball is caught or gets out of control, it is started again as at the beginning of the test.

A reliability coefficient of 0.93 was found between repeated tests by the subjects during the same testing period. For validity, a coefficient of 0.86 is reported between scores on the test and the combined judgment of four qualified observers.

Inasmuch as the Brady wall volleying test was developed for college men, other investigators have proposed changes in this type of test for other groups. For college women, Clifton[78] used restraining lines on the floor marked five and seven feet from the wall; the wall area was marked the same as for the Russell-Lange volleying test; the score was the number of times a volleyball was legally volleyed in 30 seconds from behind a given restraining line. The subjects were rated on their volleyball playing ability by five experienced judges during a volleyball game as a criterion of playing ability. Comparing results from the five-foot and seven-foot restraining lines, the seven-foot line was accepted for the test. The validity coefficient for the final test was 0.70; the test-retest reliability coefficient was 0.83.

Kronqvist and Brumbach[79] studied a number of volleyball tests for high school boys, finally selecting a volleying type similar to Brady's test. The wall target area has a five-foot line, 11 feet from the floor; from both ends of this line, lines extend toward the ceiling for at least four feet. No restraining line on the floor is used. The test consists of three 20-second trials of repetitive volleying. For validity, a correlation coefficient of 0.78 was obtained between the test and ratings of volleyball ability by three experienced judges using a rating scale; the test-retest reliability coefficient was 0.82.

An adaptation of the Brady test was made by Cummisky[80] for boys aged 11 through 14 years. The wall line is five feet long, placed eight feet above the floor; the usual four-foot vertical lines are drawn at

[77]George F. Brady, "Preliminary Investigations of Volleyball Playing Ability," *Research Quarterly*, **16**, No. 1 (March 1945), 14.

[78]Marguerite A. Clifton, "Single-Hit Volley Test for Women's Volleyball," *Research Quarterly*, **33**, No. 2 (May 1962), 208.

[79]Roger A. Kronqvist, and Wayne B. Brumbach, "A Modification of the Brady Volleyball Skill Test for High School Boys," *Research Quarterly*, **39**, No. 1 (March 1968), 116.

[80]Joseph K. Cummisky, "The Effects of Motivation and Verbal Reinforcement upon Performance and Complex Perceptual-Motor Tasks," Doctoral Dissertation, Stanford University, 1962.

the ends of this line. A backdrop is set up 15 feet from the target wall to act as a barrier in retrieving loose balls. A 15-second practice trial is allowed before the test is begun. The test consists of two volleying sessions, one for 30 seconds and the other for 45 seconds. The test-retest reliability coefficient was 0.86.

AAHPER Volleyball Test Manual

A single AAHPER Volleyball Test Manual is available for both boys and girls. Instructions and scoring tables for the following four skills are provided: volleying, serving, passing, and set-up.

Johnson Test of General Sports Skills

Johnson[81] constructed a test battery to measure skills of college men in basketball, soccer, softball, touch football and volleyball. Twenty-five test items, selected as basic skills of the five sports, were utilized as a criterion measure. A multiple correlation of 0.91 was obtained between the following five items and the criterion.

1. Football pass for distance. Same as in the Borleske tests.

2. Basketball dribble. Same as in the Johnson and Knox tests.

3. Volleyball volleying test. Same as in the Brady test.

4. Softball throw for distance. Best of three distance throws with a 12-inch softball. A run is permitted.

[81]Kenneth P. Johnson, "A Measure of General Sports Skill of College Men," Doctoral Dissertation, Indiana University, 1956.

5. Soccer repeated volleys. An outline 15 feet long and 10 feet high is drawn on a wall. A floor area 30 feet square is also marked out; a restraining line is drawn five feet from the wall. Six assistants are placed around the floor area (two on each side and two across the back line) who stop the ball when it is about to leave the area and place it on the line where it would have crossed. The test is for the subject to kick the ball against the wall as many times as possible in one minute. The score is the number of balls which strike within the target or on the line outlining the target.

The subject's total score is calculated from the following regression equation:

2.8(Basketball dribble) + 0.6(soccer repeated volley) + 1.1(softball distance throw) + 1.0(touch football distance pass) + 0.4(volleyball volleying).

The following norms indicate the student's general sports skill rating:

Score	Rating
370–up	Excellent
287–369	Good
203–286	Average
121–202	Poor
120–below	Inferior

SELECTED REFERENCES

BARROW, HAROLD M., and ROSEMARY MCGEE. *A Practical Approach to Measurement in Physical Education,* 2nd ed. Philadelphia: Lea and Febiger, 1971, Ch. 9.

JOHNSON, BARRY L., and JACK K. NELSON. *Practical Measurements for Evaluation in Physical Education,* 2nd ed. Minneapolis: Burgess Publishing Co., 1972, Ch. 18.

CHAPTER 15

In this chapter, tests of knowledge and attitudes will be presented. Such tests should play an important role in the total evaluation of health and physical education. It is of interest, however, that the commercial publication of knowledge tests has been confined mostly to those in health education.

PHYSICAL EDUCATION

In connection with the teaching of the various activities included in the physical education program, it is important to give pupils instruction not only in the skills involved, but in various types of information, such as the rules governing the activity, the requirements of the performers, the general strategy of the game, the history of the activity, and its general value to the pupil. Details describing the construction of knowledge tests appear in Chapter 2.

Objective knowledge tests have at least three important purposes in physical education:

1. To discover the pupil's level of knowledge at the beginning of a course of instruction. This

initial information permits the instructor to eliminate those phases of the course already familiar to the class and to concentrate his attention on less well known parts.

2. To determine the degree to which pupils have grasped the subject matter presented. This is the typical use of such tests in the academic classroom.

3. To motivate learning. Objective knowledge tests given from time to time acquaint students with their level of ability and with their rate of progress, which may thus motivate further effort.

When using physical education knowledge tests, the recency of their construction may well be considered. The rules of some sports, such as basketball and football, are constantly being changed by the governing bodies; thus, rules in such sports included in knowledge tests prepared some years ago may no longer be correct in this respect. The rules of other sports, such as soccer, softball, tennis, and volleyball, are quite constant, so recency in this regard need not be a concern. However, strategy does change, techniques may improve, understanding of the activity may be enhanced through research, and the histories of sports are ongoing. Such developments would obviously not be reflected in the older knowledge tests.

Comprehensive Tests

Hooks' Comprehensive Knowledge Tests. Hooks[1] constructed multiple-choice knowledge tests for college men in badminton, softball, tennis, and volleyball. Preliminary test items were derived from text and reference book statements and from personal experience. These items were evaluated by experts in each sport in relation to subject-matter content, test construction technicalities, and editorial

Knowledge Tests

[1]Edgar W. Hooks, "Hooks' Comprehensive Knowledge Test in Selected Physical Education Activities for College Men," *Research Quarterly,* **37,** No. 4 (December 1966), 506.

quality. Each test was then administered to 185 college men. As a result of item analyses based on this testing, each final test contained 50 items. Reliability coefficients, as determined by the odd-even method corrected for full test length by the Spearman-Brown prophecy formula, were 0.88 for badminton, 0.89 for softball, 0.86 for tennis, and 0.95 for volleyball. National percentile norms were developed for each of the four tests. The samples for the norms were obtained from testing freshman and sophomore men in 89 colleges and universities throughout the United States; the number of men tested were 2832, badminton; 3513, softball; 2740, tennis; and 4140, volleyball.

Walker's General Knowledge Inventory Test. Walker[2] constructed a general knowledge inventory test for a general foundations course in physical education for men and women at the University of Florida. From a review of the literature and college curricula, six content areas were identified, as follows: physiological principles of exercise and movement, kinesiological and mechanical principles, sports knowledge, motor learning, safety and first aid, and objectives of physical education. With the aid of qualified physical educators, a pool of 225 best-answer multiple-choice questions were developed. After refining these questions by utilization of a jury of five experts and following item-analysis procedures, two forms of the inventory test were proposed. Subsequent investigation, however, demonstrated that the two forms were not equivalent, as Form B was shown to be significantly more difficult.

Hennis Knowledge Tests.   Multiple-choice knowledge tests suitable for use in the college women's instructional program for

badminton, basketball, bowling, field hockey, softball, tennis, and volleyball were constructed by Hennis.[3] Preliminary to the construction of the tests, an analysis of textbooks and printed source material for each sport was made. Based largely on this analysis, checklists were prepared and sent to various types of colleges and universities throughout the United States; the item content for these tests was determined from the replies. An item analysis was made for each test following the administration of the tests at 44 institutions. Reliability coefficients for the different tests range from 0.72 to 0.81.

The revised forms of the tests contain from 33 to 37 items. In general, the types of course content sampled include the following: history of the sport, equipment, etiquette, skills and techniques, playing strategy, team tactics, and rules and scoring. Percentile norms for the tests were constructed based upon test results from a large number of women students at many colleges and universities.

Knowledge Tests by French.   French[4] constructed extensive knowledge tests for college women physical education majors in the following activities: badminton, basketball, body mechanics, canoeing, field hockey, folk dancing, golf, rhythms, soccer, softball, stunts and tumbling, swimming, track and field, volleyball, and recreational sports (aerial darts, bowling, deck tennis, handball, shuffle board, table tennis, and tetherball). Two forms of the tests were presented, a long form and a short form. The reliabilities of the tests for the long form are from 0.70 to 0.88; for the short form, they range from 0.62 to

---

[2]William P. Walker, "The Development of a General Knowledge Inventory Test and a Resource Syllabus for a General Foundation Course in Physical Education for College Freshmen," Doctoral Dissertation, University of Florida, 1965.

[3]Gail M. Hennis, "Construction of Knowledge Tests in Selected Physical Education Activities for College Women," *Research Quarterly*, **27**, No. 3 (October 1956), 301.

[4]Esther French, "The Construction of Knowledge Tests in Selected Professional Courses in Physical Education," *Research Quarterly*, **14**, No. 4 (December 1943), 406.

0.88. From 21 to 26 questions compose the various tests. Norms are available for the short forms.

Scott's Knowledge Tests. The Central Association of Physical Education for College Women, through its Research Committee with M. Gladys Scott as chairman, constructed physical education knowledge tests for college women. The purposes of this project were to develop tests that are superior to those that individual teachers have time to prepare, that will serve as an adequate measure of comprehension in the respective activities, and that will provide a pattern for the construction of other test items and examinations.

Knowledge tests for three different physical education activities were completed. These are: swimming,[5] tennis,[6] and badminton.[7] In each instance, the test battery consisted of multiple-choice and true-false statements. The procedures used in constructing the tests were similar, the steps being as follows:

1. Preparation of experimental form. Questionnaires concerning the content included and the teaching procedures used in presenting each of the activities to physical education classes were sent to a large number of college teachers in the central district. From the replies received, the members of the committee for each sport suggested questions for the experimental form of the tests. These statements were then submitted to a number of teachers of women students participating in the separate activities; the final experimental batteries were prepared from the criticisms made by these people.

2. Revision of experimental form. The experimental form for each of the tests was sent to a number of colleges and universities and there

[5]M. Gladys Scott, "Achievement Examinations for Elementary and Intermediate Swimming Classes," *Research Quarterly,* **11,** No. 2 (May 1940), 100.

[6]M. Gladys Scott, "Achievement Examinations for Elementary and Intermediate Tennis Classes," *Research Quarterly,* **12,** No. 1 (March 1941), 40.

[7]M. Gladys Scott, "Achievement Examinations in Badminton," *Research Quarterly,* **12,** No. 2 (May 1941), 242.

administered to women participating in the respective activities. Following this, the results were tabulated and analyzed, the various test items revised, and the final test battery determined. In one instance, swimming, the revised test form was again submitted to women in some 12 institutions and again revised. Test items were retained on the following bases.

(a) Index of discrimination. The index of discrimination was used as the measure of validity for each individual item included in the test. The formula is: M rights $- M$ wrongs, in which "M rights" is the total score of all cases answering the item correctly, and "M wrongs" is the total score of those answering the item incorrectly. The minimum difference considered significant was arbitrarily selected and varied somewhat for the different tests. The following were chosen: elementary swimming, 6.5; intermediate swimming, 5.5; badminton, 4.0.

(b) Difficulty rating. The difficulty rating of each test item is the percentage of subjects who passed the item. The easiest item (those with difficulty ratings over 95) were omitted. In general, the tests for all three activities are overbalanced on the easy end.

(c) Elimination of choices. Choices in the multiple-choice items that were never selected by the experimental subjects were eliminated.

3. Reliability. The reliability of the test batteries was computed by correlating the odd-numbered items against the even-numbered items and the full test length estimated by use of the Spearman-Brown Prophecy Formula. The results were as follows:

Test	*r*
Swimming:	
Elementary test	0.89
Intermediate test	0.88
Tennis:	
Elementary test	0.87
Intermediate test	0.78
Badminton	0.72–0.79

For each test, scoring tables based on letter grades were prepared. These follow a percentage distribution based roughly upon equal segments of the normal probability curve. In Scott's reports, the complete knowledge tests are given, together with scoring keys and tables.

Badminton

In addition to the Scott tests mentioned above, two other badminton knowledge tests have been constructed for use with college women.

Phillips Test. In a test constructed by Marjorie Phillips,[8] the questions consist of multiple-choice and true-false types. Validity was based upon three criteria: questions were constructed from a table of specifications developed from course outlines, texts, statements of objectives, and opinions of 14 experienced badminton teachers; indices of discrimination were computed; and the Votaw curve applied to upper and lower halves was used. Reliability of the test as determined by the Kuder-Richardson techniques is 0.92 when corrected for guessing. Percentile and T-scales are available for beginners and intermediates.

University of Washington. A committee of the Women's Physical Education Department, University of Washington, chaired by Katharine Fox, constructed a beginning badminton knowledge test.[9] The test consists of 106 questions of different types, including multiple choice, true-false, and identification. The questions test the student's knowledge of strokes and techniques, rules and scoring, strategy and terminology. In constructing the test, the usual procedures for obtaining curricular validity and item validity were followed. The reliability coefficient for the test is 0.90. The test questions and scoring table appear in the reference.

Golf

A golf knowledge test was constructed by Waglow and Rehling[10] for use in physical education service courses for college men. The test consists of 100 true-false statements. Curricular validity was based on an analysis of prominent books on golf. The reported reliability of the test is 0.82. The test questions and T-score standards are included in the reference.

Gymnastics

Gershon[11] developed a knowledge test of apparatus gymnastics for college men in professional physical education. Curricular validity was obtained from a review of textbooks, courses of study, and periodical literature dealing with gymnastics. A check-list from this analysis was submitted to a qualified jury to obtain their estimates of the contribution of the subject matter to a course in apparatus gymnastics. The major areas included in this apparatus gymnastics knowledge test are as follows: apparatus activities, mechanical principles and coaching hints, health and safety, nomenclature, learning and motivation, competitions and exhibitions, general education values, selection and care of equipment, and history.

An experimental test was administered to 586 college men in professional physical education at 21 colleges and universities. Item analysis data obtained from this administration resulted in a revised test of 100 items. National norms were established from the results of testing 940 professional students in 40 colleges and universities representing various sections of the United States.

[8]Majorie Phillips, "Standardization of a Badminton Knowledge Test for College Women," *Research Quarterly,* **17,** No. 1 (March 1946), 48.

[9]Katharine Fox, "Beginning Badminton Written Examination," *Research Quarterly,* **24,** No. 2 (May 1953), 135.

[10]I. F. Waglow and C. H. Rehling, "A Golf Knowledge Test," *Research Quarterly,* **24,** No. 4 (December 1953), 463.

[11]Ernest Gershon, "Apparatus Gymnastics Knowl-

Handball

Phillips[12] presented a knowledge test of handball as a part of his text in this sport, but did not subject it to statistical analysis. The test consists of 50 true-false statements divided into two parts: Part I, rules and glossary; Part II, fundamental techniques.

Field Hockey

Kelly and Brown[13] constructed an objective written examination on field hockey, designed for use with women majoring in physical education who are prospective teachers, coaches, and umpires of field hockey. This test consists of 88 multiple-response questions, designed to test the following four major areas: rules, techniques, coaching procedures, and officiating. A copy of the test questions may be obtained from one of the authors. Validity of the test was established by item analysis, by comparisons of scores made by expert, major, service, and lay groups, and by correlation of test scores with extent of field hockey experience and with instructor's ratings of the competence of major students to teach field hockey. The reliability coefficient for the test is between 0.79 and 0.89.

Deitz and Freck[14] proposed a field hockey test for grades nine through twelve, composed of 77 true-false and completion statements. In preparing the test, consideration was given to comprehensiveness, administrative efficiency, and flexibility in regard to ease of alteration with changing rules. The test was formulated from the authors' teaching experiences, no validity or reliability coefficients being reported.

Ice Hockey

Brown[15] presented a brief test, composed of 18 questions and true-false statements, based upon the rules for girls' ice hockey. No attempt was made to validate the test or to determine reliability for it.

Physical Fitness

A test of physical fitness knowledge was constructed by Mood[16] to measure the physical fitness understanding of senior physical education major students. A pool of 184 multiple-choice questions was formed based on 60 physical fitness facts secured from current physical fitness literature and the opinions of 73 members of the Research Council of the American Association for Health, Physical Education, and Recreation. These test items were adminstered to 1360 physical education major students enrolled in 35 collegiate institutions in the United States. As a result of item analysis based on these data, two parallel forms of the test, each containing 60 questions, were developed. In order to determine the validity and reliability of the test forms and to establish national norms for them, they were given to 4167 students enrolled in 150 colleges

edge Test for College Men in Professional Physical Education," *Research Quarterly*, **28,** No. 4 (December 1957), 332.

[12]Bernath E. Phillips, *Fundamental Handball* (New York: A. S. Barnes & Co., Inc., 1937).

[13]Ellen D. Kelly and Jane E. Brown, "The Construction of a Field Hockey Test for Women Physical Education Majors," *Research Quarterly*, **23,** No. 3 (October 1952), 322.

[14]Dorothea Deitz and Beryl Freck, "Hockey Knowledge Tests for Girls," *Journal of Health and Physical Education*, **11,** No. 6 (June 1940), 366.

[15]Harriett M. Brown, "The Game of Ice Hockey," *Journal of Health and Physical Education*, **6,** No. 1 (January 1935), 28.

[16]Dale Mood, "Test of Physical Fitness Knowledge: Construction, Administration, and Norms," *Research Quarterly*, **42,** No. 4 (December 1971), 423.

and universities. Ten physical fitness content areas were included in the test, as follows: current status and promotion, evaluation, kinesiological aspects, nutritional aspects, programs, relation to disease, physiological aspects, psychological aspects, sociological aspects, and miscellaneous concepts.

Much earlier, a physical fitness knowledge test was proposed by Stradtman and Cureton[17] for secondary school boys and girls. A preliminary test of 184 five-item multiple-choice questions was submitted to competent persons in physical fitness, physical education, and physiology and to graduate classes in physical education. From these data, a final test of 100 questions was established. Reliability coefficients for high school boys and girls were 0.96 and 0.94 respectively, determined by the split-halves method, corrected for full test length by use of the Spearman-Brown prophecy formula. Percentile norms were prepared for high school boys and girls.

Soccer

Heath and Rodgers set up a knowledge test for fifth- and sixth-grade boys consisting of 100 true-false statements dealing with playing regulations and game situations.[18] Validity for the test is claimed on the basis of: the "choice of material suitable for the test" and differences of accomplishments between grades five and six. The coefficient of reliability of the test is 0.90. T-scales for the fifth and sixth grades are also provided.

Winn[19] developed a soccer knowledge

test for college men; two forms of true-false and multiple-choice questions are available. Curricular validity was based on an analysis of eight tests of soccer and the current periodical literature on this sport; judgments of competent persons concerned with soccer were also utilized to determine the essential objectives to be realized in a soccer course and the emphasis to be placed on each. Statistical validity was obtained by use of the Votaw formula applied to the upper and lower 27 percent. The reliability coefficient by split-half method corrected by Spearman-Brown formula for all 100 questions was 0.94; this coefficient was 0.81 for each of the short forms, A and B. The total test correlated around 0.90 with the short forms. T-scale norms are available. The tests and norms appear in the reference.

Softball

Rodgers and Heath[20] proposed a test of softball for fifth- and sixth-grade boys consisting of 100 true-false statements on game rules and game maneuvers. The reliability coefficient for the test was 0.89, utilizing the method of correlation of chance halves corrected by Spearman's formula. The questions and a T-scale table appear in the report.

A softball test for determining the extent of knowledge of college men in service courses was developed by Waglow and Stephens.[21] The test consists of 60 true-false statements, 25 completion items, 10 ball-in-play or dead-ball situations, and 5 fair-or-foul questions. Curricular validity was based on the softball course as taught at the University of Florida. The value of various items in the test were determined

[17]Alan D. Stradtman and T. K. Cureton, "A Physical Fitness Knowledge Test for Secondary School Boys and Girls," *Research Quarterly*, **21**, No. 1 (March 1950), 53.

[18]Marjorie L. Heath and Elizabeth G. Rodgers, "A Study in the Use of Knowledge and Skill Tests in Soccer," *Research Quarterly*, **3**, No. 4 (December 1932), 33.

[19]Jerome E. Winn, "Soccer Knowledge Test for College Men," Doctoral Dissertation, Indiana University, 1957.

[20]Elizabeth G. Rodgers and Marjorie L. Heath, "An Experiment in the Use of Knowledge and Skill Tests in Playground Baseball," *Research Quarterly*, **2**, No. 4 (December 1931), 113.

[21]I. F. Waglow and Foy Stephens, "A Softball Knowledge Test," *Research Quarterly*, **26**, No. 2 (May 1955), 234.

by computing difficulty ratings and indices of discrimination. The reliability of the test is 0.78. The test questions appear in the reference.

Swimming

Under the chairmanship of M. Gladys Scott,[22] the Central Association of Physical Education for College Women developed elementary and intermediate swimming tests for college women. The elementary form consists of 30 multiple-choice and 26 true-false questions; the intermediate form, 22 multiple-choice and 36 true-false statements. The questions were based on the material commonly taught in swimming classes, as revealed by a questionnaire answered by the swimming instructors at the colleges in the district. Item analysis was based on tests administered to women students in nine of the colleges. Reliability coefficients were 0.86 and 0.89, respectively, for the elementary and intermediate forms. The test questions and answers appear in the reference.

Tennis

Hewitt's Comprehensive Tennis Knowledge Test.[23] This test was first presented in 1937; complete revisions of Forms A and B were reported in 1964. During the interim, 10,000 copies were used by tennis teachers. The revised forms consist of 50 questions each, covering fundamentals of the game, rules of tennis, playing situations, history of tennis, and equipment. By item analysis and by use of Holzinger's index of discrimination, difficulty ratings were determined from the percentage of beginners, advanced, and varsity groups passing each item. By using the

Spearman-Brown prophecy formula between the odd versus even items for both forms combined (100 questions), a correlation of 0.95 was obtained. The test questions and grading norms appear in the reference.

University of Washington Test.[24] A committee of the Women's Physical Education Department, University of Washington, developed a knowledge test which is associated with their tennis test described in the preceding chapter. Five test forms are used: multiple-choice, true-false, completion, matching, and identification. Knowledge of the following phases of tennis are tested: position, timing, and footwork; fundamental and advanced strokes; strategy and court position; history and events; equipment and court markings; rules and scoring. Item validity was determined from the performances of the upper and lower thirds of the subjects on the total test. The reliability of the test for the beginning group was 0.82, and for the intermediate group was 0.92. The examinations are included in the reference.

Miller Knowledge Test. Wilma Miller's knowledge test[25] is associated with her tennis skill test described in the preceding chapter. This test is designed for use with college women who are majors in physical education. One hundred true-false, multiple response, and multiple-choice questions compose this test, designed to sample the following types of information: history, rules, equipment and facilities, technics and strokes, strategy and tactics, tournaments, terminology, and etiquette.

[22]M. Gladys Scott, "Achievement Examinations for Elementary and Intermediate Swimming Classes," *Research Quarterly,* **11,** No. 2 (May 1940), 100.

[23]Jack E. Hewitt, "Hewitt's Comprehensive Tennis Knowledge Test—Form A and B Revised," *Research Quarterly,* **35,** No. 2 (May 1964), 147.

[24]Marion R. Broer and Donna M. Miller, "Achievement Tests for Beginning and Intermediate Tennis," *Research Quarterly,* **21,** No. 3 (October 1950), 303.

[25]Wilma K. Miller, "Achievement Levels in Tennis Knowledge and Skill for Women Physical Education Major Students," *Research Quarterly,* **24,** No. 1 (March 1953), 81.

Curricular validity was established through analyses of textbooks, courses of study, and the judgment of competent persons. Statistical validity of the test was determined by use of the Votaw formula, using the highest-scoring and lowest-scoring 27 percent of the distribution of the scores of 381 students. Reliability of the test is 0.90.

Volleyball

Langston[26] constructed and standardized a test to measure the volleyball knowledge of men majoring in physical education who have completed their course of instruction in this sport. The test is composed of 100 statements, Part I consists of 70 true-false questions, Part II of 30 multiple-choice questions. The phases of volleyball tested are history, pass, set-up, spike, net recovery, block, service, offensive strategy, defensive strategy, rules, and officiating. Curricular validity was accomplished through analysis of published material followed by the judgment of competent volleyball instructors. The usual item validity and discrimination analyses were employed. The questions were coded for IBM scoring.

Professional Students

While other tests presented in this chapter are useful in courses for physical education major students, some tests have been developed specifically for the professional student. Two of these tests will be presented here.

Cowell's Principles Tests.[27] Cowell designed a 50-item multiple-choice test to evaluate the general background of senior physical education students and their ability to recognize the operation of certain principles and generalizations from a number of disciplines from which physical education draws its basic principles. It may also be used as one of several screening tests to indicate readiness for graduate study in physical education. The principles and generalizations are drawn from the areas of scientific method, philosophy of education, sociology, biology, growth and development, psychology, curriculum development, methods, physiology of activity, cultural anthropology, and evaluation. The construction of this test involved item analysis and index of discrimination. The subjects were 200 physical education undergraduate and master's candidates from seven universities. Separate scales were constructed for freshman men and women combined and senior and graduate men and women combined.

Rhoda's Vocabulary Test.[28] Rhoda developed a technical vocabulary test for senior and graduate students in the three physical education areas of physiological sciences, measurement and evaluation, and adapted and corrective physical education. Each area of the test consists of 30 multiple-choice questions. The words selected for definition were based on an analysis of leading textbooks in each of the three areas. Only words which occurred in two-thirds of the textbooks in each area were included; definitions were taken from standard dictionaries and textbooks. Reliability coefficients for the total text were 0.85 for seniors and 0.90 for graduate students. Norms were constructed from testing 295 seniors and 417 graduate students in 14 leading physical education schools. Subsequently, Monahan[29] ob-

[26]Dewey F. Langston, "Standardization of a Volleyball Knowledge Test for College Men Physical Education Majors," *Research Quarterly,* **26,** No. 1 (March 1955), 60.

[27]Charles C. Cowell, "Cowell Test of Ability to Recognize the Operation of Certain Principles Important to Physical Education" (Lafayette, Ind.: Purdue University, 1961).

[28]William P. Rhoda, "The Construction and Standardization of a Test of Technical Vocabulary in Selected Areas of Physical Education for Senior and Graduate Levels," Doctoral Dissertation, University of Oregon, 1951.

[29]Russell D. Monahan, "The Relationship Between the Miller Analogies Test and the Technical Vocabu-

tained a correlation of 0.62 between Rhoda's vocabulary test and the Miller Analogies Test, with graduate students as subjects. This test is available through the author, University of Oregon, Eugene, Oregon.

ATTITUDE SCALES

As can be readily recognized, positive attitudes toward physical education are vital in effective motivation for present and future participation in physical activities. Many studies have been conducted to assess the attitude of college men and women toward local physical education. Some attention has also been given to the scientific construction of attitude scales; certain of these scales are presented here.

Kenyon's Scales. Based upon a multidimensional model for characterizing physical activity, Kenyon[30] developed two forms of an attitude inventory, one for college women and the other for college men. Items held to be representative of six dimensions were studied; the six dimensions are social experience, health and fitness, pursuit of vertigo (thrills and excitement), aesthetic experience, catharsis (relaxation and recreation), and ascetic experience (meeting physical challenge). Student response of each statement was made on a seven-alternative Likert-type scale. The selected statements were evaluated by factor and item analyses using data obtained from preliminary forms. Reliability coefficients ranged between 0.72 and 0.89 for the two forms of the six scales. These scales differentiated significantly between high and low preference groups for various types of physical activities, except for the "catharsis" scale. The

stability of the instrument was demonstrated by comparing measures of central tendency, variability, and reliability of the original sample with a second sample drawn from the same population.

Sonstroem Scales. Sonstroem[31] developed "Physical Estimation and Attraction Scales," constructed to contain two scores, estimation of one's physical ability and attraction to vigorous physical activity. These scales were extensions of earlier work by the author and of Kenyon's six attitude instrumentations for physical activity. An item pool of 155 attitude statements was administered to 710 boys in grades nine through twelve. Factor analysis revealed seven factors including one massive factor composed almost entirely of attraction statements. These factors were named, as follows.

1. Endorsement of Sports Value. Expresses a generalized appreciation of physical activity and benefits often accorded sports participation.

2. Physical Ascendance. Affirms the possession of physical endowments, such as strength, athletic ability, and leadership, often expressed in comparison with peers.

3. Confidence and Physical Potential. Affirms confidence at performing physical skills.

4. Attraction to Robust Activity. Expresses a desire to experience satisfaction from participating in strenuous, sometimes dangerous, most often noncompetitive activities, such as mountain climbing, calisthenics, judo, etc.

5. Interest and Ability in Running. Expresses attraction for and ability in activities that require running endurance and speed.

6. Recreational Skill Potential. Affirms possession of skill potential at bowling, golf, and tennis.

7. Attraction to Tennis. Expresses a preference for tennis as compared to other recreational and sports skills.

Further item analysis produced a final battery of 89 items. Preferred responses

---

lary Test," Master's Thesis, University of Oregon, 1965.

[30]Gerald S. Kenyon, "Six Scales for Assessing Attitude Toward Physical Activity," *Research Quarterly,* **39,** No. 3 (October 1968), 566.

[31]Robert J. Sonstroem, "Attitude Testing Examining Certain Psychological Correlates of Physical Activity," *Research Quarterly,* **45,** No. 2 (May 1974), 93.

were summed to obtain scores for Estimation, Attraction, and the seven factors. Internal reliability coefficients by Kuder-Richardson method for the scales ranged from 0.70 to 0.90. Significant correlation coefficients were reported between scales composed of Estimation items and measures of height, athletic experience, self-acceptance, and the Fleishman Basic Fitness Test. Copies of the scales may be obtained from the author, University of Rhode Island, Kingston.

Wear's Attitude Scales. Wear conducted two studies in efforts to evaluate the intensity of individual and group attitudes of college men toward physical education activities. The initial attitude scale consists of 120 statements; later, two equivalent forms of 30 statements each[32] were proposed. In preparing the equivalent forms, statements were matched on the bases of discrimination and favorableness indices; similar statements were placed in opposite forms, and statements on the two forms approximated the same expected objectives or outcomes of physical education. The reliability coefficients for the two forms were 0.94 and 0.96. The correlation between the forms was 0.96. Further, the means and standard deviations of the subjects taking the two forms were equivalent. The attitude scales appear in the references.

Kneer[33] revised the Wear Attitude Inventory in order to adapt its reading level to high school girls and to clarify statements found to be ambiguous by these girls. The correlation between the two inventories was 0.84. The correlation between the Kneer adaptation and graphic self-rating of attitude was 0.89; a reliability

coefficient of 0.95 is reported. Balshiser[34] obtained a low but significant positive correlation between the Kneer Adaptation and Scott's General Motor Ability Test, thus demonstrating that the attitude of high school girls toward physical education was highly related to their motor ability. The Kneer attitude scale appears in the reference.

The Wear Attitude Inventory was applied to junior high school boys by Campbell.[35] The mean inventory score for each grade, seven, eight, and nine, was found to be equal or superior to the mean reported in Wear's validation study with college men. In two categories of the scale, physical and social, eighth grade boys scored significantly higher than did those in the seventh and ninth grades. The investigator concluded that the Wear inventory was an appropriate instrument to assess the attitudes toward physical education of junior high school boys.

Johnson's Sportsmanship Scales. Alternate forms of a sportsmanship attitude scale were developed by Johnson[36] for junior high school boys and girls. An initial pool of 152 items pertaining to ethically critical behavior in the sports of football, basketball, and baseball provided the initial pool of attitude statements for the scales. These items were successfully treated with the equal-appearing interval, summated rating, and item analysis methods of constructing attitude scales. On these bases, 42 items were accepted for the final scale forms. These items were divided to provide two equivalent scale forms; a

[32]Carlos L. Wear, "Construction of Equivalent Forms of an Attitude Scale," *Research Quarterly,* **26,** No. 1 (March 1955), 113.

[33]Marian E. Kneer, "The Adaptation of Wear's Physical Education Attitude Inventory for Use with High School Girls," Master's Thesis, Illinois State University, 1956.

[34]Shirley Balshiser, "Relationship Between General Motor Ability and Attitude Toward Physical Education of High School Girls," Master's Thesis, Illinois State University, 1959.

[35]Donald E. Campbell, "Wear Attitude Inventory Applied to Junior High School Boys," *Research Quarterly,* **39,** No. 4 (December 1968), 888.

[36]Marion Lee Johnson, "Construction of Sportsmanship Attitude Scales," *Research Quarterly,* **40,** No. 2 (May 1969), 312.

correlation of 0.86 was obtained between the two forms. The coefficients of reproducibility were 0.81 and 0.86.

Other Scales. Other attempts have been made to develop attitude scales in physical education. Mercer[37] revised the Galloway Attitude Inventory for evaluating the attitudes of high school girls toward psychological, moral-spiritual, and sociological values of physical education experiences. Adams[38] proposed two scales for evaluation of the general attitude of high school and college students toward physical education; these scales are based on the Thurston and Chave scaling processes. Edgington[39] constructed a scale to assess the attitudes of ninth grade boys toward physical education. Boys judged by physical education teachers to have the most favorable attitudes toward physical education had a significantly higher means on the scale than did boys judged to have the most unfavorable attitudes.

HEALTH EDUCATION

A common practice among health educators is to utilize the results of health education testing[40] in assigning grades in health instruction courses. However, evaluation and measurement should be much more than this. As previously mentioned, evaluation is a process of determining the effectiveness of the health program and its several phases through the measurement of its progress and the extent to which the health objectives of the school are being achieved. Such evaluation includes purely subjective judgments as well as highly objective measurement of factors affecting health. Planned approaches to health education evaluation should be established; the teacher must then decide whether to choose standardized tests or to construct his own. In either event, the test utilized should meet the criteria of reliability and of curricular and statistical validity outlined in Chapter 2.

A number of health evaluation instruments have appeared in professional journals and have been published commercially. A comprehensive list of these instruments was presented by Solleder[41] in 1961; this list was revised by the same author in 1966. In addition, a book by Beyrer, Nolte, and Solleder[42] contains a section on evaluative instruments. The AAHPER has produced an annotated bibliography of health knowledge, attitudes and behavior tests for all school grades and the first year of college.[43] In this chapter, health education tests to encompass the instructional program from elementary school through college are presented. In the selection of these tests, only comparatively new tests were considered, as older tests could logically be seriously deficient in current scientific health information (tests constructed prior to

[37]Emily L. Mercer, "An Adaptation and Revision of the Galloway Attitude Inventory for Evaluating the Attitudes of High School Girls Toward Psychological, Moral-Spiritual, and Sociological Values in Physical Education Experiences," Master's Thesis, Women's College, University of North Carolina, 1961.

[38]R. S. Adams, "Two Scales for Measuring Attitude Toward Physical Education," *Research Quarterly*, **34**, No. 1 (March 1963), 91.

[39]Charles W. Edgington, "Development of an Attitude Scale to Measure Attitudes of High School Freshman Boys Toward Physical Education," *Research Quarterly*, **39**, No. 3 (October 1968), 505.

[40]Grateful acknowledgement is made to Dr. Lorraine G. Davis, Assistant Professor of Health Education, University of Oregon, for her assistance in the selection, evaluation, and presentation of health education tests contained in this chapter.

[41]Dr. Marian K. Solleder, Professor of Health Education, University of North Carolina, Greensboro, North Carolina.

[42]Mary Beyrer, Ann Nolte, and Marian K. Solleder, *A Directory of Selected References and Resources for Health Instruction* (Minneapolis, Minn.: Burgess Publishing Co., 1966).

[43]*Evaluation Instruments in Health Education.* (Washington, D.C.: American Alliance for Health, Physical Education, and Recreation, 1969).

1960 are omitted). This compilation is not exhaustive but, rather, representative. Further, all tests were checked to determine their current availability; tests no longer readily available were omitted from the text.

Elementary and Junior High Schools

Speer and Smith Health Test.   This test was constructed for grades three through eight. The test consists of 80 true-false and multiple-choice questions designed to evaluate health attitudes through responses to problem situations. Two forms are available; scoring is by letters in a code word. Norms are provided in the form of medians for each grade. *Source:* Robert K. Speer, and Samuel Smith, *Health Test,* rev. ed. (Chicago: Psychometric Affiliates), 1963.

Elementary School Health Behavior Inventory.   This instrument is the first in the series of health behavior inventories from the California Test Bureau; these inventories were utilized as part of a nationwide School Health Survey by the Bronfman Foundation. The test is intended to determine what the pupil does in his daily health habits. It contains 40 picture-question items; each picture provides three choices. Norms are based on 7145 cases. *Source:* Sylvia Yellen, *Health Behavior Inventory, Elementary School* (Monterey, Calif.: California Test Bureau, 1963).

Junior High School Health Behavior Inventory.   Second in the California Test Bureau health behavior inventories, this instrument is designed for use at the junior high school level. It contains 100 multiple-choice questions distributed as follows: 25 on health behavior, 25 on health attitudes, and 50 on health knowledge. Norms are based on 6000 cases. *Source:* Albert D. Colebank, *Health Behavior Inventory, Junior High School* (Monterey, Calif.: California Test Bureau, 1963).

Trudys' Appraisal of Emotional Health Knowledge.   This test appraises knowledge of emotional health by elementary school pupils. It has one form consisting of cartoon-type multiple choice items. *Source:* Lawrence Trudys, "Appraising the Emotional Health Knowledge of A5 Pupils," Independent Study, University of Southern California, 1962.

Lohr's Health Knowledge Test.   Proposed for the upper elementary school grades, Lohr's test examines into 14 health areas; it contains 50 multiple-choice questions. The content of the test was determined from an analysis of current elementary health textbooks. *Source:* Ruth S. Lohr, "The Construction of a Health Knowledge Test for the Upper Elementary Grades," Master's Thesis, University of California at Los Angeles, 1961.

Harrison's Harmful Health Misconceptions.   Harrison proposed an inventory of health misconceptions based on junior high school pupils attending metropolitan public schools. The test has two forms of 90 items each; the forms reflect 70 harmful misconceptions and 29 true concepts. *Source:* E. Price Harrison, "A Determination of the Prevalence of Certain Harmful Misconceptions Among Junior High School Students Attending Public Schools in Metropolitan Areas," Doctoral Dissertation, Boston University, 1962.

Television Health Advertising.   Lowell developed a test on television health advertising as related to health attitudes at the ninth grade level; the form for the test is based on the completion of sentences. Sentence stems are identified with products dealing with relief from pain and tension, with food and nutrition, and with the preventive aspects of health. *Source:* Bernard Lovell, "Television Health Advertising and Its Relationship to Health Attitudes," Doctoral Dissertation, University of Maryland, 1962.

AAHPER Cooperative Health Education Test. This test has three forms, as follows: Forms 3A and B for junior high school, 60 multiple-choice questions each; Form 4 for upper elementary school, 50 multiple-choice questions. Questions pertain to these areas: consumer, community, international, and mental health; disease; personal health care; growth and development; nutrition; drugs; safety; first aid; and sex education (junior high school only). *Source: AAHPER Cooperative Health Education Test* (Berkeley, Calif.: Educational Testing Service, 1972).

Senior High School

Senior High School Health Behavior Inventory. The third in the series of health behavior inventories from the California Test Bureau was developed for high school students. This inventory contains 75 situation-response items; norms are based on 4476 cases. The content of the test covers personal health, safety, first aid, family health, infection, disease, mental health, nutrition, community health, exercise, drinking, smoking, narcotics, and dental health. *Source:* Harold E. LeMaistre, and Marion E. Pollock, *Health Behavior Inventory, Senior High School* (Monterey, Calif.: California Test Bureau, 1963).

Community Health Knowledge Test. This instrument is intended to test the general health knowledge of high school students, grades ten through twelve. The test consists of 120 multiple-choice questions. Basically, this test appears to be a good one; however, the manual contains neither norms nor information on its reliability and validity. *Source:* School District of Philadelphia, *Philadelphia Health Knowledge Test,* Philadelphia, Pa., 1960.

Family Life Education. This instrument is designed to determine the attitude of twelfth grade students toward "my need to learn about this." *Source:* Vernon R. Charlson, "The Need for Family Life Education on the Secondary School Level," Doctoral Dissertation, Indiana University, 1963.

Health Knowledge Examination. The New York State Council on Health and Safety Education developed this health knowledge examination for secondary school students. The test consists of 80 multiple-choice questions. *Source:* John S. Sinacore, *Health Knowledge Examination for the Secondary Level.* (Cortland, N.Y.: State University College of Education, 1962).

Secondary School and College

Kilander Health Knowledge Test. Between 1936 and 1969, Kilander repeatedly revised his health knowledge test for senior high school and college students. The test comprehensively covers the areas of nutrition, safety, first aid, community health and sanitation, communicable diseases, family living, and common errors and superstitions. It contains 100 multiple-choice questions. Percentile tables are available in the manual. *Source:* Frederick H. Kilander, *Kilander Health Knowledge Test* (East Orange, N.J.: The Author, 39 Colonial Terrace).

Fast-Tyson Health Knowledge Test. The Fast-Tyson test was designed for use as a pretest or retest instrument in a basic health course at the high school and college levels. The test evolved over several years of use with the health education tests by Kilander and Dearborn. Two forms are available, each with 100 multiple-choice questions. Ten health areas are included, as follows: personal health; exercise, relaxation, and sleep; nutrition and diet; consumer health; contemporary health problems; tobacco, alcohol, drugs, and narcotics; safety and first aid; communicable and noncommunicable diseases; mental health; sex and family life. *Source:* Charles G. Fast, *Fast-Tyson Health Knowl-*

edge Test (Kirksville, Mo.: The Author, Northwest Missouri State College, 1971).

College and University

College Health Behavior Inventory. Fourth in the health behavior test series from the California Test Bureau, this inventory was prepared for college students. It consists of descriptions of health problems upon which 100 multiple-choice test items are based. *Source:* Carmen P. Reid, *Health Behavior Inventory, College* (Monterey, Calif.: California Test Bureau).

Attitudes Toward Healthful Living. This instrument is a Likert-type scale consisting of 100 items. It was constructed to evaluate opinions in 12 health areas. *Source:* William C. Meise, *A Scale for Measuring Attitudes Toward Healthful Living* (Slippery Rock, Pa.: The Author, Slippery Rock State College, 1962).

Richardson Health Attitude Test. In this instrument, health attitudes of college students are indicated via sentence-completion statements. Fifty-one partial sentences are utilized in the areas of health education, foods and nutrition, physical fitness and exercise, sex and sex education, and physicians and medical care. *Source:* Charles E. Richardson, "A Sentence Completion Health Attitudes Test for College Students," *Journal of School Health,* **30,** No. 1 (January 1960), 32.

Engs Health Concerns Questionnaire. This questionnaire contains 50 multiple-choice questions concerning 20 health worries of college men and women. The items were validated by three qualified health educators. *Source:* Ruth C. Engs, "Health Concerns Questionnaire," Master's Thesis, University of Oregon, 1970.

Bush Health Analogies Test. This test contains 100 multiple-choice items of analogies regarding the health knowledge of college students. *Source:* Herman S. Bush, "A Health Analogies Pretest for a Basic College Health Course," Doctoral Dissertation, Indiana University, 1969.

Smoking and Drugs

Sallak Smoking Habits Questionnaire. This questionnaire was developed for and used in a study of smoking practices of junior and senior high school students in the public schools of Erie County, New York. It is chiefly concerned with the extent of tobacco use and the type of tobacco smoked; additional questions on parental smoking practices are included. *Source:* V. J. Sallak, "A Study of Smoking Practices of Selected Groups of Junior and Senior High School Students in Erie County, N.Y.," *Journal of School Health,* **31** (November 1961), 307.

Thompson Smoking Knowledge Test. This 25-item multiple-choice test was constructed from the concepts which had previously been established as important facts in the physiological, psychological, and socio-economic areas of smoking and tobacco. The difficulty of the test is suitable at and above the seventh grade level. *Source:* Clem W. Thompson, *Thompson Smoking and Tobacco Knowledge Test* (Mankato, Minn.: The Author, Mankato State College, 1963).

Iverson Drug Knowledge Test. This test was developed for and used in a survey of the drug knowledge of college students selected from colleges and universities throughout the United States for the purpose of establishing national norms. *Source:* Donald D. Iverson, "A Drug Knowledge Survey of College Students Selected from Colleges and Universities Throughout the United States," Doctoral Dissertation, University of Oregon, 1971.

Sex and Venereal Disease

Sex Education Attitudes. Segal developed a scale in order to compare the sex attitudes of graduate students in elementary and in secondary education. Following a review of college textbooks in health, family life, and sex education, a Likert-type scale consisting of 80 items was constructed. Eleven areas of sex education are represented in the scale. *Source:* Zen Segal, "A Comparison of Sex Education Attitudes of Graduate Students in Elementary and Secondary Education," Doctoral Dissertation, New York University, 1962.

Smith Venereal Disease Knowledge Test. This instrument was designed to evaluate the level of knowledge about venereal disease attained by high school students. The test contains 77 statements that are answered by indications of agreement, disagreement, or undecided. *Source:* Byron C. Smith, "A Study of the Venereal Disease Knowledge Held by Promiscuous and Non-promiscuous Teenagers 15–18 Years of Age in Oregon," Master's Thesis, University of Oregon, 1960.

Vencel Venereal Disease Test. This test consists of 30 multiple-choice questions pertaining to the venereal disease knowledge of senior high school students. *Source:* Steve A. Vencel, "Venereal Disease Education in Indiana Secondary Schools," Doctoral Dissertation, Indiana University, 1964.

Other Health Topics

Dental Health Knowledge Questionnaire. This questionnaire contains 15 multiple-choice items to evaluate the health knowledge of sixth grade pupils. *Source:* Douglas Koch, Gonan Koch, and Gunilla Tynelius, "Comparison of Three Methods of Teaching Oral Hygiene to School Children," *Journal of Dental Education,* March 1970.

Traffic Safety Attitude Scale. Fulton developed a traffic study attitude scale for ninth grade students consisting of situation-response statements. *Source:* Martin W. Fulton, "A Traffic Safety Attitude Scale for Ninth Grade Students," Doctoral Dissertation, Indiana University, 1964.

Bicycle Safety Quiz. Designed for elementary school pupils, this 20-item true-false quiz can be used independently or in conjunction with showing of the film, "Safe on Two Wheels." *Source:* Information and Education Department, Aetna Life Affiliated Co., Hartford, Conn.

Bicycle Safety Information Test. Suitable for elementary school children, this test contains 20 true-false statements related to bicycle safety. *Source:* National Safety Council, 425 North Michigan Avenue, Chicago, Ill.

Harmful Safety Misconceptions. Designed for seventh and eighth grade pupils, this instrument contains 200 statements of safety misconceptions. Following a review of previous studies and publications, the items were validated by 20 safety experts. *Source:* Phyllis L. Douglas, "A Determination of the Prevalence of Certain Harmful Safety Misconceptions Among Seventh and Eighth Grade Children," Doctoral Dissertation, Boston University, 1961.

General Health Program Evaluation

The general evaluation of a health program should encompass school health services and healthful school environment as well as health instruction. The task of maintaining the health status of the school child is a cooperative, multidisciplinary one. School boards, administrators, teachers, physicians, and nurses have roles to play in this process. The school should do all in its power to protect the health of the student as well as to provide him with a knowledge of sound health practices.

A number of scales are available for use in evaluating the over-all health program in schools and colleges. In applying these instruments, greatest value results when related personnel in a given school situation engage in comprehensive self-study. Self-study can be accomplished under local leadership or under the guidance of outside experts or visiting teams.

Examples of instruments available for conducting such evaluations follow.

National Evaluative Criteria.   The National Study of Secondary School Evaluation prepared evaluative criteria for most programs of study in secondary schools. Included in this series are criteria for both health education and physical education and for health services and school plant. Checklists require the use of five letters; the general evaluations utilize five numbers. *Source: Evaluative Criteria, 1960 Edition* (Washington, D.C.: National Study of School Evaluation).

College Health Service Evaluation.   Kirk developed an instrument for evaluating college health service programs, which consists of descriptive items, utilizing a quantative gradation of scores. *Source:* Robert H. Kirk, *An Instrument for Evaluating College and University Health Service Programs,* rev. ed. (Washington, D.C.: American Alliance for Health, Physical Education, and Recreation, 1964).

New York State Health and Safety Education Review Guide.   The New York State Cooperative Review Service, a joint effort of the State Education Department and local school systems, has developed guides for the review of elementary and secondary school programs in health and safety education. A majority of items in the guides are related to general and specific objectives and organization of the program. Provisions are made for checking curriculum, quality of instruction, facilities, and evaluation techniques. Responses are recorded by checkmarks under two headings: strong aspect or needs improvement. Space for general comments is provided following each section. *Source: A Guide for the Review of a Health and Safety Education Program* (Al-

bany, N.Y.: Cooperative Review Service, State Education Department, 1963).

Washington   Self-Evaluation   Instrument. The Washington State Department of Public Instruction has provided an instrument for administrators to evaluate their school health programs. Five aspects of the health program are considered: personnel, inservice training, community involvement, written guidelines, and evaluation. The instrument was prepared by the state's Program Evaluation Task Force. *Source: Self-Evaluation Instrument for School Health Programs* (Olympia, Wash.: State Superintendent of Public Instruction, 1973).

Dalis Health Education Appraisal Instrument.   The purpose of this instrument is to evaluate the effectiveness with which the objectives of health education have been met. By checking an inventory, students are asked to indicate what they have learned in various health areas, and whether they believe additional instruction would be helpful. *Source:* Gus T. Dalis, "Development and Application of a New Health Appraisal Instrument," Master's Thesis, University of California at Los Angeles, 1961.

Wilkes Analysis of Health Practices.   Wilkes developed an instrument for analyzing the health practices of junior high school pupils. Nine different health areas are included in this 56 multiple-choice inventory. *Source:* Dorothy J. Wilkes, "An Analysis of Health Practices of Junior High School Pupils with Implications for School Health Instruction," Master's Thesis, University of California at Los Angeles, 1960.

Drake Tuberculosis Appraisal Inventory.   The purpose of this inventory is to appraise the progress of junior high school students in tuberculosis education. The test items are related to nine health areas. The inventory contains 60 items designed to indicate health knowledge, attitudes, and behavior in the area of tuberculosis and respiratory disease education. *Source:* Florence K. Drake, "An Evaluative Instrument for Appraising Student Progress in Tuberculosis Education for Grades 7–8–9," Master's Thesis, University of California at Los Angeles, 1960.

SELECTED REFERENCES

BARROW, HAROLD M., and ROSEMARY McGEE. *A Practical Approach to Measurement in Physical Education*, 2nd ed. Philadelphia: Lea and Febiger, 1971, Ch. 11.

MATHEWS, DONALD K. *Measurement in Physical Education*, 4th ed. Philadelphia: W. B. Saunders Company, 1973, Ch. 12.

PART FIVE

ADMINISTRATIVE PROBLEMS

Measurement programs are not easy to conduct. They require hard work and close attention to detail. These factors, coupled with the usual heavy load of physical educators, make the problem of inaugurating and conducting such programs difficult. Many directors and teachers, however, are attempting it, feeling that the benefits derived by the pupils in increased physical fitness, social efficiency, cultural attainments, and recreational competency, and by themselves in professional growth, are well worth the effort and attendant sacrifices.

An efficient measurement program depends upon a balanced teaching and administrative load for the physical educator, administrative adjustments in scheduling pupils for classes, and an adequate budget for meeting the costs entailed. Over-worked personnel, haphazard scheduling of classes, and lack of funds are not conducive to effective physical education programs. In many instances, nevertheless, these conditions are accepted at the start, in the belief that a thorough demonstration of the value of the program will convince administrative authorities, boards of education, and the community that the program is needed

Measurement Programs

and will result in the necessary adjustments to guarantee its effective functioning. This chapter considers problems arising in conducting a well-rounded measurement program in the schools.

INAUGURATING MEASUREMENT PROGRAMS

When conditions are other than ideal, the physical educator may be well advised to proceed slowly and to do a thorough job of each step as it comes up when inaugurating a measurement program. This means, first of all, thorough and accurate testing; then, proper and adequate use of test results. As has been stressed before, the only justification for testing rests in the utilization of test results to aid health and physical educators in the realization of effective programs. Measurement is functional—it is directed toward the realization of basic objectives. The whim of the moment should not dictate the program for the hour.

It is better judgment, therefore, to start with only as many pupils as can be conveniently and efficiently handled, rather than to include the entire school in the testing program at once. This procedure has several advantages.

1. Time enough can be taken by the physical educator for a complete follow-up of each pupil included in the measurement program.

2. An opportunity is provided to try out procedures and to routinize desirable ones with a limited number of cases, rather than to become confused and frustrated with a great many all at once.

3. Successful accomplishments with fewer pupils can frequently be used to convince administrative superiors of the necessity for measurement.

4. Measurement programs are more apt to be attempted on this basis, the physical educator having more confidence in his ability to handle them without becoming so deeply involved that the task becomes hopeless.

5. Efficient programs, needed assistance, necessary supplies, equipment, and facilities, and desirable arrangements may logically be expected as outcomes of such a procedure if properly handled and the results effectively presented.

A successful suggestion for inaugurating a measurement program when the physical educator wishes to make a gradual beginning and to do effective work is to limit the number of pupils tested. The purposes to be achieved by testing and the practical limitations imposed by local situations will necessarily dictate how this suggestion is implemented.

In relation to purposes to be achieved, a larger number of pupils can be included if testing is for classification purposes, for motivation, or for determining program results. For these situations, the limitations imposed are mostly related to the number that can be tested. However, the number must necessarily be smaller if individual needs are to be met, as this process requires more time. Individuals with needs must be identified, the causes of needs must be determined, and individual programs must be provided.

The general principle involved in a gradual beginning is to include only as many pupils as can be properly tested and the test results satisfactorily utilized. One possibility is to test only one grade the first year, and concentrate all the follow-up work on this group. A new grade may be added each year. If the lowest grade in the school participated at first and the entering grade is added each year, the entire school will be included in the program within a relatively short time.

Suggestions for administering tests

Medical Examinations

Medical examinations should precede the administration of strenuous physical tests. Pupils subject to hernia, those with cardiac defects, or those recovering from recent accidents, illnesses, or operations should be exempt from such testing. Others who in the opinion of the physician might be harmed by the tests should not take them. Generally speaking, however, it is safe for any individual who is able to participate in the regular physical education program of the school to take vigorous activity tests. If there is any doubt in individual cases, however, the subject should be excused until a careful check can be made.

Testing Personnel

"Many hands make light work" is a truism as far as the administration of testing programs is concerned. Four ways of handling the personnel problem follow:

1. Staff and students. The use of student leaders as testers has been advocated frequently and has considerable merit. Students can be utilized in recording and in scoring tests, with little more than the proper directions; but in the actual giving of tests, they should be well trained and carefully supervised. In initiating student testing, it is advisable to utilize underclassmen as much as possible, thus providing experienced testers for a number of years. The physical education staff may also be augmented by using the services of other members of the faculty.

2. Classroom teachers and housewives. In the elementary schools of Ellensburg, Washington, classroom teachers and housewives have been utilized in the administration of the Washington Motor Fitness Test to children in the primary grades and the Oregon Simplification of the Physical Fitness Index to girls and boys in the intermediate grades. These individuals aided in giving tests with the least difficult techniques. Also, they were carefully trained prior to the testing and were supervised during the administration of the tests.

3. "Trading works." A common practice in some rural areas during the summer months is to "trade works" in order to get the threshing done, one farmer helping all those neighbors who assist him. This idea may well be utilized in conducting measurement programs, the physical educators in several nearby schools "trading works" with each other, and doing the testing in each of the schools on successive days. The cost of testing apparatus might also be shared in the same manner, a practice which has been utilized successfully in several situations. In one instance, a county athletic association purchased strength-testing equipment for the use of its member schools.

4. Teacher-training students. School systems located near teachers colleges or professional schools often have opportunities to develop cooperative educational projects. Such projects are mutually beneficial: for the school system, they can play a vital part in the educational curriculum by providing services that might otherwise be difficult to obtain; for the teacher in training, they can provide practical experiences in thinking through professional problems and applying appropriate procedures in local situations. Such projects may include, but need not be limited to, the administration and scoring of tests.

Time for Testing

Various authorities have agreed that the total amount of program time spent in testing should not exceed 10 percent annually. In some schools, it may be necessary, at least in the beginning, to cut the amount of teacher and pupil testing time to an absolute minimum. The following suggestions, based upon a reduction of the number to be tested each year, may prove helpful to those faced with this problem:

1. Gradual beginning. This procedure coincides with the suggestions made above for physical educators who wish to make a small beginning with their measurement work and to broaden out as time goes on. If the pupils in only one or two grades were tested the first year, and a new grade added annually, the amount of testing required would be kept small and provisions would be made for expansion from year to year.

2. Alternate testing. Instead of testing every pupil in the school each year, pupils may be tested every second year. For example, the seventh, ninth, and eleventh grades may be tested annually. Referred cases, of course, should be tested more often.

3. Retests. Considerable time can be saved each year by retesting only those pupils who were found to have deficiencies at the time of the preceding tests, thus testing the entire student body once a year only.

Economy of Testing Time

Frequently, the use of certain tests has been condemned on the ground that they are excessively time-consuming in their administration. In some instances this criticism is justified. However, before the physical educator abandons desirable tests for this reason, he should study ways and means for their economical administration in order to staisfy himself that the test cannot be given in a reasonable length of time. The application of good administration to all testing projects should be followed as a matter of course. But physical educators should remember that academic teachers test almost constantly. There are daily quizzes, weekly papers, monthly formal examinations, quarterly reviews, semester "finals." Taking good tests is positively developmental; for example a high-jumping test is excellent practice. Similarly, a PFI test is strength-developing, a test of information in hygiene serves to fix facts in mind, and so on.

Strength Testing. As an example of efficient test administration, the procedure for administering and scoring the Physical Fitness Index tests at the rate of 50 per hour and faster is described in Chapter 7.

Track and Field Testing. Individual timing in track events is obviously a slow process. An economical procedure for timing dashes, in which the participants run at full speed for the entire distance, is to record the distances they can run in a set time, rather than record the times they can run a set distance. For a selected dash, the track would be marked off in two-yard zones, beginning at the finish and working back toward the start to the point that the slowest runner will reach. As many runners as there are lanes are started, an observer being assigned to each one. When the finish gun or whistle is sounded (in 10 seconds for 100 yards and in 6 seconds for 60 yards, for example), each observer spots the zone reached by his runner. The distance for each may then be corrected into time for the entire distance or scored directly in points, depending upon the scoring system used.

Shuttle runs, as in the "potato" race, may be timed in a similar manner. Six lines, two yards apart, are drawn on the floor or ground. The runners shuttle forward and back for a set time, say 12 seconds, and the distance traveled by the end of the time is noted by an observer. The zones are numbered 1, 2, 3, 4, and 5 going forward; and 6, 7, 8, 9, and 10 when returning. Thus, three round trips and four zones would be recorded as 34. Swimming events may be handled by using a similar scheme.

Zones for the standing broad jump, at two-inch intervals, can also be used to reduce testing time, the jumper taking three consecutive jumps, of which the best is recorded. Markings in this instance would be two inches apart and the tester would estimate the distance between markers. The shot-put and various other throws may be administered in a similar manner, utilizing arcs drawn at convenient intervals with the center of the throwing circle as the center of the arc. In the shot-put, these arcs may be one foot apart, beginning at a distance that can be exceeded by the poorest performer and continuing beyond the distance expected from the best performer. In the case of the discus throw or the basketball throw, these marks may be from 5 to 10 feet apart, the judge estimating the distance between arcs at which the object lands.

In this type of marking, it is usually most economical to have the markings made from both ends of the testing area, as was done with the football punt and pass for distance in Borleske's touch football test. Thus, the football is punted or passed from the second line, making it unnecessary to return it for each subject.

In such events as the high jump and pole vault, the most effective way to reduce the amount of time required is to increase the number of standards and jumping pits. Some time can be saved, however, by utilizing the following procedures: (a) permit the subject to choose the height at which he wishes to start; and (b) permit each subject to jump once at each height, but to continue to jump after he has knocked the bar off. Record the best height cleared.

Posture Testing.   Considerable time can be saved in testing posture by utilizing rough subjective screening tests to select those pupils who will be given complete posture examinations. In such screenings, each pupil is quickly inspected by the examiner, who decides subjectively whether or not he should be included in the posture corrective program. Those so selected should then be given either a detailed objective test, like the Cureton, the Wickens-Kiphuth, or the Wellesley test, or a careful subjective test, like that proposed by Phelps and Kiphuth.

Skill Tests.   Each skill test proposed for use in physical education should be studied individually for ways in which it can be economically administered. As these tests vary so greatly in their testing requirements, set methods to be applied in all situations cannot be given.

Routine Procedures

There are a number of routine procedures that should be followed in the administration of any testing program if efficiency is to be achieved. Among these procedures are the following:

1. Plan, if possible, to have pupils report for testing in a continuous, unbroken procession. Stops, starts, and waits in the testing process cause losses of time and should be avoided. The physical educator, however, should utilize pupils assigned to his physical education classes first; study halls, second. He should disrupt classroom schedules last, and then only if necessary and permissible.

2. Have all necessary testing equipment set up and organized for the efficient administration of the tests to be given. All floor or field markings required should also be made before the testing time. Careful planning in this respect is essential if tests are to be given quickly and with a minimum of confusion. The physical educator should set down on paper the complete layout of and details for the testing. He should exercise as much care in this respect as he customarily gives to planning track meets and other athletic events. The arrangement of testing stations for the Rogers Physical Fitness Index test proposed in Chapter 7 will serve as an example of test organization.

3. Provide for the required number of qualified examining and recording assistants. Assistants who are to help with the testing, whether they be pupils or other staff and faculty members, should be carefully instructed in their duties and in the testing techniques they are to perform. Nothing should be left to chance, as it is better not to test at all than to permit unqualified testers to assist. In fact, it is best to have a testing staff in which all members are qualified to take charge of any testing station and carry on in an efficient manner. Written instructions covering all phases of the testing might logically be prepared and at least one organization meeting held so that a complete understanding of the entire process may be given all testers.

4. Give students an explanation of the reason for the test at the outset so that they will understand in general what it is they are striving to do and what outcomes they may expect. This procedure is of considerable help in securing the full cooperation of pupils and in obtaining an all-out effort on their part in taking the tests. The use of visual aids, such as photographs, motion pictures, lantern slides, or filmstrips, would be particularly valuable in motivating the measurement program.

5. "Use Evaluation Positively" is the title of an article by Finke,[1] in which he stresses: "If the

key function of evaluation takes place within the learner it seems essential that evaluation must not destroy the learner's individuality or confidence in himself as a learner. On the contrary, evaluation must build up the learner's self-reliance; it must increase his desire and ability to move on to next goals and tasks." The learner needs constant feedback to better know himself and to see more clearly the desirable goals ahead; he must see for himself his progress toward these goals, goals he must accept if they are to be realized. Continuous evaluation is essential as a basis for further progress, but evaluation must be specific to facilitate this progress. Evaluation must pinpoint specific understandings and competencies as well as needed next steps. The greater understanding and insight the pupil has of himself in relation to evaluation, the greater is his ability to evaluate himself and the more certain will be his full participation in the measurement program and in appropriate follow-up procedures suggested to him.

6. Inform pupils of the results of their own tests. Not only should this information be told to the pupils, but a complete interpretation of what the scores mean should be given. For the most part, such information and such explanations should be made privately, in order to protect the pupil psychologically. Such information constitutes the best form of motivation possible, and provides an excellent opportunity for improving the pupil's understanding of physical education.

Test Records

Some method of recording the test scores of pupils is, of course, necessary. Such scores may be kept as class records or as individual records. Individual records have the advantage of maneuverability and alphabetizing, and can be used to accompany the pupil from class to class or school to school.

The class record has the names of all class members; opposite the names are spaces for their test scores and other necessary data. As an illustration of this type of score sheet, the form proposed for the California Physical Performance Test is presented in Figure 16.1. This method of

[1]Charles W. Finke, "Use Evaluation Positively," *Journal of Health, Physical Education, and Recreation,* **43,** No. 9 (November–December 1972), 16.

SCORE SHEET
for California Physical Performance Tests

School _____

Teacher _____ Grade _____

Squad number _____ Leader _____

Date: _____
month   year

Boys ☐   Girls ☐

Student	Age	Standing Broad Jump[1]			Pull-up	Knee Push-up	Knee Bent Sit-up	Dash[1]		Softball Throw for Distance	Comments
		Trial 1	Trial 2	Trial 3				Trial 1	Trial 2		
	Years	Inches	Inches	Inches	Number	Number	Number	Seconds	Seconds	Feet	

[1] Circle best score.

FIGURE 16.1. *California Physical Performance Record, 1962 edition*

recording scores may be unwieldy if more than one tester administers tests at the same time; either the score sheet must be passed back and forth between testers or scores must be transferred after testing. The California test is described in Chapter 9.

An individual record card on which repeated test records are made during the year was formerly utilized in the men's physical education service program at the University of Oregon, as shown in Figure 16.2. The tests administered are the Oregon Simplification of the Rogers Strength and Physical Fitness Indices and the 600-yard run. The Rogers indices are described in Chapter 7.

A cumulative record system is proposed

for the Oregon Motor Fitness Test; this score card is shown in Figure 16.3. These cards are available for both boys and girls from the fourth grade through high school. Rating norms for this test and its component parts are included on the test record. On the back of this score card, T-scale norms are given. The Oregon test is presented in Chapter 9.

Computerized Reporting

Charles T. Avedisian, Director of Physical Education in the Darien, Connecticut, Public Schools, has developed a computerized approach to recording data from AAHPER Youth Fitness Test, with the assistance of Donald K. Mathews at

Physical Fitness Index Record

Name: Lewis, Allen L.
Class (circle Fr) So. Jr. Sr. Gr.

High School: Corvallis — Corvallis, Oregon

Birth Date: 9 Mar. 1947 — Can You Swim: (circle Yes) No — 293

No	Item	Raw Score (9-22-65, Age 18 Mos. 6½)	Converted Score	Raw Score (11-3-65, Age 18 Mos. 8)	Converted Score	Raw Score (12-9-65, Age 18 Mos. 9)	Converted Score	Raw Score	Converted Score
1.	Weight	138		142		142			
2.	Height	70		70		70			
3.	Pull Ups	7½		7		8½			
4.	Push Ups	8		10		15			
5.	Total (No. 3 + No. 4)	15½		17		23½			
6.	Multiplier W/10 + Ht. − 60	24		24		24			
7.	Arm Strength (No. 5 × No. 6)	372	440	408	488	564	666		
8.	Lift, Legs	910	1156	1250	1588	1400	1778		
9.	Constant		544		544		544		544
10.	Strength Index Total No. 7 thru No. 9		2140		2620		2988		
11.	Normal S.I.		2291		2374		2374		
12.	Physical Fitness Index	93	47	110	57	126	65		
13.	600 Yard Run	2:00	33	1:46	47	1:43	50		
	Total Score		80		104		115		

FIGURE 16.2. *University of Oregon Physical Fitness Record*

OREGON MOTOR FITNESS TEST SCORE CARD—GIRLS GRADES 4, 5, AND 6

NAME ....

SCHOOL .... COUNTY ....

DATE	Month Sept. 19......			Month 19......			Month 19......			Month 19......			Month 19......			Month 19......			Month 19......			Month 19......			Month 19......		
GRADE																											
AGE																											
HEIGHT																											
WEIGHT																											
OBJECTIVE TESTS	Test Score	Rating	Std. Pts.	Test Score	Rating	Std. Pts.	Test Score	Rating	Std. Pts.	Test Score	Rating	Std. Pts.	Test Score	Rating	Std. Pts.	Test Score	Rating	Std. Pts.	Test Score	Rating	Std. Pts.	Test Score	Rating	Std. Pts.	Test Score	Rating	Std. Pts.
Hanging in Arm-Flexed Position																											
Standing Broad Jump																											
Crossed-Arm Curl-Ups																											
TOTAL STANDARD POINTS																											

RATING NORMS FOR GIRLS GRADES 4, 5, AND 6

TEST ITEMS	Superior	Good	Fair	Poor	Inferior	Grade
Hanging in Arm-Flexed Position	30-Up	20- 29	5- 19	1- 4	0	
Standing Broad Jump	65-Up	58- 64	49- 57	39- 48	0- 38	4
Crossed-Arm Curl-Ups	66-Up	50- 65	26- 49	2- 25	0- 1	
Hanging in Arm-Flexed Position	31-Up	22- 30	10- 21	2- 9	0- 1	
Standing Broad Jump	75-Up	68- 74	57- 67	46- 56	0- 45	5
Crossed-Arm Curl-Ups	68-Up	52- 67	28- 51	4- 27	0- 3	
Hanging in Arm-Flexed Position	37-Up	27- 36	12- 26	1- 11	0	
Standing Broad Jump	73-Up	66- 72	55- 65	44- 54	0- 43	6
Crossed-Arm Curl-Ups	71-Up	55- 70	31- 54	1- 30	0	
TOTAL STANDARD POINTS	204-Up	180-203	144-179	112-143	111-Down	

DIRECTIONS FOR RECORDING AND SCORING TESTS

1. Record the actual test score for each item in the column marked "Test Score" on this side of the score card.
2. Using test score, check rating norms and record superior, good, fair, poor, or inferior for each test item in the rating column.
3. Find standard point score corresponding to each actual test score in the "Scoring Table" on the back of the card and record in column marked "Standard Points".
4. Add "Standard Points" for all test items and record total at bottom of card in space on line marked "Total Standard Points".
5. Using total standard points, check rating norms to determine fitness rating of superior, good, fair, poor, or inferior. Record this rating in the space provided at the bottom of the rating column.
6. Repeat the test at the end of the school year; it is recommended that a mid-year test also be given. Below-standard individuals should be tested more frequently.

FIGURE 16.3. *Oregon Motor Fitness Record*

Ohio State University. The physical education teachers in the schools record the obtained scores on all test items for each student tested on a print-out sheet and send them to the school system's data processing center. The processing center reads results cumulatively each successive year from fifth through tenth grades. Four copies are printed by the computer to be distributed as follows: central cumulative file, current physical education teacher, next year's physical education teacher, and parents. A column is provided on the report form for awards: Presidential, Gold, and Silver for those scoring on all tests at the 85th, 80th, and 50th percentiles, respectively. The advantages of this system are that a time consuming phase of record keeping is drastically reduced, cumulative records are provided, research data are readily available via the computer, and up-dated local norms may be readily constructed.

In the 1971 Revision of the California Physical Performance Test, methods for processing test scores are proposed.

Machine processing, hand processing, or a combination of machine and hand processing may be utilized. These methods with illustrated data-processing cards are presented in the test manual. The California test is described in Chapter 9.

A Lesson from Field-Testing Conditions

As a project of the Eastern District Research Council, American Association for Health, Physical Education, and Recreation, Appleton[2] conducted a field trial of physical performance tests, in order to establish national norms for entering college students. Two batteries of six items each, a total of 12 tests, were administered at 17 colleges and universities. Each institution was requested to follow a common set of directions. Similar data were collected by the physical education staff at the United States Military Academy under controlled testing conditions. These data were obtained from six training centers throughout the country by testers trained at the Academy.

The data from each college were compared with the West Point results and with those from the other institutions. Consistency was evident in the West Point data, but was definitely lacking in the colleges. Critical ratios between the means of the various institutions for the different tests were found to range from +8 to −20, as the most extensive difference, and from +5 to −5, as the smallest difference. It was concluded that the differences between colleges were due, not to differences in the degree of ability, but rather to the testing conditions.

The final observation made by Appleton can be applied to all physical educators engaged in testing boys and girls in their

[2]Lloyd O. Appleton, *The Practicability of Standardized Procedures for Physical Performance Tests* (West Point: Office of Physical Education, United States Military Academy, April 15, 1949, mimeographed).

programs: Motivation, proper interpretation of written procedures, and extreme care by scorers are very important factors in the administration of tests; every care should be taken to see to it that these factors are properly accomplished if comparable results are to be obtained at different institutions and under varying testing situations and to be valid for norms provided with tests.

PREPARATION OF REPORTS

An essential finale of measurement programs is the preparation of a report of testing results and the progress made in conducting these programs. Such reports might logically include statements of the nature, objectives, and scope of the program; nontechnical descriptions of the tests used; interpretations of the significance of test scores; explanations of the use made of the test results and follow-up procedures; and reports of pupils' progress in terms of average improvement, significant case-study data, and other pertinent findings resulting from the program.

In the preparation of these reports, it is necessary to make various tabulations and to prepare significant graphs that may be used in effectively portraying the results obtained. The final selection of tabulations and graphs to be used in the report will depend primarily upon two factors: the essential ideas to be stressed, that is, the actual results obtained, or the method of arriving at the results; and the interests and abilities of the group for whom the report is prepared, that is, whether laymen or technically trained personnel.

The object of presenting tabular materials and graphs is, of course, to portray basic facts in condensed form so that outstanding points to be stressed will be evident to those for whom the report is prepared. However, much of the effectiveness of such presentations has been destroyed because tabular materials have often been presented in such form that they could not be read and interpreted with ease. In order to aid in improving these reports, therefore, the following suggestions for the preparation of tabulations and graphs are given.

Construction of Tables

Various points to keep in mind in constructing tables are as follows:

1. Emphasize only one significant fact in each table.

2. Avoid crowded tables.

3. Place each table on a single page, if possible.

4. Arrange tabulations in a logical manner.

5. Space columns of figures so that they may be easily read.

6. Construct the tables so that they may be read from left to right.

7. Arrange the points to be compared so that comparison can be made easily.

8. Rule tables as follows:
  a. Double horizontal line at top of the table.
  b. Single vertical lines to set off the main divisions of the table.
  c. Single horizontal and vertical lines to mark off minor subdivisions.
  d. Vertical lines to separate columns of figures.
  e. Omit lines at both right and left margins.
  f. Use either a double space after every fifth row of figures, or rows of dots extended from the items to the first column of figures.
  g. Horizontal line at bottom of the table.

9. Align right-hand digits in columns of figures, except when decimal points are used. Decimal points must always be aligned.

10. Label the table in sufficient detail so that it may be read and understood without supplementary explanation. Use a single phrase and avoid the use of unnecessary words.

Graphic Exhibits

A graphic exhibit is usually more easily interpreted than a tabular exhibit. As a general rule, each tabular exhibit, especially if it contains several long columns of figures, should be accompanied by a graphic presentation of the same data. The vivid portrayal of test data and their easier understanding by the public make the use of this device especially effective in reporting the results of measurement programs. Points to keep in mind in the logical construction of graphs are as follows:

1. Select the type of graph that will best show the points to be emphasized.

2. Emphasize only one significant point in each graph.

3. Arrange the graph so that it may be read from left to right.

4. As a general rule, show the zero line on the graph. If the nature of the data is such that the presentation of the zero line gives the graph a long-drawn-out and unbalanced appearance, show the zero line and then place at a small distance above it two wavy lines extending horizontally across the body of the graph and indicating a break in it.

5. Place the scale line at the left, except in especially wide graphs, when it may be placed on both sides.

6. Distinguish clearly the line of the graph from other rulings on the graph.

7. Construct graphs that are pleasing in appearance, well spaced and well proportioned, and centered on the page.

8. Title the graph as clearly and completely as possible, using a single phrase and avoiding unnecessary words.

9. As a rule, place the title of the graph below the body of the graph.

PURPOSES OF REPORTING

Test scores and other evaluative data should be tabulated and prepared for presentation to school administrators, boards of education, pupils and parents, and the public as justification for the continued support of physical education. Such data may be used for the following purposes:

1. To portray the results of the physical education program *in general.*

2. To justify *particular phases* of the program.

3. To prove the worth of a *change in methodology.*

4. To indicate the need for *expanded* programs.

5. To show the necessity for *redirected* programs.

In certain instances, a series of tables or graphs will be necessary to support completely the conclusions reached. For example, it is very doubtful whether one can portray the results of the entire physical education program in one table and still maintain clarity. Proving the worth of a *particular phase* of the program, however, may be done with one table, as shown in the next section of this chapter. Following are several illustrations of the use of tabular presentation.

Justification of Particular Phases of the Program

To induce boys to participate in a wide variety of physical education skills, a decathlon was conducted at the Melrose, Massachusetts, High School.[3] Twenty events were scheduled, with points awarded for each of 35 levels of performance. No other pressure was exerted to encourage boys to participate. All but ten boys in the school participated in one or more events, 641 boys in all. The total number of activity participations was 4064—an average of nearly six and a half different events for each boy. Of consid-

[3]Frederick Rand Rogers, *An Admirable New England High School Physical Education Program* (Newton, Mass.: Pleiades Company, April 18, 1938), p. 16.

TABLE 16.1 *Number of Participants in Melrose High School Decathlon*

Events	Participants
1. 100 Yards	319
2. 50 Yards	292
3. High Jump	73
4. Running Broad Jump	190
5. Shot-Put	245
6. Half-Mile	299
7. Hop-Step-Jump	253
8. Standing Broad-Jump	202
9. Fence Vault	34
10. Snap-Under-Bar	227
11. 5-Potato-Race	155
12. 8-Potato-Race	175
13. Half-Lever	33
14. Pull-Ups	158
15. Push-Ups	148
16. Rope-Climb	152
17. Free Throws	371
18. Baskets (one minute)	372
19. Football-Punt	178
20. Football-Pass	188
Total	4064

erable significance was the half-mile: 299 boys ran in this event—a real record of participation.[4] Table 16.1 reports the events included in the decathlon and the number of participants in each event.

Need for Expanded Program

In determining the swimming ability of undergraduate students at the University of Illinois, Cureton administered tests to 621 men classified as the "basic group" by his Motor Fitness Test.[5] Fifty-nine percent, or 368 men, could not pass the 100-yard test in the pool; 84 percent could not swim 440 yards; only 3 percent of this basic group could qualify for lifesaving. The results of this testing appear in Table 16.2.

[4]For a method of tabulating intramural participation, see H. Harrison Clarke, "The Use of Intramural Participation Statistics," *Research Quarterly*, **6**, No. 3 (October 1935), 27.

[5]Thomas K. Cureton, "The Unfitness of Young Men in Motor Fitness," *Journal of the American Medical Association*, **123** (September 11, 1943), 69.

TABLE 16.2 *Swimming Classification of "Basic Group" University of Illinois Men*

	Classification	Number	Percent
NS	Unable to swim 75 feet after jumping into deep water feet first (nonswimmers)	235	37.84
PS	Unable to swim 100 yards, any way at all (poor swimmers)	133	21.42
AS	Able to swim 100 yards but unable to demonstrate crawl, back crawl, breast and side stroke 75 feet each (average swimmers)	159	25.60
SS	Able to swim 440 yards and demonstrate four strokes as named (superior swimmers)	73	11.76
LS	Qualified in life-saving with one or more of the national life-saving organizations (life-savers)	21	3.38
		621	100.00

Worth of a Change in Methodology

In experimenting with methods of equating groups for basketball competition, Oestreich recorded the number of games won, lost, and tied (at the close of regular playing time) for teams equated on the basis of *Strength Indices* and for teams arranged by the "choose-up sides" method.[6] In Table 16.3, three groups appear as follows: (a) Initial League: a preliminary trial with teams equated by Strength Indices; (b) Berry League: four teams equated by Strength Index scores; (c) Choose-up League: three teams organized by choosing sides.

Eighteen games were played by teams in the Initial League and 26 by those in the Berry League. The results of the two leagues were comparable: the median

[6]Harry G. Oestreich, "Strength Testing Program Applied to Y.M.C.A. Organization and Administration," *Supplement to the Research Quarterly,* **6,** No. 1 (March 1935), 197.

point differences in scores were 3.5 and 3.4 points, respectively. In the Choose-up League, the median point difference was 6 points.

COOPERATIVE MEASUREMENT PROJECTS

The formulation and conduct of measurement programs are difficult functions. They require complete rethinking and re-evaluation of physical education. Numerous problems appear—to be solved eventually in respect to particular local situations. In many instances, follow-up procedures (the use of test results) have not been well considered and need to be studied carefully, tried out locally, and adopted, modified, or rejected according to the results of this trial under actual school conditions. Also, many physical educators hesitate to take the plunge into measurement because of lack of time due to heavy schedules and large classes. If they are truly interested in measurement, such individuals need encouragement and assistance in planning their local programs.

For these reasons, a cooperative measurement project, in which not only physical educators, but also administrative

TABLE 16.3 *Comparative Scores of Basketball Games Played by Differently Organized Teams and Leagues*

Point Difference in Score	Initial League (percent)	Berry League (percent)	Choose-up League (percent)
0–4	61	72	44
5–9	28	20	28
10–14	11	4	17
15–19		4	
20–24			5.5
25–29			5.5
Total	100	100	100
Median Difference	3.5 points	3.4 points	6 points

officers, assist each other, would be of great value. Such a project involves an organization of physical educators who are convinced of the value of and the need for measurement and who reside in the same geographical area. The organization need not be especially formal in its construction, although it is desirable to designate one individual to act as chairman and to assume responsibility for the necessary administrative work entailed. A secretary would also be helpful in recording the minutes of meetings held and in preparing reports on the results of the project. If possible, a few principals and a superintendent or two should be induced to attend regularly. Measurement projects of this sort will be described briefly.

Central New York State Project

A joint physical fitness project was organized by nine schools in central New York State[7] and continued to function for several years. The project was planned and conducted in cooperation with physical educators at Syracuse University and in the New York State Bureau of Physical Education. Quarterly meetings of involved personnel from all project schools were held to report progress, exchange experiences, and explore problems encountered. Before a program was started in each school, the university and state department representatives met with local personnel to orient all concerned with the purpose of the program, with the test to be used to evaluate physical fitness and its validity, and with the proposed follow-up procedures based on test results. Local adaptations were thus made in conference with the school's physical educators, administrators, physicians, nurse, counselors, and health education specialists. Assistance in administering semiannual

[7]C. R. Robbins, "Central New York State Demonstration," *School Activities,* **11,** No. 7 (March 1940), 296.

tests was provided by undergraduate students from the university.

The purpose of the project was to try out, modify as found desirable, and improve under practical school conditions procedures for meeting the physical fitness objective of physical education. Among these procedures were: organization of the testing process for rapid, yet accurate, administration of tests; the use of physical fitness test data, case study, and follow-up procedures, with emphasis on pupil program adjustment and general program organization pursuant thereto; ways and means of simplifying procedures and eliminating inefficiency in record-keeping; and the development of simple and efficient report that would be used in informing school authorities concerning the nature, scope, problems, and progress of this program and that would also be used to inform parents and the public regarding the physical fitness program and results achieved.

The Central New York State Physical Fitness Project proved successful. Not only did the physical educators participating receive considerable encouragement and assistance, but the pupils in the schools benefited greatly, as indicated by improved individual test scores and by higher school averages. In terms of the test used in this project, which was the Rogers Physical Fitness Index, the following significant results were obtained.

1. At the end of the first two years, the median PFI for the nine schools participating was 112, an increase of 15 points. All schools had median PFI's above 100 at this time; only two schools had medians this high at the start.

2. Average increases of 12 to 15 PFI points per year were typically reported for boys selected for special follow-up work. In one school, the average annual increase over a three-year period was 19.5 points, an improvement of 25 percent in physical power and strength (during a fourth year, the average increase was 25 points), results that cannot fail to be significant for the present and future well-being of these individuals.

Project Broadfront

Under the direction of Lloyd J. Rowley, Project Broadfront was planned and conducted over a five year period in the Ellensburg, Washington, School District. The project was supported by a grant under Title III of the Elementary and Secondary Education Act of 1965, which authorized funds for Projects to Advance Creativity in Education. The overall consultant for the Project was John E. Nixon, Stanford University; health education consultant was Harold Cornacchai, San Francisco State College; physical fitness consultant was the author of this book; physical fitness testing guidance and assistance was provided by Everett A. Irish, Robert N. Irving, and their physical education students at Central Washington College; and consultation was had with Howard Schaub, Washington State Supervisor of Health, Physical Education, and Recreation. Identified with Broadfront in various capacities were: State Department of Public Instruction, State Forestry Department, Northern Pacific Railroad, Camp Illahee Board, State Game Department, State Health Department, Kittitas Medical Association, State Department of Parks and Recreation, Bureau of Outdoor Education, and Lifetime Sports Foundation.

Project Broadfront had many facets: a process involving elementary classroom teachers, with curriculum associate assistance, assuming primary responsibility for planning and conducting physical education for their pupils; a perceptual-motor program for grades one through three; developmental programs for boys and girls of subpar physical fitness; a community-school program in three schools; an Outdoor Education Project for grades four and five and all special education pupils; and a unique cost analysis

project in health education and in elementary school physical education. The project produced a wide variety of educational materials, including brochures, pictures, reports, slide-tape presentations, 16 mm. colored film reports, and newspaper and magazine articles. Many visitors from other schools viewed various phases of the project. The director made numerous lay and professional presentations related to Project Broadfront, its purposes, programs and results. At its 1970 meeting, the American Academy of Physical Education cited Lloyd Rowley for his directorship of the project and the Ellensburg School District for its support.[8]

The physical fitness program had two purposes: to conduct developmental programs for boys and girls who were below accepted standards on basic physical fitness components; and to provide maintenance programs for those who met such standards. The physical fitness tests employed were the Washington Motor Fitness Test for children in the first three grades and the Oregon Simplification of Rogers' Physical Fitness Index for boys and girls in grades four through ten. An interesting indication of early results is shown by the percentages of pupils above the averages expected from the norms for these tests: in 1967, only five grades exceeded these averages, while, in 1969, all grades did so. In 1969, 75 percent of pupils in four of the grades were above the average.

Other progress data are too numerous to mention here, but the physical fitness averages for the school grades did increase from year to year, a logical expectation under the circumstances. Fewer and fewer boys and girls were candidates for developmental classes as they progressed through school. An example of the end result of this effect is shown with tenth grade

[8]Awards and Citations, "Lloyd Rowley and the Ellensburg, Washington, School District," *The Academy Papers*, No. 5 (March 31–April 1, 1971), p. 86.

boys in 1971: only 13 percent had PFI's below 100; the first quartile was 110, well above the average of 100 for the norms; the median was 123, exceeding considerably the expected 115 according to the norms; and the third quartile was an exceptional 138. Similar results were obtained for the tenth grade girls: first quartile, 100; median, 115; third quartile, 142.

Oregon Pilot Physical Fitness Project

During the academic year 1954–1955, the Oregon Association for Health, Physical Education, and Recreation carried out a pilot physical fitness project,[9] through a Central Physical Fitness Committee. The following three basic premises for creating an effective physical fitness program for boys and girls in Oregon schools were adopted.

1. The program should be directed toward boys and girls who are sub-par in fundamental physical fitness elements.

2. The program should be based upon the identification of such individuals through the use of valid tests.

3. The program should be designed to meet the individual needs of each low fitness individual.

Eleven high schools in different parts of the state agreed to participate in the project. Testing teams from the University of Oregon and Southern Oregon College assisted in the establishment of the pilot programs. Initially, one day was spent in each school, at which time approximately 100 boys and girls, preferably from the sophomore class, were given the Physical Fitness Index (PFI) test. At this visit, too, clinics were conducted to train testers and seminars were held to consider appro-

priate follow-up procedures for those with low scores, as applied to the local situation.

Three months later, the testing teams returned to the schools to retest the same students to evaluate the progress made. At this time, the local physical educators were able to help with the testing; assistance was also provided by the faculty and physical education major students of other colleges and universities when the testing was done in their respective areas of the state. The following additional institutions participated: Oregon State University, Willamette University, Portland State College, and Lewis and Clark College.

The results of this pilot project, as indicated by the test scores, were as follows:

1. The median PFI for the boys in all schools was 108 at the time of the final test; this was a gain of 10 points over the initial tests. The highest median for a single school was 120 at Roseburg, up 18 points over the first test; the median at Medford was 118, a gain of 15 points. Only one school had a median PFI for boys below 100 at the close of the project.

2. The girls' median PFI reached 106 on the retests, a substantial gain of 13 points. The highest median was 118 at Coos Bay, an increase for this school of 22 points. The girls in only one school retested below median 100. It was generally agreed that the girls displayed some hesitancy in taking the tests the first time; however, this had mostly disappeared on the retests, the girls showing much greater interest and effort.

In the high scoring and/or large-gain schools, special attention in physical education was given to the low-scoring boys and girls. In several instances, all pupils below 90 were given individual exercise assignments. Time was provided during the regular physical education class period to practice their special exercises; daily working at home with the exercises was encouraged. The nature of the individual programs was vigorous body-building activity, including conditioning and progressive-resistance exercises, apparatus and tumb-

[9]H. Harrison Clarke, "Oregon Pilot Physical Fitness Project," *The Physical Educator,* **14,** No. 2 (May 1957), 55.

ling, and track work. Careful orientation was provided these pupils on the PFI test, the meaning of each individual's score, and the activity program to follow.

In the low-scoring schools with small gains, very little time was spent in helping individual pupils. The special conditioning activities and the differentiation of class activities found in the high-scoring schools were not in evidence. At two such schools, both boys and girls were in health education classes for six weeks after the first tests were administered; and the following six weeks were devoted to preparation for a physical education exhibition. Thus, only a very few class periods of vigorous physical activity were possible between tests.

Moses Lake Project

The Washington State Fitness Committee, composed of representatives from the Washington Association for Health, Physical Education, and Recreation, the State Department of Public Health, and the State Department of Public Instruction, sponsored a pilot physical fitness study at the Moses Lake Junior High School.[10] Planning meetings were held with Moses Lake school personnel, including the superintendent of schools, public health nurse, school physician, guidance staff, home economists, and physical education administrators. The objectives adopted for the project were: to evaluate the fitness status of the junior high school boys and girls, to select sub-fit children for further study, and to provide individual programs based upon the pupils' needs.

The Rogers Physical Fitness Index and the Kraus-Weber Tests of Minimum Muscular Fitness were administered to approximately 1000 boys and girls. Individual studies of the 40 lowest scoring

[10]Donald K. Mathews, Virginia Shaw, and Philip Risser, "The Moses Lake Project," *Journal of Health, Physical Education, and Recreation,* **29,** No. 4 (April 1958), 18.

children on the PFI were selected as the sub-fit group. A team-approach to the study of these low fitness pupils was made, including the physician, nurse, guidance staff, home economics teacher, and physical educators. The main purpose of this pilot project was to study the group approach to meeting the individual needs of the sub-fit child; the consensus of the participants was that such an approach was feasible and successful. Specialists in the school were "amazed" at the many factors of common interest and how scattered information, when pooled, gave a much broader and deeper understanding of each child's problems.

New Britain, Connecticut

Charles C. Avidisian conducted a cooperative physical fitness program for a number of years in schools of New Britain, Connecticut. Especially effective was the joint relationship with the guidance staff. This program was initiated with the assistance of Donald K. Mathews and professional physical education students from Springfield College. Over 5000 boys were given the Physical Fitness Index test. The subsequent extensive approach to the physical fitness program included staff orientation, developmental and remedial program, and education of the public.

Each year, a summation record was prepared showing the PFI means for boys in each grade in all junior and senior high schools. A PFI card was sent home both in the fall and spring; this card is kept by the parents when their son reaches his senior year. An "Adapted Physical Education" booklet was developed for use at Washington Junior High School. The classification scheme used in New Britain, based on PFI scores, is as follows: A, Gifted, 127 and above; B, Superior, 107–126; C+, High Average, 96–106; C, Average, 85–95; C−, Low Average, 72–84; D, Sub-Strength, 55–71; E, Referrals, 55 and below. This type of classification should, of course, be adapted to local situations.

Springfield College, under the leadership of Clayton T. Shay and utilizing professional students as testers, has cooperated with nearby schools in inaugurating and conducting physical fitness programs, especially at Longmeadow and Holyoke, Massachusetts, and in continuing the program at New Britain.

SELECTED REFERENCES

CLARKE, H. HARRISON, "Oregon Pilot Physical Fitness Project," *The Physical Educator,* **14,** No. 2 (May 1957), 55.

CLARKE, H. HARRISON, "Physical Fitness Testing for the Professional Physical Educator," *The Physical Educator,* **12,** No. 1 (March 1955), 23.

FINKE, CHARLES W., "Use Evaluation Positively," *Journal of Health, Physical Education, and Recreation,* **43,** No. 9 (November-December 1972), 16.

MATHEWS, DONALD K., VIRGINIA SHAW, and PHILLIP RISSER, "The Moses Lake Project," *Journal of Health, Physical Education, and Recreation,* **29,** No. 4 (April 1958), 18.

ROBBINS, C. R., "Central New York Demonstration," *School Activities,* **11,** No. 7 (March 1940), 296.

CHAPTER 17

As has been stressed throughout the text, the *use* of test results in physical education is fundamental. Test results may be used to present important facts to school administrators, boards of education, and the public. This was considered in the preceding chapter. Test results may also be used to motivate boys and girls to greater efforts and for continued practice of desirable habits of exercise, healthful living, and desirable social conduct. This is essential in conducting health and physical education programs.

Tests, however, are essentially the *means of measurement.* They should not constitute the program itself. Testing is a particular phase of administration, as tests should be used to obtain essential information about pupils so that programs can be planned effectively and conducted efficiently. The follow-up procedures constitute "the program" and are of greatest importance for the physical educator as a teacher. To study the *application* of this function of measurement is the purpose of the present chapter.

INDIVIDUALS DIFFER

Individuals differ in their mental, physical, and social make-up. Some have great intelligence and learn quickly; others are slow in their mental processes and have difficulty in keeping up with schoolwork. Some are "alive" physically; others are weak and unfit. Some are capable of being great athletes; others will always be mediocre and below average. Some get along well with people and are liked and respected by their peers; others are obnoxious and unsportsmanlike in their social relationships. Some learn physical skills with great facility; others will probably always be a bit awkward and clumsy at sports and games.

Clarke[1,2] has documented the nature and extent of individual differences, as related to the maturity, physique type, body size, gross and relative muscular strength and endurance, and motor ability elements of boys, and their significance for participation in physical education activities and in interscholastic athletics from elementary school through high school. Some of the conclusions reached were as follows.

Maturity. The more mature boys determined by skeletal age measurement, were larger, stronger, and had greater potential for success in athletics; they were prone to higher levels of aspiration and better psychological adjustment, and had higher levels of academic achievement.

Physique Type. Endomorphic boys were handicapped by excessive body bulk, by low strength relative to weight, by inability to perform muscular endurance exercises involving moving the body, and by inability to make and be successful on interscholastic athletic teams; they had negative self-images but seemed fairly well ad-

[1]H. Harrison Clarke, "Characteristics of Athletes," *Physical Fitness Research Digest,* President's Council on Physical Fitness and Sports, **3,** No. 2 (April 1973).

[2]H. Harrison Clarke, "Individual Differences, Their Nature, Extent, and Significance, *Physical Fitness Research Digest,* President's Council on Physical Fitness and Sports, **3,** No. 4 (October 1973).

Application of Measurement

justed psychologically. Mesomorphic boys had advantages related to greater gross and relative strength, muscular endurance, successful athletic participation, peer status, and psychological adjustment. Ectomorphic boys had disadvantages related to less body bulk and gross strength; they had advantages in relative strength and muscular endurance; they demonstrated some lack of peer status and psychological adjustments and some favorable self-image characteristics.

Body Bulk. Weight was positively related to gross strength and negatively related to relative strength and muscular endurance; except in obese boys, weight was an advantage in making and being successful on interscholastic athletic teams; heavier boys enjoyed greater peer status and higher levels of aspiration (again excepting the obese).

Gross Strength. Gross strength was among the best differentiators of athletic ability at all school levels and in all sports; stronger boys showed better psychological adjustment, greater peer status, and enhanced self-image; some low, but significant, positive correlations were found with academic achievement measures.

Relative Strength. Outstanding athletes in football, basketball, and track had superior relative strength scores as indicated by the Physical Fitness Index, especially at the elementary and junior high school levels; the PFI showed positive relationships to motor ability tests; high PFI boys had greater peer status, positive self-image and positive psychological adjustment on some traits.

Some of the physical and motor traits underlying the individual's total effectiveness are not subject to appreciable improvement through exercise; these traits include maturity, physique type, and body size. However, such traits need to be considered in forming judgments of each

child's capabilities. Other physical traits related to the person's effectiveness as a total being are improvable through appropriate utilization of exercise. These traits include muscular strength, muscular endurance, and circulatory-respiratory endurance, all basic components of physical fitness. Tests of these traits should be included in the physical education program. Appropriate activities should be selected and presented so that boys and girls can reach and maintain appropriate standards on such tests.

As a consequence of these observations, each child, as far as possible, should be treated differently in school programs. The old emphasis in education passed every child through the same educative process. The new emphasis adapts the educational program to the individual's capacities and needs—and necessarily after those capacities and needs have been determined by examinations, tests, and analyses by teachers. Such a program as the one just mentioned brings out and develops the inherent ability of each student in the school.

Procedures necessary for adjusting physical education programs to the capabilities of students and meeting their individual needs follow. These procedures are definitely related to the various objectives of physical education as discussed in Chapters 3, 10, and 13. Particular consideration is given to physical fitness, social adjustment, homogeneous grouping, and sports and athletic activities.

PHYSICAL FITNESS NEEDS

In meeting individual physical fitness needs, pupils with special deficiencies must first be discovered through examinations and tests. The best tests, of course, should be selected (preferably those that have proved practicably usable in schools), so that physically unfit students may be selected for study and treatment. Such a selection of tests might logically include the following types.

1. Medical examination and various sensory tests. Pupils with serious conditions who, in the opinion of physicians, should receive a modified physical education program, should be discovered.

2. Posture and foot tests. Pupils with remedial postural and foot defects may be selected for special exercise prescriptions.

3. Tests of body build. Somatotyping, or other methods of assaying body build, will furnish an important framework of reference for interpreting many test scores and for understanding those limitations and expectations traceable to body type and structure.

4. Nutrition tests. Especially for younger children, a determination of nutritional status is especially important for understanding growth demands.

5. Tests of general physical condition. To discover those pupils whose general fitness either is below par or is declining is the most fundamental phase of physical fitness testing. These tests should be ones that physical educators are trained to administer and the results of which they are competent to interpret.

The Individual Approach

In early editions of this text, considerable attention was given to the steps considered essential in meeting the individual physical fitness needs of students. A separate book has been published by the author and an associate[3] which presents this problem in detail. Reference, therefore, is made to this text; a summarization only will be given here.

After pupils with special needs have been discovered, it is then necessary to assign specific reasons for each pupil's lack of fitness. This identification of causes is a prime concern of the physical educator in successfully meeting the individual needs

of unfit boys and girls. Once causes are discovered, appropriate follow-up procedures for each unfit subject can be properly determined. In "The Case Study Approach," Clarke and Clarke[4] present the following "Ten Essential Steps" for improving the fitness status of pupils who are below accepted standards.

1. Discover boys and girls with special deficiencies revealed by medical, sensory, nutritional, and psychological tests and examinations. An adequate health appraisal by a physician is the starting point of any physical fitness program.

2. Select those who are below predetermined standards of strength, stamina, and other basic physical fitness elements through the administration of valid tests available to the physical educator.

3. For the sub-fit group, conduct physical activities selected to improve their condition (strength and stamina). These activities should be presented progressively within each individual's exercise tolerance and by application of proper principles of exercise.

4. After about six weeks, retest the sub-fit group in order to determine progress and to identify those who do not respond favorably to exercise. For example, those whose test scores decrease or do not increase appreciably should be retested. For students who improve at a satisfactory rate, the exercise program should continue with progressive increases in dosage until minimum standards are reached, or, preferably, exceeded.

5. Identify the cause or causes of the sub-fit condition for those who do not improve scores satisfactorily on retests. These causes may be located by use of case-study procedures, living-habit surveys, personal interviews, and supplementary tests. (Clarke and Clarke present a "Case-Study Form" and a "Health-Habit Questionnaire" to aid this process.)

6. Refer to other specialists, such as the physician, guidance officer, home economist, or school nurse, when physical defects, organic lesions, personality maladjustments, or nutri-

---

[3]H. Harrison Clarke and David H. Clarke, *Developmental and Adapted Physical Education* (Englewood Cliffs, N.J.: Prentice-Hall, Inc., 1963).

[4]Ibid., p. 131.

tional disturbances are suspected as a result of the case-study process. Actually, case-study procedures should be instituted after initial physical fitness tests in some instances, as in the case of obese boys and girls or other easily recognized atypical conditions.

7. Provide individually planned physical fitness programs utilizing the following, as appropriate in each case: proper kind and amount of exercise, health guidance, relaxation procedures, methods and activities applied to improve social and personal adjustment, and medical attention.

8. Relate all factors accumulated in the case study to the individual's somatotype, mental aptitude, and scholastic success. Frequently, these are related, so an understanding of the configuration of the total personality is desirable.

9. Repeat physical fitness tests at intervals of about six weeks, in order to continue checking on the progress made by each sub-fit boy and girl.

10. Re-direct programs in individual cases as found desirable in the light of retest and re-study results.

The procedures presented for improving the fitness status of students who are subpar in basic physical fitness components are more than just theories. They have evolved by use over four decades in school and college physical education. Further, they do not preclude participation by these individuals in the regular activities of physical education. If the physical condition warrants it, sub-fit students should participate in the full physical education program, as they need to learn the skills and to benefit from the social opportunities of these regular classes. For them, however, emphasis on their fitness needs should be primary.

Administrative Adjustments

The physical educator who plans to adopt a program designed to improve effectively the physical fitness of boys and girls who are below acceptable standards in basic components must have an opportunity to supervise case studies, to survey health habits, to interview pupils concerning their psycho-social relationships and other problems, and to conduct classes designed to meet the needs of the individuals. The school administrator who sincerely approves and seriously supports such a program should be ready and willing to provide the necessary time and assistance as rapidly as the needs are demonstrated. In the main, two administrative adjustments should be made if the program is to be conducted effectively and efficiently: extra class time should be arranged for the physical educator to devote to case-study supervision and pupil interviews, and pupils should be scheduled for fitness classes at periods during the week designated for development and relaxation work. Following are a number of suggestions that may prove helpful in arranging for these administrative adjustments.

The Physical Educator's Time. To expect the physical educator to undertake a measurement program on a comprehensive scale when his teaching assignments are already extensive and possibly greater than he should normally be expected to fulfill is unreasonable. The school should expect to pay for this service and should provide sufficient personnel for its administration. The following suggestions for providing this assistance may be considered.

1. In those small school systems where the physical educator is required to teach academic subjects and to perform study-hall duty, relief from these responsibilities would allow him needed extra time for the measurement program.

2. Several phases of the physical education program could be handled by other faculty members under the supervision of the physical educator, thus releasing him for additional

work with pupils in need of special care. Certain academic teachers could either be paid extra for assisting with the intramural and noon-hour programs or for coaching interscholastic teams, for example, or, when faculty members are engaged, such duties may be included in their service contracts.

3. A number of institutions train teachers of physical education who are also prepared and may be certified to teach in an academic field, such as mathematics, history, science, or social studies. If certain academic teachers are carrying exceptionally heavy loads, or if the principal needs relief from teaching duties because of an expanding school program, they may be relieved and the physical educator provided with the help he should have by the addition to the faculty of a combination physical education-academic subject man or woman.

4. In the larger schools, the need will soon be felt for the addition of full-time physical education men and women. These individuals should be selected for their understanding of and ability to conduct measurement programs and to follow them up effectively.

Scheduling Pupils for Classes.   The scheduling of those in need of developmental, postural, or relaxation programs for the same physical education classes is a desirable administrative adjustment if best results are to be obtained in meeting individual physical fitness needs. It permits the physical educator to concentrate his attention on the individual needs of the pupils in the class to the exclusion of other responsibilities. In small schools, this is not an easy task. Nevertheless, if two or three periods can be set aside for this work, the majority of pupils may be accommodated if their academic programs are carefully studied. It is essential, however, for the principal or scheduling officer to have during the summer the physical education classification of each pupil in the school. In order to supply this information, *the annual physical fitness tests must be conducted in the spring.*

When there are physical education teachers for both boys and girls in the school, two methods of scheduling for physical education are possible, depending on whether or not a special exercise room is available.

1. With a special exercise room. Boys may be scheduled for physical fitness work in the special exercise room while the regular girls' classes are being held in the gymnasium, and the girls in the same manner when the boys are in the gymnasium. While specially constructed special exercise rooms are to be preferred, vacant classrooms, or even storage rooms, have been equipped and utilized for this purpose. In large schools, where there are separate gymnasiums and corrective rooms for both boys and girls, and where staff members are assigned to corrective work only, the matter of scheduling students for these special classes is a comparatively simple one.

2. Without a special exercise room. Boys and girls may be scheduled for individual classes at the same period, and the gymnasium divided for class work. This procedure has proved successful in several schools. The physical education teachers can thus concentrate their efforts on the special needs of their pupils. Time for case studies, posture correction, and interviews is also possible, the boys' physical education teacher doing this work while regular girls' classes are in progress, and the girls' director while the boys are in classes.

Where there is only one physical education teacher in the school, definite periods should be set aside for physical fitness work only. Of course, in many situations, ideal arrangements are, for the time being, impossible, and in such instances the next best thing should be done. Following are several suggested makeshifts, arranged in preferential order: (a) the physical educator may hold both physical fitness and regular physical education classes simultaneously, and attempt to shuttle back and forth between the two groups; the use of well-trained pupil leaders is a great help in this situation; (b) only one day each week may be set aside for individual work; (c) the pupils in each physical education class who need developmental and remedial programs may be noted and singled out for special work during regular class; and (d) the physical fitness program may be conducted either during the school's activity period or as an after-school class.

SOCIAL ADJUSTMENT

Will lessons in team play and willingness to sacrifice one's personal advantages for the good of the team result in better citizenship? Will good sportsmanship on the athletic field be reflected in good business ethics? Will the ability to face difficult situations and the necessity to fight through to the very end be reflected in life situations requiring the individual to face odds and not give in—to stand for the right against ridicule—to fight on when the going becomes difficult? Will the ability to accept adverse decisions from officials in athletic contests result in ability to accept adverse decisions from classroom teachers and from other duly constituted authorities?

These are realistic questions in the development of social efficiency as applied to physical education. Physical educators may develop desirable social characteristics in boys and girls as they apply to their own activities, *but* do these same qualities carry over into life situations? The problem of transfer of training is, therefore, a vital one—one that is too frequently neglected in the school.

Transfer of character traits takes place when the individual is able to generalize concerning them. When problems are similar in nature and method of solution, transfer may take place provided the similarities are recognized by the pupil. If he experiences a number of situations that have common elements throughout, he may be brought to generalize. To be most effective, generalizations should be those of the pupil himself. Too frequently, they are the teacher's, and as such are imposed upon the pupil. Under these conditions

they may remain relatively meaningless, and there may be little transfer.

Some method, therefore, must be used that will cause learnings in the physical education field to have a wider sphere of influence. The common elements in the various types of situations covered by the same general trait-name must be utilized in order that their applications may be recognized. For example, the trait "courtesy" covers many different situations. It connotes courtesy in athletics (sportsmanship), in the schoolroom, in business, within one's own family, with one's own group, and with outside individuals and groups. The pupil must be guided in forming generalizations concerning this and other traits. The entire school may very logically cooperate in this effort, using physical education experiences as the bases upon which transfer takes place.

It should be pointed out, however, that there is danger in overemphasizing traits in the development of social efficiency. Attention may be centered upon self, and the act and its consequences obscured. Also, situations will arise in which desirable traits are opposed to each other and the individual must make a choice, sacrificing one virtue for another. Here a total situation must be evaluated and the best decision made. The trait-conditioned person may be in severe conflict with himself and thus unable to do this easily and efficiently. Trait conditioning may develop a conformative rather than a creative society. The total-situation approach, with well-established general principles as guides upon which to base decisions, and with the will to act for the greatest good of the greatest number over the greatest period of time, is the only sound answer to this problem.

Selection of Social Tests

In the selection of tests to measure social efficiency, the physical educator may logically consider such instruments related to his field as the Blanchard Behavior Rating Scale, the Cowell Social Behavior Trend Index, the Cowell Personal Distance Ballot, or a sociometric questionnaire. However, he may also use the various character and personality tests constructed in education and psychology, provided the traits measured in these tests conform to the traits developed through the physical activity program. The latter selection of tests can have value in securing the transfer of social traits from physical education to school and life situations. The aim of the physical educator thus is directed toward life problems rather than toward the limited field of conduct and relationships in sports and athletics only. A consideration of both types of tests appears in Chapter 11.

Meeting Individual Needs

Once those individuals with social problems are discovered, either through general observation or by objective measurement, the physical educator should take such steps as necessary to assist these pupils in making proper adjustments. The general approach is similar to the one outlined above for meeting individual physical fitness needs: a determination of "causes" through case-study and interview techniques, instigating appropriate remedies for removing such causes, and including in individual physical education programs the types of activities that will best develop the boy or girl socially.

Causes of social maladjustment will vary considerably from the conditions sought in studying low physical fitness. A partial list of such causes follows.

1. Peculiarities or differences in student's physique, including physical weakness, defects, or extreme variations in body structure, facial features, or skin color, may cause him to avoid other students or to seek compensation through antisocial bids for attention.

2. Unhealthy mental attitudes, such as feelings of inferiority and inadequacy, are often caused by undesirable parental and school relationships, financial insecurity, and marked deviations from other pupils in dress, speech, popularity, and success.

3. Oversolicitous parents, who may shield pupils from all difficulties and harshness and who may dominate and restrict their activities, may cause submissiveness, selfishness, aggressiveness, domineering social habits, and inability to meet new situations.

4. Attitude of teachers who emphasize mistakes and blunders of their pupils and try to be clever and witty at their expense, or who tactlessly and bluntly belittle their achievements and ability to achieve, frequently produces feelings of inferiority, resentment, lack of interest, truancy, and ineffective efforts to achieve.

5. Inability to achieve in the academic field may result in attempts to compensate for this failure by assuming an attitude of bravado, destructiveness, and bullying to hide the pupil's sensitiveness and thwarted desire for social approval, or to adopt fantasy, romancing, or boasting, or to seek companionship in groups where his talents will be appreciated.

6. Physical aspects of the home, such as appearance, location, comfort, and cultural resources, often arouse feelings of inferiority, shame, rebellion, and frustration, and cause students to avoid social contacts.

7. Awkwardness in students clumsy in movement and deficient in motor skills results in social unacceptability among their peers, especially during adolescence.

8. Insufficient social experiences of the right type result in social maladjustment when the individual attempts to establish new relationships.

9. Poor recreational experiences may result in social difficulties and other personality defects.

It is extremely difficult to get at the underlying causes of social maladjustment in many instances, partly because pupils are inclined to hide these facts from others, partly because these causes may be so obscure and involved with extraneous factors that the student may feel fully justified in attributing his difficulty to some source far removed from the real

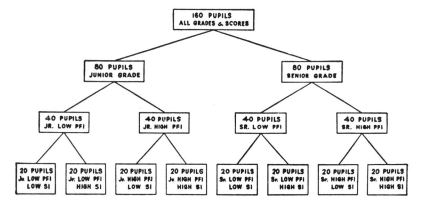

FIGURE 17.1. *Chart for Securing Homogeneity on Multi-Variable Bases*

one, and partly because the student may be entirely ignorant of the causes of his difficulty. The physical educator needs to gain experience in the use of counseling procedures, and may wish to confer with psychologists, psychiatrists, or the regular guidance personnel in the school.

The remedy, of course, should fit the cause. General procedures for meeting the social objective in physical education are discussed in Chapter 10.

HOMOGENEOUS GROUPING

The values and purposes of homogeneous grouping in physical education are given in Chapter 10; tests for equating groups on the basis of general physical abilities are presented in Chapter 12; and tests of specific activities in physical education, which may be used for such grouping on the basis of individual sport skills, appear in Chapter 14. The present section will consider methods of securing homogeneity.

Homogeneous grouping can be secured on the basis of only one quality at a time. Several measures of unlike traits when combined into a single rating tend to destroy homogeneity rather than to provide it. For example, the following individuals are not comparable:

	PFI	I.Q.	Total
Pupil A	125	75	200
Pupil B	75	125	200
Pupil C	100	100	200

Here are three boys, A, B, and C, with equal total scores. Are they homogeneous in any quality disclosed? One is physically strong, another is not; one is intelligent, another is not; the third is average in both qualities.

The proper method for securing homogeneity on a multiple basis is first to divide the group on one basis, and then to divide the new groups on a second basis. If three bases for differentation are used, the subdivision should be redivided, making eight different groups. For example, if the divisions are on the basis of grade in school, Physical Fitness Index, and Strength Index, the groupings are illustrated in Figure 17.1.[5]

Two groups are most effective when the test scores involved have a narrow range and/or when the number of pupils is small. When the range is extensive, as when the Strength Index is used as the test for group formations, and the number of subjects is large, the number of groups will

[5]Adapted from Frederick Rand Rogers, *Fundamental Administrative Measures in Physical Education* (Newton, Mass.: Pleiades Company, 1932), p. 66.

logically be increased. Still, some experience in trying out various arrangements in practice may be desirable. For example, Cox and DuBois[6] reported several years of experience in equating secondary school groups with the Strength Index. They recommended a 200-point range for each group. They found that, if a 300-point range in SI is permitted within any single division, the strongest boys in each division almost always win, whereas the weakest almost never win in track and field events. Reducing the spread to 200 points for junior high school boys seems to guarantee a more equitable distribution of winning and losing experiences: a satisfactory teaching and learning adjustment. Judgment, however, should be used in working out these classifications, for, when the groups to be divided into teams or squads are small, levels must be determined by the number to be included on each team. For regular classwork in physical education, squads of 12 pupils each are most convenient, as this number will serve for two basketball teams within the group or a single baseball, soccer, touch football, or track team.

When the divisions have been determined, the next step is to form teams within each level. To do this, the most satisfactory method is to *match* the scores. That is, it is necessary not only to have the total scores of competing teams equal, but to have the variability of the pupils alike as well. Thus, if John has an SI of 1522 and is placed on Team *A,* Henry, who is on Team *B,* should have approximately the same Strength Index. This principle for equating groups for physical activities applies not only to the Strength Index but equally well to any other test used for this purpose, whether it be Larson's, McCloy's, Cozens', and so forth, or whether it be on the basis of individual test scores, such as in basketball, soccer, or football.

[6]Walter A. Cox and Kenneth B. DuBois, "Equating Opponents in Intramural Track and Field Activities," *Supplement to the Research Quarterly,* **6,** No. 1 (March 1935), 219.

Carson[7] described physical education class experiences from the ability grouping of girls at the Chief Sealth Junior High School, Seattle, Washington. With four teachers and 100 girls assigned to physical education each class period, three ability groups were formed in each class; each of the ability groups contained girls from freshman to senior years in school. The instrument utilized to form the groups was Scott's Motor Ability Test, described in Chapter 11. Physical education class activities were adapted to the level of each group. The low group started with body mechanics and fundamental activities, designed to help them in each sport in turn. The middle group participated in a combination of team and individual sports. The high group concentrated on individual sports, with intensive short units on team activities and recreational leadership.

At the end of the year, both students and faculty evaluated the program. Of the students, 96 percent liked the ability grouping; more than 85 percent felt they had accomplished more than they would have in the usual class. The faculty response was also enthusiastic. Characteristics of the three groups as taught under these conditions follow.

High Group. Highly competitive, rarely absent, seldom failed to shower, well coordinated, learned readily, evaluated themselves better, helped each other, greater participation in the intramural program, and made good assistants.

Middle Group. Unpredictable, difficult to handle effectively, attitudes inconsistent, short attention span, absent more than high group, forgot clothes more often and missed showers more frequently, did not help each other, tended to be critical, and less initiative.

[7]Mary Carson, "Chief Sealth Junior High Groups PE Classes by Ability," *Physical Education Newsletter,* **5,** Letter 12 (February 27, 1964).

Low Group.   Health poorer, often absent from school, made more shower excuses and forgot more clothing, lower written and skill test grades, willing to practice and eager to learn, lacked confidence, poor coordination, slow moving, poor judgment and little concept of space, not critical of others, and gained satisfaction from success experiences.

Sport and athletic skills

Diagnostic analyses and remedial processes can be applied to any trait that can be evaluated or measured. Such procedures have been discussed above in relation to physical fitness and social adjustment. They may also be used in relation to sport and athletic skills. In fact, the diagnosis of skill difficulties and the application of remedial measures are everyday practices of the physical education teacher; they are as nearly second nature to him as anything he does. True, these processes are largely subjective as the physical educator watches the performance of his pupils and makes criticisms and suggestions as to how the skill may best be accomplished or be improved to the point of perfection. In teaching exercises on the apparatus, stunts in tumbling, or fundamentals of game skills, the physical educator is continually alert to correct and improve the performance of his pupils; in coaching athletic teams, the coach must be eternally vigilant to improve his players' performances if the team is to be successful in competition. These are essential functions of the physical educator.

Objective skill testing, however, is infrequently used in physical education for diagnostic and remedial purposes. Track and field is very highly objective, as times and distances become essential data in appraising the performance of the competitors. The athletic team is also objectively tested on the day of a game, when it competes in actual contest with opponents of similar abilities. The day-by-day work of the physical educator, nevertheless, is of a more subjective nature. Objective testing may be an aid to him, but will not replace his judgment in diagnosing and suggesting remedies for the improvement of skill.

In fact, the present status of skill testing in physical education does not lend it readily to diagnostic procedures. The various skill tests presented in Chapter 14 are usable more for the general evaluation of physical education activities than for a complete analysis of the activity. In diagnosing athletic ability, McCloy's batteries of general motor capacity and general motor ability, discussed in Chapter 12, are attempts in this field and indicate the possibilities of this type of testing.

The clinical approach

At the 1965 meeting of the Western College Men's Physical Education Society, N. P. Neilson proposed a clinical approach to the college physical education program. The health clinic is an accepted procedure in medicine and public health. Conditions causing or conducive to poor health are discovered and treatment is given, prescribed, or recommended. Data are kept on file for present and future use. A similar clinical approach is possible in physical education.

Neilson maintains that college students are interested in knowing their status with reference to reasonable standards and with reference to the status of other members of their group. In some cases, they are not aware of their deficiencies and so tend to select (when allowed to do so) activities about which they already have considerable knowledge and in which they have considerable skill. According to Neilson, ideally, they should be tested in various ways in order to find their strengths and weaknesses so that programs could be adapted to their individual needs.

The proposed Physical Education Clinic has the following features:

I. Test Administration

A. General health status

1. Health examination, examination by the health service. (The recorded results should be transferred for use by the physical education department before the department's clinical tests are given.)
2. Health knowledge test.

B. Developmental status in physical education

1. Interpretive development: knowledge tests on general theory of physical education and about selected physical education activities.
2. Impulsive development: tests of interests, attitudes, emotions, and ideals.
3. Neuromuscular development: strength tests of major muscle groups, and a series of skill tests in selected physical education activities.
4. Organic development: muscular endurance tests of major muscle groups, and a test of cardiovascular-respiratory endurance.

II. Activity Evaluation

An evaluation of selected physical education activities should be made in terms of their specific contributions to different aspects of development so that recommendations can be made for their use in relation to deficiencies.

III. Central Record System and Consultation Service

A central record system with a consultant should be available to each student for counseling and follow-up of test results. In the various tests of functions, the goal should be the construction of achievement scales. A card for each student would show his status upon entering the physical education program and would allow for additional test records as contemplated. The records would be used in the guidance program so that each student could be given advice and encouragement to participate in the activities best suited to his needs.

As announced by Superintendent Leon M. Lessinger, the San Mateo, California, Union High School District has established a Physical Fitness Research Laboratory as an added teaching station in physical education.[8] The laboratory contains instruments for testing neuromuscular coordination, cardiovascular endurance, respiratory capacity and endurance, posture and body mechanics, flexibility and mobility, and the strength and endurance of the muscular system. The laboratory is staffed with physical educators qualified to use the instruments and to interpret the results as applied to individuals. Students are trained in an elective high school course to assist with laboratory testing, thus providing them with experience in technical-vocational work.

The laboratory has many advantages, including the following: testing pupil status and progress as related to numerous aspects of physical fitness; providing teachers and administrators with clearer insights into the individual needs of students; giving students a better understanding of and respect for their physical fitness status and needs and for appropriate means of improving and maintaining their fitness; providing opportunities for physicians and other health-related personnel to work with physical educators in resolving various physical fitness problems encountered; and conducting special physical fitness research projects. The laboratory is used as a referral agency by nurses, doctors, counselors, and administrators. Thus, this experimental physical fitness facility becomes a direct adjunct to the guidance program. The scientific aspects of physical education demonstrated by the laboratory should build greater acceptance of the value of exercise, which needs to be adopted by all people as a way of life, and of the importance of physical education in the school.

[8]"A Physical Fitness Laboratory," *Physical Education Newsletter,* **9,** No. 12 (February 15, 1965).

SELECTED REFERENCES

CLARKE, H. HARRISON, "Individual Differences, Their Nature, Extent, and Significance," *Physical Fitness Research Digest,* President's Council on Physical Fitness and Sports, **3,** No. 2 (April 1973).

CLARKE, H. HARRISON, and DAVID H. CLARKE, *Developmental and Adapted Physical Education.* Englewood Cliffs, N.J.: Prentice-Hall, Inc., 1963.

COX, WALTER A., and KENNETH B. DUBOIS, "Equating Opponents in Intramural Track and Field Activities," *Supplement to the Research Quarterly,* **6,** No. 1 (March 1935), 219.

ROGERS, FREDERICK RAND, *Fundamental Administrative Measures in Physical Education.* Newton, Mass.: Pleiades Company, 1932.

AN EPILOGUE

As an ordinary citizen, how do you know when your automobile tires have sufficient pressure? When you have a fever, and how high it is? What your weight is and whether you have gained or lost, and how much? How fast you drive a car? The time of day? The fertility of the soil in your garden and its deficiencies? *Do you guess? or, do you measure?*

As a physical educator, how do you know the speed your star athlete ran the 100-yard dash? The record your broad-jumper made? The bacterial content of your swimming pool water? The exact second a football game is over? The layout of a tennis court? The temperature of your gymnasium? *Do you guess? or, do you measure?*

Is it not true that by measurement, you make sure rather than guess or take for granted?

If measurement is so important for so many things, is it not absolutely vital in order to determine the status of those basic growth factors in boys and girls capable of development through physical education? In determining pupil strength or physical fitness, *should you guess? or, should you measure?*

Through the use of objective, valid tests, the physical educator determines the physical, motor, and personal-social status of his pupils; he identifies those who are deficient in these essential qualities and he measures their progress toward desirable standards. His service to boys and girls is rendered effective and efficient. He not only knows the direction of his program, but is able to determine its accomplishments. He no longer justifies his work by rationalization or by facile oratory, but is able to present indisputable proof.

"To Measure or Not to Measure—
That is the Question!"

Do You Guess?
Or
Do You Measure?

APPENDIX A

An understanding of the elements of statistics is essential to the physical educator who wishes to be completely trained in the fundamentals of his profession, and is indispensable to the individual who desires to be competent in the field of measurement. Such an understanding has definite advantages, as follows.

1. To understand and interpret scientific literature. The use of statistical terms is commonplace in research journals. For example, seldom has the *Research Quarterly* of the American Alliance for Health, Physical Education, and Recreation published an article in which quantitative data are not analyzed statistically in some way. Therefore, a knowledge of statistics is essential in order to understand these articles and evaluate these researches.

2. To determine the scientific worth of tests. Although the construction of tests is a phase of research, the evaluation of tests should be a concern of all health and physical educators who use them. Statistical procedures are utilized widely in this process: to validate, to establish reliability, and to construct norms. The ability, therefore, to determine the scientific worth of tests is dependent upon a knowledge of statistics.

3. To prepare reports based on test results. The preparation of reports of the results achieved in school programs is a common responsibility of educators. An effective aspect of such reports is the inclusion of test results that show pupil progress. The use of graphs and some of the easily understood statistics, such as frequency distributions, percentiles, medians, and quartiles, are of value for this purpose.

4. To conduct research. Obviously, the conduct of scientific research requires the application of statistics in the treatment of test data in order to determine the results and significance of studies. Although the following presentation of the elements of statistics is not designed to make expert statisticians, this aspect of the work may appeal to a certain few with special interests of a scientific nature.

No attempt is made in this chapter to give a complete exposition of all statistical concepts the physical educator will encounter in his study of tests and measurements. An understanding of the elementary, basic concepts only are included. The material is such as might logically be included in a first course in tests and measurements and is needed in order to evaluate the tests appearing in the text.

Elements of Statistics

THE FREQUENCY TABLE

As statistics is a quantitative technique, dealing with large numbers of test scores, the first task is to organize the data. This is accomplished by assembling the scores into groups or classes, thus constructing a frequency table. As an illustration of this technique, the following 62 weights are given in pounds:

120	104	94	76	79	113	103
102	97	156*	115	98	139	92
119	129	93	102	116	75	84
90	75	81	109	122	59	137
79	54	116	91	67	68	72
141	131	100	147	64	60	105
83	57	89	85	110	110	108
42*	100	100	77	80	130	100
125	49	112	120	105	97	

The procedures in constructing the frequency table fall into four main headings.

First, the range of scores must be found in order to determine the distance over which the scores are spread. In the data given above, these two scores are starred, 156 being the highest and 42 the lowest; the range, therefore, is 114. In other words, all the weights fall between 156 and 42, a distance of 114 pounds.

Second, the number of groups, or step intervals (SI), must be determined. To arrive at this number, there is only one general rule to follow: the number of steps should be between 10 and 20, the final selection depending upon the range and the number of scores. With a few cases, or with a small or moderate range, the number of step intervals should be nearer 10; while with many cases, or a moderate or large range, the number should be nearer 20. In the figures above there are what might be considered a few cases and a moderate range; therefore, approximately 12 step intervals should be selected.

Third, some step interval sizes are preferable as they are more convenient for tabulation. These sizes are 1, 2, 3, 5, 10, 20, and 25. These intervals will take care of most sets of data; where greater intervals are necessary, however, 50, 100, 200, and so forth are more desirable than numbers in between. With the range of 114 in the illustrated problem, and a decision to use approximately 12 step intervals, each step would consist of 10 pounds.

Fourth, the step intervals should be in tabular form, with the largest scores at the top and the smallest at the bottom. The limits of the top "step" should be such as to include the highest score. Instead of using the highest score as the upper limit of this step, however, it is always easier and just as satisfactory to use a multiple of the size of the step selected, which in this case is 10.

Thus, as 156 is the highest score, the top step should be the interval 150–159. Each of the following 10 scores are included: 150, 151, 152, 153, 154, 155, 156, 157, 158, and 159. Scores of 149.5 to 150.4 are considered 150; scores of 158.5 to 159.4, 159. Thus, this step actually extends from 149.5 to 159.4, as it is assumed that each score is rounded off to the nearest whole number.

All step intervals, then, should be arranged in tabular form, beginning with the step 150–159 and continuing down until the lowest step includes the smallest score, 42.

Finally, each weight score should be placed in its proper step interval. For example, the first score, 120, goes in the step 120–129; the second, 102, in 100–109; and so on until all the scores are placed, each indicated by a check mark opposite the proper step interval. The number of scores in each step is then designated with the appropriate figure. This column is known as the "frequency column" and is indicated by the letter f. The total of the frequency column, indicated by N, should equal 62, the original number of weights. The details concerning this procedure are illustrated in Table A.1.

MEASURES OF CENTRAL TENDENCY

A measure of central tendency is a single score that represents all the scores in a distribution. If one asked the accomplishment of a class on an examination, the answer would not be that John received 85; Mary, 75; Jack, 82; and so on until all the individual scores had been enumerated. This would be both meaningless and confusing, as one would still wonder how well the class as a whole had performed. Instead, the answer would probably be: "The average of the class was 82," or whatever the average may have been. The answer, thus, is in terms of central tendency—a single score representing all the scores. There are three measures of central tendency in common use: the mode, the median, and the mean.

Mode

The mode is the score or measure that appears most frequently. When scores are ungrouped, but arranged in order from high to low, it is a very simple matter to determine the score appearing the greatest number of times. For example, in the 62 weights, 100 appears four times, the largest number for any single score, and consequently it is the mode.

From grouped scores, however, it is impossible to determine the most frequent score, but one can tell the step interval in which the largest number of scores lies. In the data illustrated in Table A.1, 12 scores, the largest number in any one step, appear

in the interval 100–109. When it is necessary to represent a step interval by a single score, which is true in this case, the mid-point is taken. Thus, the mode is 104.5.

To find the mid-point of a step interval, add half the size of the step to its lower limit. In the illustration, the size of the step is 10, half of which is 5, which, added to the lower limit, 99.5, makes the answer 104.5.[1]

A more reliable method of obtaining the mode from the frequency distribution is to compute it from the following formula:

$$\text{mode} = 3(\text{median}) - 2(\text{mean}).$$

Median

The median is the mid-point in a distribution, that point above which and below which lie 50 percent of the scores. When scores are ungrouped but arranged in order from high to low, it is quite easy to find the center, or middle score. For example, in the five scores 18, 17, 15, 12, and 9, the middle score is 15.

With scores grouped in a frequency table, this process is not so simple. One can, however, count up the frequency column from the bottom and find in which group the median lies. Then, by a process of interpolation, the exact point can be found. This process is illustrated in Table A.1, where the 62 weights appear in a frequency table.

With 62 scores, the mid-point is at the 31st score:

$$\frac{N}{2} = \frac{62}{2} = 31.$$

Counting off from the small end of the frequency column, there are 30 scores below the step 100–109. Thus, the point 99.5, the lower limit of the step, is reached, the 31st score being somewhere above this

TABLE A.1 *Calculation of the Mode, Median, and Mean from Data Grouped into a Frequency Table*

Scores		f	d	fd
150–159	/	1	5	5
140–149	//	2	4	8
130–139	////	4	3	12
120–129	ЖЙ	5	2	10
110–119	ЖЙ ///	8	1	8
				(+ 43)
100–109	ЖЙ ЖЙ //	12	0	0
90–99	ЖЙ ///	8 (30)	−1	−8
80–89	ЖЙ /	6	−2	−12
70–79	ЖЙ //	7	−3	−21
60–69	////	4	−4	−16
50–59	///	3	−5	−15
40–49	//	2	−6	−12
				(−84)
		$N = 62$		−41

1. Mode falls in class-interval 100–109, or at 104.5 (the mid-point).

2. Median = $\dfrac{N}{2} = \dfrac{62}{2} = 31.$

Median = $99.5 + \dfrac{1}{12} \times 10 = 100.33$

3. Mean (short method): $GA + \left(\dfrac{\Sigma fd}{N} \times SI \right) =$

$GA = 104.5$　　　$104.5 + \left(\dfrac{-41}{62} \times 10 \right) =$

$\dfrac{\Sigma fd}{N} = \dfrac{-41}{62}$　　$104.5 + (-6.61) = 97.89.$

[1] This mid-point is taken when the test scores have been recorded to the nearest unit; it would be 105, if the scores had been recorded to the last unit.

point. With 30 scores gone, therefore, one more is needed to reach the middle. As there are 12 scores in the step interval, $\frac{1}{12}$ of it should be taken, $\frac{1}{12}$ of 10, the size of the step, equals 0.83. Adding this amount to 99.5 gives the median: 100.33.

Mean

The *mean* may best be defined as the *average,* for both terms are used interchangeably. In arithmetic, the average is the sum of the scores divided by their number.

$$\text{Ave.} = \frac{\Sigma(s)}{N},$$

in which Σ means *summation* and N is the number of scores.

A short method of determining the mean, when the scores are grouped in a frequency table, is to guess an average and then apply a correction, thus: GA + C. The guessed average (GA) is taken from the mid-point of the step selected, and the correction is in terms of the deviation of the scores in step intervals from this guessed average. The formula is developed as follows:

$$\text{Mean} = \text{GA} + \text{C}$$
$$\text{C} = c \times \text{SI}$$
$$c = \frac{\Sigma fd}{N}$$
$$\text{Mean} = \text{GA} + \left(\frac{\Sigma fd}{N} \times \text{SI} \right)$$

In the sample problem given in Table A.1, the guessed average is selected at the 100–109 step. As the mid-point of the step is used, the GA equals 104.5. The only guide in choosing the guessed average is to select it somewhere near the center of the distribution, as this saves work.

The next step in computing the mean is to determine the deviation of the different mid-points from the one guessed. The mid-point of the step 110–119 deviates 10

points, or 1 step interval, from the guessed average, the 1 being used to indicate the deviation. Each mid-point above is 1 point farther removed, so in the d column the deviations are 1, 2, 3, 4, and 5. These are positive deviations, as they represent values greater than the guessed average. Below the guessed average, the same situation exists, except that the deviations are negative, as the values are less than guessed average.

Since there are more values in some steps than there are in others, it is necessary to take this fact into consideration, which is done by multiplying the number of scores contained in each step (f column) by the deviation of the step from the guessed average (d column). Thus $f \times d = fd$. The sum of this final column (the fd column) must then be computed. As there are positive and negative values in the column, they must be added separately and their difference determined. In the problem (Table A.1), the sum of the positive values is 43 and that of the negative values 84. Thus the sum of the column is -41. Substitution in the formula may now be completed.

$$\text{Mean} = \text{GA} + \left(\frac{\Sigma fd}{N} \times \text{SI} \right)$$
$$= 104.5 + \left(\frac{-41}{62} \times 10 \right) = 97.89.$$

By experimenting with several guessed averages, the student will find that the same answer is obtained each time. It will readily be seen that, if the guessed average is low, a preponderance of positive values in the fd column will pull it up to the proper point. The reverse is true if the guessed average is high, for negative values will pull it down.

Use of Mode, Median and Mean

The *mode* is a rough measure and may be quite inaccurate as a measure of central tendency, especially if a small group of scores is involved, as in the present case. The larger the number of cases and the more symmetrical (normal) the distribution, however, the more reliable it becomes as a measure of central tendency. Aside from its use as a measure of central tendency, it also has value in indicating the greatest concentration of scores.

The *median* may be computed quickly and easily, and is not affected by extreme scores in the distribution. If one wishes to avoid the influence of extremely high or extremely low scores on the measure of central tendency, the median should be used. It should also be used when the distribution is truncated, that is, cut off at the top or bottom. Truncation may be a definite problem for some physical education tests, especially when zeros are possible, or even probable, as in chinning. In this situation, a zero score does not mean that the pupil has no arm strength; rather, the test does not measure it. Further, one pupil with a zero number of chins may differ significantly in arm strength from another pupil with a zero score.

The *mean* is the most reliable of the measures of central tendency, and is the one used when advanced work in statistics is to be done. Each score in the distribution has equal weight, that is, equal to its full value, in determining the central tendency, as extreme scores at either end of the distribution affect this measure.

QUARTILES AND PERCENTILES

The use of quartiles and percentiles is valuable in making test scores meaningful and in describing the results achieved by a class or group of individuals that has been tested. It is impossible to know how well one has done on a test unless his score is shown in relationship to others taking the same test. For example, simply giving a score of 150 on an examination is meaningless. If, however, the 30th percentile score is 150, it is immediately known that this individual has exceeded 30 percent of those taking the test but is below the score achieved by 70 percent. Percentiles are also of considerable value in comparing the standing of different individuals in a number of tests. For example, how does a score of 11 seconds in the 100-yard dash compare with a score of 16 feet in the broad jump? If 11 seconds is at the 75th percentile point and 16 feet is at the 65th percentile, the comparison becomes clear.

The quartiles are of use, also, in dividing or sectioning grades or classes into quarters, based, of course, upon test results, or in determining division points for the lower 25 percent, the middle 50 percent, and the upper 25 percent.

Quartiles

The 25th percentile, or Q_1, is the first quarter or quartile point: the point below which lie 25 percent of the scores and above which lie 75 percent. Similarly, the 75th percentile, or Q_3, is the third quarter or quartile point: the point below which lie 75 percent of the scores and above which lie 25 percent. The median, by way of comparison, is the 50th percentile, or Q_2.

The method of calculating the quartiles is similar to the procedure followed in locating the median, except that different points are to be found. In finding the median, it was the middle score or 50 percent point. In finding Q_1, however, it is the one-fourth, or 25 percent point; with Q_3, it is the three-fourths, or 75 percent point. If the scores are ungrouped, counting up the necessary number of cases is all that is required. With grouped scores, however, it is necessary to interpolate, as was done in finding the median.

Table A.2 illustrates the calculation of Q_1 and Q_3 for the distribution of the 62 weights. With 62 scores, the one-fourth point is at 15.5:

$$\frac{N}{4} = \frac{62}{4} = 15.5.$$

Table A.2 *Calculation of Quartiles and Deciles (Percentiles) from Data Grouped into a Frequency Table (Data from Table A.1)*

Scores	f	Cum f	Quartiles
150–159	1	62	$Q_1 = 78.79$
140–149	2	61	$Q_3 = 115.13$
130–139	4	59	
120–129	5	55	*Deciles Table*
110–119	8	50	P_{100} 156
100–109	12	42	P_{90} 132
90– 99	8	30	P_{80} 119
80– 89	6	22	P_{70} 111
70– 79	7	16	P_{60} 106
60– 69	4	9	P_{50} 100
50– 59	3	5	P_{40} 93
40– 49	2	2	P_{30} 84
	$N = \overline{62}$		P_{20} 74
			P_{10} 63
			P_0 42

Calculation of Deciles

$$P_{10} = \frac{N}{10} = 6.2 \qquad 59.5 + \left(\frac{1.2}{4} \times 10\right) = 63$$

$$P_{20} = \frac{2N}{10} = 12.4 \qquad 69.5 + \left(\frac{3.4}{7} \times 10\right) = 74$$

$$P_{30} = \frac{3N}{10} = 18.6 \qquad 79.5 + \left(\frac{2.6}{6} \times 10\right) = 84$$

$$P_{40} = \frac{4N}{10} = 24.8 \qquad 89.5 + \left(\frac{2.8}{8} \times 10\right) = 93$$

$$P_{50} = \frac{5N}{10} = 31.0 \qquad 99.5 + \left(\frac{1}{12} \times 10\right) = 100$$

$$P_{60} = \frac{6N}{10} = 37.2 \qquad 99.5 + \left(\frac{7.2}{12} \times 10\right) = 106$$

$$P_{70} = \frac{7N}{10} = 43.4 \qquad 109.5 + \left(\frac{1.4}{8} \times 10\right) = 111$$

$$P_{80} = \frac{8N}{10} = 49.6 \qquad 109.5 + \left(\frac{7.6}{8} \times 10\right) = 119$$

$$P_{90} = \frac{9N}{10} = 55.8 \qquad 129.5 + \left(\frac{.8}{4} \times 10\right) = 132$$

Calculation of Quartiles

$$Q_1 = \frac{N}{4}, \text{ or } \frac{62}{4} = 15.5$$

$$69.5 + \frac{6.5}{7} \times 10 = 78.79$$

$$Q_3 = \frac{3N}{4} \text{ or } \frac{3 \times 62}{4} = 46.5$$

$$109.5 + \frac{4.5}{8} \times 10 = 115.13$$

Counting up from the bottom of the frequency columns, there are 9 scores below the step 70–79. The lower limit of that step, or 69.5, is thus reached, score number 15.5 lying somewhere within the step. With 9 scores gone, therefore, 6.5 more are needed. As there are 7 scores in the step interval, 6.5/7 of it is taken. The size of the step is 10, so:

$$\frac{6.5}{7} \times 10 = 9.29$$

Adding this amount to 69.5, Q_1 equals 78.79.

In like manner, Q_3 is found by counting off three-fourths of the scores from the small end of the distribution. Three-fourths of $N = 46.5$:

$$\frac{3N}{4} = \frac{3 \times 62}{4} = 46.5$$

There are 42 scores below the step 110–119. Therefore, 4.5 additional scores are needed. As there are 8 scores in the step:

$$\frac{4.5}{8} \times 10 = 5.63.$$

Adding this amount to 109.5, the beginning of the step, makes Q_3 equal 115.13.

Percentiles

It is frequently very useful to know, in addition to the median and the quartiles, the ten decile points in the distribution, that is, 10th, 20th, 30th, 40th, and the like percentile points. The method of calculating these points is similar to that used for finding the median and the quartiles except that again different points are found. For example, the 10th percentile is found by counting off one-tenth, and the 20th percentile by counting off two-tenths (one-fifth) of the scores from the small end of the distribution, rather than one-fourth, one-half, and three-fourths, as was true with Q_1, median, and Q_3, respectively.

Table A.2 illustrates the method used in calculating the percentiles in the distribution of the 62 weights. The 10th percentile (P_{10}) is located by finding one-tenth of 62 ($N/10$), or 6.2 and counting this number of scores from the small end of the distribution. Thus, the 10th percentile is 62.5. In like manner, the 20th percentile (P_{20}), which is $^2/_{10}$ of 62 ($2N/10$), or 12.4, is found by counting 12.4 scores from the small end of the distribution, and is located at 74.36. When percentile scores result in fractions, the score is usually taken

at the nearest whole number. Thus, in the above examples, the deciles are 63 and 74, respectively.

The 0 and 100th percentiles are the lowest and highest scores in the distribution. Thus, in the original data from which the frequency table was constructed, the lowest score was 42 and the highest 156. Therefore, the 0 percentile falls at 42 and the 100th at 156.

A cumulative frequency column (marked *Cum f*) appears in Table A.2. The scores in this column were obtained by adding the frequencies serially, beginning with the lowest frequency and continuing to the largest. This column is of assistance in locating the desired point when counting for any particular percentile. For example, P_{80} is 49.6 scores:

$$\frac{4N}{5} = \frac{4 \times 62}{5} = 49.6$$

from the beginning of the distribution. Hence, it is clear from the *Cum f*'s that there are 42 scores below the step 110–119, and that the lower limit of that step (109.5) has been reached.

When percentile scoring tables are constructed, all percentiles are used from 0 to 100, rather than restricting them to decile points, as shown in the above computations. To illustrate for P_{43}:

$$P_{43} = \frac{43 \times N}{100} = \frac{43 \times 62}{100} = 26.6$$

Thus, P_{43} is 26.6 scores from the low end of the distribution; from the *Cum f*'s column, there are 22 scores below the step 90–99 and its lower limit (89.5) has been reached. From this interval, 4.6 scores are needed: $26.6 - 22 = 4.6$. Thus:

$$\text{Mdn} = 89.5 + \frac{4.6 \times 10}{8} = 95.25.$$

MEASURES OF VARIABILITY

Measures of central tendency indicate typical performance for a group or for test scores as a whole. The next step is to consider the variability of these scores, that is, of the spread of the scores around the measure of central tendency. In order to show the usefulness of a measure of variability, consider the *strength indices* of the following two groups of high school boys arranged for competition with each other:

Group A: average SI = 1500
Group B: average SI = 1500

As far as can be determined from the data at hand, these two groups are alike in so far as the quality being measured is concerned. Suppose, however, that the highest SI in Group A is 2500 and the lowest is 500; in Group B the highest is 2000 and the lowest 1000. The two groups no longer seem alike, as the range of scores for Group A covers a distance of 2000 SI points, whereas for Group B, the distance is only 1000. In thus using the range, a measure of variability has been applied to indicate the spread of all the scores. *Similarity can be shown between groups only when both the central tendency and the variability of the scores are approximately the same.*

There are three measures of variability in common use: the range, the quartile deviation, and the standard deviation. These will be discussed in the order listed.

Range

In the preceding illustration, the range was used to indicate the variability of all the scores. Its use as a measure of variability, however, is unreliable when frequent or extreme gaps occur in the distribution, as it takes into account only the extreme scores. In the illustration above, for example, one or two extreme scores in Group A could distort the picture and make the variability appear greater than it actually is for the bulk of the scores. In order to avoid this condition, the other measures of variability cut off the extreme scores and consider only the scatter or spread of those in the center of the distribution.

Quartile Deviation

The quartile deviation, or Q, indicates the scatter or spread of the middle 50 percent of the scores taken from the median. Thus, in an effort to eliminate the effect of extreme scores on the measure of variability, this measure cuts 25 percent from each end. The formula for calculating Q is as follows:

$$Q = \frac{Q_3 - Q_1}{2}.$$

As both Q_3 and Q_1 were calculated in the preceding section, the additional mathematical process is quite simple. Table A.3 indicates this procedure with the 62 weights. The third and first quartiles, 115.13 and 78.79 respectively, are taken from Table A.2. The distance between the two, or the distance from the first to the third quartile, is 36.34, a distance frequently referred to as the *interquartile range*. Half of this distance, or Q, is 18.17. This relationship is shown in Figure A.1, using the quartiles, median, and quartile

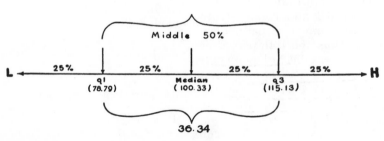

FIGURE A.1 *Relationships of Interquartile Range*

deviation found in the sample problem. In interpreting the quartile deviation, or Q, this value is marked off in plus and minus distances from the median. It will be noted that 100.33, the median, plus 18.17, the quartile deviation, does not equal the actual Q_3; nor does 100.33 minus 18.17 equal the actual Q_1. Only in absolutely normal or symmetrical distributions will this occur.

Standard Deviation

Like the mean, as a measure of central tendency, the standard deviation, or SD (also designated by the Greek sigma sign, σ), is the most reliable of the measures of variability and consequently is usually employed in advanced statistics and in research. The SD, or σ, may be defined as that measure which indicates the spread of the middle 68.26 percent of the scores taken from the mean.

The formula for calculating the standard deviation by the short method, that is, in calculating it from a guessed average in a frequency table rather than from the actual average, is:

$$\sigma = \sqrt{\frac{\Sigma f d^2}{N} - \left(\frac{\Sigma f d}{N}\right)^2} \times SI$$

It will readily be seen from the formula and from Table A.3, where the standard deviation is computed, that the only computation that is new at this point is $\Sigma f d^2$. The steps to be followed in finding SD are as follows:

1. Calculate the *fd* column, as previously described in the presentation of the mean.

TABLE A.3 *Calculation of Measures of Variability from Data Grouped into a Frequency Table (Data from Table A.2)*

Scores	f	d	fd	fd²
150–159	1	5	5	25
140–149	2	4	8	32
130–139	4	3	12	36
120–129	5	2	10	20
110–119	8	1	8 (+43)	8
100–109	12	0	0	0
90– 99	8	−1	−8	8
80– 89	6	−2	−12	24
70– 79	7	−3	−21	63
60– 69	4	−4	−16	64
50– 59	3	−5	−15	75
40– 49	2	−6	−12 (−84)	72
	N = 62		−41	427

Quartile Deviation:

$$Q = \frac{Q_2 - Q_1}{2}$$

$Q_3 = 115.13$ (Table A. 2)
$Q_1 = 78.79$ (Table A. 2)

$$Q = \frac{115.13 - 78.79}{2} = \frac{36.34}{2} = 18.17$$

Standard Deviation (short method):

$$\sigma = \sqrt{\frac{\Sigma f d^2}{N} - \left(\frac{\Sigma f d}{N}\right)^2} \times SI$$

$$\frac{\Sigma f d^2}{N} = \frac{427}{62} = 6.89.$$

$$\left(\frac{\Sigma f d}{N}\right)^2 = \left(\frac{-41}{62}\right)^2 = (.66)^2 = .44$$

$$= \sqrt{6.89 - .44} \times 10$$

$$= 2.54 \times 10 = 25.4$$

2. Add another column (*fd²*), which is calculated by multiplying each figure in the *d* column by the corresponding figure in the *fd* column. Add this column serially, since all the signs are now positive. This will be Σfd^2.

3. Compute a correction $(\Sigma fd/N)^2$. This is to be subtracted from $\Sigma fd^2/N$, because the computations are being made from a guessed average rather than from the actual mean.

4. Substitute in the formula and complete the computations.

With a few cases, SD may be computed from the following formula:

$$\sqrt{\frac{\Sigma d^2}{N}}$$

(In this case, *d* is the actual deviation of each score from the calculated mean.)

Use of Measures of Variability

The *range* is a rough measure of variability and is useful when a knowledge of the total spread of the scores is wanted. It is, however, unreliable when frequent or extreme gaps occur in the distribution.

The *quartile deviation* may be computed quickly and easily, and, like the median, is not affected by extreme scores in the distribution and when the distribution is truncated. It is also valuable when only the concentration of scores around the central tendency is sought. It is used in conjunction with the median only.

The *standard deviation* should be used when the most reliable measure of variability is wanted. Like the mean, it is affected by extreme scores in the distribution.

Equating Groups

In experimental research, it is often necessary to equate two or more groups on the basis of test scores. This is usually done by a process of matching, that is, of placing individuals with like scores (approxi-

TABLE A.4 *Shay's Equation of Two Groups According to the Rogers Strength Index and the Brace Scale of Motor Ability*

	Group A	Group B
ROGERS STRENGTH INDEX:		
Mean	1800	1794
Standard Deviation	269	287
BRACE SCALE OF MOTOR ABILITY:		
Mean	64.76	64.50
Standard Deviation	10.76	10.44

mately) in opposite groups. When this process is completed, it is necessary to show statistically that the two groups are similar so far as the test scores are concerned. This similarity is usually shown by giving the mean and the standard deviation of the test scores for each group. If these are nearly alike, the equation is accepted. Thus, it can be demonstrated that not only are the central groupings the same, but that the scatter or spread of the scores in the different groups is also comparable, a fact that takes into account the possibility of extreme deviations.

To illustrate this procedure, the process of equating two groups adopted by Shay[2] in conducting an experiment on the progressive part versus the whole method of learning motor skills is cited. As one phase of the experiment, Shay equated two groups of college students, using both *Rogers Strength Index* and the *Brace Scale of Motor Ability,* with the results shown in Table A.4. From the previous discussion of the characteristics of the mean and the standard deviation, one can be very sure that the two groups involved are very well equated *in so far as the test results are concerned,* as both the means and standard deviations are approximately the same for both groups.

[2]Clayton T. Shay, "The Progressive-Part vs. Whole Method of Learning Motor Skills," *Research Quarterly,* **5,** No. 4 (December 1934), 62.

The process of equating groups is of particular significance to the physical educator, for he may frequently wish to equate the competing powers of intramural teams or of groups within a physical education class. For this purpose he can follow out the process of matching scores, checking his work by computing means and standard deviations.

NORMAL PROBABILITY CURVE

An understanding of the characteristics of the normal probability curve is essential to the student of measurement. Upon it is based an understanding of reliability, that important phase of statistics dealing with the interpretation of statistical results. It is only through measures of reliability that the true value of such obtained measures as means, standard deviations, and coefficients of correlation can be understood.

Principle of the Normal Curve

The principle of the normal curve is based upon the probable occurrence of an event when that probability depends upon chance. For example, in flipping a coin, the chances are even, or one in two, that it will come down heads, and there is the same probability that it will come down tails. If two coins are flipped, there are four possibilities as follows:

$$
\begin{array}{cccc}
(1) & (2) & (3) & (4) \\
a \quad b & a \quad b & a \quad b & a \quad b \\
H \quad H & H \quad T & T \quad H & T \quad T
\end{array}
$$

Thus, the chances of both coins falling heads is one in four; of one head and one tail, one chance in two; and of both tails, one chance in four. If this line of reasoning were to be carried still further, it would be found that there is one chance in eight of getting all heads when three coins are flipped, and one chance in 1024 when ten coins are tossed.

This same ratio of chance probabilities in flipping coins is found in the binomial expansion theorem. For example, in expanding the binomial $(H + T)^2$, we get: $H^2 + 2HT + T^2$; and for $(H + T)^{10}$: $H^{10} + 10H^9T + 45H^8T^2 + 120H^7T^3 + 210H^6T^4 + 252H^5T^5 + 210H^4T^6 + 120H^3T^7 + 45H^2T^8 + 10HT^9 + T^{10}$.

If a graph were plotted showing the chance possibilities when ten coins are tossed, the result would be a normal probability curve, as shown in Figure A.2, with ten heads and ten tails at opposite extremes of the curve and with five heads five tails in the center. This curve represents the distribution of measures which are dependent upon chance.

This theory of normal distribution, as applied to the chance occurrence of heads and tails in coin tossing, is also applied to the chance occurrence of human characteristics. Heredity, environment, and training are the factors upon which depend the amount of any human attribute: biological, anthropometrical, psychological, and social. These factors are very much a matter of chance, and the scores of those various attributes will cluster about an average and will be distributed in much the same way as were the heads and tails in tossing coins.

The occurrence of the normal curve, however, whether it be in coin tossing or in the occurrence of human attributes, depends upon two very important factors:

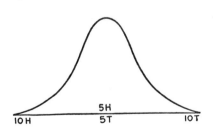

FIGURE A.2 *Theoretical Curve for Coin Tossing*

1. The occurrence of the event must depend upon *chance*. If it can be shown that skill enters into tossing coins, then a normal distribution will not result. Also the *motor ability* of physical education majors could not be used to represent the general run of students, as this particular group is a selected one physically—selection thereby not depending upon chance occurrence.

2. A *large number* of observations must be made. One would not expect an even distribution of heads and tails with only a few tosses; but, with a large number of trials, the distribution would begin to take on a normal aspect. The same rule applies to human attributes. For example, a teacher would not be justified in grading students on a normal curve when the class is small and she has only a few observations upon which to base her grades. It would be possible for the entire class to be exceptionally good, exceptionally poor, or quite a normal group. Then, too, in this instance, the teacher should consider the matter of selection as previously discussed. For example, the children of university professors or professional people would be expected to have greater intellectual ability on the whole than would the general run of children. Grading on the normal curve, however, may be justified when a large, unselected group is used, as there is a good possibility that the ability of the group is clustered around the center, with a few exceptionally

brilliant students and a like number of dull ones.[3]

Characteristics of the Normal Curve

Central Tendency. In the normal probability curve, the mean, the median, and the mode are all exactly in the center of the distribution and hence are numerically equal. This must be true, as it has been shown that the normal probability curve is perfectly symmetrical bilaterally, and, as a consequence, all of the measures of central tendency must fall in the exact middle of the curve.

Measures of Variability. In the normal curve, the measures of variability include certain constant fractional amounts of the total area of the curve. Special reference will be given to the standard deviation, as follows.

If an SD, which indicates the spread of the middle 68.26 percent of the scores, is

[3]Normality of distributions may be tested by various methods described in statistics books, particularly by measures of skewness, kurtosis, and chi-square.

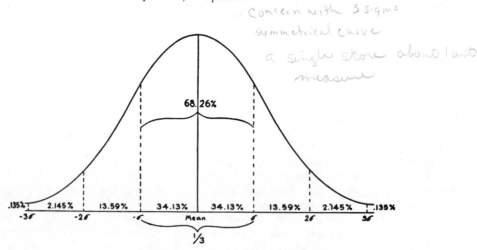

FIGURE A.3. *Properties of the Normal Curve in Terms of Standard Deviation*

laid off in plus and minus distances on a normal curve, it will take up the middle one-third of the base line; actually, two SD's are present, one on each side of the mean. Thus, as shown in Figure A.3, there are, for practical purposes, six SD's in a complete distribution. Within the limits of six standard deviations lie 99.73 percent of the scores, as will be seen.

Proportional Areas of the Normal Curve

A table is available that gives the proportion of the area between the mean and any point on the base line, measured in units of standard deviation. Table A.5 shows the fractional parts of the total area under the normal probability curve corresponding to distances on the base line between the mean and successive points from the mean in units of standard deviation.

By use of Table A.5, it is possible to relate scores to performance levels, provided normal probability of distribution can be assumed. Knowing the mean and standard deviation, the percentage of cases that would fall above or below a given score can be determined. The table shows that the area between the mean and two standard deviations is 47.72 percent of the total. An individual who is two sigmas above the mean on a tennis test, for example, will have a tennis score not only higher than the 50 percent below the mean but also higher than the 47.72 percent who fall within the mean and the two sigmas, or he will have a score that is higher than 97.72 percent of the group. Many other problems can be worked out from this table, such as those showing the percentage differences between two means or the percentage of students that should receive each mark in grading a class (marking on the normal curve).

T-Score and Sigma Score

Both the T-scale, as originated by McCall, and the sigma scale itself are based upon SD values of the distribution. Unlike the percentile scale, where the distances on the base line are close together near the mean and spread out at the extremities of the distribution, sigma values are based upon equal distances on the base line of the normal curve. Zero in the percentile table is located at the lowest score in the data from which the table is constructed, with 100 placed at the highest score. Zero in the sigma table is located at a point three sigmas below the mean, with 100 at three sigmas above the mean. Thus, the lowest score is zero, the mean is 50, and the highest sigma value is 100. Zero in the T-scale is located five sigmas below the mean, with 100 at five sigmas above the mean. The unit of measure, or one "T," is 0.1 of the sigma of the distribution. The mean T-score, therefore, is 50, and each 10 points above and below this point represent one sigma. In practice, however, T-scores will usually be found to range between 15 and 85. The T-scale technique has the advantage of placing both zero and 100 at points so far below and above what could possibly be expected in future performances that one is very unlikely to find scores that cannot be placed on the scale.

The only items needed in constructing a Sigma Table or a T-scale when distributions are normal are the mean and the standard deviation.[4] The mean is a given value of 50 in both instances (50th sigma value and 50th T-score, respectively). The standard deviation is added to and subtracted from this amount for each σ distance above and below the mean. The only difference between the two scoring tables

[4] When data are not normally distributed, other techniques are necessary to construct T-scales and sigma scales. Standard books on statistics should be consulted for this process.

TABLE A.5 *Percentage Parts of the Total Area Under the Normal Probability Curve Corresponding to Distances on the Base Line Between the Mean and Successive Points from the Mean in Units of Standard Deviation.* Example: Between the mean and a point 1.57 sigma is found 44.18 percent of the entire area under the curve.

Units	.00	.01	.02	.03	.04	.05	.06	.07	.08	.09
0.0	00.00	00.40	00.80	01.20	01.60	01.99	02.39	02.79	03.19	03.59
0.1	03.98	04.38	04.78	05.17	05.57	05.96	06.36	06.75	07.14	07.53
0.2	07.93	08.32	08.71	09.10	09.48	09.87	10.26	10.64	11.03	11.41
0.3	11.79	12.17	12.55	12.93	13.31	13.68	14.06	14.43	14.80	15.17
0.4	15.54	15.91	16.28	16.64	17.00	17.36	17.72	18.08	18.44	18.79
0.5	19.15	19.50	19.85	20.19	20.54	20.88	21.23	21.57	21.90	22.24
0.6	22.57	22.91	23.24	23.57	23.89	24.22	24.54	24.86	25.17	25.49
0.7	25.80	26.11	26.42	26.73	27.04	27.34	27.64	27.94	28.23	28.52
0.8	28.81	29.10	29.39	29.67	29.95	30.23	30.51	30.78	31.06	31.33
0.9	31.59	31.86	32.12	32.38	32.64	32.90	33.15	33.40	33.65	33.89
1.0	34.13	34.38	34.61	34.85	35.08	35.31	35.54	35.77	35.99	36.21
1.1	36.43	36.65	36.86	37.08	37.29	37.49	37.70	37.90	38.10	38.30
1.2	38.49	38.69	38.88	39.07	39.25	39.44	39.62	39.80	39.97	40.15
1.3	40.32	40.49	40.66	40.82	40.99	41.15	41.31	41.47	41.62	41.77
1.4	41.92	42.07	42.22	42.36	42.51	42.65	42.79	42.92	43.06	43.19
1.5	43.32	43.45	43.57	43.70	43.83	43.94	44.06	44.18	44.29	44.41
1.6	44.52	44.63	44.74	44.84	44.95	45.05	45.15	45.25	45.35	45.45
1.7	45.54	45.64	45.73	45.82	45.91	45.99	46.08	46.16	46.25	46.33
1.8	46.41	46.49	46.56	46.64	46.71	46.78	46.86	46.93	46.99	47.06
1.9	47.13	47.19	47.26	47.32	47.38	47.44	47.50	47.56	47.61	47.67
2.0	47.72	47.78	47.83	47.88	47.93	47.98	48.03	48.08	48.12	48.17
2.1	48.21	48.26	48.30	48.34	48.38	48.42	48.46	48.50	48.54	48.57
2.2	48.61	48.64	48.68	48.71	48.75	48.78	48.81	48.84	48.87	48.90
2.3	48.93	48.96	48.98	49.01	49.04	49.06	49.09	49.11	49.13	49.16
2.4	49.18	49.20	49.22	49.25	49.27	49.29	49.31	49.32	49.34	49.36
2.5	49.38	49.40	49.41	49.43	49.45	49.46	49.48	49.49	49.51	49.52
2.6	49.53	49.55	49.56	49.57	49.59	49.60	49.61	49.62	49.63	49.64
2.7	49.65	49.66	49.67	49.68	49.69	49.70	49.71	49.72	49.73	49.74
2.8	49.74	49.75	49.76	49.77	49.77	49.78	49.79	49.79	49.80	49.81
2.9	49.81	49.82	49.82	49.83	49.84	49.84	49.85	49.85	49.86	49.86
3.0	49.865									
3.1	49.903									
3.2	49.93129									
3.3	49.95166									
3.4	49.96631									
3.5	49.97674									
3.6	49.98409									
3.7	49.98922									
3.8	49.99277									
3.9	49.99519									

*An adaptation from Karl Pearson, *Tables for Statisticians and Biometricians* (Cambridge: Cambridge University Press, 1924).

is that Sigma Tables range between three sigmas below and three above the average and the T-scale ranges between five sigmas below and five above the average. A T-scale in decile units appears in Table A.6.[5]

Of course, if T-scales are prepared for all units between zero and 100, the T for any given score may readily be found. From the data appearing in Table A.6, however, this would be impossible. A score of 163, for example, falls between the T's of 50 and 60; interpolation thus becomes necessary. An easy and accurate method for completing such interpolations based

[5]The method described here is an approximation only. For more refined procedures, standard statistics texts should be consulted.

upon an algebraic equation appears in the table. An alternative method would be to utilize $.1\sigma$ for each T value.

A third type of scoring table based upon standard deviation distances is the Hull scale, which extends three and one-half sigmas either side of the mean. It goes beyond the somewhat narrow limits of the sigma scale, but does not leave the ends of the scale so generally unused as does the T-scale. As a result, it has considerable merit for wider use as a scale.

The stanine is a fourth scoring scale based upon the properties of the normal probability curve. In this instance, a nine-point scale is used. The standard deviation distances for points on this scale are: 1, below -1.75; 2, between -1.75 and -1.25; 3, between -1.25 and $-.75$; 4, be-

TABLE A.6 *Calculation of a T-scale from Data Given in the Table*

Mean weight = 150
Standard deviation = 20
Thus,
T-score of 50 = 150
Add or subtract 20 for each decile point.

	Decile Table	
$T_{50} = 150$	*T*	*Score*
$T_{60} = 150 + 20 = 170$	100.........	250
$T_{70} = 170 + 20 = 190$	90.........	230
$T_{80} = 190 + 20 = 210$	80.........	210
$T_{90} = 210 + 20 = 230$	70.........	190
$T_{100} = 230 + 20 = 250$	60.........	170
$T_{50} = 150$	50.........	150
$T_{40} = 150 - 20 = 130$	40.........	130
$T_{30} = 130 - 20 = 110$	30.........	110
$T_{20} = 110 - 20 = 90$	20.........	90
$T_{10} = 90 - 20 = 70$	10.........	70
$T_{0} = 70 - 20 = 50$	0.........	50

To Calculate T of a Given Score
Score given = 163

$$20 \left\{ \quad 13 \left\{ \begin{array}{|c|c|} \hline 170 & 60 \\ \hline 163 & \chi \\ \hline 150 & 50 \\ \hline \end{array} \right\} 10 \right.$$

$$13 : 20 : \chi : 10$$
$$\frac{13}{20} = \frac{\chi}{10} \text{ or } \frac{13 \times 10}{20} = \chi$$
$$\chi = 6.5$$
$$50 + 6.5 = 56.5$$

tween −.75 and −.25; 5, between −.25 and +.25; 6, between +.25 and +.75; 7, between +.75 and +1.25; 8, between +1.25 and +1.75; 9, above +1.75.

Still another method of scoring, the *standard score,* is occasionally used in testing. The standard score is the standing deviation unit above or below the mean. Thus, a standard score of 0.42 made by a given pupil can be interpreted as a score $^{42}/_{100}$ of a standard deviation distance above the mean score made by the group; a standard score of −2.00, as a score two standard deviations below the mean score.

The formula for obtaining standard scores follows directly from the definition and may be written:

$$Z = \frac{X - M}{\sigma},$$

where Z = a standard score,
X = a test score,
M = mean of the test scores.

For example, the standard score for a pupil making a score of 60 on a given test, in which the mean score is 70 and the standard deviation is 20, would be computed as follows:

$$Z = \frac{60 - 70}{20} = \frac{-10}{20} = -.5.$$

Figure A.4 is presented to compare the various scoring tables presented in this appendix.

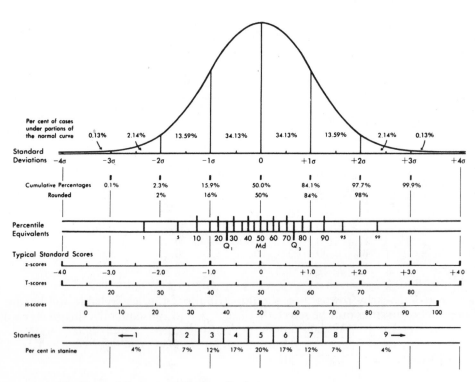

FIGURE A.4. *The Normal Curve and Various Scales*

MEASURES OF RELIABILITY

Meaning of Reliability

In statistical work, the true measure of any quality is very seldom obtained. For example, in the development of norms, it is impractical to obtain the true average upon which these norms are based. Thus, in order to determine the true average weight of 12-year-old boys, it would be necessary to measure the weight of every boy 12 years of age in the entire population. This, of course, would be impossible. The usual procedure is to depend upon random sampling, and to assume that this sample represents the whole. After this sample is taken, a measure of reliability may be applied to the mean in order to estimate how near it is to the true mean (the mean of the entire population). The reliability of the mean, therefore, indicates within what limits an obtained mean approximates the corresponding true mean. What is true for the reliability of the mean is also true for all of the measures used in statistics; consequently, there are statistical methods for determining the reliability of the mean, the median, the standard deviation, the coefficient of correlation, and so forth.

Three major factors influence the reliability of a measure, or, to express it differently, show how nearly an obtained mean approximates the true measure. The *first* of these is the sample itself. How truly random is it? As has been previously shown, normal probability is definitely lacking if the factor of *selection* enters into the picture. In a random sample, therefore, boys should not be selected from one town or from nearby towns, nor should school subjects in cities only be selected. To be truly representative, the sampling must include boys in school and out, from both urban and rural areas, and so forth. The more successful one is in securing an "unselected" group, the more nearly representative will his group be of all the boys of 12 years of age in the country.

The *second* factor influencing the reliability of a measure is the number of cases contained in the sample. It can readily be demonstrated that an obtained mean may be changed by the addition of one new case to the distribution, and that this new case will affect the mean much more when it is based upon a few scores than when a large number is involved. For example, the addition of one extreme score to a group of 10 measures will cause a greater change in the obtained mean than the addition of a similar score to a group of 1000 measures, as each case counts for less in the larger group.

It is also true that the reliability of an average will increase not in proportion to the number of measures upon which it is based, but upon the *square root* of the number. Thus, the reliability of the mean obtained from 50 cases is not twice that from 25; 100 cases would be needed to obtain twice the reliability of 25. To illustrate:

$$\sqrt{25} = 5; \sqrt{100} = 10.$$

The *third* factor affecting the reliability of a measure is the variability of the distribution. The more variable the distribution, the greater the possibility of extreme scores appearing in the untested population, or the greater the distance scores may be from the mean. It is readily seen that the farther removed scores are from the average, the greater will be the possible pull on the mean of scores not measured (which those measured represent). For example, the effect of a score of 200 is greater on a mean of 100 than is a score of 125. Therefore, the more variable the distribution, the less reliable will be the results, and consequently, the greater will be the measure of reliability. It should be pointed out, too, that this factor of variability is entirely dependent upon the nature of the variable being considered, and it can in no way be controlled by the experimenter. For example, a variable such as the weight of 12-year-old boys is naturally much greater than is the variable of height for these same boys: an unavoidable situation, as heights simply do not vary to the same extent.

Thus, the reliability of the mean, or of any other statistical concept, depends first upon the representativeness of the sample itself. When this condition has been met, the other two factors affecting the reliability of measures, the number of scores and the variability of the distribution, can be accounted for in a formula. The measure of reliability usually used today is the *standard error,* and this may be applied, with appropriate formulae, to other statistics. For the purposes of this text, however, the reliability of the mean, of the difference between means, and of the coefficient of correlation only will be considered.

Reliability of the Mean

Standard Error of the Mean.   The formula for the standard error of the mean is:

$$\sigma_M = \frac{\sigma_{\text{dist.}}}{\sqrt{N-1}}$$

Taking data from Tables A.1 and A.3, $M = 97.89$, $\sigma = 25.4$, and $N = 62$. Substituting in the formula:

$$\sigma_M = \frac{25.4}{\sqrt{62}} = 3.23$$

It will be noted in the standard error of the mean that the larger the number of scores and the smaller the deviation of the score, the less will be the measure, or the greater the reliability of the obtained mean.

Interpretation.   In interpreting the measures of reliability, it should be understood that the results obtained from calculating the mean do not give an absolutely accurate value true in all cases, but simply the

obtained figures from a random sampling of the much larger population. Random samplings are relative affairs. Returning to the illustration of the weights of 12-year-old boys, if successive samplings of these weights were taken with a different group of boys each time, the means would not always be precisely the same. Some of these means might agree, but many more would not. If additional random samplings were taken until there were, say 100 samplings, and if the means of these 100 samples were plotted on a graph, the results would approximate a normal curve, the mean of all the means would be located in the center, and the other means would be clustered around this center within the limits of the standard error of the distribution.

For example, using the figures in the sample problem calculated above, if 97.89 should have been the mean of many samples, 68.26 percent of them would fall between 97.89 ± 3.23; and nearly all of them would fall between $97.89 \pm 3 \times 3.23$, in accordance with the known qualities of normal distributions.

However, conclusions must be drawn from only *one* sample and not from many. This is done in terms of probability. The chances are 68.26 in 100, therefore, that the true mean lies between 97.89 ± 3.23; and one can be practically certain (99.73 chances in 100) that it lies between $97.89 \pm 3 \times 3.23$. For these chance relationships, consult Table A.5.

The investigator need not accept "practical certainty" as his level of reliability. Various "levels of confidence" or "accuracy limits" have been proposed. However, two such limits, called the .05 and .01 (or 5 percent and 1 percent) levels, have come into common use for most experimental work. From Table A.5, it will be seen that 95 percent of the normal distribution lies within the limits $\pm 1.96\sigma_M$ hence, the odds are 95 in 100 that any sample mean will be within these limits. This is the 0.05 level. For the 0.01 level, 99 percent of the normal distribution lies between $\pm 2.58\sigma_M$; hence, the chances are 99 in 100 that any sample mean will lie within these limits.

The preceding presentations of the normal probability curve and of reliability statistics assume large samples. As was shown, normal probability distributions occur when many chance observations are made (either in coin tossing or in drawing subjects from an infinite population). With small samples, usually utilized by most investigators, the standard deviations systematically underestimate the standard deviations of the total population. For this reason, adjustments must be made in interpreting reliability when such small samples are utilized, as explained in standard statistics textbooks.

Reliability of the Difference Between Two Means

In studying the position at which the strength of the knee extensor muscles could be applied most effectively, Harrell[6] used the tensiometer to measure the amount of strength applied when the body was placed in two different positions. The mean for Position I was 112.94 pounds; for Position 2, 147.94 pounds. The question may logically be raised: Is this difference of 35 pounds statistically significant? The answer can only be found in terms of reliability. The results were as follows:

Position 1	*Position 2*
$M_1 = 112.94$	$M_2 = 147.94$
$\sigma_{M_1} = 3.20$	$\sigma_{M_2} = 6.55$

The formula for calculating the standard error of a difference between two means is:

$$\sigma_d = \sqrt{\sigma^2{}_{M_1} + \sigma^2{}_{M_2}}$$
$$= \sqrt{3.20^2 + 6.55^2} = 7.29$$

[6] Dean U. Harrell, "Further Refinement of Objective Orthopedic Strength Tests," Master's Thesis, Springfield College, Springfield, Mass., 1949.

The actual difference between the means of the two groups is designated by d. Hence, $d = 35 \pm 7.29$. The reliability of the difference between two means is interpreted in the same way in which the reliability of the mean is interpreted. Thus, the chances are 68.26 in 100 that the true difference lies between 35 ± 7.29; and one may be practically certain that it lies between $35 \pm 3 \times 7.29$.

Also, *statistically*, one may be practically certain from the evidence given that there is a definite difference in favor of Position 2, as $\pm 3 \times 7.29 = \pm 21.87$, which, subtracted from 35, the practical lower limit of probability, does not reach zero. The ratio between the difference and its measure of reliability is known as the *critical ratio*. Of course, the larger the critical ratio, the greater is the statistical significance of the difference. However, in order for the difference to be really significant, it should be 3 times its standard error, d/σ_d, as 3 times the standard error just reaches zero, indicating a favorable difference throughout. The concept of levels of confidence, now known as levels of significance, as applied to small samples also applies here.

CORRELATION

Meaning of Correlation

Up to this point, in considering statistics, one variable only has been dealt with. The next step will consider the degree of relationship between two variables, that is, correlation. There are various methods of computing correlations, but the standard method is known as the *product-moment* method, and is signified by the symbol r, also known as the "Pearson-r," after its originator.

The range of the possible magnitude of correlations extends from a $+1.00$ through 0.00 to a -1.00, all divisions of the scale being used (such as 0.95, 0.137,

−0.17, and so forth). A +1.00 indicates a perfect positive correlation: a large amount of one variable is found with a large amount of the other; a small amount of one with a small amount of the other; and these are in direct proportion throughout all ranges of their distributions. A −1.00 is just as significant a correlation as is a +1.00, but the proportions are in reverse. A large amount of one variable is found with a small amount of the other, and these variables are in direct proportion throughout all ranges of their distribution.

In a zero (0.00) correlation, however, no relationship exists: an individual with a high score in one variable may appear anywhere on the scale for the opposite variable. With high positive or negative correlations, one could predict with considerable accuracy an individual's score in one variable by merely knowing his score in the other. With zero or near-zero correlations, such prediction would be impossible—would, in fact, be entirely a matter of guessing.

To illustrate: If a +1.00 were obtained by correlating strength and intelligence, it would mean that the strongest individuals were the most brilliant and the weakest were the least brilliant. If a −1.00 correlation were obtained from the same two variables, it would indicate that the weakest individuals were the most brilliant and the strongest individuals were low in intelligence (the old expression of "a strong back and a weak mind"). With a zero correlation, however, the strongest individual may appear anywhere on the intelligence scale and the weak individual likewise; no relationship exists.

Computing Correlations

The procedures for calculating a coefficient of correlation by the product-moment method (r) may best be described by showing the actual computations involved. The following 90 pairs of foot arch-angles of college freshmen will serve as a problem to illustrate these techniques.

The problem is to determine the correlation between the arch heights (as determined by arch-angles) of the right and left feet of college freshmen. The steps, illustrated in Table A.7, are as follows:

1. Construct a scattergram by preparing a double-entry table, as follows.

a. Decide upon the intervals to be used for each one of the variables. This is done in the manner previously described for setting up a frequency table. Care should be taken to obtain approximately the same number of in-

R	L	R	L	R	L	R	L	R	L	R	L
19	16	32	22	57	42	39	37	28	32	45	47
54	50	49	45	39	41	36	38	39	39	48	46
44	47	46	42	35	50	41	48	35	41	27	26
56	56	46	47	33	27	37	42	50	48	50	46
43	41	41	41	45	39	46	47	50	58	40	45
46	50	49	48	36	30	28	21	49	42	45	45
49	53	47	45	20	18	37	43	34	46	47	46
40	42	43	41	31	33	20	18	44	45	35	33
32	36	27	35	47	56	38	35	54	54	50	52
37	40	41	35	50	54	47	47	43	41	45	41
44	35	43	38	38	51	29	31	41	43	42	44
45	47	43	43	50	43	47	44	48	48	31	29
38	35	55	53	37	34	42	48	51	51	44	44
45	49	47	30	45	47	47	39	48	48	48	47
44	45	43	44	31	27	53	47	40	40	39	41

TABLE A.7 *Calculation of the Coefficient of Correlation by the Product-Moment Method Utilizing a Scattergram*

X-VARIABLE: LEFT FOOT

Y-VARIABLE: RIGHT FOOT

Y \ X	16-19	20-23	24-27	28-31	32-35	36-39	40-43	44-47	48-51	52-55	56-59	fy	dy	fdy	fdy²	x'−	y'+
56-59							(5) 5		(15) 15		(25) 25	2	5	10	50		30
52-55									(12)	(32) 16	(15) 20	4	4	16	64		52
48-51							(6) 3	(8) 8	(45)	(36) 12	(15) 15	14	3	42	126		120
44-47							(6) 3	(52) 4	(18) 8		(10) 10	23	2	46	92	2	86
40-43							(8)	(6)	(18)	(9)	(5)	16	1	16	16	3	20
36-39												13	0	130 / −38 / +92			
32-35					(−2) −2	(−1)	(−7) −7	(−2) −2	(−3) −3			7	−1	−7	7	6	8
28-31			(3)	(8) 4	(4) 2							6	−2	−12	24		26
24-27			(9)		(3) 3							2	−3	−6	18		12
20-23	(4) 4	(8)	(9)									2	−4	−8	32		40
16-19	(40) 20	(25) 25										1	−5	−5	25		25
fx	3	2	3	4	9	7	20	21	13	5	3	90		−38	454	−11	419 / −11 / =408
dx	−5	−4	−3	−2	−1	0	1	2	3	4	5			+487 / −49 / =438			
fdx	−15	−8	−9	−8	−9	0	20	42	39	20	15	156					
fd²x	75	32	27	16	9		20	84	117	80	75	535					

Case No. 1

$$c_y = \frac{92}{90} = 1.022$$

$$c_x = \frac{87}{90} = .967$$

$$\sigma_y = \sqrt{\frac{454}{90} - (1.022)^2} = 2.0$$

$$\sigma_x = \sqrt{\frac{535}{90} - (.967)^2} = 2.238$$

$$r = \frac{\dfrac{\Sigma x'y'}{N} - c_x c_y}{\sigma_x \sigma_y} = \frac{\dfrac{398}{90} - (.967 \times 1.022)}{2.238 \times 2.0} = .792$$

363

tervals for both variables; the size of the intervals will not necessarily be the same (although this is true in the sample problem, as the variabilities are the same), a step of 4 being used in both instances.

b. List the intervals for one variable on the left (Y-variable) of the diagram, and the other at the top (X-variable). For the Y-variable, the intervals should run from high at the top to low at the bottom, in the accepted manner for frequency tables; and for the X-variable, from low at the left to high at the right.

c. Starting with the first pair of arch-angles, 19 for the right foot and 16 for the left, make a tally in the proper square for them. The square for pair number 1 has been heavily ruled in Table A.7. The tallies are placed in the upper left-hand corners of the squares.

d. Complete the scattergram with frequency columns: *fy* at the right of the scattergram for the Y-variable (right foot, in this instance), and *fx* at the bottom of the scattergram for the X-variable (left foot).

2. Select as a guessed mean for each variable the mid-point of an interval approximately in the middle of each distribution. Rule off with heavy lines the squares in the row and the column in which these guessed averages lie, as indicated in Table A.7. Then compute the correction (*c*, or $\Sigma fd/N$) for each variable, c_x and c_y[7] and the standard deviation

$$\sqrt{\frac{\Sigma fd^2}{N} - \left(\frac{\Sigma fd}{N}\right)^2}$$

of each variable, σx and σy,[8] in terms of deviation units, that is, without multiplying by the size of the interval. In making these computations, the following columns are necessarily adjacent to the scattergram: *d, fd,* and *fd²,* placed on the right side for the Y-variable and at the bottom for the X-variable. So far, in calculating *r*, with the exception of the construction of the scattergram, no new statistical work has been presented.

3. The final step in the problem is to compute $\Sigma x'y'$. A definition of *x'y'* is the deviation of the various scores from the two guessed averages; it is obtained by multiplying the deviation of the scores from one guessed average by the deviation from the other, in terms of deviation units (that is, without considering the size of the interval). This procedure may be outlined as follows.

a. The lines representing the two guessed averages divide the scattergram into four quadrants: upper right, upper left, lower right, lower left. Squares on the right of the guessed average for the X-variable are positive; squares on the left, negative. Squares above the guessed average for the Y-variable are positive; squares below, negative. Therefore, all squares in the upper right and lower left quadrants are positive, as plus times plus and minus times minus equal plus, or positive. All squares in the upper left and lower right quadrants are negative, as plus times minus equals minus, or negative.

b. In case number 1, the square deviation, or product deviation from the two guessed averages, is $(-5 \times -5) = 25$, as the square deviates five squares from both guessed averages, the final deviation being the product of these two distances. The figure 25, therefore, represents the value of the square, and is placed in its lower right corner, as shown in Table A.7. The values of all the squares are determined in like manner.

c. As there are more scores in some squares than in others, this fact must now be taken into account. For example, in the square representing case number 1, there is one frequency. Its product-moment, therefore, will be 1×25, or 25. If, however, there had been two frequencies in the square, its product-moment would be 2×25, or 50. In the square immediately above case number 1, there are two frequencies and a square deviation value of 20; its product-moment, therefore, is 2×20, or 40.

d. When the product-moments of all the squares have been computed, with due regard for plus and minus signs, the entries in the *x'y'* column can be made. It will be noted that all the product-moments in Table A.7 have been circled to facilitate addition. Add the product-moments for each step of the Y-variable, placing the sum of the positive values under the plus sign, and the sum of the negative values under the minus sign. The algebraic sum of this column, then, is the difference between positive and negative values, 408 for the problem in question. This procedure may be duplicated for the

---

[7]See the computation of the mean.

[8]See the computation of the standard deviation.

X-variable columns to check the work; the two answers should agree.

4. Compute the coefficient of correlation, *r*, by means of the formula:

$$r = \frac{\dfrac{\Sigma x'y'}{N} - c_x c_y}{\sigma_x \sigma_y}$$

The corrections, $c_x c_y$, and the standard deviations, $\sigma_x \sigma_y$, are in terms of deviation units and are not multiplied by the size of the step interval.

Interpreting Coefficients of Correlation

Coefficients of correlation should not be confused with percent relationships. A correlation of $+0.50$ is not halfway to perfect correlation; nor is a correlation of 0.80 only twice as significant as one of 0.40. Actually, there are three ways of interpreting correlations:

1. *General terms.* The correlation may be considered in such general terms as "good," "fair," "poor," "no correlation," or, "high, "low," "insignificant," and so forth, depending upon the size of *r*. Although this method is frequently used, it is obviously a very rough one and lacking in precise definition.

2. *Predictive Index.* Coefficients of correlation may be reduced to "percentages," or *Predictive Indices,* by the following formula:

$$PI = 1 - \sqrt{1 - r^2}.$$

When this formula is applied, the following results are obtained:

r	*P.I.*
0.10	0.005
0.20	0.020
0.30	0.046
0.40	0.083
0.50	0.134
0.60	0.200
0.70	0.286
0.80	0.400
0.90	0.564
0.95	0.688
0.99	0.859
1.00	1.000

Predictive Indices are interpreted in terms of their percent of prediction value better than pure chance. Thus, a correlation of 0.50 is 13.4 percent better than chance in predicting performance.

In physical education, the Predictive Index has been used to compare the significance of two or more coefficients. For example, *r*'s of 0.40 and 0.80 have PI's of 0.083 and 0.400, respectively. By comparing the PI's, therefore, a coefficient of 0.80 is seen to be nearly five times as significant as one of 0.40.

3. *Statistical significance.* With low correlations, it often becomes important to determine whether or not a significant relationship actually exists. The concept of significance at the .05 and .01 levels, mentioned previously in connection with the difference between means, is applicable to coefficients of correlation as well; furthermore, it is the method in common use today to indicate statistical significance.

Tables are included in statistics textbooks which provide the amount of the correlation necessary for significance, depending on the number of cases in the computations. For example, with 102 cases, an *r* of 0.195 is significant at the .05 level; an *r* of 0.254 is significant at the .01 level. Thus, only correlations as high as these could occur by sampling error 5 times in 100 at the .05 level and once in 100 at the .01 level.

Special Correlation Methods

Various methods of computing correlation have been devised for special conditions. Several of the more commonly used ones are described briefly below.

Rank-Difference Method. The rank-difference method, designated as rho, is designed to correlate two variables when the scores are arranged as ranks, when the number of cases is small, and when it would be cumbersome and impractical to use the more detailed product-moment method described above.

Biserial r. Occasionally it is useful to ascertain a relationship existing between two variables when one of them is expressed in two categories. This method was utilized by Larson and McCurdy, for example, when they correlated the results of their "Organic Efficiency Test" with a criterion consisting of two groups, infirmary patients, and varsity swimmers.

Tetrachoric Correlation. This method of correlation is used when both variables are dichotomies (two categories each).

Contingency Coefficient. Whenever a relationship exists between two distributions, either one of which is not a variable, the usual methods of correlation are unsatisfactory. As an illustration: to determine the relationship between the extracurricular activities of college students and the type of position held five years after graduation. The coefficient of contingency indicates whether resultant frequencies are distributed as might be expected from mere chance or whether there is a tendency for certain characteristics in the one distribution to be associated with the characteristics in the other.

Modified Spearman-Brown Prophecy Formula. The Spearman-Brown Prophecy Formula is used frequently in the construction of objective written tests. In securing reliability for these tests, the answers to the odd questions may be correlated with the answers to the even questions. However, as the length of a test affects its reliability, and the odd-even correlation represents only half of the entire test, a correction for the full-length test becomes necessary. The Prophecy Formula is designed to make this correction. A modified formula proposed by Wert[9] is as follows:

$$r = \frac{2r_{oe}}{1 + r_{oe}}.$$

r = coefficient of reliability;
r_{oe} = correlation: odds and evens

[9]James E. Wert, *Educational Statistics* (New York: McGraw-Hill Book Company, 1938), p. 211.

With an odd-even correlation of 0.60,

$$r = \frac{2(0.60)}{1 + 0.60} = 0.75.$$

Wert also proposed an *Index of Reliability,* which is the square root of the coefficient of reliability. Thus,

$$\sqrt{0.75} = 0.87.$$

Multiple and Partial Correlation. So far, all measures of relationship that have been considered deal with two variables only. It is not only possible but often quite useful to estimate relationships when three or more variables are concerned.

The coefficient of multiple correlation has been developed for the purpose of indicating the degree to which values of one variable may correlate with two or more other variables. For example, how well does broad-jumping ability correlate with sprinting ability and leg strength?

The coefficient of partial correlation determines the net relationship between two variables when the influence of one or more other factors is excluded.

SELECTED REFERENCES

CLARKE, DAVID H., and H. HARRISON CLARKE, *Research Processes in Physical Education, Recreation, and Health.* Englewood Cliffs, N.J.: Prentice-Hall, Inc., 1970, Ch. 7–11.

CLARKE, H. HARRISON, and DAVID H. CLARKE, *Advanced Statistics with Applications to Physical Education.* Englewood Cliffs, N.J.: Prentice-Hall, Inc., 1972.

APPENDIX B

Scoring Tables

TABLE B.1 *Wellesley Weight Prediction Table for College Women**

Sum of Skeletal Measures	Predicted Weight in Pounds	Sum of Skeletal Measures	Predicted Weight in Pounds	Sum of Skeletal Measures	Predicted Weight in Pounds
88.0	74.5	103.0	113.5	118.0	152.5
88.5	76.0	103.5	115.0	118.5	154.0
89.0	77.0	104.0	116.0	119.0	155.0
89.5	78.5	104.5	117.5	119.5	156.5
90.0	79.5	105.0	118.5	120.0	157.5
90.5	81.0	105.5	120.0	120.5	159.0
91.0	82.5	106.0	121.5	121.0	160.5
91.5	83.5	106.5	122.5	121.5	161.5
92.0	85.0	107.0	124.0	122.0	163.0
92.5	86.0	107.5	125.0	122.5	164.0
93.0	87.5	108.0	126.5	123.0	165.5
93.5	89.0	108.5	128.0	123.5	167.0
94.0	90.0	109.0	129.0	124.0	168.0
94.5	91.5	109.5	130.5	124.5	169.5
95.0	92.5	110.0	131.5	125.0	170.5
95.5	94.0	110.5	133.0	125.5	172.0
96.0	95.5	111.0	134.5	126.0	173.5
96.5	96.5	111.5	135.5	126.5	174.5
97.0	98.0	112.0	137.0	127.0	176.0
97.5	99.0	112.5	138.0	127.5	177.0
98.0	100.5	113.0	139.5	128.0	178.5
98.5	102.0	113.5	141.0	128.5	180.0
99.0	103.0	114.0	142.0	129.0	181.0
99.5	104.5	114.5	143.5	129.5	182.5
100.0	105.5	115.0	144.5	130.0	183.5
100.5	107.0	115.5	146.0	130.5	185.0
101.0	108.5	116.0	147.5	131.0	186.5
101.5	109.5	116.5	148.5	131.5	187.5
102.0	111.0	117.0	150.0		
102.5	112.0	117.5	151.0		

*F. E. Ludlum, and Elizabeth Powell, "Chest-Height-Weight Tables for College Women, *Research Quarterly*, **11,** No. 3 (October 1940), 55.

TABLE B.2 *Obesity Standards for Caucasian Americans: Skinfold over Triceps Muscle**

Age (Years)	Minimum Skinfold Thickness Indicating Obesity (Millimeters)	
	Males	Females
5	12	14
6	12	15
7	13	16
8	14	17
9	15	18
10	16	20
11	17	21
12	18	22
13	18	23
14	17	23
15	16	24
16	15	25
17	14	26
18	15	27
19	15	27
20	16	28
21	17	28
22	18	28
23	18	28
24	19	28
25	20	29
26	20	29
27	21	29
28	22	29
29	22	29
30–50	23	30

*C. C. Selzer and J. Mayer, "Simplified Criterion of Obesity," *Postgraduate Medicine,* **38,** 2 (1965), A-101.

TABLE B.3 *Strength Index Norms*
A. *Boys*

Weight	8	8-6	9	9-6	10	10-6	11	11-6	12	12-6	13	13-6	14	14-6	15	15-6	16	16-6	17	17-6	18	Weight
180															2664	2813	2917	2993	3056	3105	3159	180
178															2632	2778	2880	2954	3016	3064	3118	178
176															2601	2743	2843	2916	2976	3023	3077	176
174														2363	2569	2708	2805	2877	2936	2983	3035	174
172														2336	2537	2674	2768	2838	2896	2942	2994	172
170														2308	2505	2639	2731	2799	2856	2901	2953	170
168														2280	2474	2604	2694	2761	2816	2860	2911	168
166													2067	2253	2442	2569	2657	2722	2776	2819	2870	166
164													2043	2225	2410	2534	2620	2683	2736	2779	2829	164
162													2020	2198	2378	2499	2583	2645	2696	2738	2787	162
160												1848	1996	2170	2346	2465	2546	2606	2656	2607	2746	160
158												1827	1972	2142	2315	2430	2509	2567	2616	2656	2704	158
156											1718	1807	1949	2115	2283	2395	2472	2528	2576	2615	2663	156
154											1699	1786	1925	2087	2251	2360	2435	2490	2536	2575	2622	154
152											1680	1766	1902	2060	2219	2325	2398	2451	2496	2534	2580	152
150										1610	1661	1745	1878	2032	2188	2291	2361	2412	2456	2493	2539	150
148										1591	1642	1724	1854	2004	2156	2256	2324	2373	2416	2452	2498	148
146										1573	1623	1704	1831	1977	2124	2221	2287	2335	2376	2411	2456	146
144									1525	1554	1604	1683	1807	1949	2092	2186	2250	2296	2336	2371	2415	144
142									1506	1536	1585	1663	1784	1922	2060	2151	2213	2257	2296	2330	2374	142
140								1470	1487	1517	1566	1642	1760	1894	2029	2116	2176	2219	2256	2289	2332	140
138								1451	1468	1498	1547	1621	1736	1866	1997	2082	2139	2180	2216	2248	2291	138
136							1401	1431	1449	1480	1528	1601	1713	1839	1965	2047	2102	2141	2176	2207	2249	136
134							1382	1412	1430	1461	1509	1580	1689	1811	1933	2012	2065	2102	2136	2167	2208	134
132							1362	1392	1411	1443	1490	1560	1666	1784	1901	1977	2028	2064	2096	2126	2167	132
130						1318	1343	1372	1392	1424	1471	1539	1642	1756	1870	1942	1991	2025	2056	2085	2125	130
128					1273	1299	1324	1353	1373	1405	1452	1518	1618	1728	1838	1907	1954	1986	2016	2044	2084	128
126				1227	1255	1280	1304	1333	1354	1387	1433	1498	1595	1701	1806	1873	1917	1948	1976	2003	2043	126
124			1185	1209	1236	1261	1285	1314	1334	1368	1414	1477	1571	1673	1774	1838	1879	1909	1936	1963	2001	124
122		1146	1169	1192	1218	1242	1266	1294	1315	1342	1395	1457	1548	1646	1743	1803	1842	1870	1896	1922	1960	122
120		1130	1152	1174	1199	1223	1246	1275	1296	1331	1376	1436	1524	1618	1711	1768	1805	1831	1856	1881	1919	120
118	1092	1114	1135	1156	1181	1204	1227	1255	1277	1312	1357	1415	1500	1590	1679	1733	1768	1793	1816	1840	1877	118
116	1077	1098	1119	1139	1162	1185	1208	1235	1258	1294	1338	1395	1477	1563	1647	1699	1731	1754	1776	1799	1836	116
114	1061	1082	1102	1121	1144	1166	1188	1216	1239	1275	1319	1374	1453	1535	1615	1664	1694	1715	1736	1759	1795	114
112	1046	1066	1085	1104	1125	1146	1169	1196	1220	1257	1300	1354	1430	1508	1584	1629	1657	1677	1696	1718	1753	112
110	1030	1050	1069	1086	1107	1127	1150	1177	1201	1238	1281	1333	1406	1480	1552	1594	1620	1638	1656	1677	1712	110
108	1014	1034	1052	1068	1088	1108	1130	1157	1182	1219	1262	1312	1382	1452	1520	1559	1583	1599	1616	1636	1670	108
106	999	1018	1035	1051	1070	1089	1111	1138	1163	1201	1243	1292	1359	1425	1488	1524	1546	1560	1576	1595	1629	106
104	983	1002	1018	1033	1051	1070	1092	1118	1144	1182	1224	1271	1335	1397	1457	1490	1509	1522	1536	1555	1588	104
102	968	986	1002	1016	1033	1051	1072	1099	1125	1164	1205	1251	1312	1370	1425	1455	1472	1483	1496	1514	1546	102
100	952	970	985	998	1014	1032	1053	1079	1106	1145	1186	1230	1288	1342	1393	1420	1435	1444	1456	1473	1505	100
98	936	954	968	980	995	1013	1034	1059	1087	1126	1167	1209	1264	1314	1361	1385	1398	1405	1416	1432	1464	98
96	921	938	952	963	977	994	1014	1040	1068	1108	1148	1189	1241	1287	1329	1350	1361	1367	1376	1391	1422	96
94	905	922	935	945	958	975	995	1020	1049	1089	1129	1168	1217	1259	1298	1316	1324	1328	1336	1351		94
92	890	906	918	928	940	956	976	1001	1030	1071	1110	1148	1194	1232	1266	1281	1287	1289	1296	1310		92
90	874	890	902	910	921	937	956	981	1011	1052	1091	1127	1170	1204	1234	1246	1250	1251	1256			90
88	858	874	885	892	903	918	937	962	992	1033	1072	1106	1146	1176	1202	1211	1213	1212	1216			88
86	843	858	868	875	884	898	918	942	973	1015	1053	1086	1123	1149	1171	1176	1176	1173	1176			86
84	827	842	851	857	866	879	898	923	954	996	1034	1065	1099	1121	1139	1141	1139	1134	1136			84
82	812	826	835	840	847	860	879	903	935	978	1015	1045	1076	1094	1107	1107	1102	1096				82
80	796	810	818	822	829	841	860	883	916	959	996	1024	1052	1066	1075	1072	1065	1057				80
78	780	794	801	804	810	822	840	864	897	940	977	1003	1028	1038	1043	1037	1028	1018				78
76	765	778	785	787	792	803	821	844	878	922	958	983	1005	1011	1012	1002	991					76
74	749	762	768	769	784	802	825	858	903	939	962	981	983	980	967	953						74
72	734	746	751	752	755	765	782	805	839	885	920	942	958	956	948	933						72
70	718	730	735	734	736	746	763	786	820	866	901	921	934	928	916	898						70
68	702	714	718	718	727	744	766	801	847	882	900	910	900	885								68
66	687	698	701	699	699	708	724	746	782	829	863	880	887	873								66
64	671	682	684	681	689	705	727	763	810	884	859	863	845									64
62	656	666	668	664	662	669	686	707	744	792	825	839	840									62
60	640	650	651	646	644	650	666	688	725	773	806	818										60
58	624	634	634	628	625	631	647	668	706	754	787	797										58
56	609	618	618	611	607	612	628	649	687	736	768											56
54	593	602	601	593	588	593	608	629	668	717	749											54
52	578	586	584	576	570	574	589	610	649	699												52
50	562	570	568	668	551	555	570	590	630	680												50
*	7.80	8.00	8.35	8.80	9.26	9.54	9.67	9.78	9.52	9.30	9.50	10.30	11.80	13.80	15.89	17.41	18.52	19.36	20	20.40	20.68	

*Weight Deviation Multiplier.

Reproduced with permission of Frederick Rand Rogers.

1. Norms for individuals whose weights are above limits for which norms are included are calculated by adding to the norm for any chosen weight the pound difference between that weight and the individual's weight *times* the Weight Deviation Multiplier.

B. *Men*

Weight	18	19	20	21	22	23	24	25	26	27	28	29	30	31	32	33	34	35	36	37	38	Weight
230													3845	3796	3755	3722	3690	3664	3642	3621	3601	230
228													3808	3759	3719	3686	3653	3628	3606	3585	3565	228
226													3771	3723	3682	3649	3617	3592	3570	3549	3529	226
224													3734	3686	3646	3613	3581	3555	3534	3513	3493	224
222													3697	3650	3609	3577	3545	3519	3498	3477	3457	222
220												3706	3660	3613	3573	3541	3509	3483	3462	3441	3421	220
218												3669	3623	3576	3537	3504	3473	3447	3426	3405	3385	218
216												3632	3586	3540	3500	3468	3437	3411	3390	3369	3349	216
214											3650	3595	3549	3503	3464	3432	3401	3375	3354	3333	3313	214
212											3613	3557	3512	3467	3427	3396	3365	3339	3318	3297	3277	212
210										3626	3575	3520	3476	3430	3391	3359	3329	3303	3282	3261	3241	210
208										3588	3538	3483	3439	3393	3255	3323	3292	3267	3246	3225	3205	208
206										3550	3500	3446	3402	3357	3318	3287	3256	3231	3210	3189	3169	206
204									3567	3512	3462	3408	3365	3320	3282	3251	3220	3195	3174	3153	3133	204
202								3580	3529	3474	3425	3371	3328	3284	3245	3214	3184	3159	3138	3117	3097	202
200							3594	3541	3490	3436	3387	3334	3291	3247	3209	3178	3148	3123	3102	3081	3061	200
198						3603	3554	3502	3451	3398	3349	3297	3254	3210	3173	3142	3112	3087	3066	3045	3025	198
196					3596	3562	3514	3462	3413	3360	3312	3260	3217	3174	3136	3105	3076	3051	3030	3009	2989	196
194				3564	3554	3521	3474	3423	3374	3322	3274	3222	3180	3137	3100	3069	3040	3015	2994	2973	2953	194
192			3515	3522	3512	3480	3433	3384	3335	3284	3236	3185	3143	3101	3063	3033	3004	2979	2958	2937	2917	192
190			3473	3480	3471	3439	3393	3344	3297	3246	3199	3148	3107	3064	3027	2997	2968	2943	2922	2901	2881	190
188		3412	3431	3438	3429	3398	3353	3305	3258	3208	3161	3111	3070	3027	2991	2960	2931	2907	2886	2865	2845	188
186	3283	3371	3389	3396	3387	3357	3313	3265	3220	3170	3124	3073	3033	2991	2954	2924	2895	2871	2850	2829	2809	186
184	3242	3329	3347	3354	3345	3316	3273	3226	3181	3132	3086	3036	2996	2954	2918	2888	2859	2835	2814	2793	2773	184
182	3201	3287	3306	3312	3304	3275	3233	3187	3142	3094	3048	2999	2959	2918	2881	2852	2823	2799	2778	2757	2737	182
180	3159	3246	3264	3270	3262	3234	3192	3147	3104	3056	3011	2962	2922	2881	2845	2815	2787	2763	2742	2721	2701	180
178	3118	3204	3222	3228	3220	3193	3152	3108	3065	3018	2973	2924	2885	2844	2809	2779	2751	2727	2706	2685	2665	178
176	3077	3162	3180	3187	3179	3152	3112	3069	3026	2980	2935	2887	2848	2808	2772	2743	2715	2691	2670	2649	2629	176
174	3035	3121	3138	3146	3137	3112	3072	3029	2988	2942	2898	2850	2811	2771	2736	2707	2679	2654	2634	2613	2593	174
172	2994	3079	3096	3102	3095	3071	3032	2990	2949	2904	2860	2813	2774	2735	2699	2670	2643	2618	2598	2577	2557	172
170	2953	3037	3055	3060	3054	3030	2992	2951	2910	2866	2822	2775	2738	2698	2663	2634	2607	2582	2562	2541	2521	170
168	2911	2996	3013	3018	3012	2989	2951	2911	2872	2828	2785	2738	2701	2661	2627	2598	2570	2546	2526	2505	2485	168
166	2870	2954	2971	2976	2970	2948	2911	2872	2833	2790	2747	2701	2664	2625	2590	2562	2534	2510	2490	2469	2449	166
164	2829	2912	2929	2934	2928	2907	2871	2833	2794	2752	2709	2664	2627	2588	2554	2525	2498	2474	2454	2433	2413	164
162	2787	2871	2887	2892	2887	2866	2831	2793	2756	2714	2672	2626	2590	2552	2517	2489	2462	2438	2418	2397	2377	162
160	2746	2829	2845	2850	2845	2825	2791	2754	2717	2676	2634	2589	2553	2515	2481	2453	2426	2402	2382	2361	2341	160
158	2704	2788	2804	2808	2803	2784	2751	2714	2679	2638	2597	2552	2516	2478	2445	2417	2390	2366	2346	2325	2305	158
156	2663	2746	2762	2766	2762	2743	2710	2675	2640	2600	2559	2515	2479	2442	2408	2380	2354	2330	2310	2289	2269	156
154	2622	2704	2720	2724	2720	2702	2670	2636	2601	2562	2521	2477	2442	2405	2372	2344	2318	2294	2274	2253	2233	154
152	2580	2663	2678	2682	2678	2661	2630	2596	2563	2524	2484	2440	2405	2369	2335	2308	2282	2258	2238	2217	2197	152
150	2539	2621	2636	2640	2637	2620	2590	3557	2524	2486	2446	2403	2369	2332	2299	2272	2246	2222	2202	2181	2161	150
148	2498	2579	2594	2598	2595	2579	2550	2518	2485	2448	2408	2366	2332	2295	2263	2235	2209	2186	2165	2145	2125	148
146	2456	2538	2553	2556	2553	2538	2510	2478	2447	2410	2371	2329	2295	2259	2226	2199	2173	2150	2129	2109	2089	146
144	2415	2496	2511	2514	1511	2497	2470	2439	2408	2372	2333	2291	2258	2222	2190	2163	2137	2114	2093	2073	2053	144
142	2374	2454	2469	2472	2470	2456	2429	2400	2369	2334	2295	2254	2221	2186	2153	2126	2101	2078	2057	2037	2017	142
140	2332	2413	2427	2430	2428	2415	2389	2360	2331	2296	2258	2217	2184	2149	2117	2090	2065	2042	2021	2001	1981	140
138	2291	2371	2385	2388	2386	2374	2349	2321	2292	2258	2220	2180	2147	2112	2081	2054	2029	2006	1985	1965	1945	138
136	2249	2330	2343	2346	2345	2333	2309	2281	2254	2220	2183	2142	2110	2076	2044	2018	1993	1970	1949	1929	1909	136
134	2208	2288	2301	2304	2303	2292	2269	2242	2215	2182	2145	2105	2073	2039	2008	1981	1957	1934	1913	1893	1873	134
132	2167	2246	2260	2262	2261	2251	2229	2203	2176	2144	2107	2068	2036	2003	1971	1945	1921	1898	1877	1857	1837	132
130	2125	2205	2218	2220	2220	2210	2188	2163	2138	2106	2070	2031	2000	1966	1935	1909	1885	1862	1841	1821	1801	130
128	2084	2163	2176	2178	2178	2169	2148	2124	2099	2068	2032	1993	1963	1929	1899	1873	1848	1826	1805	1785	1765	128
126	2043	2121	2134	2136	2136	2128	2108	2085	2060	2030	1994	1956	1926	1893	1862	1836	1812	1790	1769	1749	1729	126
124	2001	2080	2092	2094	2088	2087	2068	2045	2022	1992	1957	1919	1889	1856	1826	1800	1776	1753	1733	1713	1693	124
122	1960	2038	2050	2052	2053	2047	2028	2006	1983	1954	1919	1882	1852	1820	1789	1764	1740	1717	1697	1677	1657	122
120	1919	1996	2009	2010	2011	2006	1988	1967	1944	1916	1881	1844	1815	1783	1753	1728	1704	1681	1661	1641	1621	120
118	1877	1955	1967	1968	1969	1965	1947	1927	1906	1878	1844	1807	1778	1746	1717	1691	1668	1645	1625	1605	1585	118
116	1836	1913	1925	1926	1928	1924	1907	1888	1867	1840	1806	1770	1741	1710	1680	1655	1632	1609	1589	1569		116
114	1795	1871	1883	1884	1886	1883	1867	1849	1828	1802	1768	1733	1704	1673	1644	1619	1596	1573	1553			114
112	1753	1830	1841	1842	1844	1842	1827	1809	1790	1764	1731	1695	1667	1637	1607	1583	1560	1537				112
110	1712	1788	1799	1800	1803	1801	1787	1770	1751	1726	1693	1658	1631	1600	1571	1546	1524					110
108	1670	1747	1758	1758	1761	1760	1747	1730	1713	1688	1656	1621	1594	1563	1535	1510						108
106	1629	1705	1716	1716	1719	1719	1706	1691	1674	1650	1618	1584	1557	1527	1498							106
104	1588	1663	1674	1674	1677	1678	1666	1652	1635	1612	1580	1546	1520	1490								104
102	1546	1622	1632	1636	1637	1626	1612	1597	1574	1543	1509	1483	1454									102
100	1505	1580	1590	1590	1594	1596	1586	1573	1558	1536	1505	1472	1446									100
*	20.68	20.82	20.92	21	20.85	20.48	20.08	19.68	19.32	19	18.82	18.62	18.45	18.30	18.20	18.13	18.05	18.02	18.01	18	18	

*Weight Deviation Multiplier.   *Reproduced with permission of Frederick Rand Rogers.*

1. Norms for individuals whose weights are above limits for which norms are included are calculated by adding to the norm for any chosen weight the pound difference between that weight and the individual's weight *times* the Weight Deviation Multiplier.

2. Norms for men over 38 years of age may be calculated roughly by subtracting twenty points from the 38-year norm for each year over 38.

C. Girls

Age

Weight	8	8-6	9	9-6	10	10-6	11	11-6	12	12-6	13	13-6	14	14-6	15	15-6	16	16-6	17	17-6	18	Weight
180															2840	2933	2990	2984	2960	2912	2835	180
178														2721	2796	2885	2940	2934	2912	2865	2790	178
176													2598	2681	2752	2837	2890	2884	2863	2819	2745	176
174												2492	2560	2640	2707	2789	2840	2835	2815	2772	2700	174
172											2364	2457	2523	2600	2663	2741	2790	2785	2766	2726	2655	172
170										2250	2332	2422	2486	2559	2619	2693	2740	2735	1718	2679	2610	170
168										2220	2300	2387	2449	2518	2575	2645	2690	2685	2670	2632	2565	168
166									2085	2190	2268	2352	2412	2478	2531	2597	2640	2635	2621	2586	2502	166
164									2058	2160	2236	2318	2374	2437	2486	2549	2590	2586	2573	2539	2475	164
162								1923	2030	2130	2204	2283	2337	2397	2442	2501	2540	2536	2524	2493	2430	162
160							1818	1897	2002	2100	2172	2248	2300	2356	2398	2453	2490	2486	2476	2446	2385	160
158							1793	1871	1974	2070	2140	2213	2263	2315	2354	2405	2440	2436	2428	2399	2340	158
156						1736	1769	1845	1946	2040	2108	2178	2226	2275	2310	2357	2390	2386	2379	2353	2295	156
154						1711	1744	1818	1919	2010	2076	2144	2188	2234	2265	2309	2340	2337	2331	2306	2250	154
152					1681	1687	1720	1792	1891	1980	2044	2109	2151	2194	2221	2261	2290	2287	2282	2260	2205	152
150				1625	1657	1663	1695	1766	1863	1950	2012	2074	2114	2153	2177	2213	2240	2237	2234	2213	2160	150
148			1524	1602	1633	1639	1670	1740	1835	1920	1980	2039	2077	2112	2133	2165	2190	2187	2186	2166	2115	148
146			1502	1578	1609	1615	1646	1714	1807	1890	1948	2004	2040	2072	2089	2117	2140	2137	2137	2120	2070	146
144		1419	1479	1555	1584	1590	1621	1687	1780	1860	1916	1970	2002	2031	2044	2069	2090	2088	2089	2073	2025	144
142	1340	1398	1457	1531	1560	1566	1597	1661	1752	1830	1884	1935	1965	1991	2000	2021	2040	2038	2040	2027	1980	142
140	1319	1376	1435	1508	1536	1542	1572	1635	1724	1800	1852	1900	1928	1950	1956	1973	1990	1988	1992	1980	1935	140
138	1298	1354	1413	1485	1512	1518	1547	1609	1696	1770	1820	1865	1891	1909	1912	1925	1940	1938	1944	1933	1890	138
136	1278	1333	1391	1461	1488	1494	1523	1583	1668	1738	1788	1830	1854	1869	1868	1877	1890	1888	1895	1887	1845	136
134	1257	1311	1368	1438	1463	1469	1498	1556	1641	1710	1756	1796	1816	1828	1823	1829	1840	1839	1847	1840	1800	134
132	1237	1290	1346	1414	1439	1445	1474	1530	1613	1680	1724	1761	1779	1788	1779	1781	1790	1789	1798	1794	1755	132
130	1216	1268	1324	1391	1415	1421	1449	1504	1585	1650	1692	1726	1742	1747	1735	1733	1740	1739	1750	1747	1710	130
128	1195	1246	1302	1368	1391	1397	1424	1478	1557	1620	1660	1691	1705	1706	1691	1685	1690	1689	1702	1700	1665	128
126	1175	1225	1280	1344	1367	1373	1400	1452	1529	2590	1628	1656	1668	1666	1647	1637	1640	1639	1653	1654	1620	126
124	1154	1203	1257	1321	1342	1348	1375	1425	1502	1560	1596	1622	1630	1625	1602	1589	1590	1590	1605	1607	1575	124
122	1134	1182	1235	1297	1318	1324	1351	1399	1474	1530	1564	1587	1593	1585	1558	1541	1540		1556	1561	1530	122
120	1113	1160	1213	1274	1294	1300	1326	1373	1446	1500	1532	1552	1556	1544	1514	1493	1490	1490	1908	1514	1485	120
118	1092	1138	1191	1251	1270	1276	1301	1347	1418	1470	1500	1517	1519	1503	1470	1445	1440	1440	1460	1467	1440	118
116	1072	1117	1169	1227	1246	1252	1277	1321	1390	1440	1468	1482	1482	1463	1426	1397	1390	1390	1411	1421	1395	116
114	1051	1095	1146	1204	1221	1227	1252	1294	1363	1410	1436	1448	1444	1422	1381	1349	1340	1341	1363	1374	1350	114
112	1031	1074	1124	1180	1197	1203	1228	1268	1335	1380	1404	1413	1407	1382	1337	1301	1290	1291	1314	1328	1305	112
110	1010	1052	1102	1157	1173	1179	1203	1242	1307	1350	1372	1378	1370	1341	1293	1253	1240	1241	1266	1281	1260	110
108	989	1030	1080	1134	1149	1155	1178	1216	1279	1320	1340	1343	1333	1300	1249	1205	1190	1191	1218	1234	1215	108
106	969	1009	1058	1110	1125	1131	1154	1190	1251	1290	1308	1308	1296	1260	1205	1157	1140	1141	1169	1188	1170	106
104	948	987	1035	1087	1100	1106	1129	1163	1224	1260	1276	1274	1258	1219	1160	1109	1090	1092	1121	1141	1125	104
102	928	966	1013	1063	1076	1082	1105	1137	1196	1230	1244	1239	1221	1179	1116	1061	1040	1042	1072	1095	1080	102
100	907	944	991	1040	1052	1058	1080	1111	1168	1200	1212	1204	1184	1138	1072	1013	990	992	1024	1048	1035	100
98	886	922	969	1017	1034		1055	1085	1140	1170	1180	1169	1147	1097	1028	965	940	942	976	1001	990	98
96	866	901	947	993	1004	1010	1031	1059	1112	1140	1148	1134	1110	1057	984	917	890	892	927	955	945	96
94	845	879	924	970	979	985	1006	1032	1085	1110	1116	1100	1072	1016	939	869	840	843	879	908	900	94
92	825	858	902	946	955	961	982	1006	1057	1080	1084	1065	1035	976	895	821	790	793	830	862	855	92
90	804	836	880	923	931	937	957	980	1029	1050	1052	1030	998	935	851	773	740	743	782	815	810	90
88	783	814	858	900	907	913	932	954	1001	1020	1020	995	961	894	807	725	690	693	734	768	765	88
86	763	793	836	876	883	889	908	928	973	990	988	960	924	854	763	677	640	643	685	722	720	86
84	742	771	813	853	858	864	883	901	946	960	956	926	886	813	718	629	590	594	637	675	675	84
82	722	750	791	829	834	840	859	875	918	930	924	891	849	773	674	581	540	544	588	629	630	82
80	701	728	769	806	810	816	834	849	890	900	892	856	812	732	630	533	490	494	540	582	585	80
78	680	706	747	783	786	792	809	823	862	870	860	821	775	691	586	485	440	444	492	535		78
76	660	685	725	759	762	768	785	797	834	840	828	786	738	651	542	437	390	394	443	489		76
74	639	663	702	736	737	743	760	770	807	810	796	752	700	610	497	389	340	345	395			74
72	619	642	680	712	713	719	736	744	779	780	764	717	663	570	453	341	290	295	346			72
70	598	620	658	689	689	695	711	718	751	750	732	682	626	529	409	293	240	245				70
68	577	598	636	666	665	671	686	692	723	720	700	647	589	488	365	245	190					68
66	557	577	614	642	641	647	662	666	695	690	668	612	552	448	321	197	140					66
64	536	555	591	619	616	622	637	639	668	660	636	578	514	407	276	149						64
62	516	534	569	595	592	598	613	613	640	630	604	543	477	367	232							62
60	495	512	547	572	568	574	588	587	612	600	572	508	440	326								60
58	474	490	525	549	544	550	563	561	584	570	540	473	403									58
56	454	469	503	525	520	526	539	535	556	540	508	438										56
54	433	447	480	502	495	501	514	508	529	510	476											54
52	413	426	458	478	471	477	490	482	501	480												52
50	392	404	436	455	447	453	465	456	473													50
	8	8-6	9	9-6	10	10-6	11	11-6	12	12-6	13	13-6	14	14-6	15	15-6	16	16-6	17	17-6	18	
*	10.3	10.8	11.1	11.7	12.1	12.1	12.3	13.1	13.9	15	16	17.4	18.6	20.3	22.1	24	25	24.9	24.2	23.3	22.5	

*Weight Deviation Multiplier.

Reproduced with permission of Frederick Rand Rogers.

D. *Women*

Age

Weight	18	19	20	21	22	23	24	25	26	27	28	29	30	31	32	33	34	35	36	37	38	Weight
220													3035	3017	3000	2994	2978	2975	2972	2969	2955	220
218												3017	2998	2981	2964	2958	2942	2939	2936	2933	2919	218
216											3001	2980	2962	2944	2928	2922	2906	2903	2900	2897	2883	216
214										2985	2964	2944	2925	2908	2891	2885	2870	2867	2864	2861	2848	214
212										2948	2927	2907	2889	2871	2855	2849	2834	2831	2828	2825	2812	212
210									2946	2911	2890	2870	2852	2835	2819	2813	2798	2795	2792	2789	2776	210
208								2943	2908	2874	2853	2833	2815	2799	2783	2777	2762	2759	2756	2753	2740	208
206								2905	2871	2837	2816	2796	2779	2762	2747	2741	2726	2723	2720	2717	2704	206
204							2913	2867	2833	2799	2779	2760	2742	2726	2710	2704	2690	2687	2684	2681	2669	204
202							2875	2829	2796	2762	2742	2723	2706	2689	2674	2668	2654	2651	2648	2645	2633	202
200						2873	2836	2791	2758	2725	2705	2686	2669	2653	2638	2632	2618	2615	2612	2609	2597	200
198						2834	2797	2753	2720	2688	2668	2649	2632	2617	2602	2596	2582	2579	2576	2573	2561	198
196					2844	2795	2759	2715	2683	2651	2631	2612	2596	2580	2566	2560	2546	2543	2540	2537	2525	196
194					2804	2756	2720	2677	2645	2613	2594	2576	2559	2544	2529	2523	2510	2507	2504	2501	2490	194
192				2822	2765	2717	2682	2639	2608	2576	2557	2539	2523	2507	2493	2487	2474	2471	2468	2465	2454	192
190				2782	2725	2678	2643	2601	2570	2539	2520	2502	2486	2471	2457	2451	2438	2435	2432	2429	2418	190
188			2808	2742	2685	2639	2604	2563	2532	2502	2483	2465	2449	2435	2421	2415	2402	2399	2396	2392	2382	188
186			2766	2701	2646	2600	2566	2525	2495	2465	2446	2428	2413	2398	2385	2379	2366	2363	2360	2357	2346	186
184		2804	2725	2661	2606	2561	2527	2487	2457	2427	2409	2392	2376	2362	2348	2342	2330	2327	2324	2321	2311	184
182	2880	2761	2683	2620	2567	2522	2489	2449	2420	2390	2372	2355	2340	2325	2312	2306	2294	2291	2288	2285	2275	182
180	2835	2718	2642	2580	2527	2483	2450	2411	2382	2353	2335	2318	2303	2289	2276	2270	2258	2255	2252	2249	2239	180
178	2790	2675	2601	2540	2487	2444	2411	2373	2344	2316	2298	2281	2266	2253	2240	2234	2222	2219	2216	2213	2203	178
176	2745	2632	2559	2499	2448	2405	2373	2335	2307	2279	2262	2244	2230	2216	2204	2198	2186	2183	2180	2177	2167	176
174	2700	2590	2518	2459	2408	2366	2334	2297	2269	2241	2224	2208	2193	2180	2167	2161	2150	2147	2144	2141	2132	174
172	2655	2547	2476	2418	2369	2327	2296	2259	2232	2204	2187	2171	2157	2143	2131	2125	2114	2111	2108	2105	2096	172
170	2610	2504	2435	2378	2329	2288	2257	2221	2194	2167	2150	2134	2120	2107	2095	2089	2078	2075	2072	2069	2060	170
168	2565	2461	2394	2338	2289	2249	2218	2183	2156	2130	2113	2097	2083	2071	2059	2053	2042	2039	2036	2033	2024	168
166	2520	2418	2352	2297	2250	2210	2180	2145	2119	2093	2076	2060	2047	2034	2023	2017	2006	2003	2000	1997	1988	166
164	2475	2376	2311	2257	2210	2171	2141	2107	2081	2055	2039	2024	2010	1998	1986	1980	1970	1967	1964	1961	1953	164
162	2430	2333	2269	2216	2171	2132	2103	2069	2044	2018	2002	1987	1974	1961	1950	1944	1934	1931	1928	1925	1917	162
160	2385	2290	2228	2176	2131	2093	2064	2031	2006	1981	1965	1950	1937	1925	1914	1908	1898	1895	1892	1889	1881	160
158	2340	2247	2187	2136	2091	2054	2025	1993	1968	1944	1928	1913	1900	1889	1878	1872	1862	1859	1856	1853	1845	158
156	2295	2204	2145	2095	2052	2015	1987	1955	1931	1907	1891	1876	1864	1852	1842	1836	1826	1823	1820	1817	1809	156
154	2250	2162	2104	2055	2012	1976	1948	1917	1893	1869	1854	1840	1827	1816	1805	1799	1790	1787	1784	1781	1774	154
152	2205	2119	2062	2014	1973	1937	1910	1879	1856	1832	1817	1803	1791	1779	1769	1763	1754	1751	1748	1745	1738	152
150	2160	2076	2021	1974	1933	1898	1871	1841	1818	1795	1780	1766	1754	1743	1733	1727	1718	1715	1712	1709	1702	150
148	2115	2033	1980	1934	1893	1859	1832	1803	1780	1758	1743	1729	1717	1707	1697	1691	1682	1679	1676	1673	1666	148
146	2070	1990	1938	1893	1854	1820	1794	1765	1743	1721	1706	1692	1681	1670	1661	1655	1646	1643	1640	1637	1630	146
144	2025	1948	1897	1853	1814	1781	1755	1727	1705	1683	1669	1656	1644	1634	1624	1618	1610	1607	1604	1601	1595	144
142	1980	1905	1855	1812	1775	1742	1717	1689	1668	1646	1632	1619	1608	1597	1588	1582	1574	1571	1568	1565	1559	142
140	1935	1862	1814	1772	1735	1703	1678	1651	1630	1609	1595	1582	1571	1561	1552	1546	1538	1535	1532	1529	1523	140
138	1890	1819	1773	1732	1695	1664	1639	1613	1592	1572	1558	1545	1534	1525	1516	1510	1502	1499	1496	1493	1487	138
136	1845	1776	1731	1691	1656	1625	1601	1575	1555	1535	1521	1508	1498	1488	1480	1474	1466	1463	1460	1457	1451	136
134	1800	1734	1690	1651	1616	1586	1562	1537	1517	1497	1484	1472	1461	1452	1443	1437	1430	1427	1424	1421	1416	134
132	1755	1691	1648	1610	1577	1547	1524	1499	1480	1460	1447	1435	1425	1415	1407	1401	1394	1391	1388	1385	1380	132
130	1710	1648	1607	1572	1537	1508	1485	1461	1442	1423	1410	1398	1388	1379	1371	1365	1358	1355	1352	1349	1344	130
128	1665	1605	1566	1530	1497	1469	1446	1423	1404	1386	1373	1361	1351	1343	1335	1329	1322	1319	1316	1313	1308	128
126	1620	1562	1524	1489	1458	1430	1408	1385	1367	1349	1336	1324	1315	1306	1299	1293	1286	1283	1280	1277	1272	126
124	1575	1520	1483	1449	1418	1391	1369	1347	1329	1311	1299	1288	1278	1270	1262	1256	1250	1247	1244	1241	1236	124
122	1530	1477	1441	1408	1379	1352	1331	1309	1292	1274	1262	1251	1242	1233	1226	1220	1214	1211	1208	1205	1201	122
120	1485	1434	1400	1368	1339	1313	1292	1271	1254	1237	1225	1214	1205	1197	1190	1184	1178	1175	1172	1169	1165	120
118	1440	1391	1359	1328	1299	1274	1253	1233	1216	1200	1188	1177	1168	1161	1154	1148	1142	1139	1136	1133	1129	118
116	1395	1348	1317	1287	1260	1235	1215	1195	1179	1163	1151	1140	1132	1124	1118	1112	1106	1103	1100	1097	1093	116
114	1350	1306	1276	1247	1220	1196	1176	1157	1141	1125	1114	1104	1095	1088	1081	1075	1070	1067	1064	1061	1058	114
112	1305	1263	1234	1206	1181	1157	1138	1119	1104	1088	1077	1067	1059	1051	1045	1039	1034	1031	1028	1025	1022	112
110	1260	1220	1193	1166	1141	1118	1099	1081	1066	1051	1041	1030	1022	1015	1009	1003	998	995	992	989	986	110
108	1215	1177	1152	1126	1101	1079	1060	1043	1028	1014	1003	993	985	979	973	967	962	959	956			108
106	1170	1134	1110	1085	1062	1040	1022	1005	991	977	966	956	949	942	937	931	926	923				106
104	1125	1092	1069	1045	1022	1001	983	967	953	939	929	920	912	906	900	894	890					104
102	1080	1049	1027	1004	983	962	945	929	916	902	892	883	876	869	864	858						102
100	1035	1006	986	964	943	923	906	891	878	865	855	846	839	833	828							100
98	990	963	945	924	903	884	867	853	840	828	818	809	802	797								98
96	945	920	903	883	864	845	829	815	803	791	781	772	766									96
94	900	878	862	843	824	806	790	777	765	753	744	736										94
92	855	835	820	802	785	767	752	739	728	716	707											92
90	810	792	779	762	745	728	713	701	690													90
	18	19	20	21	22	23	24	25	26	27	28	29	30	31	32	33	34	35	36	37	38	
*	22.5	21.4	20.7	20.2	19.8	19.5	19.3	19	18.8	18.6	18.5	18.4	18.3	18.2	18.1	18.1	18	18	18	18	17.9	

*Weight Deviation Multiplier.   *Reproduced with permission of Frederick Rand Rogers.*

TABLE B.4 *Rating Table for Crampton Blood-Ptosis Test**

Heart Rate Increase					Systolic Blood Pressure					
	Increase						*Decrease*			
	+10	+8	+6	+4	+2	0	−2	−4	−6	−8	−10
0 to 4	100	95	90	85	80	75	70	65	60	55	50
5 to 8	95	90	85	80	75	70	65	60	55	50	45
9 to 12	90	85	80	75	70	65	60	55	50	45	40
13 to 16	85	80	75	70	65	60	55	50	45	40	35
17 to 20	80	75	70	65	60	55	50	45	40	35	30
21 to 24	75	70	65	60	55	50	45	40	35	30	25
25 to 28	70	65	60	55	50	45	40	35	30	25	20
29 to 32	65	60	55	50	45	40	35	30	25	20	15
33 to 36	60	55	50	45	40	35	30	25	20	15	10
37 to 40	55	50	45	40	35	30	25	20	15	10	5
41 to 44	50	45	40	35	30	25	20	15	10	5	0

*C. Ward Crampton, "A Test of Condition," *Medical News,* **87,** (September 1905), 529.

TABLE B.5 *Cardiovascular Efficiency Test Scores for Girls and Women*

	Junior H.S. Girls[1]		Senior H.S. Girls[1]		College Women[2]	
Rating	C-V Eff. Score	30-sec. Recov. Pulse	C-V Eff. Score	30-Sec. Recov. Pulse	C-V Eff. Score	30-Sec. Recov. Pulse
Excellent	72–100	44 or less	71–100	45 or less	71–100	45 or less
Very Good	62–71	45–52	60–70	46–54	60–70	46–54
Good	51–61	53–63	49–59	55–66	49–59	55–66
Fair	41–50	64–79	40–48	67–80	39–48	67–83
Poor	31–40	80–92	31–39	81–96	28–38	84–116
Very Poor	0–30	93 & above	0–30	91 & above	0–27	117–120

[1]Vera Skubic and Jean Hodgkins, "Cardiovascular Efficiency Test Scores for Junior and Senior High School Girls in the United States," *Research Quarterly,* **35,** No. 2 (May 1964), 184.

[2]Jean Hodgkins and Vera Skubic, "Cardiovascular Efficiency Test Scores for College Women in the United States," *Research Quarterly,* **34,** No. 4 (December 1963), 454.

TABLE B.6 *Queens College Step Test.* Percentile Norms for Recovery Heart Rate Following 3-Min. Step Test (N = 300)*

Percentile	5–20 Sec. Heart Rate, bpm	Percentile	5–20 Sec. Heart Rate, bpm
100	128	45	168
95	140	40	170
90	148	35	171
85	152	30	172
80	156	25	176
75	158	20	180
70	160	15	182
65	162	10	184
60	163	5	196
55	164	0	216
50	166		

*William D. McArdle, and others, "Percentile Norms for A Valid Step Test for College Women," *Research Quarterly,* **44,** No. 4 (December 1973), 498.

TABLE B.7 *Scoring Table for Schneider's Cardiovascular Test**

A. Reclining Pulse Rate		B. Pulse Rate Increase on Standing				
Rate	*Points*	*0–10 Beats, Points*	*11–18 Beats, Points*	*19–26 Beats, Points*	*27–34 Beats, Points*	*35–42 Beats, Points*
50– 60............	3	3	3	1	1	0
61– 70............	3	3	2	1	0	−1
71– 80............	2	3	2	0	−1	−2
81– 90............	1	2	1	−1	−2	−3
91–100............	0	1	0	−2	−3	−3
101–110............	−1	0	−1	−3	−3	−3

C. Standing Pulse Rate		D. Pulse Rate Increase Immediately after Exercise				
Rate	*Points*	*0–10 Beats, Points*	*11–20 Beats, Points*	*21–30 Beats, Points*	*31–40 Beats, Points*	*41–50 Beats, Points*
60– 70............	3	3	3	2	1	0
71– 80............	3	3	2	1	0	0
81– 90............	2	3	2	1	0	−1
91–100............	1	2	1	0	−1	−2
101–110............	1	1	0	−1	−2	−3
111–120............	0	1	−1	−2	−3	−3
121–130............	0	0	−2	−3	−3	−3
131–140............	−1	0	−3	−3	−3	−3

E. Return of Pulse Rate to Standing Normal after Exercise		F. Systolic Pressure, Standing, Compared with Reclining	
Seconds	*Points*	*Change in Mm.*	*Points*
0– 30.............	3	Rise of 8 or more	3
31– 60............	2	Rise of 2–7	2
61– 90............	1	No rise	1
91–120............	0	Fall of 2–5	0
After 120: 2–10 beats above normal	−1	Fall of 6 or more.................	−1
After 120: 11–30 beats above normal	−2		

*E. D. Schneider, "A Cardiovascular Rating as a Measure of Physical Fatigue and Efficiency," *Journal of American Medical Association,* **74** (May 29, 1920), 1507.

TABLE B.8 *Oregon Motor Fitness Test Norms**
A. *Rating Norms for Boys (Grades 4–6)*

Test items	Superior	Good	Fair	Poor	Inferior	Grade
Standing Broad Jump	69-Up	62–68	52–61	42–51	12–41	
Push-Ups	25-Up	18–24	7–17	1–6	0	4
Sit-Ups	64-Up	47–63	22–46	1–21	0	
Standing Broad Jump	73-Up	66–72	56–65	46–55	16–45	
Push-Ups	22-Up	16–21	7–15	1–6	0	5
Sit-Ups	70-Up	52–69	22–51	2–21	0–1	
Standing Broad Jump	77-Up	70–76	59–69	49–58	18–48	
Push-Ups	24-Up	18–23	9–17	4–8	0–3	6
Sit-Ups	75-Up	55–74	25–54	1–24	0	

(Grades 7–9)

Test items	Superior	Good	Fair	Poor	Inferior	Grade
Jump and Reach	19-Up	16–18	14–15	10–13	0–9	
Pull-Ups	8-Up	6–7	3–5	1	0	7
Potato Race	0–32	33–35	36–39	40–42	43-Up	
Jump and Reach	21-Up	18–20	15–17	13–14	0–12	
Pull-Ups	10-Up	7–9	4–6	1–3	0	8
Potato Race	0–31	32–34	35–37	38–40	41-Up	
Jump and Reach	24-Up	21–23	17–20	14–16	0–13	
Pull-Ups	10-Up	8–9	3–7	1–2	0	9
Potato Race	0–30	31–32	33–35	36–39	40-Up	

(Grades 10–12)

Test items	Superior	Good	Fair	Poor	Inferior	Grade
Jump and Reach	25-Up	23–24	19–22	15–18	0–14	
Pull-Ups	12-Up	9–11	5–8	2–4	1–0	10
Potato Race	0–30	31–32	33–35	36–38	39-Up	
Jump and Reach	27-Up	24–26	20–23	17–19	0–16	
Pull-Ups	14-Up	11–13	6–10	2–5	0–1	11
Potato Race	0–30	31	32–34	35–36	37-Up	
Jump and Reach	29-Up	26–28	22–25	17–21	0–16	
Pull-Ups	15-Up	11–44	7–10	3–6	0–2	12
Potato Race	0–30	31	32–34	35–36	37-Up	
All Grades Total Standard Points	204-Up	180–203	144–179	112–143	111-Down	

Motor Fitness Tests for Oregon Schools (Salem, Oregon: State Education Department, 1962).

B. *Oregon Motor Fitness Test Rating Norms for Girls (Grades 4–6)*

Test items	Superior	Good	Fair	Poor	Inferior	Grade
Hanging in Arm-Flexed Position	30-Up	20–29	5–19	1–4	0	
Standing Broad Jump	65-Up	58–64	49–57	39–48	0–38	4
Crossed-Arm Curl-Ups	66-Up	50–65	26–49	2–25	0–1	
Hanging in Arm-Flexed Position	31-Up	22–30	10–21	2–9	0–1	
Standing Broad Jump	75-Up	68–74	57–67	46–56	0–45	5
Crossed-Arm Curl-Ups	68-Up	52–67	28–51	4–27	0–3	
Hanging in Arm-Flexed Position	37-Up	27–36	12–26	1–11	0	
Standing Broad Jump	73-Up	66–72	55–65	44–54	0–43	6
Crossed-Arm Curl-Ups	71-Up	55–70	31–54	1–30	0	

(Grades 7–9)

Test items	Superior	Good	Fair	Poor	Inferior	Grade
Hanging in Arm-Flexed Position	44-Up	36–43	24–35	16–23	0–15	
Standing Broad Jump	76-Up	70–75	59–69	49–58	0–48	7
Crossed-Arm Curl-Ups	59-Up	47–58	29–46	15–28	0–14	
Hanging in Arm-Flexed Position	44-Up	36–43	24–35	16–23	0–15	
Standing Broad Jump	78-Up	72–77	61–71	51–60	0–50	8
Crossed-Arm Curl-Ups	59-Up	47–58	29–46	15–28	0–14	
Hanging in Arm-Flexed Position	51-Up	37–50	17–36	8–16	0–7	
Standing Broad Jump	81-Up	75–80	63–74	53–62	0–52	9
Crossed-Arm Curl-Ups	65-Up	51–64	31–50	17–30	0–16	

(Grades 10–12)

Test items	Superior	Good	Fair	Poor	Inferior	Grade
Hanging in Arm-Flexed Position	48-Up	34–40	13–33	5–12	0–4	
Standing Broad Jump	81-Up	75–80	64–74	53–63	0–52	10
Crossed-Arm Curl-Ups	65-Up	51–64	31–50	17–30	0–16	
Hanging in Arm-Flexed Position	49-Up	35–48	14–34	6–13	0–5	
Standing Broad Jump	85-Up	76–84	65–75	55–64	0–54	11
Crossed-Arm Curl-Ups	67-Up	53–66	33–52	19–32	0–18	
Hanging in Arm-Flexed Position	50-Up	36–49	14–35	7–13	0–6	
Standing Broad Jump	85-Up	76–84	65–75	56–64	0–55	12
Crossed-Arm Curl-Ups	67-Up	53–66	33–52	19–32	0–18	
All Grades Total Standard Points	204-Up	180–203	144–179	112–143	111-Down	

TABLE B.9 *Percentile Norms: California Physical Performance Test**
A. *Boys' Standing Long Jump*

	Length of Jump in Inches, According to Age								
Percentile	10	11	12	13	14	15	16	17	18
99	76	83	86	92	98	102	103	105	108
95	72	75	80	84	91	96	98	100	101
90	69	72	77	82	88	93	95	98	98
85	67	70	75	79	86	90	93	96	96
80	66	69	73	78	84	89	91	94	95
75	65	68	72	76	83	87	90	93	94
70	64	66	71	75	81	86	88	91	92
65	62	65	70	73	80	84	87	90	91
60	61	64	69	72	79	83	86	89	90
55	60	—	67	71	78	82	85	87	88
50	59	63	66	70	76	81	84	86	87
45	58	62	—	69	75	80	83	85	86
40	—	60	65	68	74	78	82	84	85
35	57	59	64	67	72	77	80	83	84
30	55	58	62	66	71	76	79	82	83
25	54	57	61	64	70	74	77	80	81
20	53	56	60	63	68	73	75	78	79
15	51	54	59	61	66	71	73	76	77
10	49	52	56	59	63	68	71	73	74
5	44	49	52	55	60	65	67	69	69

**The Physical Performance Test for California,* Rev. ed. (Sacramento, Calif.: Bureau of Physical Education, Health Education, Athletics, and Recreation, California State Department of Education, 1971).

B. *Boys' Bent-Knee Sit-ups*

	Number of Sit-ups, According to Age								
Percentile	10	11	12	13	14	15	16	17	18
99									
95	44	49	55	58					
90	39	44	50	54					
85	36	41	49	51	55	59	61	63	61
80	33	38	46	49	53	56	59	60	59
75	32	36	45	48	51	54	57	58	57
70	30	35	43	47	50	52	55	55	55
65	28	33	41	45	49	51	53	54	54
60	27	31	40	44	48	50	51	52	52
55	25	29	39	43	46	49	50	51	50
50	24	28	37	42	45	47	49	49	49
45	23	26	36	41	44	46	48	48	48
40	22	24	34	40	43	45	46	47	46
35	20	23	32	38	41	44	45	45	45
30	19	22	31	37	40	42	44	44	44
25	18	20	29	35	39	41	42	42	42
20	16	19	27	33	37	39	40	40	40
15	14	16	24	31	34	38	39	39	38
10	11	14	21	29	31	35	35	36	35
5	5	4	14	23	27	31	32	32	30

C. Boys' Chair Push-ups

Percentile	Number of Push-ups, According to Age								
	10	11	12	13	14	15	16	17	18
99	50		50	50					
95	36	39	40	49	50	50			
90	29	32	34	42	49	49	50	50	50
85	26	29	30	37	42	45	49	—	49
80	23	25	28	33	38	41	45	49	—
75	21	23	25	30	34	39	42	46	45
70	20	21	23	29	32	35	40	43	43
65	18	19	21	26	30	34	39	40	40
60	16	17	20	24	29	31	37	39	39
55	15	16	18	22	27	30	35	36	36
50	13	14	16	20	25	29	34	34	34
45	12	13	15	—	23	26	32	32	32
40	10	12	13	19	21	24	30	30	30
35	9	10	12	16	20	23	29	—	29
30	8	9	10	15	19	20	27	28	28
25	7	8	9	13	17	19	25	25	25
20	5	7	8	11	14	18	22	24	24
15	4	5	6	9	11	15	20	21	21
10	2	3	4	6	9	11	18	19	19
5	0	0	1	3	5	6	12	14	14

D. Boys' Side Step

Percentile	Number of Lines Crossed or Touched, According to Age								
	10	11	12	13	14	15	16	17	18
99	21	25	24	26	29	31	31	32	31
95	18	20	21	23	25	26	26	27	27
90	17	18	20	21	23	24	24	25	25
85	16	—	19	—	22	23	—	—	24
80	—	17	18	20	21	—	23	23	23
75	15	—	—	19	—	22	22	—	—
70	14	16	17	—	20	21	21	22	22
65	—	—	—	18	—	—	—	21	21
60	—	15	—	—	19	20	20	—	—
55	13	—	16	17	—	—	—	20	20
50	—	14	—	—	18	19	19	—	—
45	—	—	15	—	—	—	—	19	19
40	—	13	—	16	17	18	18	—	—
35	12	—	14	—	—	17	17	18	18
30	—	—	—	15	16	—	—	17	17
25	11	12	13	—	—	16	16	—	16
20	10	11	12	14	15	15	15	16	—
15	9	10	11	13	14	14	14	15	15
10	8	9	10	11	13	13	13	14	14
5	7	7	8	10	12	11	11	12	12

E. *Boys' Pull-ups*

Percentile	*Number of Pull-ups, According to Age*								
	10	*11*	*12*	*13*	*14*	*15*	*16*	*17*	*18*
99	12	13	14	17	19	23	21	20	21
95	8	9	9	10	13	15	16	17	17
90	6	7	7	9	11	12	14	15	15
85	5	5	6	7	10	11	13	14	14
80	4	—	5	6	9	10	12	—	—
75	—	4	4	—	8	—	11	12	12
70	3	3	—	5	7	9	10	11	11
65	—	—	3	4	6	8	—	10	10
60	2	—	—	—	—	7	9	—	—
55	—	2	2	—	5	—	8	9	—
50	1	—	—	3	—	6	—	—	9
45	—	1	—	—	4	5	7	8	8
40	0	—	1	2	—	—	—	7	—
35	—	0	—	—	3	4	6	—	7
30	—	—	0	1	2	—	5	6	6
25	—	—	—	0	—	3	4	—	—
20	—	—	—	—	1	—	—	5	5
15	—	—	—	—	—	2	3	4	4
10	—	—	—	—	0	1	2	3	3
5	—	—	—	—	—	0	0	1	1

F. *Boys' Jog-Walk*

Percentile	*Number of 110-Yard Segments Completed, According to Age*								
	10	*11*	*12*	*13*	*14*	*15*	*16*	*17*	*18*
99									
95									
90	15	17	15	—	16	16	16	16	16
85	14	14	—	15	—	—	—	—	—
80	13	—	14	—	15	—	—	—	—
75	—	13	—	—	—	15	15	15	—
70	12	—	—	14	—	—	—	—	15
65	—	—	13	—	—	—	—	—	—
60	—	12	—	—	14	—	—	—	—
55	11	—	—	—	—	14	14	14	14
50	—	—	12	13	—	—	—	—	—
45	—	—	—	—	—	—	—	—	—
40	—	11	—	—	13	—	—	13	—
35	10	—	11	12	—	13	13	—	13
30	—	10	—	—	—	—	—	—	—
25	—	—	—	—	12	—	—	12	12
20	9	9	10	11	—	12	12	—	—
15	8	—	9	10	11	11	—	11	11
10	6	8	8	9	10	10	11	10	10
5	0	0	2	7	7	9	10	9	8

G. *Girls' Standing Long Jump*

Percentile	Length of Jump in Inches, According to Age								
	10	*11*	*12*	*13*	*14*	*15*	*16*	*17*	*18*
99	72	79	80	85	85	87	86	84	87
95	68	71	75	79	79	79	79	78	80
90	65	69	72	75	76	76	76	76	76
85	63	67	71	73	74	74	74	74	74
80	62	65	69	72	73	72	72	72	72
75	61	64	68	70	71	71	71	71	71
70	60	63	66	69	70	70	70	70	70
65	59	62	65	68	68	69	68	69	69
60	58	60	64	67	67	68	67	68	68
55	57	59	63	65	66	66	66	67	67
50	56	58	62	64	65	65	65	66	65
45	55	—	61	63	64	64	64	65	—
40	54	57	60	62	63	63	63	64	64
35	53	56	59	61	62	62	62	63	62
30	52	54	58	60	61	61	61	61	61
25	51	53	56	59	60	60	60	60	60
20	49	52	55	57	58	58	58	59	58
15	48	50	53	56	56	57	57	57	57
10	46	48	51	53	54	54	54	54	54
5	44	45	47	50	50	50	51	50	50

H. *Girls' Bent-Knee Sit-ups*

Percentile	Number of Sit-ups, According to Age								
	10	*11*	*12*	*13*	*14*	*15*	*16*	*17*	*18*
99	50	51	50	53	52	54	52	50	51
95	39	42	44	46	47	47	45	45	46
90	35	37	40	42	43	43	42	42	42
85	33	35	38	40	41	41	40	40	41
80	31	33	36	38	39	39	39	39	39
75	29	31	35	37	38	38	37	38	38
70	28	29	33	35	36	36	36	36	36
65	26	28	32	34	35	35	35	35	35
60	25	26	31	33	34	34	34	34	34
55	24	24	30	32	33	32	32	33	33
50	22	23	29	31	32	31	31	32	32
45	21	21	28	30	30	30	30	30	31
40	19	20	26	29	29	29	29	29	30
35	18	19	25	27	28	28	28	28	29
30	17	18	23	26	26	26	26	27	27
25	15	16	21	24	25	25	25	25	25
20	14	15	20	23	23	23	24	24	23
15	12	13	18	21	21	21	21	21	21
10	10	11	15	19	18	19	18	19	19
5	7	7	10	14	13	13	13	13	15

I. *Girls' Chair Push-ups*

	Number of Push-ups, According to Age								
Percentile	10	11	12	13	14	15	16	17	18
99	45	46	40	35	36	33	35	25	38
95	25	26	24	21	21	19	17	18	20
90	20	20	19	17	17	15	12	14	15
85	17	16	15	14	14	11	10	11	12
80	14	14	12	12	12	10	9	9	10
75	12	12	11	10	10	9	8	8	9
70	11	11	10	9	9	8	6	6	7
65	10	10	9	8	8	6	5	—	6
60	9	9	7	7	6	5	—	5	5
55	8	8	6	6	5	—	4	4	—
50	7	6	5	5	—	4	3	3	4
45	6	5	4	4	4	3	—	—	3
40	5	4	—	—	3	—	2	2	—
35	4	—	3	3	2	2	1	—	2
30	3	3	2	2	—	—	—	1	—
25	—	2	—	—	1	1	0	—	1
20	2	1	1	1	—	0	—	0	0
15	1	—	0	0	0	—	—	—	—
10	0	0	—	—	—	—	—	—	—
5	—	—	—	—	—	—	—	—	—

J. *Girls' Side Step*

	Number of Lines Crossed or Touched, According to Age								
Percentile	10	11	12	13	14	15	16	17	18
99	25	22		25	23	24	24	24	24
95	18	19	20	20	20	21	21	21	21
90	16	17	19	19	—	—	20	20	20
85	15	—	18	—	—	19	19	19	19
80	—	16	—	18	18	18	18	—	—
75	—	—	17	—	—	—	—	18	18
70	14	15	—	17	17	17	17	—	—
65	—	—	16	—	—	—	—	17	17
60	13	14	—	—	—	—	—	—	—
55	—	—	—	16	16	—	16	16	16
50	—	—	15	—	—	16	—	—	—
45	12	13	—	15	15	15	15	—	—
40	—	—	14	—	—	—	—	15	15
35	—	12	—	—	—	—	—	—	—
30	11	—	13	14	14	14	14	—	—
25	—	11	—	—	—	—	—	14	14
20	10	10	12	13	13	13	13	13	13
15	9	9	11	12	12	12	—	—	—
10	7	8	10	11	11	11	12	12	12
5	5	7	8	9	10	10	10	11	10

K. *Girls' Pull-ups*

	Number of Pull-ups, According to Age								
Percentile	*10*	*11*	*12*	*13*	*14*	*15*	*16*	*17*	*18*
99	37	36	20	30	28	26	14	6	11
95	8	5	4	4	4	4	2	2	2
90	3	3	3	2	2	1	1	1	1
85	2	2	2	1	1	—	—	0	—
80	1	1	1	—	—	0	0	—	0
75	—	—	—	0	0	—	—	—	—
70	0	0	0	—	—	—	—	—	—
65	—	—	—	—	—	—	—	—	—
60	—	—	—	—	—	—	—	—	—
55	—	—	—	—	—	—	—	—	—
50	—	—	—	—	—	—	—	—	—
45	—	—	—	—	—	—	—	—	—
40	—	—	—	—	—	—	—	—	—
35	—	—	—	—	—	—	—	—	—
30	—	—	—	—	—	—	—	—	—
25	—	—	—	—	—	—	—	—	—
20	—	—	—	—	—	—	—	—	—
15	—	—	—	—	—	—	—	—	—
10	—	—	—	—	—	—	—	—	—
5	—	—	—	—	—	—	—	—	—

L. *Girls' Bent-Arm Hang (Alternate)*

	Number of 110-Yard Segments Completed, According to Age								
Percentile	*10*	*11*	*12*	*13*	*14*	*15*	*16*	*17*	*18*
99									
95	18	19	16	14	14	14	13	13	13
90	13	15	13	13	13	13	12	12	12
85	12	13	—	—	—	12	—	—	—
80	—	12	12	12	12	—	—	11	11
75	11	—	—	—	—	—	11	—	—
70	—	—	—	—	—	11	—	—	—
65	—	11	11	—	11	—	—	—	—
60	—	—	—	11	—	—	—	—	10
55	10	—	—	—	—	—	10	10	—
50	—	10	—	—	—	—	—	—	—
45	—	—	10	—	—	10	—	—	—
40	—	—	—	10	10	—	—	—	—
35	9	9	—	—	—	—	9	9	9
30	—	—	9	—	—	—	—	—	—
25	—	—	—	9	—	9	—	—	—
20	8	8	—	—	9	—	—	—	8
15	7	7	8	8	—	—	8	8	—
10	4	6	7	—	8	8	7	7	7
5	0	0	3	6	7	7	6	5	4

M. *Girls' Jog-Walk*

	Number of 110-Yard Segments Completed, According to Age								
Percentile	10	11	12	13	14	15	16	17	18
99									
95	18	19	16	14	14	14	13	13	13
90	13	15	13	13	13	13	12	12	12
85	12	13	—	—	—	12	—	—	—
80	—	12	12	12	12	—	—	11	11
75	11	—	—	—	—	—	11	—	—
70	—	—	—	—	—	11	—	—	—
65	—	11	11	—	11	—	—	—	—
60	—	—	—	11	—	—	—	—	10
55	10	—	—	—	—	—	10	10	—
50	—	10	—	—	—	—	—	—	—
45	—	—	10	—	—	10	—	—	—
40	—	—	—	10	10	—	—	—	—
35	9	9	—	—	—	—	9	9	9
30	—	—	9	—	—	—	—	—	—
25	—	—	—	9	—	9	—	—	—
20	8	8	—	—	9	—	—	—	8
15	7	7	8	8	—	—	8	8	—
10	4	6	7	—	8	8	7	7	7
5	0	0	3	6	7	7	6	5	4

TABLE B.10 *AAHPER Youth Fitness Test: Percentile Norms by Ages* *
A. *Flexed-Arm Hang for Girls. Percentile Scores Based on Age / Test Scores in Seconds*

	Age							
Percentile	10	11	12	13	14	15	16	17
100	66	79	64	80	60	74	74	76
95	31	35	30	30	30	33	37	31
90	24	25	23	21	22	22	26	25
85	21	20	19	18	19	18	19	19
80	18	17	15	15	16	16	16	16
75	15	16	13	13	13	14	14	14
70	13	13	11	12	11	13	12	12
65	11	11	10	10	10	11	10	11
60	10	10	8	9	9	10	9	10
55	9	9	8	8	8	8	8	9
50	7	8	6	7	7	8	7	8
45	6	6	6	6	6	6	6	7
40	6	5	5	5	5	6	5	6
35	5	4	4	4	4	4	4	4
30	4	4	3	3	3	3	3	4
25	3	3	2	2	2	2	2	3
20	2	2	1	2	1	1	1	2
15	2	1	0	1	1	0	1	0
10	1	0	0	0	0	0	0	0

*AAHPER Youth Fitness Test Manual, 2nd rev. ed. (Washington, D.C.: American Alliance for Health, Physical Education, and Recreation, 1975).

B. *Sit-up for Girls (Flexed leg) Percentile Scores Based on Age / Test Scores in Number of Sit-ups Performed in 60 Seconds*

					Age				
Percentile	10	11	12	13	14	15	16	17	18
99	50	51	50	53	52	54	52	50	51
95	39	42	44	46	47	47	45	45	46
90	35	37	40	42	43	43	42	42	42
85	33	35	38	40	41	41	40	40	41
80	31	33	36	38	39	39	39	39	39
75	29	31	35	37	38	38	37	38	38
70	28	29	33	35	36	36	36	36	36
65	26	28	32	34	35	35	35	35	35
60	25	26	31	33	34	34	34	34	34
55	24	24	30	32	33	32	32	33	33
50	22	23	29	31	32	31	31	32	32
45	21	21	28	30	30	30	30	30	31
40	19	20	26	29	29	29	29	29	30
35	18	19	25	27	28	28	28	28	29
30	17	18	23	26	26	26	26	27	27
25	15	16	21	24	25	25	25	25	25
20	14	15	20	23	23	23	24	24	23
15	12	13	18	21	21	21	21	21	21
10	10	11	15	19	18	19	18	19	19
5	7	7	10	14	13	13	13	13	15

C. *Shuttle Run for Girls. Percentile Scores Based on Age / Test Scores in Seconds and Tenths*

				Age				
Percentile	10	11	12	13	14	15	16	17
100	8.5	8.8	9.0	8.3	9.0	8.0	8.3	9.0
95	10.0	10.0	10.0	10.0	10.0	10.0	10.0	10.0
90	10.5	10.2	10.2	10.2	10.3	10.3	10.2	10.3
85	10.8	10.6	10.5	10.5	10.4	10.5	10.4	10.4
80	11.0	10.9	10.8	10.6	10.5	10.7	10.6	10.5
75	11.0	11.0	10.9	10.8	10.6	10.9	10.8	10.6
70	11.1	11.0	11.0	11.0	10.8	11.0	10.9	10.8
65	11.4	11.2	11.2	11.0	10.9	11.0	11.0	11.0
60	11.5	11.4	11.3	11.1	11.0	11.1	11.0	11.0
55	11.8	11.6	11.5	11.3	11.1	11.2	11.2	11.1
50	11.9	11.7	11.6	11.4	11.3	11.3	11.2	11.2
45	12.0	11.8	11.8	11.6	11.4	11.5	11.4	11.4
40	12.0	12.0	11.9	11.8	11.5	11.6	11.5	11.5
35	12.1	12.0	12.0	12.0	11.7	11.8	11.8	11.6
30	12.4	12.1	12.1	12.0	12.0	11.9	12.0	11.8
25	12.6	12.4	12.3	12.2	12.0	12.0	12.0	12.0
20	12.8	12.6	12.5	12.5	12.3	12.3	12.2	12.0
15	13.0	13.0	12.9	13.0	12.6	12.5	12.5	12.3
10	13.1	13.4	13.2	13.3	13.1	13.0	13.0	13.0
5	14.0	14.1	13.9	14.0	13.9	13.5	13.9	13.8
0	16.6	18.5	19.8	18.5	17.6	16.0	17.6	20.0

D. *Standing Broad Jump for Girls. Percentile Scores Based on Age* / *Test Scores in Feet and Inches*

	Age							
Percentile	10	11	12	13	14	15	16	17
100	7' 0"	7'10"	8' 2"	7' 6"	7' 4"	7' 8"	7' 5"	7' 8"
95	5' 8"	6' 2"	6' 3"	6' 3"	6' 4"	6' 6"	6' 7"	6' 8"
90	5' 6"	5'10"	6' 0"	6' 0"	6' 2"	6' 3"	6' 4"	6' 4"
85	5' 4"	5' 8"	5' 9"	5'10"	6' 0"	6' 1"	6' 2"	6' 2"
80	5' 2"	5' 6"	5' 8"	5' 8"	5'10"	6' 0"	6' 0"	6' 0"
75	5' 1"	5' 4"	5' 6"	5' 6"	5' 9"	5'10"	5'10"	5'11"
70	5' 0"	5' 3"	5' 5"	5' 5"	5' 7"	5' 9"	5' 8"	5'10"
65	5' 0"	5' 2"	5' 4"	5' 4"	5' 6"	5' 7"	5' 7"	5' 9"
60	4'10"	5' 0"	5' 2"	5' 3"	5' 5"	5' 6"	5' 6"	5' 7"
55	4' 9"	5' 0"	5' 1"	5' 2"	5' 4"	5' 5"	5' 5"	5' 6"
50	4' 7"	4'10"	5' 0"	5' 0"	5' 3"	5' 4"	5' 4"	5' 5"
45	4' 6"	4' 9"	4'11"	5' 0"	5' 1"	5' 3"	5' 3"	5' 3"
40	4' 5"	4' 8"	4' 9"	4'10"	5' 0"	5' 1"	5' 2"	5' 2"
35	4' 4"	4' 7"	4' 8"	4' 8"	5' 0"	5' 0"	5' 0"	5' 0"
30	4' 3"	4' 6"	4' 7"	4' 6"	4' 9"	4'10"	4'11"	5' 0"
25	4' 2"	4' 4"	4' 5"	4' 6"	4' 8"	4' 8"	4'10"	4'10"
20	4' 0"	4' 3"	4' 4"	4' 4"	4' 6"	4' 7"	4' 8"	4' 9"
15	3'11"	4' 1"	4' 2"	4' 2"	4' 3"	4' 6"	4' 6"	4' 7"
10	3' 9"	3'11"	4' 0"	4' 0"	4' 1"	4' 4"	4' 4"	4' 5"
5	3' 6"	3' 9"	3' 8"	3' 9"	3'10"	4' 0"	4' 0"	4' 2"
0	2' 8"	2'11"	2'11"	2'11"	3' 0"	2'11"	3' 2"	3' 0"

E. *50-yard Dash for Girls. Percentile Scores Based on Age* / *Test Scores in Seconds and Tenths*

	Age							
Percentile	10	11	12	13	14	15	16	17
100	6.0	6.0	5.9	6.0	6.0	6.4	6.0	6.4
95	7.0	7.0	7.0	7.0	7.0	7.1	7.0	7.1
90	7.3	7.4	7.3	7.3	7.2	7.3	7.3	7.3
85	7.5	7.6	7.5	7.5	7.4	7.5	7.5	7.5
80	7.7	7.7	7.6	7.6	7.5	7.6	7.5	7.6
75	7.9	7.9	7.8	7.7	7.6	7.7	7.7	7.8
70	8.0	8.0	7.9	7.8	7.7	7.8	7.9	7.9
65	8.1	8.0	8.0	7.9	7.8	7.9	8.0	8.0
60	8.2	8.1	8.0	8.0	7.9	8.0	8.0	8.0
55	8.4	8.2	8.1	8.0	8.0	8.0	8.1	8.1
50	8.5	8.4	8.2	8.1	8.0	8.1	8.3	8.2
45	8.6	8.5	8.3	8.2	8.2	8.2	8.4	8.3
40	8.8	8.5	8.4	8.4	8.3	8.3	8.5	8.5
35	8.9	8.6	8.5	8.5	8.5	8.4	8.6	8.6
30	9.0	8.8	8.7	8.6	8.6	8.6	8.8	8.8
25	9.0	9.0	8.9	8.8	8.9	8.8	9.0	9.0
20	9.2	9.0	9.0	9.0	9.0	9.0	9.0	9.0
15	9.4	9.2	9.2	9.2	9.2	9.0	9.2	9.1
10	9.6	9.6	9.5	9.5	9.5	9.5	9.9	9.5
5	10.0	10.0	10.0	10.2	10.4	10.0	10.5	10.4
0	14.0	13.0	13.0	15.7	16.0	18.0	17.0	12.0

F. 600-Yard Run-Walk for Girls. Percentile Scores Based on Age / Test Scores in Minutes and Seconds

Percentile	Age							
	10	11	12	13	14	15	16	17
100	1'42"	1'40"	1'39"	1'40"	1'45"	1'40"	1'50"	1'54"
95	2' 5"	2'13"	2'14"	2'12"	2' 9"	2' 9"	2'10"	2'11"
90	2'15"	2'19"	2'20"	2'19"	2'18"	2'18"	2'17"	2'22"
85	2'20"	2'24"	2'24"	2'25"	2'22"	2'23"	2'23"	2'27"
80	2'26"	2'28"	2'27"	2'29"	2'25"	2'26"	2'26"	2'31"
75	2'30"	2'32"	2'31"	2'33"	2'30"	2'28"	2'31"	2'34"
70	2'34"	2'36"	2'35"	2'37"	2'34"	2'34"	2'36"	2'37"
65	2'37"	2'39"	2'39"	2'40"	2'37"	2'36"	2'39"	2'42"
60	2'41"	2'43"	2'42"	2'44"	2'41"	2'40"	2'42"	2'46"
55	2'45"	2'47"	2'45"	2'47"	2'44"	2'43"	2'45"	2'49"
50	2'48"	2'49"	2'49"	2'52"	2'46"	2'46"	2'49"	2'51"
45	2'50"	2'53"	2'55"	2'56"	2'51"	2'49"	2'53"	2'57"
40	2'55"	2'59"	2'58"	3' 0"	2'55"	2'52"	2'56"	3' 0"
35	2'59"	3' 4"	3' 3"	3' 3"	3' 0"	2'56"	2'59"	3' 5"
30	3' 3"	3'10"	3' 7"	3' 9"	3' 6"	3' 0"	3' 1"	3'10"
25	3' 8"	3'15"	3'11"	3'15"	3'12"	3' 5"	3' 7"	3'16"
20	3'13"	3'22"	3'18"	3'20"	3'19"	3'10"	3'12"	3'22"
15	3'18"	3'30"	3'24"	3'30"	3'30"	3'18"	3'19"	3'29"
10	3'27"	3'41"	3'40"	3'49"	3'48"	3'28"	3'30"	3'41"
5	3'45"	3'59"	4' 0"	4'11"	4' 8"	3'56"	3'45"	3'56"
0	4'47"	4'53"	5'10"	5'10"	5'50"	5'10"	5'52"	6'40"

G. 9-minute/1-mile Run for Girls. Percentile Scores Based on Age / Test Scores in Yards/Time

	9-Minute Run Girls			1-Mile Run Girls		
Percentile	Age/Yards			Age/Time		
	10	11	12	10	11	12
100	2157	2180	2203	6:13	5:42	5:08
95	1969	1992	2015	7:28	6:57	6:23
90	1867	1890	1913	8:09	7:38	7:04
85	1801	1824	1847	8:33	8:02	7:28
80	1746	1769	1792	8:57	8:26	7:52
75	1702	1725	1748	9:16	8:45	8:11
70	1658	1681	1704	9:31	9:00	8:26
65	1622	1645	1668	9:51	9:20	8:46
60	1583	1606	1629	10:02	9:31	8:57
55	1550	1573	1596	10:15	9:44	9:10
50	1514	1537	1560	10:29	9:58	9:24
45	1478	1501	1524	10:43	10:12	9:38
40	1445	1468	1491	10:56	10:25	9:51
35	1406	1429	1452	11:07	10:36	10:12
30	1370	1393	1416	11:27	10:56	10:22
25	1326	1349	1372	11:42	11:11	10:37
20	1282	1305	1328	12:01	11:30	10:56
15	1227	1250	1273	12:25	11:54	11:30
10	1161	1184	1207	12:49	12:18	11:44
5	1059	1082	1105	13:30	12:59	12:24
0	871	894	917	14:45	14:14	13:40

H. *12-Minute/1%-Mile Run for Girls, Age 13 and Older. Percentile Scores Based on Age / Test Scores in Yards/Time*

	12-Minute Run	1.5 Mile Run
Percentile	Yards	Time
100	2693	10:20
95	2448	12:17
90	2318	13:19
85	2232	14:00
80	2161	14:34
75	2100	15:03
70	2050	15:26
65	2000	15:50
60	1950	16:14
55	1908	16:34
50	1861	16:57
45	1815	i7:19
40	1772	17:39
35	1722	18:03
30	1672	18:27
25	1622	18:50
20	1561	19:19
15	1490	19:53
10	1404	20:34
5	1274	21:36
0	1030	23:33

I. *Pull-up for Boys. Percentile Scores Based on Age / Test Scores in Number of Pull-ups*

Percentile	Age							
	10	11	12	13	14	15	16	17
100	16	20	15	24	20	25	25	32
95	8	8	9	10	12	13	14	16
90	7	7	7	9	10	11	13	14
85	6	6	6	8	10	10	12	12
80	5	5	5	7	8	10	11	12
75	4	4	5	6	8	9	10	10
70	4	4	4	5	7	8	10	10
65	3	3	3	5	6	7	9	10
60	3	3	3	4	6	7	9	9
55	3	2	3	4	5	6	8	8
50	2	2	2	3	5	6	7	8
45	2	2	2	3	4	5	6	7
40	1	1	1	2	4	5	6	7
35	1	1	1	2	3	4	5	6
30	1	1	1	1	3	4	5	5
25	0	0	0	1	2	3	4	5
20	0	0	0	0	2	3	4	4
15	0	0	0	0	1	2	3	4
10	0	0	0	0	0	1	2	2
5	0	0	0	0	0	0	0	1

J. *Sit-up for Boys (Flexed Leg). Percentile Scores Based on Age / Test Scores in Number of Sit-ups Performed in 60 Seconds*

	Age							
Percentile	10	11	12	13	14	15	16	17
99								
95	44	49	55	58				
90	39	44	50	54				
85	36	41	49	51	55	59	61	63
80	33	38	46	49	53	56	59	60
75	32	36	45	48	51	54	57	58
70	30	35	43	47	50	52	55	55
65	28	33	41	45	49	51	53	54
60	27	31	40	44	48	50	51	52
55	25	29	39	43	46	49	50	51
50	24	28	37	42	45	47	49	49
45	23	26	36	41	44	46	48	48
40	22	24	34	40	43	45	46	47
35	20	23	32	38	41	44	45	45
30	19	22	31	37	40	42	44	44
25	18	20	29	35	39	41	42	42
20	16	19	27	33	37	39	40	40
15	14	16	24	31	34	38	39	39
10	11	14	21	29	31	35	35	36
5	5	4	14	23	27	31	32	32

K. *Shuttle Run for Boys. Percentile Scores Based on Age / Test Scores in Seconds and Tenths*

	Age							
Percentile	10	11	12	13	14	15	16	17
100	9.0	9.0	8.5	8.0	8.3	8.0	8.1	8.0
95	10.0	10.0	9.8	9.5	9.3	9.1	9.0	8.9
90	10.2	10.1	10.0	9.8	9.5	9.3	9.1	9.0
85	10.4	10.3	10.0	9.9	9.6	9.4	9.2	9.1
80	10.5	10.4	10.2	10.0	9.8	9.5	9.3	9.2
75	10.7	10.5	10.3	10.1	9.9	9.6	9.5	9.3
70	10.8	10.7	10.5	10.2	9.9	9.7	9.5	9.4
65	10.9	10.8	10.6	10.3	10.0	9.8	9.6	9.5
60	11.0	10.9	10.7	10.4	10.0	9.8	9.7	9.6
55	11.0	11.0	10.9	10.5	10.2	9.9	9.8	9.7
50	11.2	11.1	11.0	10.6	10.2	10.0	9.9	9.8
45	11.4	11.2	11.0	10.8	10.3	10.0	10.0	9.9
40	11.5	11.3	11.1	10.9	10.5	10.1	10.0	10.0
35	11.6	11.4	11.3	11.0	10.5	10.2	10.1	10.0
30	11.8	11.6	11.5	11.1	10.7	10.3	10.2	10.1
25	12.0	11.8	11.6	11.3	10.9	10.5	10.4	10.4
20	12.0	12.0	11.9	11.5	11.0	10.6	10.5	10.6
15	12.2	12.1	12.0	11.8	11.2	10.9	10.8	10.9
10	12.6	12.4	12.4	12.0	11.5	11.1	11.1	11.2
5	13.1	13.0	13.0	12.5	12.0	11.7	11.5	11.7
0	15.0	20.0	22.0	16.0	16.0	16.6	16.7	14.0

L. *Standing Broad Jump for Boys. Percentile Scores Based on Age / Test Scores in Feet and Inches and Inches*

				Age				
Percentile	10	11	12	13	14	15	16	17
100	6' 8"	10' 0"	7'10"	8' 9"	8'11"	9' 2"	9' 1"	9' 8"
95	6' 1"	6' 3"	6' 6"	7' 2"	7' 9"	8' 0"	8' 5"	8' 6"
90	5'10"	6' 0"	6' 4"	6'11"	7' 5"	7' 9"	8' 1"	8' 3"
85	5' 8"	5'10"	6' 2"	6' 9"	7' 3"	7' 6"	7'11"	8' 1"
80	5' 7"	5' 9"	6' 1"	6' 7"	7' 0"	7' 6"	7' 9"	8' 0"
75	5' 6"	5' 7"	6' 0"	6' 5"	6'11"	7' 4"	7' 7"	7'10"
70	5' 5"	5' 6"	5'11"	6' 3"	6' 9"	7' 2"	7' 6"	7' 8"
65	5' 4"	5' 6"	5' 9"	6' 1"	6' 8"	7' 1"	7' 5"	7' 7"
60	5' 2"	5' 4"	5' 8"	6' 0"	6' 7"	7' 0"	7' 4"	7' 6"
55	5' 1"	5' 3"	5' 7"	5'11"	6' 6"	6'11"	7' 3"	7' 5"
50	5' 0"	5' 2"	5' 6"	5'10"	6' 4"	6' 9"	7' 1"	7' 3"
45	5' 0"	5' 1"	5' 5"	5' 9"	6' 3"	6' 8"	7' 0"	7' 2"
40	4'10"	5' 0"	5' 4"	5' 7"	6' 1"	6' 6"	6'11"	7' 0"
35	4'10"	4'11"	5' 2"	5' 6"	6' 0"	6' 6"	6' 9"	6'11"
30	4' 8"	4'10"	5' 1"	5' 5"	5'10"	6' 4"	6' 7"	6'10"
25	4' 6"	4' 8"	5' 0"	5' 3"	5' 8"	6' 3"	6' 6"	6' 8"
20	4' 5"	4' 7"	4'10"	5' 2"	5' 6"	6' 1"	6' 4"	6' 6"
15	4' 4"	4' 5"	4' 8"	5' 0"	5' 4"	5'10"	6' 1"	6' 4"
10	4' 3"	4' 2"	4' 5"	4' 9"	5' 2"	5' 7"	5'11"	6' 0"
5	4' 0"	4' 0"	4' 2"	4' 5"	4'11"	5' 4"	5' 6"	5' 8"
0	2'10"	1' 8"	3' 0"	2' 9"	3' 8"	2'10"	2' 2"	3' 7"

M. *50-Yard Dash for Boys. Percentile Scores Based on Age / Test Scores in Seconds and Tenths*

				Age				
Percentile	10	11	12	13	14	15	16	17
100	6.0	6.0	6.0	5.8	5.8	5.6	5.6	5.6
95	7.0	7.0	6.8	6.5	6.3	6.1	6.0	6.0
90	7.1	7.2	7.0	6.7	6.4	6.2	6.1	6.0
85	7.4	7.4	7.0	6.9	6.6	6.4	6.2	6.1
80	7.5	7.5	7.2	7.0	6.7	6.5	6.3	6.2
75	7.6	7.6	7.3	7.0	6.8	6.5	6.3	6.3
70	7.8	7.7	7.5	7.1	6.9	6.6	6.4	6.3
65	8.0	7.8	7.5	7.2	7.0	6.7	6.5	6.4
60	8.0	7.8	7.6	7.3	7.0	6.7	6.5	6.5
55	8.1	8.0	7.8	7.4	7.0	6.8	6.6	6.5
50	8.2	8.0	7.8	7.5	7.1	6.9	6.7	6.6
45	8.3	8.0	7.9	7.5	7.2	7.0	6.7	6.7
40	8.5	8.1	8.0	7.6	7.2	7.0	6.8	6.7
35	8.5	8.3	8.0	7.7	7.3	7.1	6.9	6.8
30	8.7	8.4	8.2	7.9	7.5	7.1	6.9	6.9
25	8.8	8.5	8.3	8.0	7.6	7.2	7.0	7.0
20	9.0	8.7	8.4	8.0	7.8	7.3	7.1	7.0
15	9.1	9.0	8.6	8.2	8.0	7.5	7.2	7.1
10	9.5	9.1	8.9	8.4	8.1	7.7	7.5	7.3
5	10.0	9.5	9.2	8.9	8.6	8.1	7.8	7.7
0	12.0	11.9	12.0	11.1	11.6	12.0	8.6	10.6

N. 9-Minute/1-Mile Run for Boys. Percentile Scores Based on Age / Test Scores in Yards/Time

	9-Minute Run Boys			1-Mile Run Boys		
	Age			Age		
Percentile	10	11	12	10	11	12
	Yards			Time		
100	2532	2535	2578	5:07	4:44	4:21
95	2294	2356	2418	5:55	5:32	5:09
90	2166	2228	2290	6:38	6:15	5:52
85	2081	2143	2205	7:06	6:43	6:20
80	2011	2073	2135	7:29	7:03	6:40
75	1952	2014	2076	7:49	7:26	7:03
70	1902	1964	2026	8:05	7:42	7:19
65	1853	1915	1977	8:22	7:59	7:36
60	1804	1866	1928	8:38	8:15	7:52
55	1762	1824	1886	8:52	8:29	8:06
50	1717	1779	1841	9:07	8:44	8:21
45	1672	1734	1796	9:22	8:59	8:36
40	1630	1692	1754	9:32	9:13	8:50
35	1581	1643	1705	9:52	9:29	9:06
30	1532	1594	1656	10:09	9:46	9:23
25	1482	1544	1606	10:25	10:02	9:39
20	1423	1485	1547	10:35	10:22	9:59
15	1353	1415	1477	11:08	10:45	10:22
10	1268	1330	1392	11:36	11:13	10:50
5	1140	1202	1264	12:19	11:56	11:33
0	901	924	927	14:07	13:44	13:21

O. 12-Minute/1¾-Mile Run for Boys. Age 13 and Older. Percentile Scores Based on Age / Test Scores in Yards/Time

	12-Minute Run	1.5 Mile Run
Percentile	Yards	Time
100	3590	7:26
95	3297	8:37
90	3140	9:15
85	3037	9:40
80	2952	10:01
75	2879	10:19
70	2819	10:34
65	2759	10:48
60	2699	11:02
55	2648	11:15
50	2592	11:29
45	2536	11:42
40	2485	11:55
35	2425	12:10
30	2365	12:24
25	2305	12:39
20	2232	12:56
15	2147	13:17
10	2044	13:42
5	1888	14:20
0	1594	15:32

TABLE B.11 *Six-Sigma Scoring Chart for NSWA Physical Performance Test**

Scale Score	Standing Broad Jump	Basket-ball Throw	Potato Race	Pull-ups	Push-ups	Sit-ups	10-Second Squat Thrust	30-Second Squat Thrust	Scale Score
100	7–9	78	8.4	47	61	65	9–1	24	100
95	7–7	75	8.6	45	58	61	9	23	95
90	7–4	72	8.8	42	54	57	8–3	22	90
85	7–2	68	9.0	39	51	54	8–1	21	85
80	6–11	65	9.4	37	47	50	8	20	80
75	6–9	62	9.6	34	43	46	7–3	19	75
70	6–7	59	10.0	32	39	43	7–1	18–2	70
65	6–4	56	10.2	29	36	39	7	18	65
60	6–2	53	10.4	26	32	36	6–2	17	60
55	6–0	50	10.6	24	28	33	6–1	16	55
50	5–9	46	11.0	21	25	29	6	15	50
45	5–7	43	11.2	18	21	25	5–2	14–2	45
40	5–5	40	11.6	16	17	22	5–1	14	40
35	5–2	37	11.8	13	13	18	4–3	13	35
30	5–0	34	12.0	10	10	15	4–2	12	30
25	4–9	31	12.4	8	6	11	4	11	25
20	4–7	27	12.6	5	2	7	3–3	10	20
15	4–4	24	13.0	3	1	3	3–2	9	15
10	4–2	21	13.2	1	0	1	3	8–2	10
5	4–0	18	13.4	0	0	0	2–3	7–2	5
0	3–9	15	13.6	0	0	0	2–2	7	0

*Eleanor Metheny, Chairman, "Physical Performance Levels for High School Girls," *Journal of Health and Physical Education,* **16,** No. 6 (June 1945).

TABLE B.12 *New York State Physical Fitness Screening Test Norms.**
A. *Boys—Beginning Grade 4*

Achieve-ment Level	Per-centile Rank	Agility	Strength	Speed	Endur-ance	Total Physical Fitness	Achieve-ment Level
10	99	20+	46+	9.5–	25+	32+	10
9	98	18–19	36–45	10.0	21–24	30–31	9
8	93	16–17	32–35	10.5	18–20	27–29	8
7	84	15	28–31	11.0	16–17	25–26	7
6	69	14	23–27	11.5	15	22–24	6
5	50	12–13	20–22	12.0	13–14	19–21	5
4	31	11	16–19	12.5	12	16–18	4
3	16	10	12–15	13.0–13.5	10–11	14–15	3
2	7	8–9	6–11	14.0	8–9	11–13	2
1	2	6–7	2–5	14.5–15.0	4–7	8–10	1
0	1	0–5	0–1	15.5+	0–3	0–7	0

New York State Physical Fitness Screening Test, rev. ed. (Albany, N.Y.: Division of Health, Physical Education, and Recreation, State Education Department, 1968).

B. *Girls—Beginning Grade 4*

Achievement Level	Percentile Rank	Agility	Strength	Speed	Endurance	Total Physical Fitness	Achievement Level
10	99	18+	35+	9.5–	25+	32+	10
9	98	17	30–34	10.0	20–24	30–31	9
8	93	16	26–29	10.5	18–19	27–29	8
7	84	14–15	23–25	11.0	16–17	25–26	7
6	69	13	20–22	11.5	15	22–24	6
5	50	12	17–19	12.0	13–14	19–21	5
4	31	11	13–16	12.5–13.0	12	16–18	4
3	16	9–10	10–12	13.5	10–11	14–15	3
2	7	7–8	7–9	14.0–14.5	8–9	11–13	2
1	2	5–6	3–6	15.0	6–7	8–10	1
0	1	0–4	0–2	15.5+	0–5	0–7	0

C. *Boys—Beginning Grade 5*

Achievement Level	Percentile Rank	Agility	Strength	Speed	Endurance	Total Physical Fitness	Achievement Level
10	99	21+	46+	9.0–	25+	32+	10
9	98	19–20	38–45	9.5	21–24	30–31	9
8	93	17–18	34–37	10.0	19–20	27–29	8
7	84	16	30–33	10.5	17–18	25–26	7
6	69	15	25–29	11.0	15–16	22–24	6
5	50	13–14	22–24	11.5	14	19–21	5
4	31	12	17–21	12.0	12–13	16–18	4
3	16	11	13–16	12.5–13.0	10–11	14–15	3
2	7	9–10	8–12	13.5	8–9	11–13	2
1	2	7–8	3–7	14.0–14.5	6–7	8–10	1
0	1	0–6	0–2	15.0+	0–5	0–7	0

D. *Girls—Beginning Grade 5*

Achievement Level	Percentile Rank	Agility	Strength	Speed	Endurance	Total Physical Fitness	Achievement Level
10	99	21+	37+	9.5–	24+	32+	10
9	98	19–20	32–36	10.0	20–23	30–31	9
8	93	17–18	28–31	10.5	18–19	27–29	8
7	84	15–16	25–27	11.0	16–17	25–26	7
6	69	14	22–24	11.5	15	22–24	6
5	50	13	19–21	12.0	13–14	19–21	5
4	31	12	15–18	12.5–13.0	12	16–18	4
3	16	10–11	11–14	13.5	10–11	14–15	3
2	7	8–9	8–10	14.0–14.5	8–9	11–13	2
1	2	5–7	3–7	15.0	6–7	8–10	1
0	1	0–4	0–2	15.5+	0–5	0–7	0

E. *Boys—Beginning Grade 6*

Achieve-ment Level	Per-centile Rank	Agility	Strength	Speed	Endur-ance	Total Physical Fitness	Achieve-ment Level
10	99	23+	46+	8.5−	25+	32+	10
9	98	20–22	39–45	9.0	21–24	30–31	9
8	93	18–19	35–38	9.5	19–20	27–29	8
7	84	17	32–34	10.0	17–18	25–26	7
6	69	16	28–31	10.5	16	22–24	6
5	50	14–15	25–27	11.0	14–15	19–21	5
4	31	13	20–24	11.5	13	16–18	4
3	16	12	15–19	12.0–12.5	11–12	14–15	3
2	7	10–11	11–14	13.0	8–10	11–13	2
1	2	8–9	8–10	13.5–14.0	6–7	8–10	1
0	1	0–7	0–7	14.5+	0–5	0–7	0

F. *Girls—Beginning Grade 6*

Achieve-ment Level	Per-centile Rank	Agility	Strength	Speed	Endur-ance	Total Physical Fitness	Achieve-ment Level
10	99	21+	38+	9.0−	23+	32+	10
9	98	19–20	33–37	9.5	20–22	30–31	9
8	93	18	29–32	10.0	18–19	27–29	8
7	84	16–17	26–28	10.5	16–17	25–26	7
6	69	15	22–25	11.0	15	22–24	6
5	50	14	19–21	11.5	13–14	19–21	5
4	31	12–13	16–18	12.0–12.5	12	16–18	4
3	16	11	12–15	13.0	10–11	14–15	3
2	7	9–10	8–11	13.5–14.0	8–9	11–13	2
1	2	7–8	4–7	14.5	6–7	8–10	1
0	1	0–6	0–3	15.0+	0–5	0–7	0

G. *Boys—Beginning Grade 7*

Achieve-ment Level	Per-centile Rank	Agility	Strength	Speed	Endur-ance	Total Physical Fitness	Achieve-ment Level
10	99	24+	70+	19.5−	40+	32+	10
9	98	21–23	65–69	20.0–20.5	37–39	30–31	9
8	93	19–20	58–64	21.0	33–36	27–29	8
7	84	17–18	51–57	21.5–22.0	30–32	25–26	7
6	69	16	45–50	22.5	27–29	22–24	6
5	50	15	38–44	23.0–23.5	25–26	19–21	5
4	31	14	31–37	24.0	22–24	16–18	4
3	16	12–13	24–30	24.5–25.5	19–21	14–15	3
2	7	10–11	16–23	26.0–27.0	15–18	11–13	2
1	2	8–9	5–15	27.5–30.0	12–14	8–10	1
0	1	0–7	0–4	30.5+	0–11	0–7	0

H. *Girls—Beginning Grade 7*

Achieve-ment Level	Per-centile Rank	Agility	Strength	Speed	Endur-ance	Total Physical Fitness	Achieve-ment Level
10	99	21+	37+	13.0−	22+	32+	10
9	98	19–20	32–36	13.5	19–21	30–31	9
8	93	18	29–31	14.0	17–18	27–29	8
7	84	16–17	25–28	14.5	16	25–26	7
6	69	15	22–24	15.0	14–15	22–24	6
5	50	14	19–21	15.5	13	19–21	5
4	31	13	16–18	16.0–16.5	11–12	16–18	4
3	16	11–12	12–15	17.0–17.5	10	14–15	3
2	7	9–10	8–11	18.0–18.5	8–9	11–13	2
1	2	7–8	5–7	19.0–19.5	6–7	8–10	1
0	1	0–6	0–4	20.0+	0–5	0–7	0

I. *Boys—Beginning Grade 8*

Achieve-ment Level	Per-centile Rank	Agility	Strength	Speed	Endur-ance	Total Physical Fitness	Achieve-ment Level
10	99	24+	78+	19.5−	41+	32+	10
9	98	21–23	71–77	20.0	38–40	30–31	9
8	93	20	63–70	20.5	34–37	27–29	8
7	84	18–19	56–62	21.0–21.5	31–33	25–26	7
6	69	17	49–55	22.0	28–30	22–24	6
5	50	16	43–48	22.5–23.0	26–27	19–21	5
4	31	15	36–42	23.5	23–25	16–18	4
3	16	13–14	29–35	24.0–25.0	20–22	14–15	3
2	7	11–12	22–28	25.5–27.0	16–19	11–13	2
1	2	9–10	14–21	27.5–30.0	13–15	8–10	1
0	1	0–8	0–13	30.5+	0–12	0–7	0

J. *Girls—Beginning Grade 8*

Achieve-ment Level	Per-centile Rank	Agility	Strength	Speed	Endur-ance	Total Physical Fitness	Achieve-ment Level
10	99	21+	34+	13.0−	22+	32+	10
9	98	20	31–33	13.5	19–21	30–31	9
8	93	18–19	28–30	14.0	17–18	27–29	8
7	84	17	25–27	14.5	16	25–26	7
6	69	16	22–24	15.0	14–15	22–24	6
5	50	15	19–21	15.5	13	19–21	5
4	31	14	15–18	16.0–16.5	11–12	16–18	4
3	16	12–13	12–14	17.0–17.5	10	14–15	3
2	7	10–11	8–11	18.0–18.5	8–9	11–13	2
1	2	8–9	5–7	19.0–19.5	6–7	8–10	1
0	1	0–7	0–4	20.0+	0–5	0–7	0

K. *Boys—Beginning Grade 9*

Achieve-ment Level	Per-centile Rank	Agility	Strength	Speed	Endur-ance	Total Physical Fitness	Achieve-ment Level
10	99	25+	79+	19.0−	41+	32+	10
9	98	22–24	72–78	19.5	38–40	30–31	9
8	93	21	65–71	20.0	35–37	27–29	8
7	84	19–20	59–64	20.5–21.0	32–34	25–26	7
6	69	18	52–58	21.5	29–31	22–24	6
5	50	16–17	46–51	22.0–22.5	27–28	19–21	5
4	31	15	39–45	23.0	24–26	16–18	4
3	16	13–14	32–38	23.5–24.5	21–23	14–15	3
2	7	11–12	26–31	25.0–27.0	17–20	11–13	2
1	2	9–10	18–25	27.5–30.0	13–16	8–10	1
0	1	0–8	0–17	30.5+	0–12	0–7	0

L. *Girls—Beginning Grade 9*

Achieve-ment Level	Per-centile Rank	Agility	Strength	Speed	Endur-ance	Total Physical Fitness	Achieve-ment Level
10	99	22+	34+	13.0−	21+	32+	10
9	98	20–21	31–33	13.5	18–20	30–31	9
8	93	19	27–30	14.0	16–17	27–29	8
7	84	17–18	25–26	14.5	15	25–26	7
6	69	16	22–24	15.0	14	22–24	6
5	50	15	19–21	15.5	12–13	19–21	5
4	31	14	15–18	16.0–16.5	11	16–18	4
3	16	12–13	12–14	17.0–17.5	10	14–15	3
2	7	10–11	8–11	18.0–18.5	8–9	11–13	2
1	2	8–9	5–7	19.0–19.5	6–7	8–10	1
0	1	0–7	0–4	20.0+	0–5	0–7	0

M. *Boys—Beginning Grade 10*

Achieve-ment Level	Per-centile Rank	Agility	Strength	Speed	Endur-ance	Total Physical Fitness	Achieve-ment Level
10	99	26+	80+	25.0−	41+	32+	10
9	98	24–25	73–79	25.5–26.5	38–40	30–31	9
8	93	22–23	67–72	27.0–27.5	35–37	27–29	8
7	84	20–21	60–66	28.0	32–34	25–26	7
6	69	19	54–59	28.5	30–31	22–24	6
5	50	17–18	48–53	29.0–29.5	27–29	19–21	5
4	31	16	41–47	30.0–31.0	24–26	16–18	4
3	16	14–15	34–40	31.5–32.5	21–23	14–15	3
2	7	12–13	28–33	33.0–34.0	18–20	11–13	2
1	2	10–11	19–27	34.5–36.5	13–17	8–10	1
0	1	0–9	0–18	37.0+	0–12	0–7	0

N. *Girls—Beginning Grade 10*

Achievement Level	Percentile Rank	Agility	Strength	Speed	Endurance	Total Physical Fitness	Achievement Level
10	99	23+	34+	13.0−	21+	32+	10
9	98	21–22	31–33	13.5	18–20	30–31	9
8	93	19–20	27–30	14.0	16–17	27–29	8
7	84	18	24–26	14.5	15	25–26	7
6	69	16–17	21–23	15.0	13–14	22–24	6
5	50	15	18–20	15.5	12	19–21	5
4	31	14	15–17	16.0–16.5	11	16–18	4
3	16	13	11–14	17.0–17.5	10	14–15	3
2	7	11–12	8–10	18.0–18.5	8–9	11–13	2
1	2	9–10	4–7	19.0–19.5	6–7	8–10	1
0	1	0–8	0–3	20.0+	0–5	0–7	0

O. *Boys—Beginning Grade 11*

Achievement Level	Percentile Rank	Agility	Strength	Speed	Endurance	Total Physical Fitness	Achievement Level
10	99	27+	81+	25.0−	44+	32+	10
9	98	25–26	75–80	25.5–26.0	39–43	30–31	9
8	93	22–24	68–74	26.5–27.0	35–38	27–29	8
7	84	21	61–67	27.5	32–34	25–26	7
6	69	20	55–60	28.0–28.5	30–31	22–24	6
5	50	18–19	49–54	29.0	27–29	19–21	5
4	31	17	42–48	29.5–30.5	24–26	16–18	4
3	16	15–16	35–41	31.0–32.0	21–23	14–15	3
2	7	13–14	28–34	32.5–33.5	18–20	11–13	2
1	2	10–12	20–27	34.0–36.0	14–17	8–10	1
0	1	0–9	0–19	36.5+	0–13	0–7	0

P. *Girls—Beginning Grade 11*

Achievement Level	Percentile Rank	Agility	Strength	Speed	Endurance	Total Physical Fitness	Achievement Level
10	99	24+	34+	13.0−	21+	32+	10
9	98	21–23	30–33	13.5	17–20	30–31	9
8	93	19–20	27–29	14.0	16	27–29	8
7	84	18	24–26	14.5	15	25–26	7
6	69	16–17	21–23	15.0	13–14	22–24	6
5	50	15	18–20	15.5	12	19–21	5
4	31	14	15–17	16.0–16.5	11	16–18	4
3	16	13	11–14	17.0–17.5	10	14–15	3
2	7	11–12	8–10	18.0–18.5	8–9	11–13	2
1	2	9–10	4–7	19.0–19.5	6–7	8–10	1
0	1	0–8	0–3	20.0+	0–5	0–7	0

Q. *Boys—Beginning Grade 12*

Achieve-ment Level	Per-centile Rank	Agility	Strength	Speed	Endur-ance	Total Physical Fitness	Achieve-ment Level
10	99	27+	81+	25.0–	44+	32+	10
9	98	25–26	75–80	25.5–26.0	39–43	30–31	9
8	93	22–24	68–74	26.5	35–38	27–29	8
7	84	21	61–67	27.0–27.5	32–34	25–26	7
6	69	20	55–60	28.0	30–31	22–24	6
5	50	18–19	49–54	28.5–29.0	27–29	19–21	5
4	31	17	42–48	29.5–30.5	24–26	16–18	4
3	16	15–16	36–41	31.0–32.0	21–23	14–15	3
2	7	13–14	29–35	32.5–33.5	18–20	11–13	2
1	2	10–12	21–28	34.0–35.5	14–17	8–10	1
0	1	0–9	0–20	36.0+	0–13	0–7	0

R. *Girls—Beginning Grade 12*

Achieve-ment Level	Per-centile Rank	Agility	Strength	Speed	Endur-ance	Total Physical Fitness	Achieve-ment Level
10	99	24+	34+	13.0–	21+	32+	10
9	98	21–23	30–33	13.5	17–20	30–31	9
8	93	19–20	27–29	14.0	16	27–29	8
7	84	18	24–26	14.5	15	25–26	7
6	69	16–17	21–23	15.0	13–14	22–24	6
5	50	15	18–20	15.5	12	19–21	5
4	31	14	15–17	16.0–16.5	11	16–18	4
3	16	13	11–14	17.0–17.5	10	14–15	3
2	7	12	8–10	18.0–18.5	8–9	11–13	2
1	2	10–11	4–7	19.0–19.5	6–7	8–10	1
0	1	0–9	0–3	20.0+	0–5	0–7	0

TABLE B.13 *Percentile Norms: Glover's Physical Fitness Test for Primary Grades.**
A. *Age Six Years*

Percentile	Broad Jump (In.)	Shuttle Race (Sec.)	Seal Crawl Test (Sec.)	Sit-ups (No.)	Percentile
95	51	41.1	7.0	12	95
90	49	42.8	7.6		90
85	48	43.5	8.1		85
80	47	44.0	8.7	11	80
75	46	44.5	9.0	10	75
70	45	44.9	9.4	9	70
65		45.4	9.8		65
60	44	45.6	10.1	9	60
55	43	46.0	10.5	8	55
50	42	46.4	10.9		50
45	41	46.7	11.3	7	45
40	40	47.4	11.7	6	40
35		47.9	12.2	5	35
30	39	48.6	12.6	4	30
25	38	49.5	13.1	3	25
20	37	50.5	14.3		20
15	36	51.3	19.0	2	15
10	35	52.3	25.1		10
5	33	54.0	33.1	1	5

*Harold M. Barrow and Rosemary McGee, *A Practical Approach to Measurement in Physical Education*, 2nd ed. (Philadelphia: Lea & Febiger, 1971), p. 215.

B. *Age Seven Years*

Percentiles	Broad Jump (In.)	Shuttle Race (Sec.)	Seal Crawl Test (Sec.)	Sit-ups (No.)	Percentiles
95	53	41.3	7.6	15	95
90	51	42.0		14	90
85	50	42.5	8.0	13	85
80	49	43.1	8.8	12	80
75		43.5	9.0		75
70	48	43.8	9.5	11	70
65	46	44.4	10.0		65
60	45	44.8	10.3	10	60
55	44	45.5	10.9	9	55
50	43	46.1	11.1		50
45	42	46.5	11.3		45
40	41	47.0	11.8	8	40
35		47.6	12.6	7	35
30	40	48.4	13.3	6	30
25	39	48.8	15.0	5	25
20	38	49.5	16.7	4	20
15		50.3	19.5	2	15
10	37	50.8	24.2		10
5	34	52.6	39.5	1	5

C. *Age Eight Years*

Percentiles	Broad Jump (In.)	Shuttle Race (Sec.)	Seal Crawl Test (Sec.)	Sit-ups (No.)	Percentiles
95	63	39.9	5.9	17	95
90	59	41.1	6.9	15	90
85	58	41.5		14	85
80	57	41.6	7.1	13	80
75	55	42.0	7.4		75
70	54	42.5	7.8		70
65	53	42.8	8.0	12	65
60	51	43.2	8.4		60
55		43.5	8.8	11	55
50	50	43.8	9.2	10	50
45	49	44.2	9.5		45
40	48	44.5	9.9	9	40
35	47	45.0	10.5	8	35
30	46	45.4	10.9	7	30
25	45	45.9	11.5	6	25
20	43	46.5	12.0	5	20
15	42	47.5	13.3	4	15
10	40	48.8	14.9	2	10
5	38	50.0	18.5	1	5

D. *Age Nine Years*

Percentiles	Broad Jump (In.)	Shuttle Race (Sec.)	Seal Crawl Test (Sec.)	Sit-ups (No.)	Percentiles
95	62	38.5	4.9	18	95
90	59	39.2	5.3	16	90
85	58	39.5	5.8		85
80		40.2	6.3	14	80
75	57	40.9	6.5		75
70	56	41.5	6.9		70
65		41.7	7.3	13	65
60	55	41.9	7.6		60
55	54		8.0		55
50	52	42.0	8.3		50
45	51	42.5	8.7		45
40	50	42.9	9.1	12	40
35	49	43.5	9.5	11	35
30	48	44.1	9.9		30
25	47	45.0	11.0		25
20	46	45.9	12.4	10	20
15	45	46.5	13.4	8	15
10	44	47.0	14.4	6	10
5	43	47.9	16.9	2	5

TABLE B.14 *Point Values: Male Marine Corps Physical Fitness Test**

Points	Pull-ups	Sit-ups	3 Mile Run	Points	Pull-ups	Sit-ups	3 Mile Run	Points	Pull-ups	Sit-ups	3 Mile Run	Points	Pull-ups	Sit-ups	3 Mile Run
100	20	80	18:00	75	15		22:10	50	10	50	26:20	25	5	25	30:30
99			18:10	74		67	22:20	49		49	26:30	24		24	30:40
98		79	18:20	73			22–30	48		48	26:40	23		23	30:50
97			18:30	72		66	22:40	47		47	26:50	22		22	31:00
96		78	18:40	71			22:50	46		46	27:00	21		21	31:10
95	19		18:50	70	14	65	23:00	45	9	45	27:10	20	4	20	31:20
94		77	19:00	69			23:10	44		44	27:20	19		19	31:30
93			19:10	68		64	23:20	43		43	27:30	18		18	31:40
92		76	19:20	67			23:30	42		42	27:40	17		17	31:50
91			19:30	66		63	23:40	41		41	27:50	16		16	32:00
90	18	75	19:40	65	13		23:50	40	8	40	28:00	15	3	15	32:10
89			19:50	64		62	24:00	39		39	28:10	14		14	32:20
88		74	20:00	63			24:10	38		38	28:20	13		13	32:30
87			20:10	62		61	24:20	37		37	28:30	12		12	32:40
86		73	20:20	61			24:30	36		36	28:40	11		11	32:50
85	17		20:30	60	12	60	24:40	35	7	35	28:50	10	2	10	33:00
84		72	20:40	59		59	24:50	34		34	29:00	9		9	33:10
83			20:50	58		58	25:00	33		33	29:10	8		8	33:20
82		71	21:00	57		57	25:10	32		32	29:20	7		7	33:30
81			21:10	56		56	25:20	31		31	29:30	6		6	33:40
80	16	70	21:20	55	11	55	25:30	30	6	30	29:40	5	1	5	33:50
79			21:30	54		54	25:40	29		29	29:50	4		4	34:00
78		69	21:40	53		53	25:50	28		28	30:00	3		3	34:30
77			21:50	52		52	26:00	27		27	30:10	2		2	35:00
76		68	22:00	51		51	26:10	26		26	30:20	1		1	36:00

*Marine Corps Order, 6100 · 3F, 17 December 1971.

TABLE B.15 *Percentile Scale: Cowell Social Behavior Trend Index**

Raw Score	Percentile Score	Raw Score	Percentile Score	Raw Score	Percentile Score
88	99.55	36	68.47	− 6	25.22
81	99.10	35	67.12	− 7	23.87
80	98.65	34	65.32	− 8	23.42
79	98.20	33	64.41	− 9	22.97
78	97.75	32	63.51	−12	22.52
77	97.30	31	61.26	−15	21.62
75	96.85	30	59.91	−16	21.17
74	96.40	29	59.01	−17	20.72
73	95.94	28	57.21	−18	19.82
72	95.50	27	56.31	−19	18.92
70	95.04	26	55.40	−20	18.47
68	94.59	25	54.95	−21	17.51
65	92.79	24	53.60	−23	16.22
63	92.34	23	52.70	−25	15.32
62	91.44	22	51.80	−26	13.96
61	90.54	21	50.90	−27	12.36
60	90.09	20	50.45	−28	12.16
59	89.19	18	48.65	−29	11.71
58	88.29	17	46.85	−35	10.81
57	86.49	16	45.94	−36	9.91
56	86.04	15	45.50	−39	8.56
55	85.14	14	45.04	−40	8.11
54	84.23	13	43.24	−42	7.66
52	83.33	12	41.44	−43	7.21
51	82.88	11	40.54	−44	6.76
50	82.43	10	40.09	−45	6.31
49	81.08	9	38.74	−46	5.40
48	80.18	8	37.84	−47	4.50
47	79.28	7	36.94	−49	4.05
46	78.38	6	35.59	−50	3.60
45	77.03	4	34.68	−54	3.15
44	74.77	3	33.33	−55	2.70
43	73.42	2	32.43	−58	1.80
42	72.97	1	30.63	−61	1.35
41	72.52	−1	29.73	−62	.90
40	72.07	−2	28.38	−71	.45
38	71.17	−3	27.48	−73	.00
37	69.37	−5	26.00		

*Charles C. Cowell and Hilda M. Schwehn, *Modern Principles and Methods in High School Physical Education* (Boston: Allyn and Bacon, Inc., 1958), p. 305.

TABLE B.16 *Percentile Scale: Cowell Personal Distance Ballot**

Raw Score	Percentile Score	Raw Score	Percentile Score	Raw Score	Percentile Score
159	99.34	321	61.59	396	31.12
161	98.68	327	60.93	398	30.46
173	98.01	329	60.26	400	29.80
196	97.35	331	59.60	405	26.49
200	96.69	333	58.94	412	25.83
205	94.04	335	57.62	415	25.16
210	93.38	336	56.29	416	24.50
211	92.71	344	54.97	417	23.84
219	92.05	347	54.30	418	23.18
220	91.39	351	53.64	419	21.19
222	90.73	352	52.98	420	20.53
233	90.07	353	51.66	421	19.87
237	89.40	354	50.33	422	19.20
240	88.74	355	49.67	423	17.22
252	88.08	357	49.01	425	16.56
256	86.75	359	48.34	426	15.89
257	84.10	361	47.68	428	15.23
259	83.44	363	47.02	429	14.57
260	82.78	366	46.36	431	13.91
265	82.12	369	45.70	433	13.24
266	81.46	371	45.03	434	12.58
267	80.79	375	44.37	435	11.92
271	79.47	376	43.71	439	11.25
274	78.81	377	43.05	445	10.60
281	76.16	378	41.06	455	9.93
282	75.50	379	40.40	457	9.27
283	74.17	380	39.74	469	7.95
284	73.51	381	38.41	470	7.28
285	72.85	382	37.75	471	6.62
289	72.18	384	37.09	482	5.96
294	70.20	385	36.76	495	5.30
295	68.87	386	35.10	496	4.64
300	68.21	389	34.44	500	3.97
311	65.56	390	33.77	503	1.99
312	64.90	391	33.11	509	1.32
315	64.24	392	32.45	541	.66
319	62.91	395	31.79	636	.00

*Charles C. Cowell and Hilda M. Schwehn, *Modern Principles and Methods in High School Physical Education* (Boston: Allyn and Bacon, Inc., 1958), p. 308.

TABLE B.17 *Carpenter's Motor Ability Test for First Three Grades**
A. *Girls*

	0	1	2	3	4	5	6	7	8	9
600	125.03	125.28	125.54	125.79	126.05	126.30	126.56	126.81	127.07	127.32
590	122.48	122.74	122.99	123.23	123.50	123.76	124.01	124.26	124.52	124.78
580	119.93	120.19	120.44	120.70	120.95	121.21	121.46	121.72	121.97	122.23
570	117.38	117.64	117.89	118.15	118.40	118.66	118.91	119.17	119.42	119.68
560	114.83	115.09	115.34	115.60	115.85	116.11	116.36	116.62	116.87	117.13
550	112.29	112.54	112.79	113.05	113.30	113.56	113.81	114.07	114.32	114.58
540	109.74	109.39	110.25	110.50	110.76	111.01	111.27	111.52	111.78	112.03
530	107.19	107.44	107.70	107.95	108.21	108.46	108.72	108.97	109.32	109.48
520	104.64	104.89	105.15	105.40	105.66	105.91	106.17	106.42	106.68	106.93
510	102.09	102.34	102.60	102.85	103.11	103.36	103.62	103.87	104.13	104.38
500	99.54	99.79	100.05	100.30	100.56	100.81	101.07	101.32	101.58	101.83
490	96.99	97.25	97.50	97.76	98.01	98.27	98.52	98.78	99.03	99.29
480	94.44	94.70	94.95	95.21	95.46	95.72	95.97	96.23	96.48	96.74
470	91.89	92.15	92.40	92.66	92.91	93.17	93.42	93.68	93.93	94.19
460	89.34	89.60	89.85	90.11	90.36	90.62	90.87	91.13	91.38	91.64
450	86.80	87.05	87.30	87.56	87.81	88.07	88.32	88.58	88.83	89.09
440	84.25	84.50	84.76	85.01	85.27	85.52	85.78	86.03	86.29	86.54
430	81.70	81.95	82.21	82.46	82.72	82.97	83.23	83.48	83.74	83.99
420	79.15	79.40	79.66	79.91	80.17	80.42	80.68	80.93	81.19	81.44
410	76.60	76.85	77.11	77.36	77.62	77.62	78.13	78.38	78.64	78.89
400	74.05	74.30	74.56	74.81	75.07	75.32	75.58	75.83	76.09	76.34

Aileen Carpenter, "Strength Testing in the First Three Grades," *Research Quarterly*, **13, No. 3 (October 1942), 332.

B. *Boys*

	0	1	2	3	4	5	6	7	8	9
600	115.94	116.24	116.54	116.84	117.14	117.44	117.75	118.05	118.35	118.65
590	112.93	113.23	113.53	113.83	114.13	114.44	114.74	115.04	115.34	115.64
580	109.92	110.22	110.52	110.82	111.13	111.43	111.73	112.03	112.33	112.63
570	106.91	107.21	107.51	107.82	108.12	108.42	108.72	109.02	109.32	109.62
560	103.90	104.20	104.51	104.81	105.11	105.41	105.71	106.01	106.31	106.61
550	100.90	101.20	101.50	101.80	102.10	102.40	102.70	103.00	103.30	103.60
540	97.80	98.19	98.49	98.79	99.09	99.39	99.69	99.99	100.29	100.59
530	94.88	95.18	95.48	95.78	96.08	96.38	96.68	97.98	97.28	97.59
520	91.87	92.17	92.45	92.77	93.07	93.37	93.67	93.97	94.28	94.58
510	88.86	89.16	89.46	89.76	90.06	90.36	90.66	90.97	91.27	91.57
500	85.85	86.15	86.45	86.75	87.05	87.36	87.96	87.96	88.26	88.56
490	82.84	83.14	83.44	83.74	84.04	84.35	84.65	84.95	85.25	85.55
480	79.83	80.13	80.43	80.73	81.04	81.34	81.64	81.94	82.24	82.54
470	76.82	77.12	77.42	77.73	78.03	78.33	78.63	78.93	79.23	79.53
460	73.81	74.11	74.42	74.72	75.02	75.32	75.62	75.92	76.22	76.52
450	70.81	71.11	71.41	71.71	72.01	72.31	72.61	72.91	73.21	73.51
440	67.80	68.10	68.40	68.70	69.00	69.30	69.60	69.90	70.20	70.50
430	64.79	65.09	65.39	65.69	65.99	66.29	66.59	66.89	67.19	67.50
420	61.78	62.08	62.38	62.68	62.98	63.28	63.58	63.88	64.19	64.49
410	58.77	59.07	59.37	59.67	59.97	60.27	60.57	60.88	61.18	61.48
400	55.76	56.06	56.36	56.66	56.96	57.26	57.57	57.87	58.17	58.47

TABLE B.18 *Achievement Scales for the Newton Motor Ability Test for High School Girls**

Point Score	Hurdles	Broad Jump	Scramble	Total Points	Point Score	Decile Score
100	7.2	83.0	10.4	275	100	
99	7.3	82.5	10.6	273	99	
98	7.4	82.0	10.7	270	98	
97			10.8	268	97	
96	7.5	81.5	10.9	265	96	
95	7.6	81.0	11.0	263	95	
94	7.7	80.5	11.2	260	94	
93		80.0	11.3	258	93	
92	7.8	79.5	11.4	255	92	I
91	7.9	79.0	11.6	253	91	
90		78.5	11.7	250	90	
89	8.0		11.8	248	89	
88	8.1	78.0	11.9	245	88	
87	8.2	77.5	12.0	243	87	
86		77.0	12.2	240	86	
85	8.3	76.5	12.3	238	85	
84	8.4	76.0	12.4	235	84	
83	8.5	75.5	12.6	233	83	
82		75.0	12.7	230	82	
81	8.6		12.8	228	81	
80	8.7	74.5	12.9	225	80	
79	8.8	74.0	13.0	223	79	
78		73.5	13.2	220	78	
77	8.9	73.0	13.3	218	77	
76	9.0	72.5	13.4	215	76	
75		72.0	13.6	213	75	
74	9.1		13.7	210	74	
73	9.2	71.5	13.8	208	73	
72	9.3	71.0	13.9	205	72	
71		70.5	14.0	203	71	
70	9.4	70.0	14.2	200	70	
69	9.5	69.5	14.3	198	69	
68	9.6	69.0	14.4	195	68	
67			14.6	193	67	II
66	9.7	68.5	14.7	190	66	
65	9.8	68.0	14.8	188	65	
64		67.5	14.9	185	64	
63	9.9	67.0	15.0	183	63	
62	10.0	66.5	15.2	180	62	
61	10.1	66.0	15.3	178	61	III
60			15.4	175	60	
59	10.2	65.5	15.6	173	59	
58	10.3	65.0	15.7	170	58	
57	10.4	64.5	15.8	168	57	
56		64.0	15.9	165	56	IV
55	10.5	63.5	16.0	163	55	
54	10.6	63.0	16.2	160	54	

*Elizabeth Powell and Eugene C. Howe, "Motor Ability Tests for High School Girls," *Research Quarterly,* **10,** No. 4 (December 1939), 86–87.

Point Score	Hurdles	Broad Jump	Scramble	Total Points	Point Score	Decile Score
53		62.5	16.3	158	53	
52	10.7		16.4	155	52	V
51	10.8	62.0	16.6	153	51	
50	10.9	61.5	16.7	150	50	
49		61.0	16.8	148	49	
48	11.0	60.5	16.9	145	48	VI
47	11.1	60.0	17.1	143	47	
46	11.2	59.5	17.2	140	46	
45		59.0	17.3	138	45	
44	11.3		17.4	135	44	
43	11.4	58.5	17.6	133	43	VII
42	11.5	58.0	17.7	130	42	
41		57.5	17.8	128	41	
40	11.6	57.0	17.9	125	40	
39	11.7	56.5	18.1	123	39	
38		56.0	18.2	120	38	VIII
37	11.8		18.3	118	37	
36	11.9	55.5	18.4	115	36	
35	12.0	55.0	18.6	113	35	
34		54.5	18.7	110	34	
33	12.1	54.0	18.8	108	33	
32	12.2	53.5	18.9	105	32	IX
31	12.3	53.0	19.1	103	31	
30			19.2	100	30	
29	12.4	52.5	19.3	98	29	
28	12.5	52.0	19.4	95	28	
27		51.5	19.6	93	27	
26	12.6	51.0	19.7	90	26	
25	12.7	50.5	19.8	88	25	
24	12.8	50.0	19.9	85	24	
23			20.1	83	23	
22	12.9	49.5	20.2	80	22	
21	13.0	49.0	20.3	78	21	
20	13.1	48.5	20.4	75	20	
19		48.0	20.6	73	19	
18	13.2	47.5	20.7	70	18	
17	13.3	47.0	20.8	68	17	
16	13.4		20.9	65	16	
15		46.5	21.1	63	15	X
14	13.5	46.0	21.2	60	14	
13	13.6	45.5	21.3	58	13	
12		45.0	21.4	55	12	
11	13.7	44.5	21.6	53	11	
10	13.8	44.0	21.7	50	10	
9	13.9	43.5	21.8	48	9	
8		43.0	21.9	45	8	
7	14.0		22.1	43	7	
6	14.1	42.5	22.2	40	6	
5	14.2	42.0	22.3	38	5	
4		41.5	22.4	35	4	
3	14.3	41.0	22.6	33	3	
2	14.4	40.5	22.7	30	2	
1			22.8	28	1	
0	14.5	40.0	22.9	25	0	

TABLE B.19 *Adams' Test of Sport Type Motor Educability for College Men**

R	S	R	S	R	S
1391 – up	100	910 – 925	71	444 – 460	43
1375 – 1390	99	893 – 909	70	428 – 443	42
1358 – 1374	98	876 – 892	69	411 – 427	41
1342 – 1357	97	860 – 875	68	395 – 410	40
1325 – 1341	96	843 – 859	67	378 – 394	39
1308 – 1324	95	827 – 842	66	361 – 377	38
1292 – 1307	94	810 – 826	65	345 – 360	37
1275 – 1291	93	793 – 809	64	328 – 344	36
1258 – 1274	92	777 – 792	63	312 – 327	35
1242 – 1257	91	760 – 776	62	295 – 311	34
1225 – 1241	90	743 – 759	61	278 – 294	33
1209 – 1224	89	727 – 742	60	262 – 277	32
1192 – 1208	88	710 – 726	59	245 – 261	31
1175 – 1191	87	694 – 709	58	230 – 244	30
1159 – 1174	86	677 – 693	57	212 – 229	29
1142 – 1158	85	660 – 676	56	195 – 211	28
1126 – 1141	84	644 – 659	55	179 – 194	27
1109 – 1125	83	627 – 643	54	162 – 178	26
1092 – 1108	82	611 – 626	53	145 – 161	25
1076 – 1091	81	594 – 610	52	129 – 144	24
1059 – 1075	80	577 – 593	51	112 – 128	23
1042 – 1058	79	561 – 576	50	96 – 111	22
1026 – 1041	78	544 – 560	49	79 – 95	21
1009 – 1025	77	528 – 543	48	62 – 78	20
993 – 1008	76	511 – 527	47	46 – 61	19
976 – 992	75	494 – 510	46	29 – 45	18
969 – 975	74	478 – 493	45	9 – 28	17
943 – 968	73	461 – 477	44	below 9	16
926 – 942	72				

R = raw score.   *S* = T-score.

*Arthur R. Adams, "A Test Construction Study of Sport-Type Motor Educability Tests," Doctoral Dissertation, Louisana State University, 1954.

TABLE B.20 *Neilson and Cozens Classification Chart for Boys and Girls**
(Elementary and Junior High School)

Exponent	Height in Inches	Age in Years	Weight in Pounds
1	50 to 51	10 to 10–5	60 to 65
2	52 to 53	10–6 to 10–11	66 to 70
3		11 to 11–5	71 to 75
4	54 to 55	11–6 to 11–11	76 to 80
5		12 to 12–5	81 to 85
6	56 to 57	12–6 to 12–11	86 to 90
7		13 to 13–5	91 to 95
8	58 to 59	13–6 to 13–11	96 to 100
9		14 to 14–5	101 to 105
10	60 to 61	14–6 to 14–11	106 to 110
11		15 to 15–5	111 to 115
12	62 to 63	15–6 to 15–11	116 to 120
13		16 to 16–5	121 to 125
14	64 to 65	16–6 to 16–11	126 to 130
15	66 to 67	17 to 17–5	131 to 133
16	68	17–6 to 17–11	134 to 136
17	69 and over	18 and over	137 and over

Sum of Exponents	Class	Sum of Exponents	Class
9 and below	A	25 to 29	E
10 to 14	B	30 to 34	F
15 to 19	C	35 to 38	G
20 to 24	D	39 and above	H

*N. P. Neilson and F. W. Cozens, *Achievement Scales in Physical Education Activities for Boys and Girls in Elementary and Junior High Schools* (New York: A. S. Barnes & Co., Inc.), 1934.

TABLE B.21 *Achievement Scales in Archery for Women**

Scale	First Columbia Total Score (Target Score)	Final Columbia Record (Target Score)			
		Total Score	50 yards	40 yards	30 yards
100	436	466	150	176	194
99	430	460	148	174	192
98	424	455	146	171	190
97	418	449	143	169	187
96	412	443	141	167	185
95	406	438	139	164	183
94	400	432	137	162	181
93	394	426	135	160	179
92	388	420	132	157	176
91	382	415	130	155	174
90	376	409	128	153	172
89	370	403	126	150	170
88	364	398	124	148	168
87	358	392	121	146	165
86	352	386	119	143	163
85	346	381	117	141	161
84	340	375	115	139	159
83	334	369	113	136	157
82	328	363	110	134	154
81	322	358	108	132	152
80	316	352	106	129	150
79	310	346	104	127	148
78	304	341	102	125	146
77	298	335	99	122	143
76	292	329	97	120	141
75	286	324	95	118	139
74	280	318	93	115	137
73	274	312	91	113	135
72	268	306	88	111	132
71	262	301	86	108	130
70	256	295	84	106	128
69	250	289	82	104	126
68	244	284	80	101	124
67	238	278	77	99	121
66	232	272	75	97	119
65	226	267	73	94	117
64	220	261	71	92	115
63	214	255	69	90	113
62	208	249	66	87	110
61	202	244	64	85	108
60	196	238	62	83	106
59	190	232	60	80	104
58	184	227	58	78	102
57	178	221	55	76	99
56	172	215	53	73	97

*Scale constructed by F. W. Cozens, University of California at Los Angeles. Reproduced from Edith I. Hyde, "An Achievement Scale in Archery," *Research Quarterly,* **7,** No. 2 (May 1937), 109.

TABLE B.21 *continued*

Scale	First Columbia Total Score (*Target Score*)	Final Columbia Record (*Target Score*)			
		Total Score	50 yards	40 yards	30 yards
55	166	210	51	61	95
54	160	204	49	69	93
53	154	198	47	66	91
52	148	192	44	64	88
51	142	187	42	62	86
50	136	181	40	59	84
49	133	178	39	58	82
48	131	174	—	57	80
47	128	171	38	56	79
46	125	167	37	55	77
45	122	164	36	53	75
44	120	160	35	52	74
43	117	157	—	51	72
42	114	153	34	50	70
41	111	150	33	49	69
40	109	146	32	47	67
39	106	143	31	46	65
38	103	139	—	45	64
37	100	136	30	44	62
36	98	132	29	43	60
35	95	129	28	42	59
34	92	125	27	40	57
33	89	122	—	39	55
32	87	118	26	38	54
31	84	115	25	37	52
30	81	111	24	36	50
29	78	108	23	34	49
28	76	104	—	33	47
27	73	101	22	32	45
26	70	97	21	31	44
25	67	94	20	30	42
24	65	90	19	28	40
23	62	87	—	27	39
22	59	83	18	26	37
21	56	80	17	25	35
20	54	76	16	24	34
19	51	73	15	23	32
18	48	69	—	21	30
17	45	66	14	20	29
16	43	62	13	19	27
15	40	59	12	18	25
14	37	55	11	17	24
13	34	52	—	15	22
12	32	48	10	14	20
11	29	45	9	13	19
10	26	41	8	12	17
9	23	38	7	11	15

TABLE B.21 *continued*

Scale	First Columbia Total Score (Target Score)	Final Columbia Record (Target Score)			
	(Target Score)	Total Score	50 yards	40 yards	30 yards
8	21	34	—	9	14
7	18	31	6	8	12
6	15	27	5	7	10
5	12	24	4	6	9
4	10	20	3	5	7
3	7	17	—	4	5
2	4	13	2	2	4
1	1	10	1	1	2

TABLE B.22 *Scale Scores for Stroup Basketball Test**

Shooting	Passing	Dribbling	Scale Score	Shooting	Passing	Dribbling	Scale Score
6	53	27	51	24	78	42	76
7	55		52				77
8	56	28	53	25	79	43	78
9	57	29	54	26	80		79
	59	30	55	27	81	44	80
10	60	31	56		82		81
11	61		57	28		45	82
12	62	32	58	29	83		83
13	64	33	59		84	46	84
14	65	34	60	30	85		85
	66		61		86	47	86
15		35	62	31	87		87
16	67		63	32	88	48	88
	68	36	64		89	49	89
17	69		65	33	90	50	90
	70	37	66	34	91		91
18			67	35	93	51	92
19	71	38	68	36	94		93
	72		69	37	95	52	94
20	73	39	70		97		95
21			71	38	98	53	96
	74	40	72	39	99		97
22	75		73	40	100	54	98
23	76	41	74	41	102	55	99
	77		75	42	103	56	100

*Frances Stroup, "Game Results as a Criterion for Validating Basketball Skill Test," *Research Quarterly,* **26,** No. 3 (October 1955), 353.

TABLE B.23 *T Scales for the Harrison Basketball Test for Boys by Grades**

T Scale	Goal Shooting				Speed Pass				Dribble				Rebounding			
	7th	8th	9th	10th	7th	8th	9th	10th	7th	8th	9th	10th	7th	8th	9th	10th
76					37	38	39	42	39	37	40	36	27	29	34	
75																
74																
73		17	18	18	35			41	38						33	32
72	14				34				37	36	39		26		32	
71					33	37			36						31	
70								40				35	25	28		31
69											38				30	29
68		16	17	17		36	38	39				35		27		
67	13				32					35		34	24	26		
66			16		31	35	38				37	34			29	28
65	12	15	16											25		
64		14		15			37	37				33	23			27
63			15	14	30	34			34		36	33			28	
62		13					36	36				32				26
61	11				29	33			33				24			
60				13			35	35				32			27	
59			14		28				31	32	35		22			
58		12				32	34							25	26	
57	10							34	31				23			
56		11	13			31	33		30	31	34		21		25	
55				12	27					33	30			24		
54	9	10				30	33						22			
53			12					32	29	30	32		20		23	24
52				11			32			32	31	29			22	
51	8	9	11					32							22	
50					26	29			28	29		28	19		23	
49			10	10			31				30			21		
48									27	28		27			21	
47		8	9	9		28	30	31					18	20		22
46	6				25		29			27	29	26	17			21
45			8	8			29				28	25		19	20	
44			8	8		27		30	26			25	16			20
43		7			24		28	29	27				16			20
42				7				29	26				15		19	
41			7			25						24	15		19	
40		6			23	26	27					26		18		19
39				6				28	24			23	14		17	
38	4	6							24	25	25			17	18	18
37			6		22	25	26					22	13			
36				5				27	23			24	12	16	17	
35		5			21		25		22			21				17
34				5	20	24					24		11	15	16	
33		4		4			24	26	23			20	10			
32	3				19					23	22	19				
31					18					23						16
30			4	3		23	23		20	22	21		9	14		
29										19		18	8			
28	2	3	3		17				18	21	20		7		15	
27					16	22	22			17	17		6	13	14	
26							21			16	14		5			
25							20	25			11					
24	1		2	2	15		19		20		9	17	4	12		15

*Edward R. Harrison, "A Test to Measure Basketball Ability of Boys," Master's Thesis, University of Florida, 1969.

TABLE B.24 *Norms for Leilich Basketball Test for Women Physical Education Majors.* *

A. Norms for Half-Minute Shoot Test			B. Norms for Bounce and Shoot Test (Accuracy)		
Raw Score	T-Score	Percentile	Raw Score	T-Score	Percentile
20	81	100	20	67	100
19	78	100	19	65	98
18	75	100	18	62	93
17	73	99	17	60	87
16	70	99	16	57	79
15	67	97	15	55	69
14	64	94	14	53	61
13	61	89	13	50	52
12	58	82	12	48	42
11	55	75	11	45	35
10	53	67	10	43	28
9	50	57	9	40	21
8	47	46	8	38	16
7	44	35	7	36	11
6	41	26	6	33	9
5	38	17	5	31	6
4	35	10	4	28	4
3	33	5	3	26	2
2	30	1	2	23	2
1	27	1	1	21	1

*Wilma K. Miller, Chairman, "Achievement Level in Basketball Skills for Women Physical Education Majors," *Research Quarterly*, **25**, No. 4 (December 1954), 450.

C. *Norms for Bounce and Shoot Test (Time in Seconds)*

Raw Score	T-Score	Perc.	Raw Score	T-Score	Perc.	Raw Score	T-Score	Perc.
41	74	100	57	61	93	73	47	34
42	73	100	58	60	91	74	46	31
43	72	100	59	59	88	75	46	28
44	71	100	60	58	86	76	45	25
45	71	100	61	57	75	77	44	23
46	70	100	62	56	72	78	43	21
47	69	100	63	56	69	79	42	19
48	68	100	64	55	66	80	41	18
49	67	100	65	54	62	81	41	15
50	66	100	66	53	58	82	40	14
51	66	99	67	52	55	83	39	13
52	65	98	68	51	51	84	38	12
53	64	98	69	51	48	85	37	11
54	63	97	70	50	44	86	36	10
55	62	96	71	49	40	87	36	9
56	61	95	72	48	36	88	35	8

TABLE B.24 *continued*

Raw Score	T-Score	Perc.	Raw Score	T-Score	Perc.	Raw Score	T-Score	Perc.
89	34	8	105	21	3	121	7	1
90	33	7	106	20	2	122	6	1
91	32	6	107	19	2	123	6	1
92	31	5	108	18	2	124	5	1
93	31	5	109	17	2	125	4	1
94	30	5	110	16	2	126	3	1
95	29	4	111	16	2	127	2	1
96	28	4	112	15	1	128	1	1
97	27	4	113	14	1	129	1	1
98	26	4	114	13	1	130	0	1
99	26	3	115	12	1	131	−1	1
100	25	3	116	11	1	132	−2	1
101	24	3	117	11	1	133	−3	1
102	23	3	118	10	1	134	−4	1
103	22	3	119	9	1	135	−4	1
104	21	3	120	8	1			

D. *Norms for Push-Pass Test*

Raw Score	T-Score	Perc.	Raw Score	T-Score	Perc.	Raw Score	T-Score	Perc.
160	97	100	142	84	100	124	70	99
159	96	100	141	83	100	123	70	99
158	96	100	140	82	100	122	69	99
157	95	100	139	81	100	121	68	99
156	94	100	138	81	100	120	67	99
155	93	100	137	80	100	119	67	97
154	93	100	136	79	100	118	66	97
153	92	100	135	78	100	117	65	96
152	91	100	134	78	100	116	64	96
151	90	100	133	77	100	115	64	96
150	90	100	132	76	100	114	63	93
149	89	100	131	76	100	113	62	93
148	88	100	130	75	100	112	61	91
147	87	100	129	74	100	111	61	91
146	87	100	128	73	100	110	60	90
145	86	100	127	73	100	109	59	86
144	85	100	126	72	100	108	58	85
143	84	100	125	71	100	107	58	82

TABLE B.24 *continued*

Raw Score	T-Score	Perc.	Raw Score	T-Score	Perc.	Raw Score	T-Score	Perc.
106	57	81	85	41	18	64	26	3
105	56	79	84	41	16	63	25	3
104	55	72	83	40	15	62	24	2
103	55	71	82	39	14	61	24	2
102	54	66	81	38	13	60	23	2
101	53	65	80	38	12	59	22	2
100	52	62	79	37	10	58	21	2
99	52	55	78	36	9	57	21	2
98	51	53	77	35	8	56	20	1
97	50	47	76	35	8	55	19	1
96	50	47	75	34	7	54	18	1
95	49	44	74	33	6	53	18	1
94	48	39	73	32	5	52	17	1
93	47	37	72	32	5	51	16	1
92	47	32	71	31	4	50	15	1
91	46	31	70	30	4	49	15	1
90	45	28	69	29	3	48	14	1
89	44	25	68	29	3	47	13	1
88	44	24	67	28	3	46	12	1
87	43	21	66	27	3	45	12	1
86	42	20	65	26	3	44	11	1

E. *Classification of Raw Scores on the Tests*

	Raw Score			
Classification	Bounce and Shoot (Accuracy)	Bounce and Shoot (Time in Seconds)	Push Pass	Half-Minute Shooting
Superior	21–above	47–below	122–above	16–above
Good	16–20	48–61	106–121	12–15
Average	10–15	62–77	89–105	7–11
Fair	6–9	78–91	72–88	3–6
Poor	5–below	92–above	71–below	2–below

TABLE B.25 *Bowling Norms for College Men and Women**

Item	Scores							
	Nonexperienced				Experienced			
	Men		Women		Men		Women	
	Initial	Final	Initial	Final	Initial	Final	Initial	Final
Superior	133[b]	157[b]	117[b]	131[b]	181[b]	182[b]	148[b]	152[b]
Good	122–132	146–156	103–116	122–130	162–180	167–181	135–147	140–151
Average	99–121	122–145	76–102	103–121	125–161	138–166	110–134	117–139
Poor	88–98	110–121	62–75	95–102	106–124	123–137	97–109	105–116
Inferior	87[c]	109[c]	61[c]	94[c]	105[c]	122[c]	96[c]	104[c]
N	38	38	67	67	139	139	76	76
Range	57–147	104–182	61–122	77–147	100–222	100–221	83–180	82–172
M	110.3	133.1	89.0	112.2	143.4	151.7	121–9	128.7
SD	17.9	19.3	22.6	14.6	30.7	23.3	19.7	18.3

[a]and above.   [b]and below.

*John Martin and Jack Reogh, "Bowling Norms for College Students in Elective Physical Education Classes," *Research Quarterly*, **35**, No. 3 (October 1964), 325.

TABLE B.26 *T-Scales for Crew's Soccer Test**

T-Score	Ball Control (Number)	Dribble (Seconds)	T-Score	Ball Control (Number)	Dribble (Seconds)	T-Score	Ball Control (Number)	Dribble (Seconds)
99	47		69			39	4	51.2
98	46		68	25		38		52.1
97			67	24	25.9	37	3	53.0
96	45		66		26.7	36	2	54.0
95	44		65	23	27.7	35		54.9
94	43		64	22	28.6	34	1	55.8
93			63	21	29.5	33		56.7
92	42		62		30.4	32		57.6
91	41		61	20	31.3	31		58.5
90		5.0	60	19	32.2	30		59.4
89	40	5.9	59		33.1	29		60.3
88	39	6.8	58	18	34.0	28		61.2
87	38	7.7	57	17	34.9	27		62.1
86		8.7	56	16	35.8	26		63.0
85	37	9.6	55		36.7	25		63.9
84	36	10.5	54	15	37.6	24		64.8
83		11.4	53	14	38.6	23		65.7
82	35	12.3	52		39.5	22		66.6
81	34	13.2	51	13	40.4	21		67.5
80	33	14.1	50	12	41.3	20		68.5
79		15.0	49	11	42.2	19		69.4
78	32	15.9	48		43.1	18		70.3
77	31	16.8	47	10	44.0	17		71.2
76		17.7	46	9	44.9	16		72.1
75	30	16.6	45		45.8	15		73.9
74	29	19.5	44	8	46.7	14		73.0
73		20.4	43	7	47.6	13		74.8
72	28	21.3	42	6	48.5	12		75.9
71	27	22.2	41		49.4	11		76.6
70	26	23.2	40	5	50.3	10		77.5

*Vernon N. Crew, "A Skill Test Battery for Use in Service Program Soccer Classes at the University Level," Master's Thesis, University of Oregon, 1968.

TABLE B.27 *Fox Swimming Power Test for College Women**
T-Scores for Crawl and Side Strokes

T-Score	Crawl (Feet)	Side Stroke (Feet)	T-Score	Crawl (Feet)	Side Stroke (Feet)
76	50	52	51	27	28
73	47–49	51	49	26	26–27
72	46	50	48	25	25
70		48–49	47		24
69	45	46–47	46	24	
68	44	45	45		23
67	43	44	44	23	22
66	40–42	43	43		21
65		42	42	22	
64	39		41	21	19–20
63		40–41	40	20	18
62	38	37–39	39		17
61	36–37	36	38	19	16
60	35	35	37		15
59	34	34	36	18	
57	33	33	35	17	14
56	32		34		9–13
55	31	32	33	16	8
54	30	31	32		7
53	28–29	30	30	15	6
52		29	27	9–14	
			24	8	5

Margaret G. Fox, "Swimming Power Test," Research Quarterly, **28, No. 3 (October 1957), 233.*

TABLE B.28 *T-Scales for Table Tennis Backboard Test for College Women**

T-Score	Raw Score	T-Score	Raw Score	T-Score	Raw Score
77	60	59	45	41	29
76		58		40	
75		57	44	39	28
74		56		38	27
73	58	55	43	37	26
72		54	42	36	
71	55	53	41	35	25
70		52	40	34	24
69	54	51		33	23
68	52	50	39	32	22
67	51	49	38	31	
66	50	48	37	30	
65	49	47	36	29	21
64	48	46	34–35	28	
63		45	33	27	
62	47	44	32	26	20
61		43	31	25	
60	46	42	30	24	16

Jane A. Mott, and Aileen Lockhart, "Table Tennis Backboard Test," Journal of Health and Physical Education, **17, No. 9 (November 1946), 552.*

TABLE B.29 *Sigma-Scale Values for Dyer Backboard Test of Tennis Ability**

Sigma Scale	Test Score	Sigma Scale	Test Score	Sigma Scale	Test Score	Sigma Scale
100	67	75	50	50	33	25
99	66	74	49	49	32	24
98	—	73	—	48	—	23
97	65	72	48	47	31	22
96	64	71	47	46	30	21
95	—	70	—	45	—	20
94	63	69	46	44	29	19
93	62	68	45	43	28	18
92	—	67	44	42	27	17
91	61	66	—	41	—	16
90	60	65	43	40	26	15
89	59	64	42	39	25	14
88	—	63	—	38	—	13
87	58	62	41	37	24	12
86	57	61	40	36	23	11
85	—	60	—	35	—	10
84	56	59	39	34	22	9
83	55	58	38	33	21	8
82	—	57	—	32	—	7
81	54	56	37	31	20	6
80	53	55	36	30	19	5
79	—	54	—	29	—	4
78	52	53	35	28	18	3
77	51	52	34	27	17	2
76	—	51	—	26	—	1

*Joanna T. Dyer, "Revision of Backboard Test of Tennis Ability," *Research Quarterly,* **9,** No. 1 (March 1938), 25.

TABLE B.30 *T-Scores for Borleske Touch Football Test.* Forward Pass for Distance*
(Distance Measures to Nearest Yard)

Score in Yards	Frequency	T-Score
56–58	1	75
53–55	0	73
50–52	3	69
47–49	1	66
44–46	8	63
41–43	8	59
38–40	16	54
35–37	15	50
32–34	12	46
29–31	9	42
26–28	6	39
23–25	3	36
20–22	1	34
17–19	3	31
14–16	0	27
11–13	1	25
	N = 87	

Running Straightway
(Time Measured to Nearest Tenth-Second)

Score in Seconds and Tenths	Frequency	T-Score
5.36–5.55	2	72.5
5.56–5.75	6	65.
5.76–5.95	8	60.5
5.96–6.15	15	56.
6.16–6.35	11	51.5
6.36–6.55	14	48
6.56–6.75	8	44.
6.76–6.95	9	40.5
6.96–7.15	2	37.5
7.16–7.35	3	35
7.36–7.55	3	31.5
7.56–7.75	0	27.5
7.76–7.95	0	27.5
7.96–8.15	0	27.5
8.16–8.35	0	27.5
8.36–8.55	0	27.5
8.56–8.75	0	27.5
8.76–8.95	0	27.5
8.96–9.15	1	00.0
	N = 82	

Punt for Distance
(Distance Measured to Nearest Yard)

Score in Yards	Frequency	T-Score
50.6–53.5	1	75
47.6–50.5	1	71
44.6–47.5	1	69
41.6–44.5	14	62
38.6–41.5	12	56
35.6–38.5	16	51
32.6–35.5	4	48
29.6–32.5	19	45
26.6–29.5	4	40
23.6–26.5	2	38
20.6–23.5	1	37
17.6–20.5	5	35
14.6–17.5	2	30
11.6–14.5	0	27
8.6–11.5	1	25
	N = 83	

*Frederick W. Cozens, "Ninth Annual Report of Committee on Curriculum Research of the College Physical Education Association: Part III," *Research Quarterly,* **8,** No. 2 (May 1937), 73.

TABLE B.31 *Sigma-Scale Values: Russell-Lange Volley Ball Test for Girls in Junior High School**

Sigma Scale	Test Scores		Sigma Scale	Test Scores	
	Serve	Repeated Volleys		Serve	Repeated Volleys
100	—	51	50	—	22
99	45	50	49	16	—
98	44	—	48	—	21
97	—	49	47	—	—
96	43	—	46	15	20
95	—	48	45	—	—
94	42	—	44	—	19
93	41	47	43	14	—
92	—	46	42	—	—
91	40	—	41	—	18
90	—	45	40	13	—
89	39	—	39	—	17
88	—	44	38	—	—
87	38	43	37	12	16
86	37	—	36	—	—
85	—	42	35	—	15
84	36	—	34	11	—
83	—	41	33	—	—
82	35	—	32	—	14
81	—	40	31	10	—
80	34	39	30	—	13
79	33	—	29	—	—
78	—	38	28	9	12
77	32	—	27	—	—
76	—	37	26	—	—
75	31	36	25	8	11
74	30	—	24	—	—
73	—	35	23	—	10
72	29	—	22	7	—
71	—	34	21	—	9
70	28	—	20	—	—
69	—	33	19	6	8
68	27	32	18	—	—
67	26	—	17	—	—
66	—	31	16	—	7
65	25	—	15	—	—
64	—	30	14	—	6
63	24	—	13	4	—
62	23	29	12	—	5
61	—	28	11	—	—
60	22	—	10	3	4
59	—	27	9	—	—
58	21	—	8	—	—
57	—	26	7	2	3
56	20	25	6	—	—
55	19	—	5	—	2
54	—	24	4	1	—
53	18	—	3	—	1
52	—	23	2	—	—
51	17	—	1	—	—

*Naomi Russell and Elizabeth Lange, "Achievement Tests in Volleyball for High School Girls," Research Quarterly, **11,** No. 4 (December 1940), 33.

Index